Suicide Assessment and Treatment: Empirical and Evidence-Based Practices

Suicide Assessment and Treatment: Empirical and Evidence-Based Practices

Editor: Chris Robinson

AMERICAN
MEDICAL PUBLISHERS
www.americanmedicalpublishers.com

AMERICAN
MEDICAL PUBLISHERS
www.americanmedicalpublishers.com

Cataloging-in-Publication Data

Suicide assessment and treatment : empirical and evidence-based practices / edited by Chris Robinson.
p. cm.
Includes bibliographical references and index.
ISBN 979-8-88740-479-0
1. Suicide. 2. Suicidal behavior. 3. Suicide--Evaluation. 4. Suicide--Treatment. 5. Suicide--Prevention.
6. Evidence-based psychiatry. I. Robinson, Chris.
RC569 .S85 2023
616.858 445--dc23

American Medical Publishers,
41 Flatbush Avenue,
1st Floor, New York,
NY 11217, USA

ISBN 979-8-88740-479-0 (Hardback)

Contents

Preface

It is often said that books are a boon to mankind. They document every progress and pass on the knowledge from one generation to the other. They play a crucial role in our lives. Thus I was both excited and nervous while editing this book. I was pleased by the thought of being able to make a mark but I was also nervous to do it right because the future of students depends upon it. Hence, I took a few months to research further into the discipline, revise my knowledge and also explore some more aspects. Post this process, I begun with the editing of this book.

Suicide is referred to as the deliberate act of causing one's own death. There are several risk factors associated with suicide, such as nihilistic beliefs, substance use disorders, physical disorders like chronic fatigue syndrome, and mental disorders like depression, schizophrenia and anxiety disorders. Suicides are impulsive acts driven by stress from financial crisis or academic difficulties, relationship problems like breakups, divorces, harassment and bullying. Various preventive measures can be adopted to decrease suicide attempts, including improving economic conditions, treating mental illness and substance misuse, restricting access to suicide methods like poisons, drugs and firearms, and careful media reporting about suicide. Its assessment involves predicting the chance of a person attempting suicide. The purpose of risk assessment is to study the conditions of an individual in relation to suicide, along with protective factors, warning signs and risk factors. This book contains some path-breaking studies the assessment and treatment of suicide. It will provide comprehensive knowledge to the readers.

I thank my publisher with all my heart for considering me worthy of this unparalleled opportunity and for showing unwavering faith in my skills. I would also like to thank the editorial team who worked closely with me at every step and contributed immensely towards the successful completion of this book. Last but not the least, I wish to thank my friends and colleagues for their support.

Editor

1

Traumatization, Loneliness and Suicidal Ideation among Former Prisoners of War: A Longitudinally Assessed Sequential Mediation Model

Jacob Y. Stein[1], Liat Itzhaky[1], Yossi Levi-Belz[2] and Zahava Solomon[1]*

[1] I-CORE Research Center for Mass Trauma, Bob Shapell School of Social Work, Tel Aviv University, Tel Aviv, Israel,
[2] Department of Behavioral Sciences, Ruppin Academic Center, Emek-Hefer, Israel

***Correspondence:**
Jacob Y. Stein
cobisari@gmail.com

Although highly researched among veterans, the underlying mechanisms of suicidal ideation (SI) among former prisoners of war (ex-POWs), especially in the long-term, have rarely been investigated. Furthermore, while posttraumatic stress symptoms (PTSS) and loneliness have been individually associated with veteran SI, and both may be differentially implicated by captivity versus war traumas, the interplay between them has yet to be examined. Filling this gap, the current longitudinal study examined a hypothetical sequential model wherein war captivity, compared with combat-induced trauma, is implicated in worse PTSS, which is then implicated in worse loneliness and PTSS, which together may explain subsequent SI. Two groups of Israeli veterans of the 1973 Yom Kippur War, 163 ex-POWs and 185 matched non-captive veterans were assessed 18 (T1) and 30 (T2) years after the war. Analyses indicated that compared with war, captivity was implicated in worse PTSS, which was implicated in worse loneliness, and these worked in tandem to implicate SI. Loneliness, however, was not directly affected by the type of trauma, nor was its relation to SI linked to its implication in subsequent PTSS. These results may inform future research and clinical practice as the study underscores the importance of both PTSS and loneliness in ex-POWs' long-term SI.

Keywords: war captivity, posttraumatic stress disorder, loneliness, suicide, veterans, suicidal ideation, POWs, trauma

INTRODUCTION

The study of suicide among military personnel and veterans is gaining prominence, as suicide rates among this population seem to be reaching epidemic levels worldwide [e.g., Ref. (1, 2)]. Suicidal ideation (SI), the contemplation of taking one's own life, is a major risk factor for suicidal behaviors, suicide attempts, and suicide completions (3). Epidemiological reviews indicate that among the general population, 90% of unplanned and 60% of planned first suicide attempts occurred within 1 year of ideation onset (4), and approximately one-third of those who contemplate suicide will eventually also make a suicide attempt (5). Although SI does not appear to be more prevalent among veterans than among the general population (6, 7), when contemplations of suicide are translated into suicide attempts, these are more likely to result in death among veterans than among non-veterans (8). Investigating the underlying mechanisms of veteran SI is then imperative.

One major factor that puts veterans at risk for suicide is the emotional distress that military experiences foster [e.g., Ref. (9)]. The burden of coping with the aftermath of war, and particularly the pivotal role that posttraumatic stress disorder (PTSD) symptomatology plays in such coping efforts, may be cardinal for understanding the process linking war experiences to subsequent SI [e.g., Ref. (10)]. Former prisoners of war (ex-POWs) may be of particular interest in this respect because of the unique features of their trauma, which may implicate SI.

War Captivity, Its Aftermath, and Subsequent SI

War captivity is one of the most severe and malicious experiences known to man [e.g., Ref. (11)], and therefore it is considered to be one of the most traumatic (12). Captors often go to great lengths to break the captive's spirit, utilizing multiple assaults on the individual's physical and mental integrities, including torture, humiliation, deprivation, solitary confinement, and capricious cruelty. Studies consistently reveal that ex-POWs exhibit worse postraumatic stress symptoms (PTSS) and PTSD than non-captive combat veterans [e.g., Ref. (13)]. Moreover, compared with non-captive combat veterans, ex-POWs exhibit more chronic and protracted PTSS, greater levels of a late-onset of symptom manifestation, and fewer indicators of symptomatic resilience or recovery (14).

Among victims of war incarceration, SI may initially appear during captivity [e.g., Ref. (15)] and might persist or reappear following repatriation [e.g., Ref. (16, 17)]. Surprisingly, although one may expect the effects of trauma to subside over time, and thus also expect a decline in SI, research indicates that ex-POWs evince an *increase* rather than a decrease in SI as time progresses, and this increase is steeper than among non-captive veterans (18). Notwithstanding, the investigation of long-term SI among this population is scarce, and the underlying mechanisms of this phenomenon remain largely uninvestigated. In this study, we worked toward filling this gap.

Loneliness, SI, and PTSD

At the center of this study is the interplay between PTSD, on the one hand, and loneliness, which is typically defined as a cognitive discrepancy between the quantity or quality of relationships one perceives as having and those that are desired [e.g., Ref. (19, 20)], on the other hand. Both factors have been theoretically (21) and empirically associated with SI. The relation between PTSD and subsequent veteran SI has been demonstrated in several studies [e.g., Ref. (10, 22–24)], as was the relation between veterans' SI with increased combat exposure, stigma, barriers to care, and decreased perceptions of social support (25).

The link between loneliness and SI is demonstrated in several contemporary models of suicide [e.g., Ref. (26–28)] and has been the subject of numerous empirical studies [for reviews, see Ref. (28, 29)]. Of particular note is Joiner's interpersonal–psychological theory of suicide (28). According to this theory, the two primary contributors to SI are the subjective perception that one is a burden on his or her surrounding, and a sense of thwarted belongingness, which is constituted by loneliness. The theory's potential utility in understanding veteran suicide has been gaining prominence [e.g., Ref. (30, 31)]. For instance, in a recent study among soldiers who had attempted suicide, Bryan and Rudd (9) found that over 62% of the sample felt lonely, isolated or abandoned 24 h before their suicide attempt. In the current study, we drew on this growing body of knowledge as our point of departure. However, we also diverged from its theoretical presuppositions in one important aspect.

While Van Orden et al. (28) view loneliness as a constituent of thwarted belongingness, with an emphasis on the latter, we view thwarted belongingness as one of several potential constituents of loneliness. Placing the emphasis on loneliness rather than belongingness, we underscore the need to view the sense of isolation that may beget veterans in a broader sense. A broader scope may enable the inclusion of modes of isolation that go beyond the lack of belongingness when considering post-war SI. The necessity of expanding the scope of investigation from thwarted belongingness to loneliness becomes clear as the multifariousness and polymorphic nature of the loneliness construct and the unique features of veterans' and ex-POWs' loneliness experiences are addressed.

The Multifariousness of Loneliness and Its Qualities among Veterans

Drawing on loneliness' cognitive conceptualization presented above, the experience is typically considered as synonymous with *perceived social isolation*. It is under this conceptualization that loneliness' detrimental ramifications and clinical significance have been established (32, 33), including its association with SI [e.g., Ref. (34, 35)]. Nevertheless, loneliness is multifarious and polymorphic in nature and may manifest itself in different forms [e.g., Ref. (36, 37)]. For instance, loneliness may imply a perceived absence of care, assistance, empathy, intimacy, or any other provision that a meaningful relationship may offer (38, 39). The different sources of loneliness may be implicated in distinct psychopathologies and suicide outcomes (40), and thus its specific form in any given context must be taken into consideration.

Studies suggest that military loneliness is different from civilian loneliness (41), and that veteran loneliness is different still (42, 43). Specifically, combat veterans may feel that they belong in the military, where their capabilities are valued, but at the same time feel alienated and estranged from civilian society [e.g., Ref. (44–46)]. Furthermore, veterans may feel lonely in the sense that no one back home shares their experience or can understand what they have been through—neither family and friends, nor society at large (42, 43). This phenomenon has been conceptualized as "experiential loneliness," connoting the sensation of being undesirably alone with one's experiences. In a similar vein, research has shown that often traumatized veterans' most pressing reintegration challenges include interpersonal difficulties, particularly in overcoming the challenge of confiding or sharing personal thoughts and feelings with others, keeping up non-military friendships, and belonging in "civilian" society (47). Nevertheless, a lack of belongingness is but one of several facets of veterans' stratified experience of loneliness (42, 48).

Captivity may result in even greater degrees of loneliness than combat. First, isolation is often an inherent part of captivity. POWs spend protracted periods of time in solitary confinement, awaiting the unknown while anticipating unavoidable torture (49). Furthermore, a large portion of the traumatic experience of captivity occurs in the interpersonal domain. For instance, Laub and Auerhahn (50) underscore the experience of *failed empathy*—a person's capacity to ignore the suffering of another and deliberately inflict it—as a central element of torture that impedes interpersonal connections thereafter. According to betrayal trauma theory (51, 52), interpersonal betrayals of basic human conduct exacerbate the effect of traumatic experiences and further hinder survivors' capacity to trust others. Thus, not only is the POWs' trauma typically considered to be more severe than that of non-captive combat veterans but due to the interpersonal aspects of captivity ex-POWs are also susceptible to additional interpersonal impediments, particularly insecure attachment orientations and loneliness (53–55). Similarly, recent research among incarcerated populations has indicated that past traumas may be implicated in more loneliness and less perceived social support (56).

This may be particularly the case with PTSD, the symptoms of which may include "feelings of detachment or estrangement from others" [(57), p. 272]. Indeed, Veterans' PTSD has been found to hinder intimate relations [e.g., Ref. (58)] and potentially impede interactions among family [e.g., Ref. (59, 60)] and friends (61). Among ex-POWs, impediments to marital satisfaction were significantly associated with PTSD after repatriation, and this association was mediated by the loneliness related to their PTSS (62). Nevertheless, to the best of our knowledge, the mutual effects of PTSD and loneliness in relation to SI have not been investigated in this population.

This dearth is especially pertinent due to the findings suggesting that the association between loneliness and PTSS may be reciprocal and bidirectional (63, 64). Particularly, this reciprocal relation may be rooted in the consistent finding that the lack of social support after a traumatic episode is among the strongest risk factors for the development of PTSD (65, 66). According to Rook (67), social support and loneliness are two sides of the same coin and must be studied together. Conversely, a study among combat veterans suggests that social support may mitigate PTSD only if it also counters the veterans' loneliness (68). This suggests that loneliness may underlie PTSS as well as contribute to its maintenance (64). Investigating the interplay between captivity trauma, loneliness, and PTSS may therefore be pertinent when trying to understand the underpinnings of ex-POWs' SI. Altogether, it would seem that a more severe man-made traumatic experience (e.g., captivity vs. war) may be implicated in more severe PTSS or PTSD, more loneliness, and more SI. Therefore, in this study, we set out to examine the relations between these three factors.

The Current Study

Drawing on our former investigations with this cohort (16, 62), we hypothesized that ex-POWs would evince higher PTSS, more loneliness, and more SI than non-captive veterans (H1). Furthermore, we hypothesized a sequential mediation model (H2), wherein the type of trauma (i.e., captivity vs. combat) was expected to contribute to the prediction of PTSS (H2a), which was expected to contribute to the prediction of the severity of loneliness (H2b), which was expected to contribute to the prediction of subsequent PTSS (H2c) and SI (H2d).

MATERIALS AND METHODS

Participants and Procedure

This study is part of a longitudinal study among Israeli ex-POWs and comparable control veterans from the 1973 Yom Kippur War [for full details, see Ref. (14)], with assessments in 1991 (T1), 2003 (T2), and 2008 (T3). The ex-POWs fell captive during combat and were either held captive in Egypt for 6 weeks or in Syria for 8 months, approximately. The control group was matched for military assignment, unit and military duty as well as for scores on military performance prediction tests administered when first drafted. For this study, because loneliness was assessed only at T1, we used data only from that measurement and the following one (i.e., T1 and T2). At T1, assessment took place at a centrally located hospital, and at T2 questionnaires were administered at the participants' homes or other locations of their choice. Participants' informed consent was obtained. The ethics committees of the IDF and Tel Aviv University Institutional Review Board approved the study.

According to the Israeli Ministry of Defense, 240 soldiers in the IDF land forces were taken prisoner in the 1973 Yom Kippur War. Of the 240 ex-POWs, 164 ex-POWs participated at T1 (68.33% participation rate). At T2, 10 could not be located or refused to participate—4 were deceased and 6 could not participate due to mental deterioration—of the remaining 144, 103 agreed to participate at T2 (71.5% participation rate).

The control group consisted of 185 participants at T1 (out of 280 who were identified *via* the IDF computerized data banks). At T2, 41 of these could not be located, and 1 was deceased. Of the remaining 143 controls, 106 agreed to participate (74% participation rate).

Handling Missing Data

To decide whether the data were missing at random (MAR), we conducted analyses of differences between these groups in all variables using Little's Missing Completely at Random test (69). The analysis revealed that the data were not MAR, χ^2 (45) = 76.076, p = 0.003, as the mechanism was shown to be related to the observed data (MAR). Under the erroneous assumption of MAR, missing data are proven to be better handled with maximum likelihood (ML), this method was therefore utilized in this study. Compared with conventional methods such as arithmetic mean, listwise, or pairwise deletion, and given the longitudinal design of this study, ML method is recommended as an optimal method for computing missing data to avoid bias [e.g., Ref. (70)]. This method uses all the available relevant data for each participant as well as over time because missing information can then be recovered from earlier or later waves. We, therefore, used the data of those who participated in the first wave as an anchor for data completion. The final sample after data completion included 163 ex-POWs and 185 controls.

Measures

Suicidal Ideation

Suicidal ideation was assessed using two items from the Symptom Checklist-90 (71). The two items were as follows: (a) "*thoughts about ending your life*" and (b) "*thoughts about death*." Participants were asked to indicate how frequently they experienced each symptom during the last 2 weeks on a 5-point scale (0 = not at all and 5 = very much). Due to the strong correlations between the two items (r = 0.56), we calculated the mean score of the two items as an SI index. The use of two items as indicators of SI is commonly utilized in the literature [e.g., Ref. (18, 72–74)]. Moreover, the use of a single item as well as two items for assessing SI has been compared with the utility of the gold standard for measuring SI [i.e., Scale for Suicide Ideation (75)] and was empirically established as a valid method of SI assessment (76).

PTSD and PTSS

Posttraumatic stress disorder inventory (PTSD-I; 77, 78) was used to measure PTSS. This instrument is based on the PTSD criteria in the DSM-IV (79), which was the standard at the time the research commenced. The questionnaire consists of 17 statements describing different expressions of PTSD following war. Items comprised of following three subscales: intrusion, avoidance, and arousal. The scale was found to have high convergent validity when compared with diagnoses based on structured clinical interviews, reaching 85% agreement (77, 78). Respondents were required to rate each statement according to the frequency they experienced it during the last month. Ratings appear on a 4-point scale ranging from "never" to "very often." The total score for the scale was computed based on the total number of symptoms endorsed. In this study, the PTSD-I was found to have high internal consistency [α(T1) = 0.90, α(T2) = 0.95].

Loneliness

UCLA Revised Loneliness Scale (80) was used to measure loneliness. The scale consists of 20 items—10 reflecting satisfaction with social relationships and 10 reflecting dissatisfaction. The questionnaire targets perceived social isolation and connectedness in three main domains: general or intimate isolation (e.g., "I feel isolated from others"), relational disconnectedness (e.g., "There are people who really understand me"), and collective disconnectedness [e.g., "I have a lot in common with the people around me" (36)]. Participants were asked to indicate how often they experienced these feelings on a 4-point Likert scale (0 = *not at all*, 3 = *very often*). The scale has high internal reliability (α = 0.94) and concurrent and convergent validity (80). The total score is the sum of all items after reversing the positively worded items (maximum score is 60). High scores reflect more feelings of loneliness. The scale possesses good psychometric properties, in both its English (80) and Hebrew [e.g., Ref. (64)] versions. In this study, high internal consistency was found (α = 0.88).

RESULTS

Demographics and PTSD

Former prisoners of war and controls did not differ in age, education, or income. At T2, the mean age of the participants was 53.4 (SD = 4.4), and mean years of schooling was 13.94 (SD = 3.45). Regarding income, 17% reported their income as lower than the average, 24% as average, 38% as slightly higher than average, and 21% as much higher than average. Significantly more ex-POWs (N = 23 of 99, 23.2%) met the DSM-IV symptom criteria for PTSD 30 years after the Yom Kippur War than non-POW controls (N = 4, 3.8%) (N = 205, χ^2 = 16.70, df = 1, $p < 0.001$).

To assess the differences between ex-POWs and controls, we conducted t-test analyses for independent groups. As hypothesized (H1), results indicated that the ex-POW group scored significantly higher than controls on SI at T2 (M = 0.75, SD = 0.84, and M = 0.30, SD = 0.44, respectively; $t(237) = 6.15$, $p < 0.001$), loneliness at T1 (M = 18.79, SD = 10.43, and M = 15.80, SD = 9.59, respectively; $t(346) = 13.27$, $p < 0.01$) as well as PTSS at T1 (M = 3.48, SD = 4.50, and M = 1.85, SD = 2.90, respectively; $t(269) = 3.98$, $p < 0.001$) and T2 (M = 9.01, SD = 5.01, and M = 3.80, SD = 3.71, respectively; $t(295) = 10.90$, $p < 0.001$).

Sequential Mediational Model

To test our hypothesized mediation model, we conducted a sequential mediational model assessment using SPSS macro PROCESS [Model 6 (81)] with 95% bias corrected confidence interval based on 5,000 bootstrap samples. Study group (ex-POWs = 1, controls = 0) served as the independent variable. PTSS at T1, loneliness at T1, and PTSS at T2 served as the mediators; SI at T2 was the outcome variable. Throughout the analysis, we controlled for the effect of SI at T1 on SI at T2.

As hypothesized (H2), the analysis yielded a significant model, $F(5, 343) = 115.53$, $p < 0.001$, $R^2 = 0.57$ (see **Figure 1**), wherein the direct effect of captivity on SI at T2 was not significant when all of the mediators and hypothesized indirect effects were entered into the model. Notably, three indirect effects were found to be significant (see **Table 1**). First, we found a single 1-step mediation, wherein captivity indirectly affected PTSS at T2, which was then related to higher SI at T2. In other words, ex-POWs' higher levels of PTSS, compared with controls, were related to increments in SI over time. In addition, we found two 2-step mediations. Captivity indirectly affected SI at T2 *via* PTSS and loneliness at T1. In other words, among ex-POWs, higher PTSS at T1 predicted higher loneliness cross-sectionally; loneliness predicted an increase in SI at T2. In the second 2-step mediation, captivity indirectly affected SI at T2 *via* PTSS at T1 and T2. Meaning that among ex-POWs, there were higher levels of PTSS at T1 that resulted in higher PTSS at T2; this was related to higher SI at T2. The remaining indirect effects were non-significant (**Table 1**). The ratio of indirect effects to total effects supported the results, thus indicating that the indirect effects identified in the analysis contributed significantly to the entire total effect.

DISCUSSION

In a previous study, we found that captivity was linked to SI *via* PTSS (18). Building on this, we set out to investigate whether this effect may be better understood when the interplay between ex-POWs' PTSS and their post-repatriation loneliness are considered (H2). Results mostly confirmed our hypotheses,

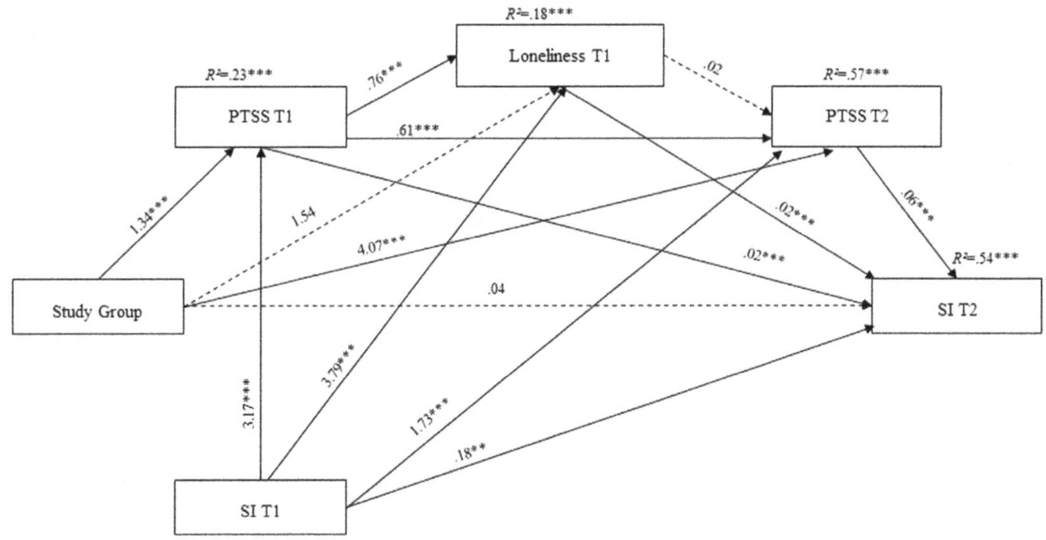

FIGURE 1 | Statistical model of the sequential meditational model for the prediction of SI. Note: Study group is a dummy-coded variable (0 = controls veterans; 1 = ex-POWs); PTSS, posttraumatic stress symptoms; SI, suicide ideation; ex-POWs, former prisoners of war; SI at T1 is a covariate; coefficients are unstandardized; dashed lines represent non-significant paths; $^{*}p < 0.05$, $^{**}p < 0.01$, and $^{***}p < 0.001$.

TABLE 1 | Bootstrapped point estimates for direct and indirect effects for predicting suicidal ideation.

		b (se)	95% CI	Ratio of indirect effect to total	
	Direct effect	0.04 (0.06)	−0.0772, 0.1644		
Step 1	Indirect effects *via*				
	PTSS T1	0.03 (0.02)	−0.0075, 0.0839	0.07 (0.06)	−0.0181, 0.2042
	Loneliness T1	0.03 (0.02)	−0.0042, 0.0713	0.06 (0.04)	−0.0107, 0.1629
	PTSS T1	0.25 (0.06)	0.1512, 0.3675	0.58 (0.11)	0.3770, 0.8157
Step 2	**PTSS T1 and loneliness T1**	0.01 (0.00)	0.0080, 0.0401	0.05 (0.02)	0.0207, 0.0911
	PTSS T1 and PTSS T2	0.05 (0.02)	0.0278, 0.0948	0.13 (0.03)	0.0738, 0.2054
	Loneliness T1 and PTSS T2	0.00 (0.00)	−0.0011, 0.0096	0.00 (0.00)	−0.0026, 0.0215
	PTSS T1, loneliness T1, and PTSS T2	0.00 (0.00)	−0.0011, 0.0048	0.00 (0.00)	−0.0026, 0.0101

PTSS, posttraumatic stress symptoms; T1, 1993, 18 years after the war; T2, 2003, 30 years after the war.
Boldface indicates significant pathways.

indicating that not only was captivity implicated in higher rates of SI, compared with war participation, but also the direct relation between captivity and SI at T2 was ostensibly nullified (i.e., non-significant) once PTSS and loneliness were taken into account. Specifically, we found indirect paths between captivity and SI through PTSS at T1 (18 years after the war), PTSS at T2 (30 years after the war), and the stability of PTSS across these two time points. We found an additional indirect path running through loneliness that was related to PTSS at T1. Nevertheless, our hypothesis that the link between captivity and subsequent SI would be explained by variations in loneliness, which are directly related to the type of trauma (i.e., captivity vs. combat), was not supported by the findings. In addition, our hypothesis that the link between captivity and subsequent SI would be explained by the link between loneliness and subsequent PTSS was not supported by the findings.

The finding that PTSS play a pivotal role in veterans' posttraumatic SI is consistent with previous studies [e.g., Ref. (10, 23)]. Furthermore, the finding that ex-POWs exhibited more SI than non-captive veterans as a result of their posttraumatic reactions, supports the argument that different traumatic experiences give rise to different posttraumatic reactions (82). Extreme man-made traumas, such as captivity and torture, may be implicated in worse suicidal behaviors and ideations due to the nature of the precipitating event and its implications both for symptom manifestation and social connectedness. This finding is also consistent with studies indicating that interpersonal traumas are implicated in worse psychological consequences [e.g., Ref. (83)], less favorable interpersonal bonds [e.g., Ref. (84)], more suicide attempts [e.g., Ref. (85)], and higher degrees of SI [e.g., Ref. (86)] than non-man-made traumas (e.g., natural disasters).

The main contribution of this study, however, is that loneliness may play an important role in ex-POWs' SI. This finding adds further support for one of the primary tenets of the interpersonal–psychological theory of suicide (27, 28) and provides further evidence for its application to veteran populations (31). That is, these findings imply that in order to understand post-captivity

SI it may be paramount to consider the impediments to interpersonal connectedness, to which both captivity and subsequent PTSS may give rise.

Notably, the analysis revealed that SI at T2 was not explained by variances in loneliness that relate to variances in trauma type (i.e., captivity and non-captivity). Rather, the impact of trauma type on SI was explained only *via* its implication in PTSS, and the effect that PTSS had on loneliness. To understand this sequential effect, it is important to realize that loneliness is not merely another burdening experience but may also inhibit adaptive coping. This is because loneliness may entail maladaptive cognitions concerning other people and their intentions. Studies across phylogeny, underscore that loneliness is associated with increased awareness of social cues of potential rejection (32, 87, 88) and may be associated in reduced perceptions of social support after trauma (56). Applied to this study, it may be suggested that ex-POWs suffer from more PTSS than non-combatants, which is a burden by its own merit. Yet, due to the interpersonal nature of captivity trauma, ex-POWs often endorse maladaptive approaches toward interpersonal relationships (53, 54); and thus may be less likely to perceive others as potential support resources. The isolation embedded in the conviction that they must cope alone may give rise to hopelessness, which itself is a strong predictor of SI [e.g., Ref. (89, 90)] as well as suicide (91).

Arguably, veterans are lonely first and foremost in the sense that their experiences are theirs alone and cannot be adequately articulated and shared with others (48). Conversely, veterans may perceive themselves as being inherently different than civilians on the basis of their experiences in the war (45, 92, 93), thus thwarting belongingness and fostering alienation upon homecoming (44). This may be the case for non-captive veterans and ex-POWs alike (43). It may also explain why the difference in loneliness rates between the two study groups, while evident, was not explained by the traumatic experience alone, but rather by the PTSS it fostered. Indeed, veterans may also be lonely in the sense that they are convinced that they must cope alone with their traumatic past and posttraumatic present (48). Hence, as the psychological burden accumulates with the manifestation of PTSS, they may become lonelier, as the current findings suggest. Ultimately, when traumatic and posttraumatic burdens must be carried alone, one may wish to escape, and death by suicide may seem like an appealing way out.

As a whole, the co-manifestation and interaction of PTSS, loneliness, and SI may be related to a phenomenon that runs like a thread through these three elements, namely, mental pain. PTSS are diagnostically acknowledged as being tormenting and debilitating (57). Loneliness is depicted as an unbearably painful experience and has recently been found to share the same neural infrastructure as physical pain (94). Finally, mental pain and the desire to avoid it are prominent factors in all comprehensive theories of suicide (95) and their role in SI initiation is all but a consensus. Put otherwise, the nucleus of ex-POWs' current torment and pain is constantly traced back to the trauma and its aftermath: the nightmares, the intrusive thoughts, the hypervigilance, the incapacity to reintegrate into civilian society and the sense of alienation this fosters, the conviction that one must cope alone, and the desire to put an end to all of this *via* suicide, are all attributed to the same painful origin—the time in incarceration and the torture it entailed, which have ultimately hindered future perceptions of interpersonal relationships. Hence they all come together to explain ex-POWs' posttraumatic SI.

Clinical Implications

This bears several important clinical implications. First, the centrality of PTSS in posttraumatic SI suggests that ex-POWs who suffer from PTSS should be assessed for SI, and that preventing SI among this population may require addressing their PTSS in therapy, as other studies have previously suggested (10). Moreover, clinicians may do well to assess and treat interpersonal impediments among ex-POWs and strive to uncover whether these are associated with SI and suicide plans. It has been argued that preventing suicide involves an empathic understanding as to the circumstances that have brought the person to the edge, thus breaching the suicidal person's loneliness (96). Since the detachment at hand may be first and foremost of an experiential nature (43), clinicians might wish to employ intersubjective approaches (97, 98), which are oriented toward apprehending the subjective experience of the trauma survivor as fully as possible; or interpersonal psychotherapy [e.g., Ref. (99)], which has been found to be efficacious for treating PTSD (100). These may increase ex-POWs' capacities to draw on social resources as they cope with their posttraumatic aftermaths. Alternatively, it may be useful to initiate group-therapy interactions. Indeed, by connecting veterans with other veterans they come to learn that they are not alone and that there are others who are also dealing with the trials and tribulations germane to such traumas [e.g., Ref. (101)]. Moreover, the commonality found in groups (e.g., the mutual understanding of the traumatic and posttraumatic experiences) may somewhat alleviate veterans' isolation as it relieves them of their burdening secrets (12). These interventions may ultimately reduce ex-POWs' SI by addressing both the trauma and the loneliness at its infrastructure, and thus, hopefully reduce death by suicide among this population.

Study Limitations and Future Directions

The findings in this study must be interpreted in the context of several limitations. First, the sole use of self-report measures, especially for the assessment of SI, may be subjected to reporting bias. Furthermore, the use of two items to assess SI, while common in the literature and deemed valid when compared with well-validated measures of SI (76), is nevertheless limited in its capacity to account for the richness and variability of the phenomenon. Future studies may do well to use better, and if possible objective, assessment tools.

Second, the long periods between measurements and between the first point of measurement and the end of the war, as well as the measurement of loneliness only in the first wave, may have impeded our ability to draw definitive conclusions concerning the causal and temporal relation between the study variables. Future longitudinal efforts must then be undertaken to further substantiate the preliminary yet important findings of this study. Specifically, future studies should investigate the causal relations between PTSD and loneliness, and between both phenomena and subsequent SI. More generally, since there is a striking dearth of loneliness focused trauma research, the finding that loneliness may add to the explained variance in SI beyond that which is explained by either the trauma or its subsequent psychopathology, may set the stage for more comprehensive investigations of this deleterious phenomenon and its contextualized posttraumatic manifestations.

AUTHOR CONTRIBUTIONS

JS was the main author and has conceptualized the study. LI preformed the statistical analyses and wrote the draft for Sections "Materials and Methods" and "Results." YL-B assisted in the conceptualization of the study, finalizing the manuscripts, and identifying relevant literature. ZS is the primary investigator, head of the research lab, and the initiator of data collection and research funding. She also supervised the entire study and the writing of the manuscript.

REFERENCES

1. Bossarte RM, editor. *Veterans Suicide: A Public Health Imperative*. 1st ed. Washington, DC: American Public Health Association (2013).
2. Kapur N, While D, Blatchley N, Bray I, Harrison K. Suicide after leaving the UK Armed Forces—a cohort study. *PLoS Med* (2009) 6(3):e1000026. doi:10.1371/journal.pmed.1000026
3. Silverman MM, Berman AL, Sanddal ND, O'Carroll PW, Joiner TE. Rebuilding the tower of babel: a revised nomenclature for the study of suicide and suicidal behaviors part 1: background, rationale, and methodology. *Suicide Life Threat Behav* (2007) 37(3):248–63. doi:10.1521/suli.2007.37.3.264
4. Kessler RC, Borges G, Walters EE. Prevalence of and risk factors for lifetime suicide attempts in the National Comorbidity Survey. *Arch Gen Psychiatry* (1999) 56(7):617–26. doi:10.1001/archpsyc.56.7.617
5. Nock MK, Borges G, Bromet EJ, Alonso J, Angermeyer M, Beautrais A, et al. Cross-national prevalence and risk factors for suicidal ideation, plans and attempts. *Br J Psychiatry* (2008) 192(2):98–105. doi:10.1192/bjp.bp.107.040113
6. Blosnich JR, Gordon AJ, Bossarte RM. Suicidal ideation and mental distress among adults with military service history: results from 5 US states, 2010. *Am J Public Health* (2014) 104(S4):S595–602. doi:10.2105/AJPH.2014.302064
7. Bossarte RM, Knox KL, Piegari R, Altieri J, Kemp J, Katz IR. Prevalence and characteristics of suicide ideation and attempts among active military and veteran participants in a national health survey. *Am J Public Health* (2012) 102(S1):S38–40. doi:10.2105/AJPH.2011.300487
8. Anestis MD, Bryan CJ. Means and capacity for suicidal behavior: a comparison of the ratio of suicide attempts and deaths by suicide in the US military and general population. *J Affect Disord* (2013) 148(1):42–7. doi:10.1016/j.jad.2012.11.045
9. Bryan CJ, Rudd MD. Life stressors, emotional distress, and trauma-related thoughts occurring in the 24 h preceding active duty US Soldiers' suicide attempts. *J Psychiatr Res* (2012) 46(7):843–8. doi:10.1016/j.jpsychires.2012.03.012
10. Jakupcak M, Cook J, Imel Z, Fontana A, Rosenheck R, McFall M. Posttraumatic stress disorder as a risk factor for suicidal ideation in Iraq and Afghanistan war veterans. *J Trauma Stress* (2009) 22(4):303–6. doi:10.1002/jts.20423
11. Hunter EJ. The Vietnam prisoner of war experience. In: Wilson JP, Raphael B, editors. *International Handbook of Traumatic Stress Syndromes*. New York: Springer (1993). p. 297–303.
12. Herman JL. *Trauma and Recovery*. New York, NY: Basic Books (1992).
13. Solomon Z, Greene T, Ein-Dor T, Zerach G, Benyamini Y, Ohry A. The long-term implications of war captivity for mortality and health. *J Behav Med* (2014) 37(5):849–59. doi:10.1007/s10865-013-9544-3
14. Solomon Z, Horesh D, Ein-Dor T, Ohry A. Predictors of PTSD trajectories following captivity: a 35-year longitudinal study. *Psychiatry Res* (2012) 199(3):188–94. doi:10.1016/j.psychres.2012.03.035
15. Hunt SC, Orsborn M, Checkoway H, Biggs ML, McFall M, Takaro TK. Later life disability status following incarceration as a prisoner of war. *Mil Med* (2008) 173(7):613–8. doi:10.7205/MILMED.173.7.613
16. Levi-Belz Y, Zerach G, Solomon Z. Suicide ideation and deliberate self-harm among ex-prisoners of war. *Arch Suicide Res* (2015) 19(2):231–48. doi:10.1080/13811118.2013.845123
17. Robson D, Welch E, Beeching N, Gill G. Consequences of captivity: health effects of far East imprisonment in World War II. *QJM* (2009) 102(2):87–96. doi:10.1093/qjmed/hcn137
18. Zerach G, Levi-Belz Y, Solomon Z. Trajectories of suicidal ideation and posttraumatic stress symptoms among former prisoners of war: a 17-year longitudinal study. *J Psychiatr Res* (2014) 49:83–9. doi:10.1016/j.jpsychires.2013.11.003
19. Perlman D, Peplau LA. Toward a social psychology of loneliness. *Pers Relatsh* (1981) 3:31–56.
20. Russell DW, Cutrona CE, McRae C, Gomez M. Is loneliness the same as being alone? *J Psychol* (2012) 146(1–2):7–22. doi:10.1080/00223980.2011.589414
21. Bryan CJ, Grove JL, Kimbrel NA. Theory-driven models of self-directed violence among individuals with PTSD. *Curr Opin Psychol* (2017) 14:12–7. doi:10.1016/j.copsyc.2016.09.007
22. Guerra VS, Calhoun PS, Mid-Atlantic Mental Illness Research, Education and Clinical Center Workgroup. Examining the relation between posttraumatic stress disorder and suicidal ideation in an OEF/OIF veteran sample. *J Anxiety Disord* (2011) 25(1):12–8. doi:10.1016/j.janxdis.2010.06.025
23. Krysinska K, Lester D. Post-traumatic stress disorder and suicide risk: a systematic review. *Arch Suicide Res* (2010) 14(1):1–23. doi:10.1080/13811110903478997
24. Oquendo M, Brent DA, Birmaher B, Greenhill L, Kolko D, Stanley B, et al. Posttraumatic stress disorder comorbid with major depression: factors mediating the association with suicidal behavior. *Am J Psychiatry* (2005) 162(3):560–6. doi:10.1176/appi.ajp.162.3.560
25. Pietrzak RH, Goldstein MB, Malley JC, Rivers AJ, Johnson DC, Southwick SM. Risk and protective factors associated with suicidal ideation in veterans of Operations Enduring Freedom and Iraqi Freedom. *J Affect Disord* (2010) 123(1):102–7. doi:10.1016/j.jad.2009.08.001
26. Gvion Y, Horesh N, Levi-Belz Y, Apter A. A proposed model of the development of suicidal ideations. *Compr Psychiatry* (2015) 56:93–102. doi:10.1016/j.comppsych.2014.09.019
27. Joiner TE. *Why People Die by Suicide*. Cambridge, MA: Harvard University Press (2005).
28. Van Orden KA, Witte TK, Cukrowicz KC, Braithwaite SR, Selby EA, Joiner TE Jr. The interpersonal theory of suicide. *Psychol Rev* (2010) 117(2):575–600. doi:10.1037/a0018697
29. Stravynski A, Boyer R. Loneliness in relation to suicide ideation and parasuicide: a population-wide study. *Suicide Life Threat Behav* (2001) 31(1):32–40. doi:10.1521/suli.31.1.32.21312

30. Anestis MD, Bryan CJ, Cornette MM, Joiner TE. Understanding suicidal behavior in the military: an evaluation of Joiner's interpersonal-psychological theory of suicidal behavior in two case studies of active duty post-deployers. *J Mental Health Counsel* (2009) 31(1):60–75. doi:10.17744/mehc.31.1.u394h1470248844n
31. Anestis MD, Khazem LR, Mohn RS, Green BA. Testing the main hypotheses of the interpersonal–psychological theory of suicidal behavior in a large diverse sample of United States military personnel. *Compr Psychiatry* (2015) 60:78–85. doi:10.1016/j.comppsych.2015.03.006
32. Cacioppo S, Grippo AJ, London S, Goossens L, Cacioppo JT. Loneliness: clinical import and interventions. *Perspect Psychol Sci* (2015) 10(2):238–49. doi:10.1177/1745691615570616
33. Heinrich LM, Gullone E. The clinical significance of loneliness: a literature review. *Clin Psychol Rev* (2006) 26(6):695–718. doi:10.1016/j.cpr.2006.04.002
34. Chang EC, Sanna LJ, Hirsch JK, Jeglic EL. Loneliness and negative life events as predictors of hopelessness and suicidal behaviors in Hispanics: evidence for a diathesis-stress model. *J Clin Psychol* (2010) 66(12):1242–53. doi:10.1002/jclp.20721
35. Lasgaard M, Goossens L, Elklit A. Loneliness, depressive symptomatology, and suicide ideation in adolescence: cross-sectional and longitudinal analyses. *J Abnorm Child Psychol* (2011) 39(1):137–50. doi:10.1007/s10802-010-9442-x
36. Hawkley LC, Browne MW, Cacioppo JT. How can I connect with thee? Let me count the ways. *Psychol Sci* (2005) 16(10):798–804. doi:10.1111/j.1467-9280.2005.01617.x
37. Mikulincer M, Segal J. A multidimensional analysis of the experience of loneliness. *J Soc Pers Relat* (1990) 7(2):209–30. doi:10.1177/0265407590072004
38. Dykstra PA. The differential availability of relationships and the provision and effectiveness of support to older adults. *J Soc Pers Relat* (1993) 10(3):355–70. doi:10.1177/0265407593103004
39. Stein JY, Tuval-Mashiach R. The social construction of loneliness: an integrative conceptualization. *J Construct Psychol* (2015) 28(3):210–27. doi:10.1080/10720537.2014.911129
40. Lasgaard M, Goossens L, Bramsen RH, Trillingsgaard T, Elklit A. Different sources of loneliness are associated with different forms of psychopathology in adolescence. *J Res Pers* (2011) 45(2):233–7. doi:10.1016/j.jrp.2010.12.005
41. Cacioppo JT, Cacioppo S, Adler AB, Lester PB, McGurk D, Thomas JL, et al. The cultural context of loneliness: risk factors in active duty soldiers. *J Soc Clin Psychol* (2016) 35(10):865–82. doi:10.1521/jscp.2016.35.10.865
42. Stein JY. The meaning of "loneliness" for traumatized veterans: a semiotic investigation of veterans' written narratives. *J Vet Stud* (2017) 2(2).
43. Stein JY, Tuval-Mashiach R. Loneliness and isolation in life-stories of Israeli veterans of combat and captivity. *Psychol Trauma* (2015) 7(2):122–30. doi:10.1037/a0036936
44. Ahern J, Worthen M, Masters J, Lippman SA, Ozer EJ, Moos R. The challenges of Afghanistan and Iraq veterans' transition from military to civilian life and approaches to reconnection. *PLoS One* (2015) 10:e0128599. doi:10.1371/journal.pone.0128599
45. Brewin CR, Garnett R, Andrews B. Trauma, identity and mental health in UK military veterans. *Psychol Med* (2011) 41(108):1733–40. doi:10.1017/S003329171000231X
46. Figley CR, Leventman S. *Strangers at Home: Vietnam Veterans since the War*. Philadelphia, PA: Brunner/Mazel (1980).
47. Sayer NA, Noorbaloochi S, Frazier P, Carlson K, Gravely A, Murdoch M. Reintegration problems and treatment interests among Iraq and Afghanistan combat veterans receiving VA medical care. *Psychiatr Serv* (2010) 61(6):589–97. doi:10.1176/ps.2010.61.6.589
48. Stein JY. The veteran's loneliness: emergence, facets and implications for intervention. In: Lázár R, editor. *Psychology of Loneliness: New Research*. Hauppauge, NY: Nova Science Publishers (2017). p. 1–36.
49. Lieblich A. *Seasons of Captivity: The Inner World of POWs*. New York, NY: New York University Press (1994).
50. Laub D, Auerhahn NC. Failed empathy – a central theme in the survivor's holocaust experience. *Psychoanal Psychol* (1989) 6(4):377. doi:10.1037/0736-9735.6.4.377
51. Freyd JJ. *Betrayal Trauma: The Logic of Forgetting Childhood Abuse*. Cambridge, MA: Harvard University Press (1996).
52. Gobin RL, Freyd JJ. The impact of betrayal trauma on the tendency to trust. *Psychol Trauma* (2014) 6(5):505. doi:10.1037/a0032452
53. Mikulincer M, Solomon Z, Shaver PR, Ein-Dor T. Attachment-related consequences of war captivity and trajectories of posttraumatic stress disorder: a 17-year longitudinal study. *J Soc Clin Psychol* (2014) 33(3):207–28. doi:10.1521/jscp.2014.33.3.207
54. Solomon Z, Dekel R, Mikulincer M. Complex trauma of war captivity: a prospective study of attachment and post-traumatic stress disorder. *Psychol Med* (2008) 38(10):1427–34. doi:10.1017/S0033291708002808
55. Stein JY, Snir A, Solomon Z. When man harms man: the interpersonal ramifications of war captivity. In: Cherry KE, editor. *Traumatic Stress and Long-Term Recovery*. New York, NY: Springer (2015). p. 113–32.
56. Kao JC, Chuong A, Reddy MK, Gobin RL, Zlotnick C, Johnson JE. Associations between past trauma, current social support, and loneliness in incarcerated populations. *Health Justice* (2014) 2(1):7. doi:10.1186/2194-7899-2-7
57. American Psychiatric Association. *Diagnostic and Statistical Manual of Mental Disorders*. 5th ed. Arlington, VA: American Psychiatric Association (2013).
58. Monson CM, Taft CT, Fredman SJ. Military-related PTSD and intimate relationships: from description to theory-driven research and intervention development. *Clin Psychol Rev* (2009) 29:707–14. doi:10.1016/j.cpr.2009.09.002
59. Lester P, Peterson K, Reeves J, Knauss L, Glover D, Mogil C, et al. The long war and parental combat deployment: effects on military children and at-home spouses. *J Am Acad Child Adolesc Psychiatry* (2010) 49(4):310–20. doi:10.1097/00004583-201004000-00006
60. Sayers SL, Farrow VA, Ross J, Oslin DW. Family problems among recently returned military veterans referred for a mental health evaluation. *J Clin Psychiatry* (2009) 70(2):163–70. doi:10.4088/JCP.07m03863
61. Lyons JA. The returning warrior: advice for families and friends. In: Figley CR, Nash WP, editors. *Combat Stress Injury: Theory, Research and Management*. London, England: Routledge (2007). p. 311–24.
62. Solomon Z, Dekel R. The contribution of loneliness and posttraumatic stress disorder to marital adjustment following war captivity: a longitudinal study. *Fam Process* (2008) 47(2):261–75. doi:10.1111/j.1545-5300.2008.00252.x
63. Shevlin M, McElroy E, Murphy J. Loneliness mediates the relationship between childhood trauma and adult psychopathology: evidence from the adult psychiatric morbidity survey. *Soc Psychiatry Psychiatr Epidemiol* (2015) 50(4):591–601. doi:10.1007/s00127-014-0951-8
64. Solomon Z, Bensimon M, Greene T, Horesh D, Ein-Dor T. Loneliness trajectories: the role of posttraumatic symptoms and social support. *J Loss Trauma* (2015) 20(1):1–21. doi:10.1080/15325024.2013.815055
65. Brewin CR, Andrews B, Valentine JD. Meta-analysis of risk factors for post-traumatic stress disorder in trauma-exposed adults. *J Consult Clin Psychol* (2000) 68(5):748–66. doi:10.1037/0022-006X.68.5.748
66. Ozer EJ, Best SR, Lipsey TL, Weiss DS. Predictors of posttraumatic stress disorder and symptoms in adults: a meta-analysis. *Psychol Bull* (2003) 129(1):52–73. doi:10.1037/0033-2909.129.1.52
67. Rook KS. Research on social support, loneliness, and social isolation: toward an integration. *Rev Personal Soc Psychol* (1984) 5:239–64.
68. Solomon Z, Waysman M, Mikulincer M. Family functioning, perceived societal support, and combat-related psychopathology: the moderating role of loneliness. *J Soc Clin Psychol* (1990) 9(4):456–72. doi:10.1521/jscp.1990.9.4.456
69. Collins LM, Schafer JL, Kam C-M. A comparison of inclusive and restrictive strategies in modern missing data procedures. *Psychol Methods* (2001) 6(4):330–51. doi:10.1037/1082-989X.6.4.330
70. Schafer JL, Graham JW. Missing data: our view of the state of the art. *Psychol Methods* (2002) 7(2):147. doi:10.1037/1082-989X.7.2.147
71. Derogatis LR. *Manual I: Scoring, Administration and Procedures for the SCL-90*. Baltimore, MD: Johns Hopkins University School of Medicine, Clinical Psychometrics Unit (1977).
72. Angst J, Hengartner MP, Rogers J, Schnyder U, Steinhausen H-C, Ajdacic-Gross V, et al. Suicidality in the prospective Zurich study: prevalence, risk factors and gender. *Eur Arch Psychiatry Clin Neurosci* (2014) 264(7):557–65. doi:10.1007/s00406-014-0500-1
73. Meng H, Li J, Loerbroks A, Wu J, Chen H. Rural/urban background, depression and suicidal ideation in Chinese college students: a cross-sectional study. *PLoS One* (2013) 8(8):e71313. doi:10.1371/journal.pone.0071313

74. Srisurapanont M, Likhitsathian S, Chua HC, Udomratn P, Chang S, Maneeton N, et al. Clinical and sociodemographic correlates of severe insomnia in psychotropic drug-free, Asian outpatients with major depressive disorder. *J Affect Disord* (2015) 186:26–31. doi:10.1016/j.jad.2015.06.032
75. Beck AT, Kovacs M, Weissman A. Assessment of suicidal intention: the Scale for Suicide Ideation. *J Consult Clin Psychol* (1979) 47(2):343. doi:10.1037/0022-006X.47.2.343
76. Desseilles M, Perroud N, Guillaume S, Jaussent I, Genty C, Malafosse A, et al. Is it valid to measure suicidal ideation by depression rating scales? *J Affect Disord* (2012) 136(3):398–404. doi:10.1016/j.jad.2011.11.013
77. Solomon Z, Benbenishty R, Neria Y, Abramovitz M, Ginzburg K, Ohry A. Assessment of PTSD: validation of the revised PTSD inventory. *Israel J Psychiatry Relat Sci* (1993) 30:110–5.
78. Solomon Z, Horesh D. Changes in diagnostic criteria for PTSD: implications from two prospective longitudinal studies. *Am J Orthopsychiatry* (2007) 77(2):182–8. doi:10.1037/0002-9432.77.2.182
79. American Psychiatric Association. *Diagnostic and Statistical Manual of Mental Disorders*. 4th ed. Washington, DC: American Psychiatric Association (1994).
80. Russel D, Peplau LA, Cutrona CE. The revised UCLA Loneliness Scale: concurrent and discriminant validity evidence. *J Pers Soc Psychol* (1980) 39(3):472–80. doi:10.1037/0022-3514.39.3.472
81. Hayes AF. *Introduction to Mediation, Moderation, and Conditional Process Analysis: A Regression-Based Approach*. New York, NY: Guilford Press (2013).
82. Stein JY, Wilmot DV, Solomon Z. Does one size fit all? Nosological, clinical, and scientific implications of variations in PTSD Criterion A. *J Anxiety Disord* (2016) 43:106–17. doi:10.1016/j.janxdis.2016.07.001
83. Ford JD, Stockton P, Kaltman S, Green BL. Disorders of extreme stress (DESNOS) symptoms are associated with type and severity of interpersonal trauma exposure in a sample of healthy young women. *J Interpers Violence* (2006) 21(11):1399–416. doi:10.1177/0886260506292992
84. Charuvastra A, Cloitre M. Social bonds and posttraumatic stress disorder. *Annu Rev Psychol* (2008) 59:301–28. doi:10.1146/annurev.psych.58.110405.085650
85. Belik S-L, Stein MB, Asmundson GJ, Sareen J. Relation between traumatic events and suicide attempts in Canadian military personnel. *Can J Psychiatry* (2009) 54(2):93–104. doi:10.1177/070674370905400207
86. Borges G, Benjet C, Medina-Mora ME, Orozco R, Molnar BE, Nock MK. Traumatic events and suicide-related outcomes among Mexico City adolescents. *J Child Psychol Psychiatry* (2008) 49(6):654–66. doi:10.1111/j.1469-7610.2007.01868.x
87. Cacioppo JT, Cacioppo S, Cole SW, Capitanio JP, Goossens L, Boomsma DI. Loneliness across phylogeny and a call for comparative studies and animal models. *Perspect Psychol Sci* (2015) 10(2):202–12. doi:10.1177/1745691614564876
88. Cacioppo JT, Hawkley LC. Perceived social isolation and cognition. *Trends Cogn Sci* (2009) 13(10):447–54. doi:10.1016/j.tics.2009.06.005
89. Chang EC. Hope and hopelessness as predictors of suicide ideation in Hungarian college students. *Death Stud* (2017) 41(7):455–60. doi:10.1080/07481187.2017.1299255
90. Qiu T, Klonsky ED, Klein DN. Hopelessness predicts suicide ideation but not attempts: a 10-year longitudinal study. *Suicide Life Threat Behav* (2017) 47(6):718–22. doi:10.1111/sltb.12328
91. McMillan D, Gilbody S, Beresford E, Neilly L. Can we predict suicide and non-fatal self-harm with the Beck Hopelessness Scale? A meta-analysis. *Psychol Med* (2007) 37(06):769–78. doi:10.1017/S0033291706009664
92. Orazem RJ, Frazier PA, Schnurr PP, Oleson HE, Carlson KF, Litz BT, et al. Identity adjustment among Afghanistan and Iraq war veterans with reintegration difficulty. *Psychol Trauma* (2017) 9(S1):4–11. doi:10.1037/tra0000225
93. Smith RT, True G. Warring identities identity conflict and the mental distress of American veterans of the wars in Iraq and Afghanistan. *Soc Mental Health* (2014) 4(2):147–61. doi:10.1177/2156869313512212
94. MacDonald G, Leary MR. Why does social exclusion hurt? The relationship between social and physical pain. *Psychol Bull* (2005) 131(2):202–23. doi:10.1037/0033-2909.131.2.202
95. Selby EA, Joiner TE, Riberio JD. Comprehensive theories of suicidal behaviors. In: Nock MK, editor. *The Oxford Handbook of Suicide and Self-injury*. New York, NY: Oxford University Press (2014). p. 286–307.
96. Orbach I. How would you listen to the person on the roof? A response to H. Omer and A. Elitzur. *Suicide Life Threat Behav* (2001) 31(2):140–3. doi:10.1521/suli.31.2.140.21518
97. Carr RB. Combat and human existence: toward an intersubjective approach to combat-related PTSD. *Psychoanal Psychol* (2011) 28(4):471–96. doi:10.1037/a0024174
98. Stolorow RD. Undergoing the situation: emotional dwelling is more than empathic understanding. *Int J Psychoanal Self Psychol* (2014) 9(1):80–3. doi:10.1080/15551024.2014.857750
99. Weissman MM, Markowitz JC, Klerman GL. *Comprehensive Guide to Interpersonal Psychotherapy*. New York, NY: Basic Books (2000).
100. Markowitz JC, Petkova E, Neria Y, Van Meter PE, Zhao Y, Hembree E, et al. Is exposure necessary? A randomized clinical trial of interpersonal psychotherapy for PTSD. *Am J Psychiatry* (2015) 172(5):430–40. doi:10.1176/appi.ajp.2014.14070908
101. Hundt NE, Robinson A, Arney J, Stanley MA, Cully JA. Veterans' perspectives on benefits and drawbacks of peer support for posttraumatic stress disorder. *Mil Med* (2015) 180(8):851–6. doi:10.7205/MILMED-D-14-00536

2

Diffusion of a Peer-Led Suicide Preventive Intervention Through School-Based Student Peer and Adult Networks

Trevor A. Pickering[1], Peter A. Wyman[2], Karen Schmeelk-Cone[2], Chelsey Hartley[2], Thomas W. Valente[1], Anthony R. Pisani[2], Kelly L. Rulison[3], Charles Hendricks Brown[4] and Mark LoMurray[4]*

[1] Department of Preventive Medicine, Keck School of Medicine, University of Southern California, Los Angeles, CA, United States, [2] Department of Psychiatry, School of Medicine and Dentistry, University of Rochester, Rochester, NY, United States, [3] Department of Public Health Education, University of North Carolina at Greensboro, Greensboro, NC, United States, [4] Department of Psychiatry and Behavioral Sciences, Feinberg School of Medicine, Sources of Strength, Inc., Chicago, IL, United States

***Correspondence:**
Peter A. Wyman
peter_wyman@urmc.rochester.edu

Background: Peer-led interventions have been applied to prevent various health behavior problems and may be an important complement to individual-level suicide prevention approaches. Sources of Strength trains student "peer leaders" in secondary schools to conduct prevention activities that encourage other students to build healthy social bonds and strengthen help-seeking norms. Prior work examining diffusion of peer-led programs has focused on youths' closeness to peer leaders but minimally on other factors such as connections to adults and suicidal behavior.

Methods: We examined implementation and dissemination of Sources of Strength in 20 schools. Over 1 year 533 students were trained as peer leaders and 3,730 9th–12th graders completed baseline surveys assessing friendships and adults at school, and suicidal thoughts/behaviors; and end-of-year surveys reporting intervention exposure: viewed poster/video, attended presentation, direct peer communication, and activity participation. Chi-square tests compared exposure rates by student and network characteristics. Multi-level logistic regression models tested predictors of exposure across individual and school-level characteristics.

Results: Exposure to the intervention varied greatly by school and by individual student characteristics and network position. Training more peer leaders increased school-wide exposure for all modalities except presentation (Bs 0.06–0.10, *p's* < 0.05). In multivariate models, exposure was consistently higher for students closer to peer leaders in the friendship network (ORs 1.13–1.54, *p's* < 0.05) and students who named more trusted adults (ORs 1.08–1.16, *p's* < 0.001); and lower for males (ORs 0.56–0.83, *p's* < 0.05). In multivariate models, training more students as peer leaders predicted exposure to poster-video and direct peer communication in larger schools (OR = 3.34 and 2.87, respectively). Network characteristics influenced exposure similarly for students with suicidal thoughts and behaviors.

Discussion: Our findings confirm prior work showing the importance of personal affiliations to peer leaders and natural networks as a medium for diffusion of peer-led prevention efforts. We build on that work by showing independent effects of closeness to adults at school and number of peer leaders trained. There is a need to strategically select peer leaders to maximize closeness to students school-wide, particularly in larger schools. Additional work is required for Sources of Strength to devise messaging strategies to engage males and students isolated from adults at school.

Keywords: suicide prevention, peer leaders, social networks, diffusion of innovations, social connectedness, school intervention, peer messaging, social support

INTRODUCTION

School-based suicide prevention programs have utilized a narrow range of approaches along the continuum of public health interventions. Current programs focus on individual-level risk factors. The most widely used programs employ strategies—screening (1) and gatekeeper training (2)—to expand recognition and referral of adolescents at elevated risk for suicide due to psychiatric and/or behavioral problems (3). School-based educational programmes (4) are another approach designed to increase students' self-disclosure of suicide risk, identification of at-risk peers, and management of distress and depression symptoms (5–8). Despite widespread use of individual-focused interventions (9), youth suicide rates are increasing. Among those 15–19 years of age the U.S., suicide rates increased from 8.0 per 100,000 in 2000 to 9.76 per 100,000 in 2015, a 22% increase (10). Consensus is emerging among researchers and leading policy groups that a broader range of population-focused prevention approaches is needed to reduce suicide rates (11).

This study focuses on another type of public health preventive approach: preparing key opinion leaders to modify social-ecological protective factors, including healthy bonds to peers and adults, within their schools and social networks. Specifically, we examined implementation and dissemination of Sources of Strength, a peer-led suicide prevention program for secondary schools, typically encompassing individuals 14–18 years of age (12, 13). Our prior work identified Sources of Strength as the first intervention involving peer leaders to enhance protective factors associated with reduced suicidal behavior at the school population level (13). However, like nearly all other interventions employing key opinion leaders, minimal research attention has focused on identifying key implementation components of Sources of Strength and processes of dissemination through a population. To develop a more complete model for Sources of Strength, it is necessary to clarify the mechanisms behind intervention diffusion in a schoolwide context. Such knowledge is critical for determining how to maximize the intervention's efficiency and impact, especially considering that participating high schools may have widely different patterns of student social affiliations. We evaluated how characteristics of students' peer affiliation and adult networks influenced exposure to the Sources of Strength intervention messaging. A specific objective was to examine the extent to which messaging reached students who are isolated from peers and adults, as well as those at high risk for suicide due to suicidal thoughts and behaviors in the prior year.

Key Opinion Leader Interventions: Evidence and Research Needs

Peer leaders' delivering prevention programming has been applied to a variety of adolescent health problems but only recently to school-based suicide prevention (13). School-based programs incorporating peer leaders and student-to-student exercises are more effective than lecture-style programs, according to meta-analyses of substance abuse interventions (14, 15). Peer leaders have been effective in reducing HIV risk behaviors (16–18), in other health promotion programs (19), and in tobacco use prevention (20–24). Variability in how peer-led programs are implemented is extensive. Peer-led tobacco prevention interventions, for example, range from preparing older students to deliver structured classroom lessons (23) to training influential students to encourage their peers not to smoke through informal interactions (20).

Adolescents influence their peers' prosocial and antisocial behaviors including drug use and health (25, 26), and the effectiveness of peer leaders is congruent with the fact that this influence occurs through individuals' social networks. Recent social network modeling indicates that many health behaviors, including smoking cessation and obesity, reflect person-to-person spread of behaviors within social clusters (27), and the proximity of individuals within a social network determines the degree to which they will influence each over time (28, 29). That evidence is also congruent with research showing that individuals closely tied through affiliation groups influence each other's adoption of new practices (30), and evidence regarding importance of peer norms on behavior (30–32). Regarding suicide risk, peer suicidal behavior may promote a norm that suicide is a common response to distress, and adolescents are more susceptible to suicide imitation than are other age groups (33).

Work on mechanisms of peer-led programs is limited. Several studies have examined closeness to trained peer leaders to elucidate how intervention effects diffuse through a population. For example, a study of a peer health advocate program showed that individuals in a drug using community who were closest to one of the trained peer health advocates were more likely to be exposed to the intervention and adopt risk avoidance strategies (34). Valente and colleagues found that adolescents benefitted more from a tobacco prevention curriculum the more closely they were affiliated in friendship groups to those adolescents who were peer leaders delivering the intervention (24). Stoebenau and Valente (35) showed that people in one Madagascar village had higher contraceptive knowledge and use when they were directly tied to community-based contraceptive deliverers. However, many questions remain unaddressed. Work is needed to identify factors that promote dissemination of different peer leader messaging strategies, which range from informal communication to structured presentations (36). Evidence that overall school social network structure influences diffusion of substance use prevention effects (37) also points to the need for more research examining school characteristics. To systematize school programs, work is also needed to identify how the proportion of a school population trained as peer leaders influences dissemination effects. A question of specific interest to Sources of Strength is how students' ties to adults influence their receptivity to peer leader messaging.

Sources of Strength

Sources of Strength recruits and trains key opinion leaders (i.e., peer leaders) along with school staff members as advisors. Peer leaders learn a model of health and resilience that emphasizes growing healthy social bonds (i.e., trusted adults, family support, positive friends) and resources to manage adversity, such as healthy activities and medical/mental health resources for suicide concerns. With ongoing adult mentoring, peer leaders conduct activities to disseminate "sources of strength," with the aim of modifying peer norms regarding coping and help-seeking and increasing youth-adult connections, particularly among students isolated from adults. The rationale stems from evidence that suicidal behavior is lower among youth with stronger social bonds to family, peers and other adults; strong bonds may reduce suicide risk through protective mechanisms including enhanced psychological well-being (38), increased help-seeking (39), and normative social influences that encourage adaptive coping (13).

Our prior work testing Sources of Strength through a cluster randomized trial (18 high schools, 2,000 students) showed that within 3 months after adolescent peer leaders were trained and began implementing prevention messaging activities (i.e., presentations, posters, peer communication), norms about help-seeking and perceptions of adult support were changed among students throughout their schools (13). However, this study employed traditional survey methods in which social network information was not collected. In a subsequent study we contrasted peer leader messaging activities (36 classrooms; 700 students) (36) and showed that peer leader presentations based on modeling of healthy coping increased other students' positive coping attitudes and perceptions of adult support; the addition of student audience involvement in identifying their own trusted adults increased students' expectations of adult support (36). Our findings suggest that peer leaders' involving classmates in interactive "sources of strength" messaging will increase impact of their messaging, congruent with communication theories emphasizing personal engagement (40).

Current Study

The current study primarily aimed to examine the diffusion of peer leaders' messaging activities across the student populations of 20 high schools over one school year, as part of a larger randomized controlled trial of Sources of Strength (clinicaltrials.gov #02043093). We sought to use students' nominations of friends at school (collected prior to training peer leaders) to identify individual student's network position, as well as overall school network properties. Students' nominations of their trusted adults at school helped inform the presence of youth-adult networks. The principal outcome of interest was exposure to Sources of Strength messaging modalities along a continuum of engagement that ranged from viewing posters/videos to participation in interactive exercises (e.g., naming a trusted adult).

We expected that peer leaders would reach more students who had closer friendship ties to peer leaders and more ties to other students overall (i.e., higher "centrality"). In contrast, we expected that students with fewer direct ties to peer leaders and to other students would have fewer opportunities for exposure to Sources of Strength. Prior work by Valente and colleagues showed that (a) individuals with exposure to external influences were critical in the diffusion of innovative practices, and (b) although external exposure played a role in bringing innovations to individuals' attention, the interpersonal persuasion of trusted others was crucial in convincing individuals to adopt (41–43). Thus, Valente's social network threshold model would predict that having social ties facilitates exposure to influences such as Sources of Strength messages, and close ties to peer leaders may be necessary for students to become more deeply involved such as participating in a Sources of Strength activity.

At the school level, we sought to examine the proportion of students trained as peer leaders, as well as characteristics of the school-wide peer network. A finding that schools with denser friendship networks had overall greater exposure to Sources of Strength among their students would be consistent with the network thresholds model that emphasizes diffusion through natural networks. We expected that the impact of school-level factors on exposure would be greater in schools with more students, since larger networks tend to be more fragmented.

A final set of questions focused on determining the extent to which peer leader messaging reached suicidal students and students who are isolated from peers and adults at school. In other analyses examining these school networks, we found that students with recent suicide attempts were more likely to be part of affiliation groups that were less cohesive and on the periphery of the school network (44), which are network positions that may reduce opportunities for exposure to Sources of Strength messaging. We were also interested if exposure varied by student sex. In our prior examination of peer-led classroom messaging, we found greater benefit for females vs. males in terms of perceptions that adults are capable of helping suicidal youth (36).

METHODS

Schools and Student Enrollment

The 20 schools in this study were part of an effectiveness trial of Sources of Strength involving a total of 40 high schools located in predominantly rural, small town, and micropolitan communities of New York State and North Dakota. Schools in both states were recruited from counties or public health regions with past 5-year youth suicide rates above the state average (24.40 per 100,000 in North Dakota and 5.19 in New York for youth 15–19 in 2009–2011) (45). The 40 high schools were enrolled in four cohorts (2010–2013), with schools stratified by size and location; matched pairs were subsequently randomized into condition. The 20 high schools randomized to begin immediate implementation of Sources of Strength are included in this study (16 in New York, four in North Dakota). The schools ranged in size from 63 to 1,207 students ($M = 366$). Two schools served American Indian reservations.

Student recruitment occurred in two phases: (a) in early fall for participants in school-wide evaluation of Sources of Strength, and (b) immediately following for student peer leaders. For the school-wide assessments, all 9–12th graders were invited to enroll in the study evaluating Sources of Strength by completing fall and spring web-based assessments over two school years; a small portion (<1%) without language ability to independently complete web assessments were excluded. Information letters sent to parents included an option to decline their child's participation. This study was carried out in accordance with the University of Rochester Institutional Review Board who approved the study protocol. Information letters were sent to parents that included an option to decline participation. Research personnel collected opt-out forms and conducted verbal assent with eligible students followed immediately by web-based assessments. All students received information about how to access help or support for themselves or a peer if needed.

Sources of Strength Intervention

Implementation of Sources of Strength in each school followed three standardized phases: (1) School community preparation, including training several staff members as advisors; (2) Recruitment and training of student peer leaders (PLs); and (3) peer leader messaging. Schools did not begin peer leader recruitment and training until baseline assessments of the student population were completed. Adult advisors facilitated standard recruitment procedures by distributing nomination forms school-wide and each staff member was asked to nominate up to 6 students whose "voices are heard" by other students. Nominations were reviewed to invite 5–10% of the student population across diverse groups within the school. Given 5–10% of the school population were invited, peer leader teams were dependent on school size. Of the 959 invited (19–86 per school), 798 (83.2%) enrolled with parent permission and youth assent/consent across two school years.

The training for peer leaders (along with their adult advisors) emphasized interactive learning about eight protective "sources of strength" (family support, positive friends, mentors, healthy activities, generosity, spirituality, medical access, and mental health access). Each school received half-day training [standardized curriculum of 15 modules (12) led by the program developer, co-author ML]. In the training peer leaders learned skills to increase protective resources in themselves, encourage peers to grow these resources, and connect suicidal peers with resources, especially trusted adults.

During the messaging phase, adult advisors led peer leader team meetings (bi-weekly to monthly) where they fostered the 8 protective strengths, built community within the peer leaders, and planned messaging activities for dissemination. The curriculum included student activities aimed at raising awareness of Sources of Strength, generating conversations with peers, providing presentations for peer leaders to share personal examples of using strengths, and engaging other students to identify their own trusted adults. Peer leaders were encouraged to tailor the messaging style to their school, with adult advisor monitoring to ensure safe messaging.

Measures

Students completed questionnaires measuring: (a) suicidal thoughts and behaviors and (b) social networks, in the fall before peer leader training (baseline, Time 1). Students completed a questionnaire covering several modalities of exposure to Sources of Strength at the end of the school year (Time 2).

Suicidal Behaviors

Suicidal ideation and attempts were assessed using the Youth Risk Behavior Survey measure (46) that has well-established reliability and validity for population-based assessments (47, 48). Each student was asked whether in the preceding 12 months she/he had: seriously considered suicide; planned suicide; made one or more suicide attempts; and made an attempt that resulted in medical injury requiring treatment. Suicide attempt was classified as having one or more attempts regardless of injury or ideation. Suicide ideation-only was classified as having suicide ideation with no suicide attempts.

Network Measures

Students were asked to name up to seven of their closest friends at school, a peer network standard. Students nominated friends by typing in their names, a nomination method that yields fewer, closer relationships compared to selecting friends from a roster of names (49). A novel aspect of the network assessment was that students were also asked to name up to seven "adults in your school who you trust and feel you can talk to about personal things" (trusted adults).

Variables measuring the centrality of students in the network and closeness to peer leaders included: (a) Out-degree: the number of friends the student named. (b) Peer isolate: Students who named no friends and received no friendship nominations from others. (c) Coreness: An individual's coreness value k is the largest value that satisfies the following condition: the individual has at least k friends who also have at least k friends. For example, if a student is connected to 4 friends who each has at least 4 friends, that student would have a coreness value of 4. Coreness therefore reflects the extent to which an individual is a part of an interconnected friendship group and indicates the size of that group. (d) Closeness to peer leader: the number of steps in the shortest path to a peer leader, categorized into 1, 2, 3 or more steps, and not connected (i.e., there was no friendship path that connected to a peer leader). (d) Adult out-degree: total number of trusted adults named. Students who named no trusted adults were considered adult isolates.

Variables at the network level were normalized across 20 schools to have a mean of 0 and standard deviation of 1. These variables included: (a) School size: total school enrollment at Time 1. For analyses, school size was log-transformed to better fit a normal distribution. (b) School percent peer leaders: percent of school trained as a peer leader. (c) School scaled density: percent of total nominations made out of total nominations possible (maximum of 7 per student, or 7N for a school of size N).

Intervention Exposure

Exposure to Sources of Strength was categorized into four different dichotomous exposure modalities corresponding to various levels of engagement. The student survey contained a section asking about exposures, preceded by the phrase, "Some students in your school have been trained as Peer Leaders in a program called Sources of Strength." Students were subsequently asked about:

(1) Exposure to a *presentation or assembly* consisted of answering "yes" to either: Have you seen a presentation or assembly about... (a) strengths that help teens get through hard times?, or (b) helping suicidal teens by getting adults involved? Example presentations included peer leaders leading presentations in their class about the "Sources of Strength wheel" and a source they felt they were strong in.
(2) Exposure to *posters or videos* was assessed by answering "yes" to: Have you seen posters or videos at school about strengths? Example posters included pictures of the Sources of Strength wheel displaying the eight different sources.
(3) *Direct peer communication* was measured by answering "yes" to either: Has a friend or other student... (a) told you about Sources of Strength?, or (b) talked to you about using strengths?
(4) Participation in an *activity* consisted of answering "yes" to either: (a) Have you participated in a Sources of Strength activity such as adding your trusted adult to a poster?, or (b) Has a friend or other student asked you to name adults you can go to for help?

Statistical Analysis

Descriptive analyses were conducted in SPSS (V23). Creation and analyses of network variables were conducted in R v3.4.2 (50) with the igraph package (51). Gephi v0.9.2 (52) was used to graph network diagrams. Chi-square tests of proportions were used to determine if suicide ideation-only, suicide attempt, peer isolation, and adult isolation varied by demographic characteristics. This approach was also used to determine if demographic characteristics, suicidality, or network variables were associated with the four exposure modalities to Sources of Strength.

To examine the simultaneous effect of hypothesized individual- and school-level influences on Sources of Strength exposures, we fit multi-level logistic regression models using the lme4 package in R (53). These models included level-1 variables (sex, ethnicity, out-degree, coreness, closeness to a peer leader, trusted adults, suicide attempt, suicide ideation-only), level-2 variables (schoolwide density, schoolwide percent students trained as peer leaders, and school size), and a random intercept for school. To determine if the effect of closeness to a peer leader on exposure was moderated by having a more cohesive friendship group, an interaction between coreness and closeness to peer leaders was included. Similarly, an interaction between school size and school percent peer leaders was included as we hypothesized the effect of percent peer leaders would be greater in larger schools. We tested the significance of these interaction terms in each model and if the interaction was non-significant ($p > 0.05$) then it was excluded from the model.

Lastly, we examined if having suicide attempt or ideation moderated the effects of network variables on exposure. After evaluating each of the previous models, an interaction term was added for each predictor with (1) suicide attempt and (2) suicide ideation, individually. Predictors that had a significant interaction with either suicide attempt or suicide ideation-only were retained in the model.

RESULTS

Sample Participation and Demographics

Student Participants in School-Wide Assessments

Across the 20 schools, average school population enrollment was 82.2% (range 65.9–98.3%). A total of 5,677 students completed the assessments (baseline; Time 1) before training of student peer leaders (see **Table 1**). Participants included roughly equivalent proportion of males and females and grade levels. The enrolled sample was predominantly white and non-Hispanic, consistent with the rural and micropolitan communities of New York State and North Dakota. In the prior 12 months, 7.0% had made one or more suicide attempts (see **Table 1**, column 2) and 8.4% had suicidal ideation without attempt (see **Table 1**, column 3). Females had higher rates of suicide attempts and ideation, consistent with national norms (54). On the social network assessment, 194 students (3.4%) were peer isolates (i.e., students who neither made nor received a friendship nomination; see **Table 1**, column 4). A total of 2,082 students (36.1%) did not name a trusted adult at their school (see **Table 1**, column 5). Males were more likely to be isolated from peers and adults at school. More black/African American and other race students were peer isolates compared to white students. All minority race/ethnic groups were significantly more isolated from adults vs. white, non-Hispanic youth.

Among the enrolled non-peer leader students, 70.4% ($n = 3,730$) participated again at Time 2 and provided data on their exposure to Sources of Strength messaging. We examined if students who participated at both Time 1 and Time 2 were

TABLE 1 | Characteristics of students participating in school-wide assessments at Time 1.

		N (%)	Suicide attempt *N* (%)	Suicidal ideation *N* (%)	Isolate from friends *N* (%)	Isolate from adults *N* (%)
Total		5,677	397 (7.0)	502 (8.8)	194 (3.4)	2,082 (36.1)
Sex	Male†	2,874 (49.9)	139 (4.8)	172 (6.0)	116 (4.0)	1,213 (42.3)
	Female	2,803 (48.6)	278 (9.9)*	325 (11.7)*	73 (2.6)*	829 (29.6)*
Grade	9th†	1,486 (25.8)	121 (8.4)*	118 (8.0)	39 (2.6)	629 (42.4)*
	10th	1,501 (26.0)	115 (8.0)	135 (9.1)	52 (3.5)	552 (36.8)
	11th	1,315 (22.8)	93 (7.3)	125 (9.6)	46 (3.5)	454 (34.6)
	12th	1,306 (22.7)	81 (6.4)	112 (8.7)	48 (3.7)	380 (29.2)
Race	Asian	133 (2.3)	9 (7.2)	14 (10.6)	3 (2.3)	65 (48.9)*
	Black/AA	588 (10.2)	47 (8.3)	34 (5.9)*	35 (6.0)*	268 (45.8)*
	Am. Indian	270 (4.7)	26 (9.9)+	17 (6.3)	7 (2.6)	117 (43.3)*
	White†	4,248 (73.7)	285 (6.9)	390 (9.5)	117 (2.8)	1,347 (31.8)
	Other	408 (7.1)	40 (10.4)*	37 (9.1)	22 (5.4)*	218 (53.6)*
Ethnicity	Hispanic†	503 (8.7)	61 (12.9)	54 (10.9)	27 (5.4)	268 (53.5)
	Non-Hisp.	5,147 (89.3)	357 (7.2)*	443 (8.7)+	159 (3.1)*	1,761 (34.3)*

$^*p < 0.05$. $^+p < 0.10$, for difference in proportions between/among groups. †Reference group. Categories may not add to 100% due to missing data.

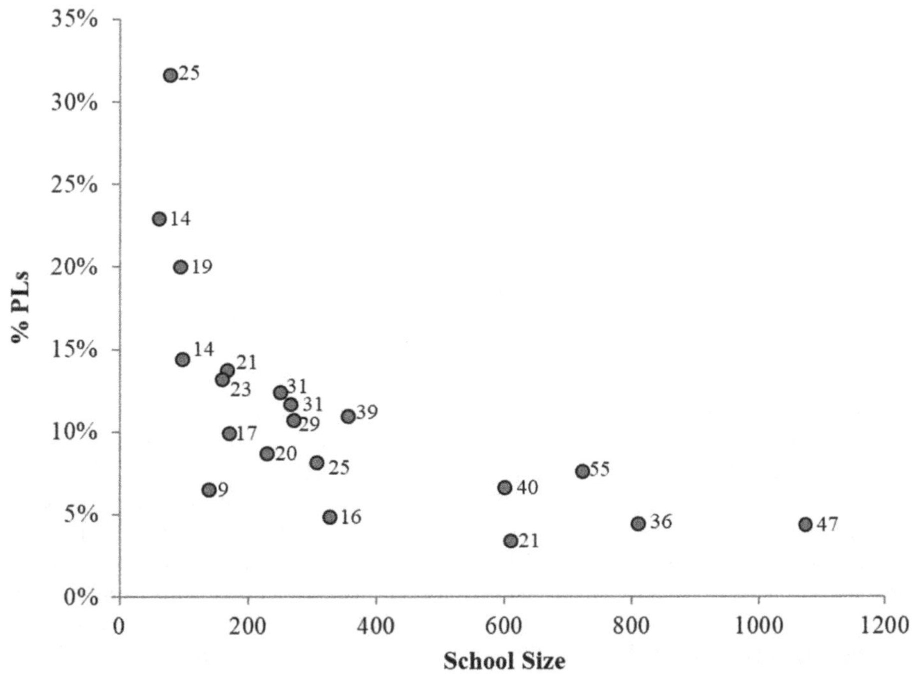

FIGURE 1 | Percent of school trained as a peer leader by school size. Nodes are labeled with total number of peer leaders.

different from those who only participated at Time 1 (i.e., differential attrition). The groups were comparable by student sex and presence of suicidal ideation. However, white students were more likely to participate in both assessments vs. all minority race students. There were also fewer suicide attempts among those with both surveys (6.4%) than those with only Time 1 data (10.8%). Those who did not take the Time 2 survey were more likely to be isolated from peers vs. those who took both surveys (4.8 vs. 2.1%, respectively) and isolated from adults (44.8 vs. 31.8%). An additional 711 students participated at Time 2 only but were not included in analyses for this study.

Student Peer Leaders

A total of 533 students enrolled and trained as peer leaders across the 20 schools (range 9–55 per school; see **Figure 1**, nodes labeled total PLs). The mean percent of total students trained as peer leaders was 9.2% (range 3–32%). The percent of students trained

TABLE 2 | Sources of Strength exposure by modality for non-peer leader students after one school year.

Group		*N*	Poster/video (%)	Presentation (%)	Direct peer (%)	Activity (%)
Total Non-PL		3,730	57.9	51.6	56.6	48.7
DEMOGRAPHICS						
Sex	Males[†]	1,908	51.2	48.9	49.9	43.5
	Females	1,778	64.9*	54.5*	63.8*	54.4*
Grade	9th	993	57.5	54.1*	57.7*	49.7
	10th	990	60.4	53.7*	61.1*	51.4*
	11th	848	55.2	50.7	55.8*	47.1
	12th[†]	809	58.0	48.0	50.8	45.9
STB	None[†]	3,105	58.5	52.5	56.8	49.4
	Ideation	310	56.4	52.7	58.2	49.7
	Attempt	235	49.6*	45.3*	56.4	45.7
SOCIAL NETWORK						
PL proximity	PL friend[†]	1,528	68.0	56.0	68.6	54.0
	No PL friend	2,194	52.7*	51.0*	50.4*	47.2*
Peer	Isolate[†]	80	38.8	35.0	43.8	40.0
	Non-isolate	3,642	58.3*	52.0*	56.9*	48.9
Adult	Isolate[†]	1,240	48.1	44.6	46.5	40.8
	Non-isolate	2,483	62.7*	55.1*	61.7*	52.7*
SCHOOL-LEVEL						
Mean of schools	20	63.0	52.7	59.3	51.3	
Range		23.4–85.1	30.7–84.3	20.3–76.5	25.0–83.0	
School size	Sm (<150)[†]	8	69.8	55.5	61.8	62.5
	Md (150–500)	7	66.5	50.7	62.8	41.4*
	Lg (500+)	5	47.3*	50.9	50.4*	47.2

*STB, suicidal thoughts/behaviors. Subgroup sample sizes may not equal total sample size due to missing data. [†]Reference group *p < 0.05 for difference in proportions.*

was sharply higher for smaller vs. larger schools, as shown in **Figure 1**. Schools with fewer than 200 students generally trained between 15 and 30% of students. Schools with more than 400 students did not train more than 10%. Peer leaders were made up of more females (56.5%). Regarding race, peer leaders had fewer black/African American members (3.7%) than non-peer leaders (5.8%); otherwise the groups were similar by race. Across grades, peer leaders had more 10th (28.5%) and 11th graders (30.1%) vs. non-peer leaders (27.2 and 23.3%, respectively). Peer leaders and non-peer leaders were similar in likelihood of reporting suicide attempts and suicidal ideation.

Exposure to Sources of Strength by Student and School Characteristics

Overall, exposure to the intervention varied by messaging modality (see **Table 2**), i.e., 48.7 (activity participation) to 57.9% (poster/video exposure). Females consistently had greater exposure to the intervention across all modalities (p's < 0.001). Students with suicide attempt were less likely than those with no suicidal thoughts/behaviors (STB) to have seen a presentation or a poster/video (p's < 0.05). Having a friend who was a peer leader systematically led to higher exposure rates across all modalities (p's < 0.01). Students who named any friend at the beginning of the year had higher exposure rates for all modalities except participation in a Sources of Strength activity (p's < 0.05). Being isolated from adults was detrimental to exposure; being an isolate from adults consistently resulted in lower exposure rates across all modalities (p's < 0.001).

Exposure was greater when students were closer to peer leaders and named more friends and trusted adults (i.e., an exposure-response relationship). That is, individuals who were closer in steps to a peer leader had even greater likelihood of exposure (**Figure 2A**). This effect was most pronounced for direct peer communication and poster/video (OR = 1.80 and 1.65, respectively, p's < 0.001) than for presentation and activity (OR = 1.16 and 1.19, respectively, p's < 0.001). For example, direct peer communication exposure for students who named a peer leader friend was 68.6%, decreased to 55% for having a peer leader as a friend of a friend, and 40% for being three or more steps away. Likewise, naming more friends modestly and incrementally increased likelihood of exposure for each additional friend named (**Figure 2B**; ORs ranged across exposure modalities from 1.05 to 1.07 per friend named, p's < 0.001) and naming more trusted adults increased the likelihood of exposure for each additional adult named (**Figure 2C**; ORs ranged across exposure modalities from 1.10 to 1.18 per adult named, p's < 0.001).

To determine if the lower exposure rates for males was explained by fewer friendship ties between males and peer leaders, we stratified this analysis by gender (**Figure 2D**). The relationship between exposure and closeness to peer leaders was similar for males and females, although uniformly lower for

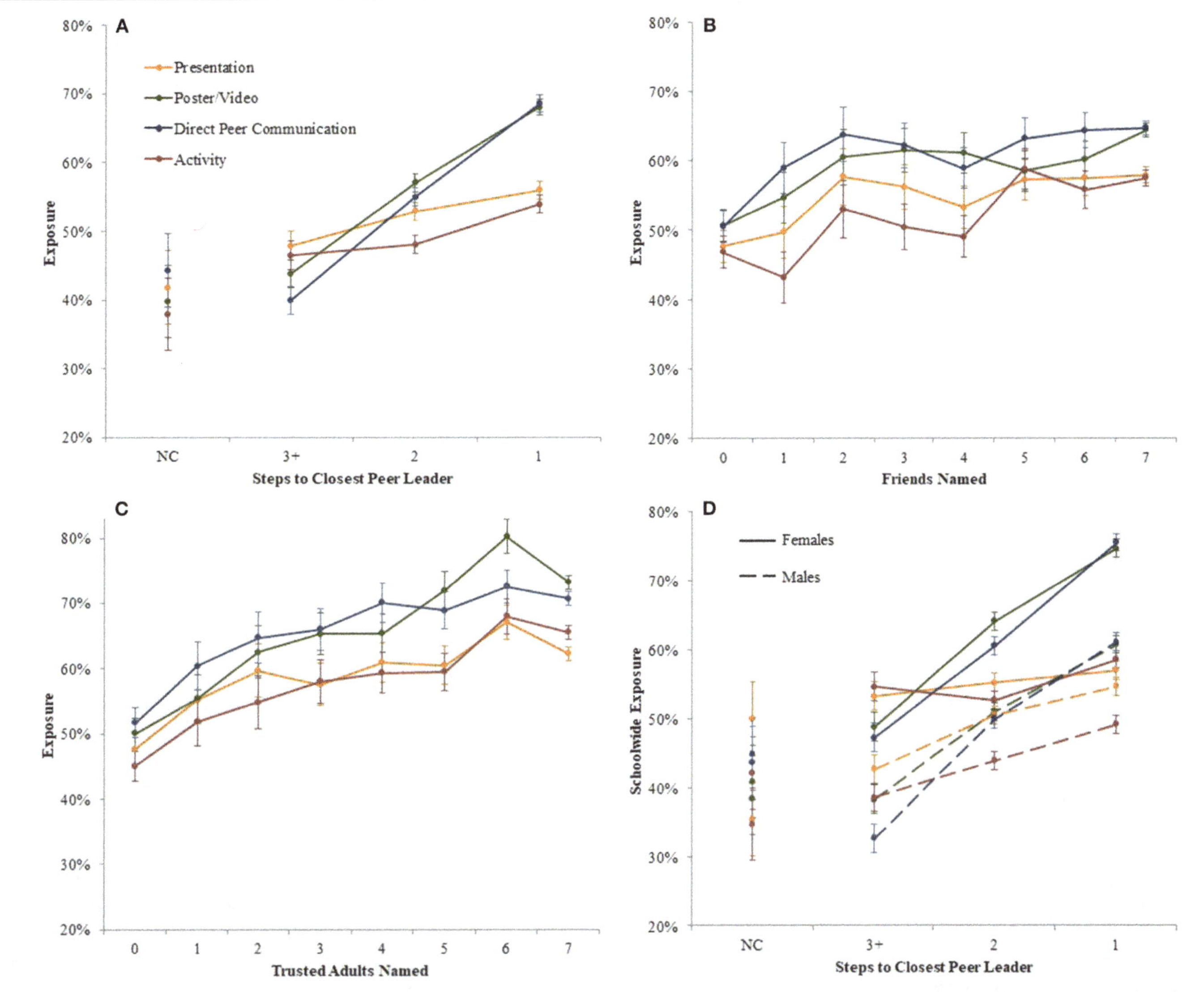

FIGURE 2 | School-wide intervention exposure by **(A)** steps to closest peer leader, **(B)** number of friends named, **(C)** number of trusted adults named, and **(D)** steps to closest peer leader, stratified by gender (female = solid lines, male = dashed lines). Error bars represent one standard error.

males. And males had lower exposure even when they named a peer leader friend. For example, direct peer communication exposure for females and males who named a peer leader as a friend was 76 and 61%, respectively.

Intervention exposure varied greatly among schools. The range of schoolwide exposure proportion was 23.4–85.1% for poster/video, 30.7–84.3% for presentation, 25.0–83.0% for direct peer communication and 20.3–76.5% for activity (see **Table 2**). Exposure to the intervention trended lower in larger schools, though this effect reached traditional significance levels only for poster/video exposure in large schools vs. small schools and for presentation exposure in medium vs. small schools (p's < 0.05). Schoolwide percent of students trained as a peer leader was generally associated with exposure (**Figure 3**). A linear regression showed significant relationships between percent of students trained as peer leaders and having seen a poster/video ($B = 1.57$, $p = 0.008$), participating in an activity ($B = 1.47$, $p = 0.01$), and having direct peer communication ($B = 0.98$, $p = 0.04$), but not having seen a presentation ($B = 0.70$, $p = 0.22$).

Correlations of school-wide and individual-level variables are presented in **Table 3**. At the school level, students' mean closeness to a peer leader was related to several variables including intervention exposures (all modalities except having seen a presentation), percent of students trained as peer leaders, school size, and school density. Schoolwide suicide attempt and ideation-only rates were not correlated with any other variables at the school level. At the individual level, network characteristics were modestly related among each other and were all related to an individual intervention exposure across all modalities. Suicide attempt was inversely related to individual network centrality measures such as out-degree, coreness, and closeness to a peer leader. Number of trusted adults named was positively correlated

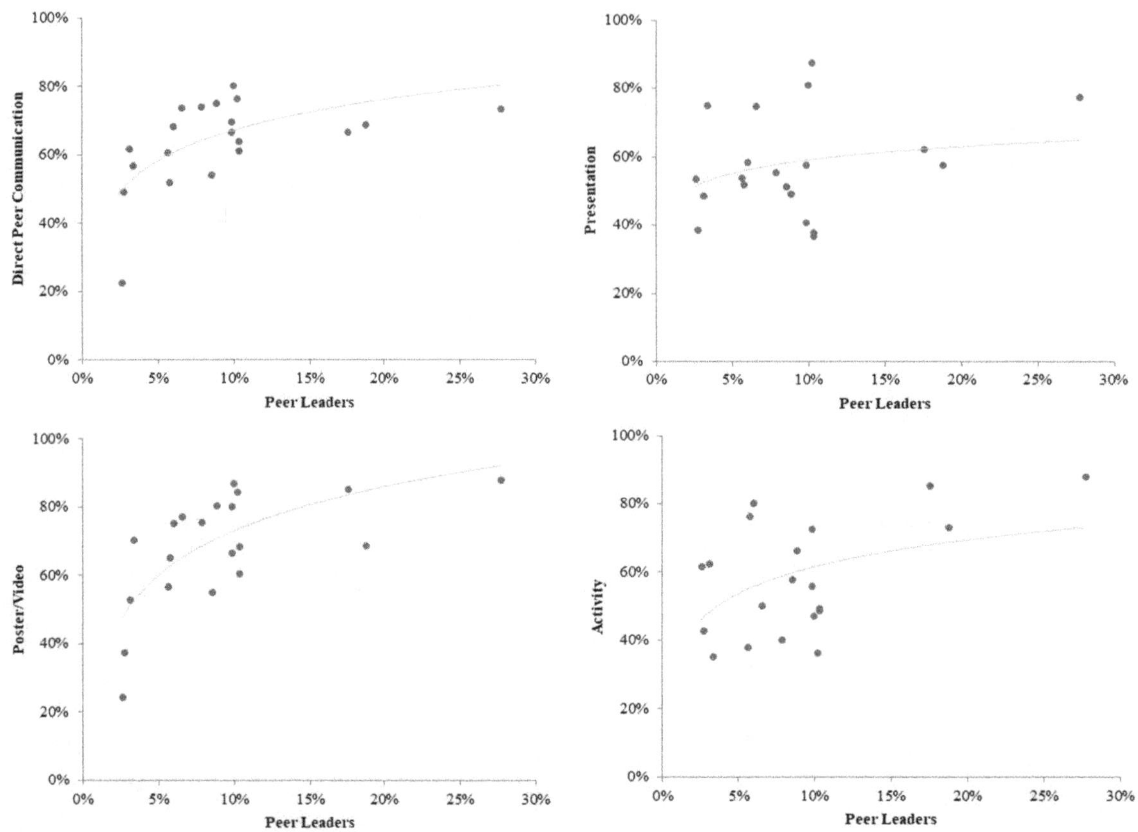

FIGURE 3 | Exposure to the Sources of Strength intervention by percent peer leaders at school.

with all individual exposure measures and all individual network centrality measures, and inversely related to suicide attempt and ideation-only.

Multivariate Analysis

The multi-level logistic regression model indicated substantial variability in random intercept among schools (random intercept SD ranged from 0.44 to 0.62 by exposure modality), reflecting the differing school-wide exposure rates (**Table 4a**). Male gender was associated with lower exposure across all modalities (**Table 4b**; ORs ranged from 0.83 to 0.56, p's < 0.05). Two network variables were consistently associated with higher likelihood of intervention exposure: closeness to a peer leader and number of trusted adults named. Even when adjusting for all other individual-level network metrics, naming more trusted adults increased exposure to the intervention (ORs ranged from 1.08 to 1.16, p's < 0.001). Students with suicide attempt were less likely to have seen a poster/video (OR $= 0.69$, $p < 0.001$) and were less likely to have seen a presentation (OR $= 0.76$, $p = 0.07$). Ego's coreness moderated the effect of closeness to a peer leader on exposure to peer communication (interaction logit $= 0.05$, $p < 0.05$). That is, the effect of being close to a peer leader on peer communication was even stronger if the student was a part of a more dense, cohesive friendship group (see **Table 4b**; ORs ranged from 1.40 for low coreness to 1.68 for high coreness, p's < 0.05).

Percent of students trained as a peer leader (a level-2 variable) still predicted poster/video exposure and direct peer communication with student closeness to a peer leader in the model (noting that percent of students trained as peer leaders was highly correlated with schoolwide closeness to a peer leader). The effect of schoolwide percent of students trained as peer leaders on exposure varied by school size for all exposures other than presentation. The effect of percent students trained as peer leader was greater for larger schools on poster/video and peer communication (interaction logit ranged from 0.38 to 0.43, p's < 0.05). Evaluated at the mean of school size, a one standard deviation increase in the percent of students trained as peer leaders was associated with a 2.17 likelihood of having seen a poster/video and a 1.97 likelihood of having direct peer communication ($p < 0.05$). This effect was greater in magnitude and significant for larger schools (+1 SD size) and nonsignificant for smaller schools (−1 SD size). Unexpectedly, this interaction was also significant for activity participation but the effects were in the opposite direction (interaction logit $= -0.56$, $p = 0.007$). The effect of schoolwide percent students trained as peer leaders was nonsignificant for schools of mean size or less, but was significant for larger schools (OR $= 0.32$, $p = 0.04$). To determine if this was an artifact of covariates an additional analysis was performed: school-level activity participation rate was regressed on school size, percent students trained as peer leaders, and their

TABLE 3a | Correlations among network and intervention exposure variables.

(A) Level-2 (schoolwide) variables ($N = 20$)

S.no	Measure	1	2	3	4	5	6	7
1	Presentation	–						
2	Poster/video	**0.57**	–					
3	Direct peer com.	0.40	**0.88**	–				
4	Activity	−0.03	0.22	0.01	–			
5	% PLs	0.29	**0.58**	**0.47**	**0.54**	–		
6	Size	−0.28	**−0.63**	−0.40	**−0.55**	**−0.73**	–	
7	Density	0.05	0.24	0.23	0.30	**0.70**	−0.26	–
8	Mean closeness to PL	0.27	**0.72**	**0.60**	**0.49**	**0.92**	**−0.80**	**0.67**
9	Trusted adults	0.12	0.33	0.35	0.05	**0.43**	−0.20	**0.66**
10	Suicide attempt	0.00	−0.13	−0.10	−0.16	−0.25	0.19	−0.40
11	Ideation-only	−0.13	0.10	0.11	−0.24	0.02	−0.12	0.02

Variables in bold are significant at $p < 0.05$. Variables 8–11 are individual-level metrics aggregated at the school level.

TABLE 3b |

(B) Level-1 (individual) variables ($N = 3,621–5,746$)

S.no	Measure	1	2	3	4	5	6	7	8	9
1	Presentation‡	–								
2	Poster/video‡	**0.39**	–							
3	Direct peer‡	**0.30**	**0.44**	–						
4	Activity‡	**0.50**	**0.35**	**0.33**	–					
5	Out-degree	**0.06**	**0.08**	**0.09**	**0.09**	–				
6	Coreness	**0.05**	**0.11**	**0.10**	**0.08**	**0.70**	–			
7	Closeness to PL	**0.06**	**0.18**	**0.20**	**0.07**	**0.44**	**0.60**	–		
8	Trusted adults	**0.11**	**0.14**	**0.18**	**0.14**	**0.45**	**0.36**	**0.27**	–	
9	Suicide attempt‡	**−0.03**	**−0.05**	−0.01	−0.02	**−0.09**	**−0.11**	**−0.04**	**−0.07**	–
10	Suicide ideation‡	0.00	0.01	0.00	−0.01	**−0.04**	**−0.04**	−0.01	−0.03	**−0.08**

‡Dichotomous variable; the correlation coefficient displayed is the point-biserial correlation. Variables in bold are significant at $p < 0.05$.

interaction. In this school-level OLS regression model ($N = 20$), the interaction term was marginally significant ($B = -0.08$, $p = 0.08$).

We included suicide attempt and suicide ideation-only individually into each of these models as interaction terms. There was no evidence that the individual and school predictors had a different impact on exposure for suicidal students, as shown by no significant interaction of suicide attempt or suicide ideation with any of the predictors (p's > 0.05).

DISCUSSION

After 1 year of Sources of Strength implementation in 20 high schools, exposure to the intervention varied widely across schools and as a function of individual student characteristics. Our findings regarding predictors of exposure build upon previous work on peer leader intervention diffusion by examining several indicators of students' connections to peers as well as adults. We found support for our hypothesis that students who were friends with peer leaders trained in Sources of Strength would have greater exposure to the intervention, across all messaging modalities. Students with peer leader friends had greater exposure to poster/video presentations, were more likely to have had direct communication about Sources of Strength from another student, and were more likely to have participated in an activity. These findings are consistent with prior research on peer-led programs (16–18) and with theoretical models (30, 41) that emphasize the importance of natural networks and direct personal affiliations as the medium through which peer leader prevention efforts are disseminated.

In addition to direct friendship ties with student peer leaders, our findings also showed that students who were closer in steps away from a peer leader in the friendship network also had greater intervention exposure. This suggests that peer leaders' social influence extends beyond their immediate friendship ties. Having a friend who is a friend of a peer leader may increase the social value of participating in Sources of Strength and attending to the intervention messaging. Interestingly, this effect was seen even for the exposure modalities such as posters that rely less on peer influence (e.g., students have an equal opportunity to see

TABLE 4a | Logit coefficients and standard errors (A) and odds-ratios (B) from a multi-level logistic regression model in 20 schools.

(A) Logit parameter estimates and standard errors

	M (SD)	Exposure modality			
		Presentation	**Poster/Video**	**Peer comm.**	**Activity**
Analytic Sample Size		3,418	3,445	3,439	3,425
Intercept		−0.20 (0.31)	−0.15 (0.29)	−0.74 (0.29)	0.08 (0.30)
LEVEL-1 (INDIVIDUAL)					
Gender (Male v. Female)	50.6%	−0.19 (0.07)*	−0.57 (0.08)**	−0.58 (0.08)**	−0.42 (0.07)**
Ethnicity (White v. Nonwhite)	72.1%	−0.16 (0.10)	0.01 (0.11)	−0.03 (0.11)	−0.01 (0.10)
Out-Degree	4.8 (2.7)	0.03 (0.02)	0.01 (0.02)	−0.04 (0.02)+	0.01 (0.02)
Coreness	5.0 (0.7)	−0.02 (0.03)	0.03 (0.03)	−0.08 (0.05)	−0.04 (0.03)
Closeness to PL	2.8 (0.8)	0.13 (0.06)*	0.22 (0.06)**	0.43 (0.06)**	0.14 (0.06)*
Trusted Adults	2.3 (2.4)	0.08 (0.02)**	0.09 (0.02)**	0.15 (0.02)**	0.10 (0.02)**
Suicide Attempt	7.61%	−0.27 (0.15)+	−0.36 (0.15)*	−0.02 (0.15)	−0.17 (0.15)
Suicide Ideation	8.81%	−0.10 (0.14)	−0.07 (0.15)	−0.06 (0.15)	−0.09 (0.15)
Coreness x Closeness to PL		-	-	0.05 (0.02)*	–
LEVEL-2 (SCHOOL)					
Density	0.60 (0.09)	−0.19 (0.18)	−0.22 (0.17)	−0.27 (0.15) +	0.17 (0.18)
Percent PLs	9.2% (6.1%)	0.17 (0.28)	0.77 (0.37)*	0.68 (0.32)*	−0.57 (0.38)
Size	5.3 (0.8)	−0.04 (0.24)	−0.26 (0.21)	0.04 (0.19)	−0.29 (0.22)
Size x Percent PLs		-	0.43 (0.20)*	0.38 (0.17)*	−0.56 (0.21)**
Random Intercept SD		0.62	0.52	0.44	0.55

All level-2 variables are normalized to mean 0 and SD 1. $^{+}p < 0.10$, $^{*}p < 0.05$, $^{**}p < 0.01$.

TABLE 4b |

(B) Odds ratios from estimates in (a) with interactions evaluated at the mean, −1 SD, and +1 SD

	Exposure modality			
	Presentation	**Poster/video**	**Peer comm.**	**Activity**
LEVEL-1				
Gender	**0.83**	**0.56**	**0.56**	**0.65**
Ethnicity	0.86	1.00	0.97	1.00
Out-degree	1.03	1.00	0.97	1.01
Coreness	0.98	1.03	0.92	0.96
Closeness to PL	**1.13**	**1.25**	-	**1.15**
−1 SD coreness	-	-	**1.40**	-
Mean coreness	-	-	**1.54**	-
+1 SD coreness	-	-	**1.68**	-
Trusted adults	**1.08**	**1.09**	**1.16**	**1.11**
Suicide attempt	0.76	**0.69**	0.98	0.84
Suicide ideation	0.91	0.93	0.93	0.91
LEVEL-2				
Density	0.82	0.80	0.76	1.18
Percent PLs	1.18	-	-	-
−1 SD size	-	1.41	1.35	0.99
Mean size	-	**2.17**	**1.97**	0.57
+1 SD size	-	**3.34**	**2.87**	**0.32**
Size	0.96	-	-	-

$p < 0.05$ *in bold.*

posters hung publicly). Having a friend or a friend of a friend who is a peer leader may make the intervention more salient in students' minds if, for example, they know they have friends involved in the program or they see a poster depicting a peer they know.

We found mixed support for our hypothesis that students with more overall friendship ties would have greater exposure to the intervention, as a function of having more social opportunities for new information. In univariate analyses, having more friends was modestly associated with intervention exposure, but

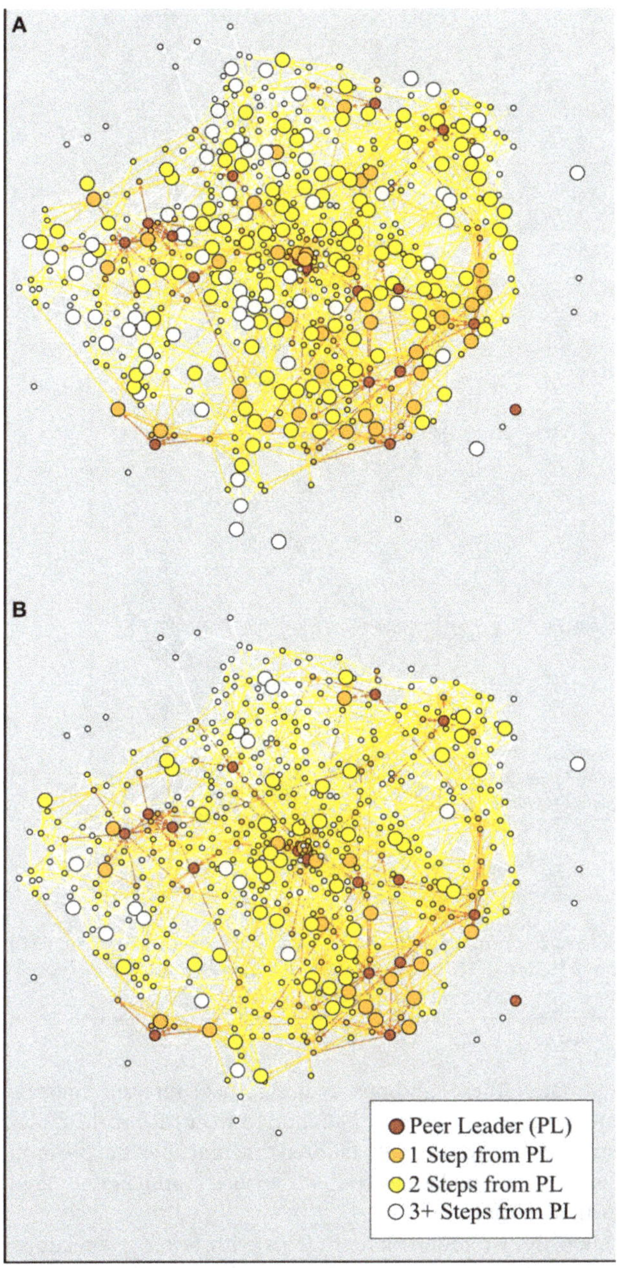

FIGURE 4 | Comparison of two Sources of Strength exposures in a large school with few peer leaders. Nodes are colored by the distance to a peer leader. Large nodes have had exposure to the intervention through either a presentation **(A)** or direct peer communication **(B)**. This school has one of the lowest percentages of students trained as peer leaders (3.2%) and consequently has a low peer communication rate (20.3%) but a modest presentation exposure (53.7%).

this effect was not significant in the multivariate model that included closeness to peer leaders and other student and school characteristics. However, the effect of closeness to peer leaders on increasing exposure to direct peer communication was greater when students were part of a denser, more cohesive friendship network. This may arise as students in more dense friendship groups are more likely to have several friendship paths to a peer leader in contrast to a peer with a sparse friendship group.

As expected, the relationship between closeness to a peer leader and exposure varied in strength based on messaging modality. Being close to a peer leader was more beneficial for exposure to a poster/video and direct peer communication, and less so for presentation and activity participation. **Figure 4** illustrates this finding with one of the largest schools in the study. This school—with low closeness to a peer leader and low percent of students trained as peer leaders—has one of the lowest peer communication rates of all schools in the study (**Figure 4B**). However, when examining the presentation exposure modality, which relies less on social connectedness, this school nonetheless has a modest proportion of students who have viewed a presentation (**Figure 4A**). While presentations may not have the ability to influence students' opinions as much as direct peer communication from a friend, they may have utility to disseminate awareness about the program to students in larger schools.

Our findings have especially relevant intervention implications for larger schools. We generally found that the greatest increases in intervention exposure occurred as the percent of students trained as peer leaders increased up to about 15% of the student population (after which the effect appeared to level off), a finding consistent with other studies (43, 55). Training this many peer leaders may be a more daunting task in larger schools, which we found generally had a lower proportion of students trained as peer leaders. In addition to logistical challenges posed when training more peer leaders, larger communities tend to form distinct sub-communities of segmented friendship groups which may hinder diffusion from the outside (56). Therefore, in larger schools it may be especially important to have more informed peer leader selection in order to distribute them in strategic areas of the network, thus using limited resources more effectively.

We also found that training more of the student population as peer leaders led to greater exposure to a poster/video and direct peer communication in medium to large schools (i.e., >150 students), adjusting for closeness to a peer leader. This finding—having an additional effect of peer leaders that doesn't act through closeness of direct friendship ties—may in part be due to the strength of so-called weak ties (i.e., acquaintances). These acquaintances are not typically captured by friendship surveys but have the ability to connect clusters of tightly-knit friendship groups and introduce new information to these social circles (57). The influence peer leaders exert on students may be largely explained by friendship ties in smaller, cohesive schools. At larger schools, though, training additional peer leaders could lead to increased opportunities for intervention exposure for individuals who are simply acquainted with these peer leaders (e.g., a peer leader taking the initiative to talk to a classmate). Indeed, weak ties' influence is stronger for message exposure than for behavior adoption, which may explain why this effect is not present for activity participation.

Closeness to a peer leader was one of the strongest predictors of intervention exposure, but there may be different ways to achieve this closeness as several network variables were correlated

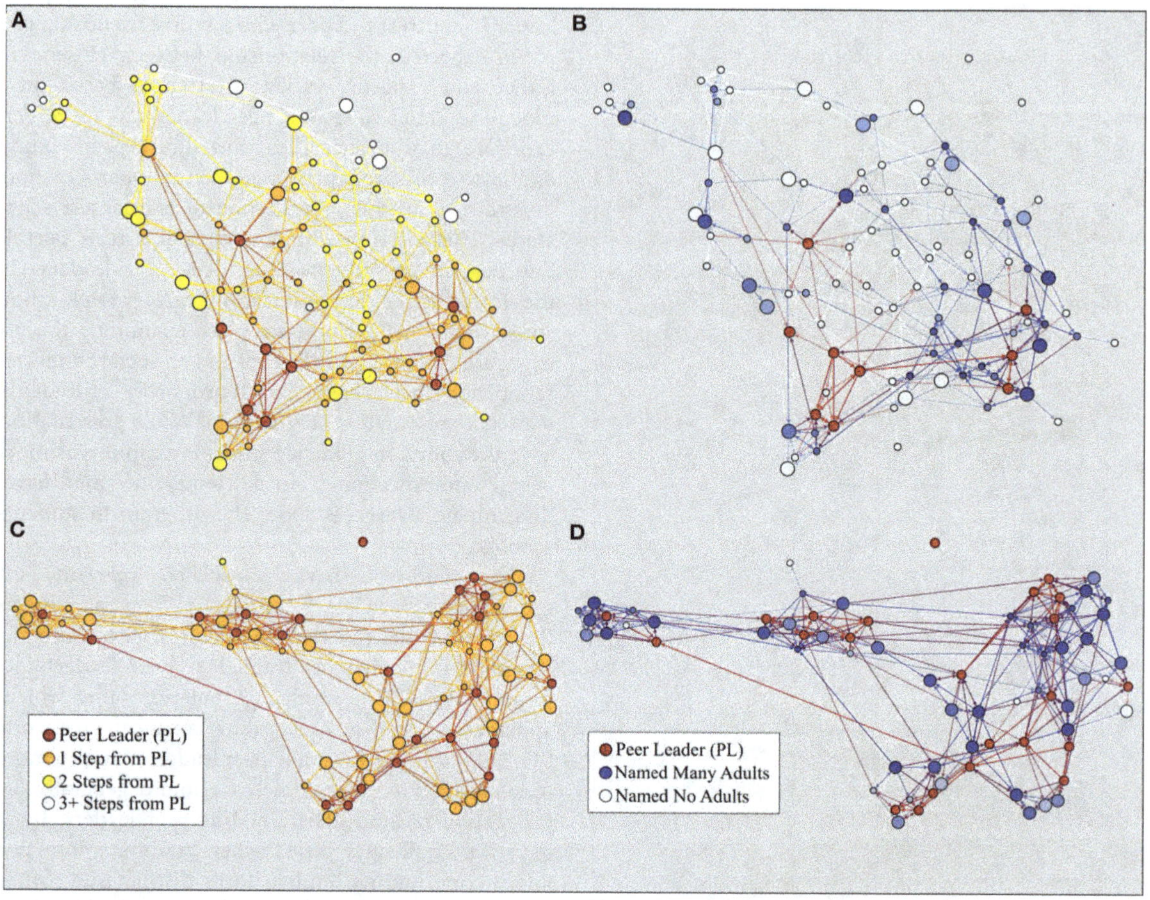

FIGURE 5 | Two networks from schools of comparable sizes. Nodes are colored by the distance to a peer leader **(A,C)** or by number of trusted adults named **(B,D)**. Large nodes have had direct peer communication while small nodes have not. School A is size 103 with 8.7% peer leaders and 52.0% peer communication exposure, while School B is size 73 with 31.3% peer leaders and 73.5% peer communication exposure.

with the measure of closeness. **Figure 5** illustrates two schools that are similar in size but have differing proportions of peer leaders and differing peer leader placement. The school in **Figures 5C,D** has higher network density, more students with ties to adults, more peer leaders, and peer leaders that appear to be more evenly placed through the network in comparison to the school in **Figures 5A,B**; it subsequently has a higher peer communication exposure (73.5 vs. 52.0%). This work demonstrates that messaging exposure is the greatest when peer leaders can reach most students with the shortest distance. Future work should address what combinations of network approaches can most effectively increase schoolwide closeness to peer leaders, or find new ways of engaging students in schools with more limited numbers of peer leaders.

Special efforts may be needed to reach male students and higher-risk youth than are currently being used in Sources of Strength. Male students in the study had consistently lower exposure to the intervention across modalities, even when males were directly tied by friendship to a student peer leader. Combined with our previous study showing that peer leader classroom messaging benefited females more than males, these findings indicate that different messaging strategies and content may be required to engage male students. Results from testing of tailored mental health promotion messaging to males in public service campaigns may be informative (58).

Likewise, we found that students with fewer connections to adults at school had consistently less exposure to the intervention across modalities. This gap is concerning given that absence of adult ties is a risk factor for a range of emotional and behavioral problems (59, 60). Additional methods of engaging youth to connect with adults at school—such as through text messaging—may provide unexplored opportunities for creating youth-adult communication and bonds.

Another at-risk group, students with suicide attempt, had modestly lower exposure to poster/video and presentation modalities, but had similar exposure to peer communication. This may suggest that students with suicide attempts are less engaged with regard to the modalities that rely less on interpersonal communication, perhaps due to other emotional or cognitive demands. On the other hand, students with prior suicidal behavior were found to engage in peer communication with others—a possible indicator of the effectiveness of the intervention's messaging activities in reaching this important sub-population.

Our finding that students' network characteristics increased intervention exposure similarly for suicidal and non-suicidal youth is promising (i.e., absence of a moderating effect of suicide attempt or ideation). This suggests that techniques used to increase exposure to the intervention (e.g., by creating denser friendship groups, fostering ties to adults, choosing peer leaders strategically to maximize closeness) will be effective for suicidal students as well as the general student population. More work is needed to clarify student attitudes—especially for higher-risk youth—and determine behaviors that appear to be discouraging their participation in the intervention.

Strengths and Limitations

We were able to examine the spread of the Sources of Strength intervention through 20 schools after 1 year. This study benefited from a large sample size, high response rates in each school, and being situated within a larger randomized controlled trial. Because the scope of this study is on dissemination of intervention messaging through the network, it is necessary to further determine how messaging exposure translates into behavior change and prevention effects.

There are some limitations to our study; namely, we cannot be sure that the intervention was spread only through peer-to-peer contact and we cannot be certain that the exposure questions assessed only messaging related to the Sources of Strength intervention. While it is reasonable to assume that messaging exposure is a key part of the intervention's impact, it is nonetheless possible that diffusion of the intervention may come about in other ways including social modeling of adaptive coping and help-seeking behaviors. And, while the student survey primed subjects to think about Sources of Strength, it is possible that some students may have provided false positive responses to exposure questions. For example, students may have found mental health information online, such as on YouTube, and reported that they had seen a video on suicide prevention even if that video was not a part of the Sources of Strength activities.

Sources of Strength was designed to be delivered over 2 years, yet our data come from the conclusion of the first school year. Within this 1-year period there may have been varying degrees of schoolwide and individual participation that could have influenced the effectiveness of the program. Future work should address how peer leaders' participation and engagement in delivering activities affects diffusion and the program's efficacy. Our findings should be interpreted cautiously, as it may take more time for peer leader training and messaging to reach its full effect in some schools.

We also found that, while percent of students trained as peer leaders was positively related to activity participation, there was a negative interaction with school size such that percent students trained as peer leaders led to lower activity participation in larger schools (>500 students). This may be due to an implementation issue where training more peer leaders exhausted resources that could have been devoted to planning activities. There was also less variation in the proportion of students trained as peer leaders in large schools; future work should attempt to replicate this effect with more variability in the proportion of students trained as peer leaders.

CONCLUSION

In the first year of a 2-year intervention study, our findings show that peer leaders across 20 schools were able to disseminate the Sources of Strength intervention within a few months to substantial portions of their school population. Peer leaders reached students at high risk for suicide (due to past year suicide attempt), with regard to direct peer communication about Sources of Strength and through an interactive activity, similarly to other students. These findings suggest that a peer-led intervention may be an important complement to other intervention strategies designed at reaching higher-risk youth. Network information analyzed in this study underscores the challenges involved with reaching youth who are more disconnected from peer friendship networks and from adults at school.

Future work with the intervention can take this information into account. One important priority is to determine how to leverage information on school friendship network structure to optimize how peer leaders are able to diffuse the intervention in schools with different patterns of connectedness.

AUTHOR CONTRIBUTIONS

PW originated the study and supervised all aspects of its implementation, reviewed data analyses, and co-led writing of the article. TP conducted all network data analyses and co-led writing of the article. KS-C and CH conducted descriptive analyses and contributed to the writing of the article. TV, AP, and CB contributed to study design, reviewed analyses and contributed to writing of the article. KR contributed to interpretation of the findings and contributed to the writing of the article. ML originated the intervention and led the implementation of the intervention.

ACKNOWLEDGMENTS

We gratefully acknowledge the support of students, school administrators and staff in this study.

REFERENCES

1. Gould MS, Marrocco FA, Kleinman M, Thomas JG, Mostkoff K, Cote J, et al. Evaluating iatrogenic risk of youth suicide screening programs: a randomized controlled trial. *JAMA* (2005) 293:1635–43. doi: 10.1001/jama.293.13.1635
2. Wyman PA, Brown CH, Inman J, Cross W, Schmeelk-Cone K, Guo J, et al. Randomized trial of a gatekeeper program for suicide prevention: 1-year impact on secondary school staff. *J Consult Clin Psychol.* (2008) 76:104. doi: 10.1037/0022-006X.76.1.104
3. Goldston DB, Walrath CM, McKeon R, Puddy RW, Lubell KM, Potter LB, et al. The Garrett lee smith memorial suicide prevention program. *Suicide Life Threat Behav.* (2010) 40:245–56. doi: 10.1521/suli.2010.40.3.245
4. Brent DA, Brown CH. Effectiveness of school-based suicide prevention programmes. *Lancet* (2015) 385:1489–91. doi: 10.1016/S0140-6736(14)61586-5
5. Aseltine RH, James A, Schilling EA, Glanovsky J. Evaluating the SOS suicide prevention program: a replication and extension. *BMC Public Health* (2007) 7:161. doi: 10.1186/1471-2458-7-161
6. Aseltine Jr RH, DeMartino R. An outcome evaluation of the SOS suicide prevention program. *Am J Public Health* (2004) 94:446–51. doi: 10.2105/AJPH.94.3.446
7. Schilling EA, Aseltine RH, James A. The SOS suicide prevention program: further evidence of efficacy and effectiveness. *Prev Sci.* (2016) 17:157–66. doi: 10.1007/s11121-015-0594-3
8. Wasserman D, Hoven CW, Wasserman C, Wall M, Eisenberg R, Hadlaczky G, et al. School-based suicide prevention programmes: the SEYLE cluster-randomised, controlled trial. *Lancet* (2015) 385:1536–44. doi: 10.1016/S0140-6736(14)61213-7
9. Walrath C, Garraza LG, Reid H, Goldston DB, McKeon R. Impact of the garrett lee smith youth suicide prevention program on suicide mortality. *Am J Public Health* (2015) 105:986–93. doi: 10.2105/AJPH.2014.302496
10. Caine ED. Suicide and attempted suicide in the United States during the 21st century. *JAMA Psychiatry* (2017) 74:1087–8. doi: 10.1001/jamapsychiatry.2017.2524
11. U.S. Department of Health and Human Services. Office of the surgeon general and national action alliance for suicide prevention. In: *2012 National Strategy for Suicide Prevention: Goals and Objectives for Action.* Washington, DC: U.S. Department of Health and Human Services (2012).
12. LoMurray M. *Sources of Strength Facilitators Guide: Suicide Prevention Peer Gatekeeper Training.* Bismarck, ND: North Dakota Suicide Prevention Project (2005).
13. Wyman PA, Brown CH, LoMurray M, Schmeelk-Cone K, Petrova M, Yu Q, et al. An outcome evaluation of the Sources of Strength suicide prevention program delivered by adolescent peer leaders in high schools. *Am J Public Health* (2010) 100:1653–61. doi: 10.2105/AJPH.2009.190025
14. Black DR, Tobler NS, Sciacca JP. Peer helping/involvement: an efficacious way to meet the challenge of reducing alcohol, tobacco, and other drug use among youth. *J Sch Health* (1998) 68:87–93. doi: 10.1111/j.1746-1561.1998.tb03488.x
15. Tobler NS, Stratton HH. Effectiveness of school-based drug prevention programs: a meta-analysis of the research. *J Prim Prev.* (1997) 18:71–128.
16. Kelly JA, St Lawrence JS, Diaz YE, Stevenson LY, Hauth AC, Brasfield TL, et al. HIV risk behavior reduction following intervention with key opinion leaders of population: an experimental analysis. *Am J Public Health* (1991) 81:168–71. doi: 10.2105/AJPH.81.2.168
17. Latkin CA. Outreach in natural settings: the use of peer leaders for HIV prevention among injecting drug users' networks. *Public Health Rep.* (1998) 113(Suppl. 1):151.
18. Sikkema KJ, Kelly JA, Winett RA, Solomon LJ, Cargill VA, Roffman RA, et al. Outcomes of a randomized community-level HIV prevention intervention for women living in 18 low-income housing developments. *Am J Public Health* (2000) 90:57. doi: 10.2105/AJPH.90.1.57
19. Valente TW. Network interventions. *Science* (2012) 337:49–53. doi: 10.1126/science.1217330
20. Campbell R, Starkey F, Holliday J, Audrey S, Bloor M, Parry-Langdon N, et al. An informal school-based peer-led intervention for smoking prevention in adolescence (ASSIST): a cluster randomised trial. *Lancet* (2008) 371:1595–602. doi: 10.1016/S0140-6736(08)60692-3
21. Elder JP, Wildey M, de Moor C, Sallis Jr JF, Eckhardt L, Edwards C, et al. The long-term prevention of tobacco use among junior high school students: classroom and telephone interventions. *Am J Public Health* (1993) 83:1239–44. doi: 10.2105/AJPH.83.9.1239
22. Klepp K-I, Halper A, Perry CL. The efficacy of peer leaders in drug abuse prevention. *J Sch Health* (1986) 56:407–11. doi: 10.1111/j.1746-1561.1986.tb05783.x
23. Perry CL, Telch MJ, Killen J, Burke A, Maccoby N. High school smoking prevention: the relative efficacy of varied treatments and instructors. *Adolescence* (1983) 18:561–6.
24. Valente TW, Hoffman BR, Ritt-Olson A, Lichtman K, Johnson CA. Effects of a social-network method for group assignment strategies on peer-led tobacco prevention programs in schools. *Am J Public Health* (2003) 93:1837–43. doi: 10.2105/AJPH.93.11.1837
25. Dishion TJ, McCord J, Poulin F. When interventions harm: Peer groups and problem behavior. *Am Psychol.* (1999) 54:755. doi: 10.1037/0003-066X.54.9.755
26. Rice RE, Donohew L, Clayton R. Peer network, sensation seeking, and drug use among junior and senior high school students1. *Connections* (2003) 25:5–19.
27. Valente TW. *Social networks and health: Models, Methods, and Applications.* Volume 1. New York, NY: Oxford University Press (2010).
28. Christakis NA, Fowler JH. The spread of obesity in a large social network over 32 years. *N Engl J Med.* (2007) 357:370–9. doi: 10.1056/NEJMsa066082
29. Christakis NA, Fowler JH. The collective dynamics of smoking in a large social network. *N Engl J Med.* (2008) 358:2249–58. doi: 10.1056/NEJMsa0706154.
30. Rogers EM. Elements of diffusion. *Diffus Innov.* (2003) 5:130–5.
31. Cialdini RB, Reno RR, Kallgren CA. A focus theory of normative conduct. *J Pers Soc Psychol.* (1990) 58:1015–26. doi: 10.1037/0022-3514.58.6.1015
32. Rimal RN, Real K. Understanding the influence of perceived norms on behaviors. *Commun Theory* (2003) 13:184–203. doi: 10.1111/j.1468-2885.2003.tb00288.x
33. Insel BJ, Gould MS. Impact of modeling on adolescent suicidal behavior. *Psychiatr Clin.* (2008) 31:293–316. doi: 10.1016/j.psc.2008.01.007
34. Li J, Weeks MR, Borgatti SP, Clair S, Dickson-Gomez J. A social network approach to demonstrate the diffusion and change process of intervention from peer health advocates to the drug using community. *Subst Use Misuse* (2012) 47:474–90. doi: 10.3109/10826084.2012.644097
35. Stoebenau K, Valente TW. Using network analysis to understand community-based programs: a case study from highland Madagascar. *Int Fam Plan Perspect.* (2003) 29:167–73. doi: 10.2307/3181045
36. Petrova M, Wyman PA, Schmeelk-Cone K, Pisani AR. Positive-themed suicide prevention messages delivered by adolescent peer leaders: proximal impact on classmates' coping attitudes and perceptions of adult support. *Suicide Life Threat Behav.* (2015) 45:651–63. doi: 10.1111/sltb.12156
37. Rulison KL, Feinberg M, Gest SD, Osgood DW. Diffusion of intervention effects: the impact of a family-based substance use prevention program on friends of participants. *J Adolesc Health* (2015) 57:433–40. doi: 10.1016/j.jadohealth.2015.06.007
38. Whitlock J, Wyman PA, Moore SR. Connectedness and suicide prevention in adolescents: pathways and implications. *Suicide Life Threat Behav.* (2014) 44:246–72. doi: 10.1111/sltb.12071
39. Pisani AR, Schmeelk-Cone K, Gunzler D, Petrova M, Goldston DB, Tu X, et al. Associations between suicidal high school students' help-seeking and their attitudes and perceptions of social environment. *J Youth Adolesc.* (2012) 41:1312–24. doi: 10.1007/s10964-012-9766-7
40. Petty RE, Cacioppo JT. The elaboration likelihood model of persuasion. In: *Communication and Persuasion.* New York, NY: Springer (1986) p. 1–24.
41. Valente TW. Social network thresholds in the diffusion of innovations. *Soc Netw.* (1996) 18:69–89.
42. Valente TW, Chou CP, Pentz MA. Community coalitions as a system: effects of network change on adoption of evidence-based substance abuse prevention. *Am J Public Health* (2007) 97:880–6. doi: 10.2105/AJPH.2005.063644

43. Valente TW, Davis RL. Accelerating the diffusion of innovations using opinion leaders. *Ann Am Acad Pol Soc Sci.* (1999) 566:55–67.
44. Wyman P, Valente T, Pickering T, Pisani A, Brown C. Effects of ego network structure and peer influence on suicide risk in the sources of strength suicide prevention program. In: *Poster session presented at the XXXIV Sunbelt Conference of the International Network for Social Network Analysis (INSNA)* St. Pete Beach, FL. (2014).
45. *Centers for Disease Control and Prevention NC for IP and C.* Web-based injury statistics query and reporting system (WISQARS). (2014). Available online at: https://www.cdc.gov/injury/wisqars/index.html
46. Eaton DK, Kann L, Kinchen S, Shanklin S, Ross J, Hawkins J, et al. Youth risk behavior surveillance—United States, 2009. *MMWR Surveill Summ.* (2010) 59:1–142.
47. Brener ND, Simon TR, Anderson M, Barrios LC, Small ML. Effect of the incident at Columbine on students' violence-and suicide-related behaviors. *Am J Prev Med.* (2002) 22:146–50. doi: 10.1016/S0749-3797(01)00433-0
48. Eaton DK, Kann L, Kinchen S, Shanklin S, Ross J, Hawkins J, et al. Youth risk behavior surveillance-United States, 2007. *MMWR Surveill Summ.* 2002. (2008) 57:1–131.
49. Valente TW, Fujimoto K, Chou C-P, Spruijt-Metz D. Adolescent affiliations and adiposity: a social network analysis of friendships and obesity. *J Adolesc Health* (2009) 45:202–4. doi: 10.1016/j.jadohealth.2009.01.007
50. Team RC. *R: A Language and Environment for Statistical Computing* Vienna: R Foundation for Statistical Computing. (2013).
51. Csardi G, Nepusz T. The igraph software package for complex network research. *InterJ Complex Systems 1695* (2006) 5:1–9.
52. Bastian M, Heymann S, Jacomy M. Gephi: an open source software for exploring and manipulating networks. *Icwsm* (2009) 8:361–2.
53. Bates D, Maechler M, Bolker B, Walker S, Christensen RHB, Singmann H, et al. *Package 'lme4.' R Package Version.* (2017) 1–1.
54. Lowry R, Crosby AE, Brener ND, Kann L. Suicidal thoughts and attempts among US high school students: trends and associated health-risk behaviors, 1991–2011. *J Adolesc Health* (2014) 54:100–8. doi: 10.1016/j.jadohealth.2013.07.024
55. Kelly J, Stevenson L. *Opinion Leader HIV Prevention Training Manual.* Milwaukee WI: Center AIDS Intervention Research Medical College Wisconsin (1995).
56. Fischer CS. Toward a subcultural theory of urbanism. *Am J Sociol.* (1975) 80:1319–41.
57. Granovetter M. The strength of weak ties: a network theory revisited. *Sociol Theory* (1983) 1:201–33. doi: 10.2307/202051
58. Rochlen AB, McKelley RA, Pituch KA. A preliminary examination of the" Real Men. Real Depression" campaign. *Psychol Men Masculinity* (2006) 7:1–13. doi: 10.1037/1524-9220.7.1.1
59. McNeely C, Falci C. School connectedness and the transition into and out of health-risk behavior among adolescents: a comparison of social belonging and teacher support. *J Sch Health* (2004) 74:284–92. doi: 10.1111/j.1746-1561.2004.tb08285.x
60. Scales PC, Benson PL, Mannes M. The contribution to adolescent well-being made by nonfamily adults: An examination of developmental assets as contexts and processes. *J Community Psychol.* (2006) 34:401–13. doi: 10.1002/jcop.20106

3

Springtime Peaks and Christmas Troughs: A National Longitudinal Population-Based Study into Suicide Incidence Time Trends in the Netherlands

Emma Hofstra[1,2*], *Iman Elfeddali*[1,2], *Marjan Bakker*[3], *Jacobus J. de Jong*[1,2], *Chijs van Nieuwenhuizen*[2,4] *and Christina M. van der Feltz-Cornelis*[1,2]

[1] *Academic Department of Specialised Mental Health Care, GGz Breburg, Tilburg, Netherlands,* [2] *Tranzo—Scientific Center for Care and Welfare, Tilburg University, Tilburg, Netherlands,* [3] *Department of Methodology and Statistics, Tilburg University, Tilburg, Netherlands,* [4] *Institute for Mental Health Care, GGzE, Eindhoven, Netherlands*

***Correspondence:**
Emma Hofstra
e.hofstra@ggzbreburg.nl

Background: Time trends are one of the most studied phenomena in suicide research; however, evidence for time trends in the Dutch population remains understudied. Insight into time trends can contribute to the development of effective suicide prevention strategies.

Methods: Time trends in national daily and monthly data of 33,224 suicide events that occurred in the Netherlands from 1995 to 2015 were examined, as well as the influence of age, gender, and province, in a longitudinal population-based design with Poisson regression analyses and Bayesian change point analyses.

Results: Suicide incidence among Dutch residents increased from 2007 until 2015 by 38%. Suicide rates peak in spring, up to 8% higher than in summer ($p < 0.001$). Suicide incidence was 42% lower at Christmas, compared to the December-average (IRR = 0.580, $p < 0.001$). After Christmas, a substantial increase occurred on January 1, which remained high during the first weeks of the new year. Suicide occurred more than twice as often in men than in women. For both genders, the results indicated a spring time peak in suicide incidence and a trough at Christmas. Suicide rates were highest in the elderly (age group, 80+), and no evidence was found of a differential effect by season in the age groups with regard to suicide incidence. No interaction effect was found with regard to province of residence for both season and Christmas, indicating that no evidence was found that these time trends had differential effects in the Dutch provinces in terms of suicide incidence.

Conclusion: Evidence was found for time trends in suicide incidence in the Netherlands. It is recommended to plan (mental) health care services to be available especially at high-risk moments, at spring time, and in the beginning of January. Further research is needed to explore the protective effect of Christmas in suicide incidence.

Keywords: suicide, time trends, seasonality, Christmas, Netherlands, gender, age, province

INTRODUCTION

Worldwide, annual suicide rates are rising. Consequently national and international suicide prevention strategies have been developed, and there is also ample scientific attention to this issue (1, 2). In 2015, almost 800,000 people lost their lives due to suicide, which is equivalent to a suicide rate of 10.7 per 100,000 people (3). Suicide is now one of the leading causes of death, especially among young people between the ages of 15 and 29 years (2, 4–6). In the Netherlands, the annual suicide number has increased since 2007 from 1,353 to 1,871 in 2015: an increase of 38% (7). The tragedy of suicide concerns not only the premature loss of a human life but also its impact on family members, friends, bystanders, railway professionals, and communities (2, 6, 8, 9). Due to increasing suicide rates and the large impact on the individual and society, it is important to gain more knowledge on predictive factors of suicide. Several risk factors of suicide have already been identified. With regard to psychopathology, the risk of suicide is almost 50 times higher in in-patients—and particularly in persons with personality and affective disorders—than in the general population (10). Furthermore, time trends in suicide incidence have gained broad international consideration (11, 12). Still, evidence remains understudied for the Dutch population, and a better understanding of predictors of suicide is needed for developing more appropriate suicide prevention strategies. Insight into high-risk time frames in suicide might contribute to the refining of these strategies, such as setting up help lines and health care services available at the right moments. In this study, we examined time trends in suicide incidence in the Netherlands from 1995 to 2015. To this end, we will first give an overview of what is already known and we will end by giving the objectives of this study.

Evidence for daily and weekly patterns in suicide incidence were found (13–19). Regarding seasonal patterns in suicide incidence, Durkheim already suggested in the early 19th century that suicide incidence shows seasonal variation (20), and seasonality is now one of the most studied phenomenon in suicide research (18, 21–28). However, studies show conflicting evidence of seasonal patterns (15, 16, 29, 30). Several studies indicated one single peak in spring or (early) summer (21–23, 25–27), while others described two peaks: one in spring and another one in autumn (16, 18). Ajdacic-Gross and colleagues assessed the long-term change of seasonality in suicide and found that seasonality is about to fade away (31). With regards to the Netherlands, one would expect to find seasonality in suicide incidence, as the Netherlands is located at a latitude of 52°23′ N and therefore has pronounced seasons. However, two studies about seasonal patterns in suicide in Dutch residents showed significant seasonal variation in suicide incidence, with a peak in spring (32, 33), but this could not be replicated in a more recent study on train suicides (13). Therefore, the literature on seasonal patterns in suicide rates in the Netherlands is ambiguous in this respect.

As for winter-holiday trends in suicide, legend has it that suicide rates are increased at Christmas. The Annenberg Public Policy Center of the University of Pennsylvania found that many news stories in the past 17 years supported this belief (34). People may indeed experience a worsened general mood during the Christmas days because of family strains, loneliness, or seasonal affective disorder, and increased alcohol use might aggravate this (11, 35–37). On the other hand, two literature reviews reported lower suicide rates at Christmas (11, 38), and this was also reported in multiple retrospective database studies (18, 19, 39–43). A remarkable finding in these studies is that suicide rates seem to be higher on New Year's Day and January 2, suggesting that suicides may be delayed until after the Christmas-holidays (18, 19, 40–43). Christmas is a Christian holiday, and in countries with other predominant religions, one would expect other trends. Indeed, in Turkey—where 99% of the population is Muslim—fewer suicides were observed in the Islamic holy month of Ramadan (44). However, Christians have become a minority of about one-third of the Dutch population due to secularization and the increase of immigrant religions in the Netherlands (45). The Christmas festivities might still play a protective role since Christmas is also a popular holiday in the non-religious population. The association between Christmas and suicide incidence in the Netherlands therefore yet remains unclear.

Seasonal trends in suicide and the association with gender report either no association (21, 23, 25) or a stronger association in men (16, 22, 27, 46). Some studies indicate one single peak in spring/summer for men and one peak in spring and a second minor peak in autumn for women (24, 29, 46). This "bimodal distribution" in suicide among women is, however, not found by others (22, 26, 47). Findings regarding age and seasonality are ambiguous as well, finding no association (23) or a stronger association in younger age groups (16, 25) or in older age groups (24). Evidence also suggests that the seasonal effect on suicide incidence differs across specific regions, as it is has been found that seasonality is more pronounced in rural settings than in urban settings (20, 25, 46). Furthermore, especially rural Catholic regions show seasonal patterns in suicide incidence as urban Protestant regions showed a larger decline in suicide seasonality over the last years (31). As far as the researchers know, seasonality in suicide across the provinces in the Netherlands has not yet been studied. Concerning Christmas trends, gender differences remain unclear. One study found that only men showed significant fewer suicides on Christmas day (19), while others reported a greater reduction in women (40, 43). Obviously, such data may depend on the degree to which the region where the study is performed holds religions that have Christmas celebrations. In the Netherlands, the Western and Northern areas of the Netherlands are most secularized and the percentage of immigrants is greater in the area "the Randstad," so there is more religious plurality in this area (45). Therefore, provinces in the Netherlands may differ in terms of religion-related popularity of Christmas.

In conclusion, it remains unclear whether season and Christmas are associated with suicide incidence in the Netherlands, and if so, whether these associations differ for gender, age group, and province of residence. More knowledge of time trends is essential to refine suicide prevention strategies. These strategies are highly needed as the annual suicide rate in the Netherlands keeps rising. Therefore, this study examines time trends in suicide incidence in the Netherlands over the time period of 1995–2015. This study has four objectives:

1. To examine annual suicide incidence over the study period.
2. To examine seasonal trends in suicide incidence.
3. To examine if suicide incidence at Christmas differs from other days in December.
4. To explore if any associations differ in relation to gender, age, and province of residence.

MATERIALS AND METHODS

Study Design

This is a retrospective longitudinal population-based study on the national register of natural and unnatural deaths data, as registered by Statistics Netherlands, a Dutch governmental institution. Statistics Netherlands receives all death certificates about injury deaths from the police and coroners, i.e., medical doctors who work in the municipal health service. In the Netherlands, a death certificate after a suicide is certified based on strict guidelines involving several professionals (48, 49). Daily and monthly data about all suicide events between 1995 and 2015, as well as age, gender, and province, were included.

Variables

This study included four variables: (1) the occurrence of a completed suicide, and the persons' (2) gender, (3) age group, and (4) province of residence. In this study, a completed suicide was defined as an act performed by the person him/herself with the specific purpose of taking his/her own life that indeed led to death (48). Thus, euthanasia and non-fatal suicide attempts were not included. Suicides are assigned in the StatLine registrar according to the International Statistical Classification of Diseases and Related Health Problems (ICD) of the World Health Organization as "intentional self-harm" (codes X60–X84). The 10th revision of the ICD is currently being used (48–50). Three characteristics of people who have died by suicide, and are related to suicide incidence, were also included as variables: gender, age group at time of death, and province of residence at time of death.

Data Sources/Measurements

The data comprise 33,224 suicide events over 21 years in a population of 15.5 million in 1995 and 16.9 million in 2015. All variables were obtained from Statistics Netherlands in an Excel database and were transposed by the researchers to Statistical Package for the Social Sciences (SPSS) and R. Daily and monthly data about completed suicides that occurred in the time period of 1995 to 2015 were operationalized into seven variables: (1) total numbers of suicide for each month of each year, (2) mean number of suicide per day for each month of each year, (3) suicide rates per 100,000 residents for each month of each year, (4) daily suicide numbers by season, (5) total suicide number per day for all 21 years together, (6) daily suicide numbers at Christmas, and (7) daily suicide numbers at all other days in December (excluding Christmas). To form the total number of suicide variable, a total number of suicides was calculated for each month in each year (for example, January 1995). To form the mean number of suicides per day variable, the total number of completed suicides for each month per year was divided by the number of days in that specific month (i.e., 31 for January, March, May, July, August, October and December; 30 for April, June, September and November; and 28 or 29 for February and 29 in leap years; which were 1996, 2000, 2004, 2008, and 2012). To form the suicide rate variable, the total number of suicides was divided by that years' mean population,[1] which was then multiplied by 100,000. A season variable was created on all daily data according to the meteorological calendar of the Northern Hemisphere in which winter includes December, January, and February; spring includes March, April, and May; summer includes June, July, and August; and autumn includes September, October, and November. A daily total number for all 21 years taken together was created by summing all daily totals per year (for example, all January 1 of all years together).

In the Netherlands, Christmas is celebrated on December 25 and 26. Therefore, to form the Christmas variable, the daily data on December 25 and 26 were allocated to the Christmas variable and daily data on all other days in December to the non-Christmas variable. This minimizes potential seasonal variation bias when the rest of the year would be used as a control period (42). In addition to data about completed suicides, data about gender, age group, and province of residence were received. Gender was classified by Statistics Netherlands into two variables: male and female. Statistics Netherlands classified age at the time of death in the following age groups: 0–19, 20–29, 30–39, 40–49, 50–59, 60–69, 70–79, and 80+. Statistics Netherlands classified province of residence into the 12 provinces of the Netherlands.

Bias

Since suicide is a sensitive issue, a challenge might be to obtain true incidence statistics due to the possibility of underreporting (2, 49, 51–54). The efforts that have been made to minimize this potential bias are strict methodological death registration procedures that are carried out by coroners and government institutions in the Netherlands after injury deaths. This increases the classification of suicides and decreases classification of undetermined deaths, which are the most common alternative verdicts in case of a probable suicide (49, 54). Indeed, the Netherlands belongs to the European countries with the lowest ratio of suicide to "undetermined death" (49). Hence, this possible bias is deemed to be low in this study.

Ethics

The anonymity of the people who died by suicide was of great importance in this study. We only received and examined anonymous data of Statistics Netherlands. Consequently, we only analyzed monthly data for the age groups, as daily suicide incidences were too low within age groups. As a result, we were not able to analyze Christmas trends for age groups.

[1] Example how we calculated the mean population for 2015: the population at January 1, 2015, and the population at January 1, 2016, were summed and then divided by two.

Statistical Methods

Data preparation and statistical analyses were performed in SPSS and R. The Statement of the Strengthening the Reporting of Observational Studies in Epidemiology (STROBE) was used to transparently and completely report about our observational research study (55). Poisson regression analysis, Bayesian change point analysis, Mann–Whitney *U* test, and Kruskal–Wallis test were used to explore time trends in suicide incidence. Independent variables were day, month, year, season, Christmas days, and non-Christmas days. Dependent variables were the number of completed suicides. Demographics examined were gender, age group, and province. Gender and province were examined for yearly, seasonal, and Christmas trends, and age group was only examined for yearly and seasonal trends, as discussed in the previous paragraph. The level of significance was adjusted by Bonferroni correction. In this correction, the alpha of 0.05 was divided by the number of tests (five tests to main effects and five tests to interaction effects), resulting in an alpha of 0.005.

RESULTS

National Suicide Incidence over the Period 1995 to 2015

In the time period of 1995 to 2015, a total number of 33,224 residents of the Netherlands lost their lives due to suicide. The relative mean annual suicide rate in the Netherlands for all years together is 9.72 per 100,000 residents. The year with the lowest suicide rate was 2007 (8.26), and the year with the highest suicide rate was 2013 (11.05), which represents an increase of 37%. The increase in absolute suicide numbers from 2007 till 2015 was 38%, as can be seen in **Figure 1**.

Seasonal Trends

A Poisson Regression Analysis on the 21-year study period taken together indicated an effect by season on suicide incidence in the population in general ($\chi^2(3) = 33.250, p < 0.001$). The mean number of suicides per day (M = 4.57, SD = 2.20) was 7–8% higher in spring than in summer (M = 4.25, SD = 2.10), autumn (M = 4.26, SD = 2.20), and winter (M = 4.25, SD = 2.16), as is shown in **Table 1**.

Christmas Trends

An effect by Christmas was found in the population in general, as indicated by Poisson regression analysis on the total study period taken together ($\chi^2(1) = 27.876$, IRR = 0.580, 95% CI = 0.474–0.710, $p < 0.001$). Suicide incidence was 42% lower at Christmas (M = 2.33, SD = 1.39), in comparison to other days in December (M = 4.02, SD = 2.02). This effect was also indicated by Bayesian change point analysis on the daily distribution of suicide for the 21-year study period taken together. Bayesian change point analysis identified three large peaks in the posterior probabilities (PPs) of change points. First, a peak in the PP of change points on December 25 was found (*PP* = 0.608), indicating a substantive decrease in mean daily suicides. Second, a peak in the PP of change points on December 27 was found (*PP* = 0.600), indicating a substantive increase to the average daily suicide incidence in December. Third, a peak in the PP change points on January 1 was found (*PP* = 0.712), indicating a substantive increase that remained high during the first weeks of the new year, as can be seen in **Figures 2** and **3**.

Associations with Age, Gender, and Province

Associations of suicide incidence with gender, age group, and province were examined. The results are provided in **Tables 2–4** and discussed per demographic variable.

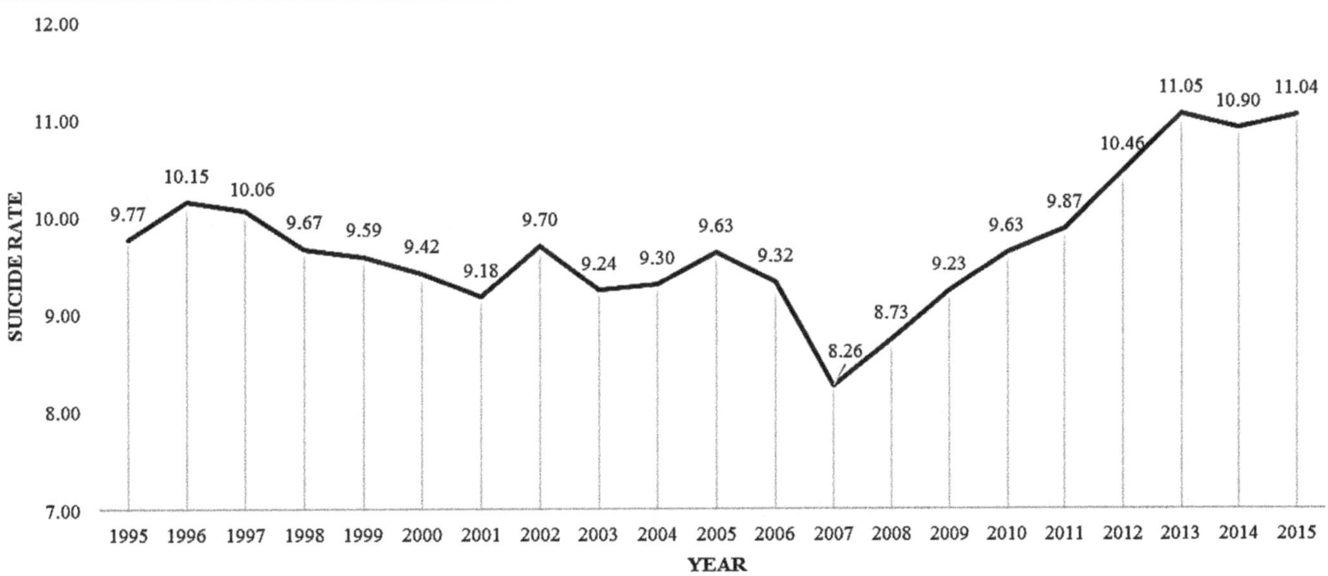

FIGURE 1 | Mean suicide rates per 100,000 residents per year.

TABLE 1 | Poisson regression analysis outcomes on seasonal trends in suicide.

	χ^2	IRR	95% CI for IRR		p
			Lower	Upper	
Spring-Summer	22.636	1.076	1.044	1.109	0.000
Spring-Autumn	21.101	1.073	1.041	1.106	0.000
Spring-Winter	21.365	1.074	1.042	1.107	0.000
Summer-Autumn	0.023	0.998	0.968	1.029	0.880
Summer-Winter	0.012	0.998	0.968	1.029	0.911
Autumn-Winter	0.001	1.001	0.970	1.032	0.969

IRR, incidence rate ratio.

Gender

First, over the 21 years together, men had significant higher mean suicide rates (M = 13.37) than women (M = 6.16) ($U = 0.000$, $p < 0.001$), as can be seen in **Table 2**. The subgroup effects of season on suicide incidence by gender are presented in **Table 3**. The interaction term, season by gender, was non-significant ($\chi^2(3) = 6.634$, $p = 0.085$), indicating that no evidence for a differential effect of season in the two genders with regard to suicide incidence was found. In **Table 4**, the subgroup effects of Christmas on suicide incidence by gender are given. The interaction term, Christmas by gender, was non-significant

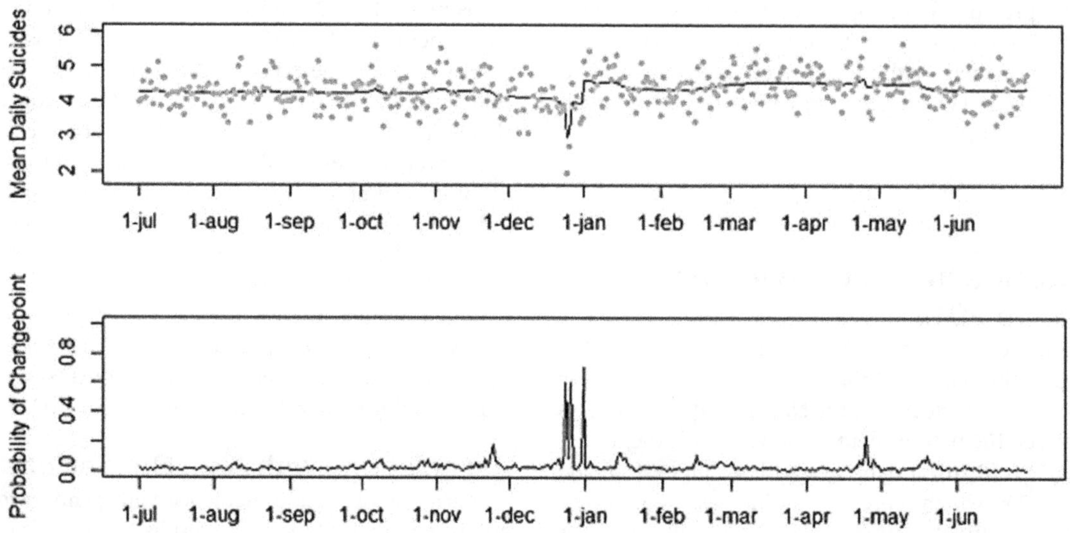

FIGURE 2 | Mean numbers of suicide per day and posterior probabilities of Bayesian change point analysis (1995–2015).

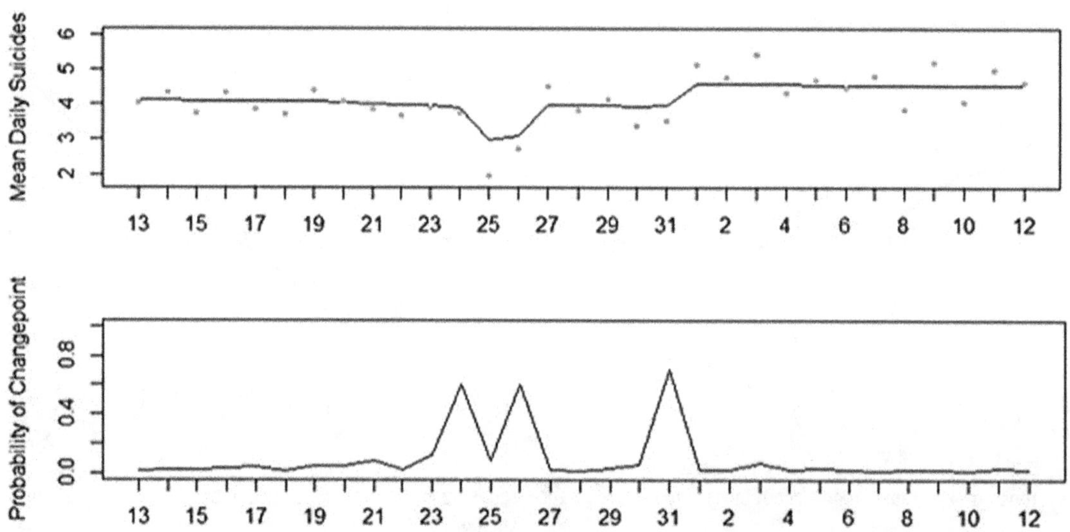

FIGURE 3 | Mean numbers of suicide per day and posterior probabilities of Bayesian change point analysis for December 13 to January 12 (1995–2015).

TABLE 2 | Suicide incidence and significance levels by gender, age group, and province.

	Total numbers		Mean rates[a]	Test[b]	
	N	%	M	Value	*p*
Gender				0.000	0.000
Males	22,609	68.05	13.37		
Females	10,615	31.95	6.16		
Age group				133.295	0.000
0–19	981	2.95	1.20		
20–29	3,677	11.07	8.32		
30–39	5,532	16.65	11.00		
40–49	7,502	22.58	14.47		
50–59	6,830	20.56	14.98		
60–69	4,181	12.58	12.24		
70–79	2,655	7.99	11.85		
80+	1,866	5.62	15.37		
Province				89.730	0.000
Groningen	1,388	4.18	11.55		
Friesland	1,391	4.19	10.40		
Drenthe	1,051	3.16	10.42		
Overijssel	2,157	6.49	9.29		
Flevoland	551	1.66	7.36		
Gelderland	3,905	11.75	9.46		
Utrecht	2,179	6.56	8.88		
Noord-Holland	5,708	17.18	10.44		
Zuid-Holland	6,410	19.29	8.82		
Zeeland	797	2.40	10.06		
Noord-Brabant	5,206	15.67	10.30		
Limburg	2,481	7.47	10.45		

[a]*Per 100,000 residents.*
[b]*Mann–Whitney U test and Kruskal–Wallis test were executed on the rates.*

($\chi^2(1) = 0.100$, $p = 0.751$), suggesting that–with regard to suicide incidence—there is no evidence for a differential effect of Christmas in men and women.

Age

As shown in **Table 2**, a significant age difference in mean suicide rates was found ($\chi^2(7) = 133.295$, $p < 0.001$). People in the age group 0–19 years (M = 1.20) and people in the age group 20–29 years (M = 8.32) had the lowest mean suicide rates. The age groups with the second highest mean suicide rates were 30–39 years (M = 11.00), 60–69 years (M = 12.24), and 70–79 years (M = 11.85). People in the age groups 40–49 years (M = 14.47), 50–59 years (M = 14.98), and older than 80 years (M = 15.37) had the highest mean suicide rates. Subgroup effects of season on suicide incidence by age groups are shown in **Table 3**. No interaction effect between season and age group was found ($\chi^2(21) = 29.883$, $p = 0.094$), indicating that no evidence was found that season had a differential effect in the age groups with regard to suicide incidence.

Province

As can be seen in **Table 2**, a significant difference in mean suicide rates across provinces was found ($\chi^2(11) = 89.730$, $p < 0.001$). Groningen was the province with the highest suicide rates (M = 11.55) and Flevoland was the province with the lowest suicide rates (M = 7.36). In **Table 3**, the subgroup effects of season on suicide incidence by provinces are presented. No interaction effect was found with regard to season and province ($\chi^2(33) = 25.391$,

TABLE 3 | Mean numbers of suicide per day by season for gender, age group, and province.

	Winter		Spring		Summer		Autumn		Poisson	
	M	SD	M	SD	M	SD	M	SD	χ^2	*p*
Gender										
Males	2.90	1.78	3.10	1.77	2.93	1.75	2.86	1.76	21.098	0.000
Females	1.36	1.15	1.47	1.24	1.31	1.14	1.39	1.19	18.675	0.000
Age group[a]										
0–19	0.13	–	0.13	–	0.11	–	0.13	–	3.927	0.269
20–29	0.49	–	0.50	–	0.46	–	0.46	–	4.383	0.223
30–39	0.74	–	0.75	–	0.68	–	0.71	–	6.262	0.100
40–49	0.92	–	1.01	–	1.00	–	0.98	–	12.432	0.006
50–59	0.89	–	0.94	–	0.87	–	0.86	–	9.719	0.021
60–69	0.52	–	0.59	–	0.54	–	0.54	–	11.401	0.010
70–79	0.33	–	0.40	–	0.33	–	0.33	–	22.466	0.000
80+	0.23	–	0.25	–	0.25	–	0.24	–	3.695	0.296
Province										
Groningen	0.19	0.45	0.19	0.44	0.17	0.42	0.17	0.41	3.791	0.285
Friesland	0.18	0.41	0.19	0.44	0.19	0.43	0.17	0.42	1.596	0.660
Drenthe	0.13	0.37	0.15	0.39	0.13	0.37	0.13	0.37	5.270	0.153
Overijssel	0.27	0.53	0.30	0.54	0.27	0.52	0.28	0.52	2.857	0.414
Flevoland	0.07	0.27	0.07	0.27	0.07	0.26	0.08	0.28	2.872	0.412
Gelderland	0.52	0.71	0.53	0.71	0.51	0.71	0.49	0.70	3.351	0.341
Utrecht	0.27	0.53	0.30	0.55	0.27	0.51	0.30	0.54	6.500	0.090
Noord-Holland	0.72	0.88	0.78	0.90	0.75	0.88	0.73	0.87	5.040	0.169
Zuid-Holland	0.81	0.90	0.88	0.95	0.81	0.90	0.84	0.95	7.774	0.051
Zeeland	0.11	0.34	0.12	0.35	0.10	0.33	0.09	0.30	10.225	0.017
Noord-Brabant	0.67	0.82	0.72	0.84	0.66	0.81	0.66	0.84	6.393	0.094
Limburg	0.32	0.59	0.34	0.58	0.31	0.55	0.32	0.59	2.758	0.430

[a]*No SD is provided since we only had monthly data for age groups.*

TABLE 4 | Mean numbers of suicide per day by Christmas for gender and province.

	Christmas days		Non-Christmas days		Poisson	
	M	SD	M	SD	χ^2	p
Gender						
Males	1.55	1.17	2.73	1.73	20.084	0.000
Females	0.79	0.90	1.29	1.08	7.841	0.005
Province						
Groningen	0.05	0.22	0.19	0.44	3.635	0.057
Friesland	0.19	0.40	0.15	0.37	0.360	0.549
Drenthe	0.10	0.30	0.14	0.38	0.524	0.469
Overijssel	0.10	0.30	0.23	0.47	2.921	0.087
Flevoland	0.02	0.15	0.06	0.26	0.904	0.342
Gelderland	0.40	0.77	0.54	0.69	1.319	0.251
Utrecht	0.07	0.26	0.27	0.52	5.237	0.022
Noord-Holland	0.36	0.53	0.65	0.86	5.145	0.023
Zuid-Holland	0.43	0.63	0.73	0.83	4.841	0.028
Zeeland	0.14	0.35	0.09	0.30	1.052	0.305
Noord-Brabant	0.26	0.45	0.68	0.81	9.849	0.002
Limburg	0.21	0.47	0.29	0.59	0.856	0.355

$p = 0.825$), suggesting that no evidence was found that season had a differential effect in the provinces in terms of suicide incidence. Subgroup effects of Christmas by province are given in **Table 4**. The interaction term, Christmas by province, was non-significant ($\chi^2(11) = 16.253$, $p = 0.132$), indicating that no evidence was found for a differential effect by Christmas in the provinces with regard to suicide incidence.

DISCUSSION

Key Findings

In this study, time trends in suicide incidence in the Netherlands in 1995–2015 were examined. The first objective is to examine national suicide incidence over the total study period. The results indicated that suicide incidence among Dutch residents increased since 2007. These findings are in line with existing literature (2, 7). As suicide is associated with lower socioeconomic status, unemployment, evictions, and indebtedness, the increase in suicide rates is possibly associated with the global economic crisis, which started in 2007 (56–58). Psychiatric disorders—and in particular major depression—increases the risk of suicide and might, also during economic crisis, mediate the relationship between suicide and economic situation (56, 59). However, a relationship between economic crisis, psychiatric disorders, and suicide remains partly unexplained due to conflicting evidence. The loss of a job might, for example, lead to depression, which might lead to suicide, but it is also possible that people with certain mental illnesses are more prone for suicide and also for losing their job (56). Moreover, some studies fail to find an association between suicide rates and the economic crisis (56).

The second objective is to examine seasonal trends in suicide incidence. The results indicated seasonal trends in suicide incidence in the Netherlands with a peak in spring. Therefore, we conclude that seasonality in suicide has not (yet) faded away in the Netherlands. Compared to summer, autumn, and winter, in spring, there is one suicide almost every 3 days. This spring-peak is also found in studies in other countries (18, 21–27, 33). However, the study of van Houwelingen to seasonal trends in train suicides did not find any seasonal effects in the Dutch population (13). This may indicate that train suicides do not follow a seasonal pattern, but suicides in general do.

Two classical theories about the seasonal patterns in suicide exist. First, Durkheim had a sociological explanation. According to him, suicide incidence is higher in spring and summer because social and occupational activities—that mostly takes place at daytime—increases in spring and summer as the days grow longer (20). Indeed, suicide incidence is higher at daytime (13–17), and peaks in suicide incidence shift throughout the year in the same way as the change in timing of sunrise and sunset does (13, 16). For example, the morning peak in suicide incidence happens 3 h earlier in summer than in winter whilst the evening peak in summer happens 3 h later than in winter (16). According to Gabennesch, however, a psychological interpretation might underlie the spring-peak: people have expectations for feeling better at times that might promise a new beginning, such as spring, weekends, or holidays. If, however, these expectations for feeling better promise more than they deliver, it can have a negative effect on subjective well-being, which might become even worse than it previously was. This might result in an increased risk of suicide after the promising event (60).

Currently, seasonality is a well-studied phenomenon in suicide research. Multiple risk factors of suicide were found to be related to seasonal patterns in suicide incidence, however, evidence remains partly inconsistent. Suicide method, occupation, geographic location, allergens, allergy related asthma, rhinitis, and atopic dermatitis are risk factors of suicide that were found to be related to seasonality in suicide (61). For example, with regards to suicide method, suicide rates by violent methods were found to peak in spring and early summer months, and a trough was found in the winter months, which is the same seasonal pattern as suicide incidence (62). More research is needed to the (potential) association of mental disorders, bioclimatic factors (such as sunshine, temperature and rainfall), viruses, pollutants, and month of birth in seasonality of suicide, to better understand the underlying mechanisms of this phenomenon (61).

The third objective is to examine if the incidence of suicide at Christmas differed from other days in December. Our results indicated that nationally, suicide incidence was nearly two times lower at Christmas compared to other days in December. This is in line with international research (11, 18, 19, 38–43). It has been suggested in earlier research that people experience lowered emotional well-being and life satisfaction before Christmas, and alcohol use and psychopathology are increased at Christmas (11, 63), which are all risk factors for suicide; however, this is not confirmed in our study. It is striking that, although several risk factors for suicide are increased at Christmas, the overall utilization of psychiatric emergency services and admissions, the number of self-harm presentations, non-fatal suicide attempts, and completed suicides are all decreased (11, 64).

The broken promise theory of Gabennesch, as already discussed in the previous paragraph, might also be an explanation for this finding (60). Christmas is a holiday that can generate feelings of hope for feeling better in individuals, which might have a protective effect on suicide. However, if Christmas promises more than it actually delivers, the suicide risk might shift from before Christmas, to after (60). This study, in line with previous research, showed an increase in suicide incidence on New Year's Day and January 2, suggesting that suicides might indeed be delayed until after the Christmas-holidays (18, 19, 40–43).

A second explanation can be that clinicians, family, and friends anticipate that Christmas might be a difficult time for some, which leads to a greater awareness and availability. This increased connectedness and social support might have a protective effect as well (11, 37).

Objective four is to explore if any associations differed in relation to gender, age, and province. In this study, multiple associations between suicide incidence and gender, age, and province were found. With regard to gender, suicide among men occurs more than twice as often than in women. It is well documented that men have higher suicide rates than women (2) and the fact that men are more likely to use violent means and are less likely to seek help than women might be an explanation (65). We found no evidence for a differential effect of season across genders in suicide incidence, which is in line with other studies that found seasonal patterns in suicide incidence in both men and women (21, 23, 25). Yet, some studies found seasonality only or greater present in men (16, 22, 27, 46). Furthermore, the results of this study are in line with previous studies that also failed to find a second minor peak in suicide incidence among women (22, 26, 47), but is in contrast with research that did find a "bimodal distribution" among women (24, 29, 46). Regarding Christmas trends, no evidence for a differential effect of Christmas was found in men and women with regard to suicide incidence. Our finding is in contrast with previous research that did find any gender differences in suicide incidence at Christmas, as other studies found that only men showed significant fewer suicides on Christmas day (19) or reported a greater reduction in women (40, 43).

With regard to age, the results pointed out that suicide rates in the Netherlands are highest in the elderly (aged 80 years and above), which was already well documented (2). An explanation for these high rates in this group may be that older people are increasingly at risk for psychical disabilities, severe pain, depression, loneliness, and social isolation; which are all risk factors for suicide (66, 67). An earlier study in the Netherlands indicated that the median peak in suicide rates among age groups has shifted since 2007 from younger adults to older adults (68). Several factors are known to have a protective effect on suicidal behavior in older people, such as religiosity, life satisfaction, and marriage. Protective factors differ for the old versus the very old population (aged 80 years and above), as it has been found that marriage had no longer a protective effect in people older than 80 years (66). As the Dutch population of 80 years and older is growing since 1995 from 3.1% of the total population to 4.3% in 2015 (69), this might play a role in the rise of suicide rates in the elderly. Furthermore, we found no evidence for a differential effect of season across age groups with regard to suicide incidence. This finding is in line with a previous study from South Africa that also found seasonal variation of suicide in all age groups (23). However, this result is conflicting with multiple other studies that did find associations of age on seasonality in suicide (61).

Regarding provinces, the highest suicide rates were found in Groningen. Groningen was in 2015 the province with the highest unemployment rates (8.5%), which was even 1.6% higher than the national mean (6.9%) (70). Unemployment is a well-known risk factor for suicide (2) and therefore might explain the high suicide rates in this province. However, Zuid-Holland (7.8%) and Flevoland (7.7%) rate second and third, respectively, in 2015 in terms of unemployment rates, but showed the lowest and second-lowest suicide rates (70). We did not find evidence for a differential effect of season in suicide incidence between provinces. These findings were against expectations, since previous research did report differential effects (20, 25, 31, 46). However, previous research mainly focused on urban versus rural areas, whereas this study examined provinces without a distinction in level of urbanization. Therefore, it can be concluded that the seasonal effects on suicide incidence show the same effects in all provinces in the Netherlands. An explanation of this finding might be that the provinces in the Netherlands have too little climatic variation to show differences in seasonal patterns in suicide incidence. Furthermore, no evidence for a differential Christmas effect on suicide incidence between provinces was found. This was against expectation, because Christmas is a Christian holiday and provinces in the Netherlands differ with regards to the size of the Christian-community. An explanation might be that Christmas is also a popular holiday in the non-religious population. As a result, religious trends, such as secularization and the rise of immigrant religions, might have less influence on the extent to which Christmas is celebrated. Therefore, Christmas might be celebrated throughout the country in about the same degree.

Strengths and Limitations

A strength of this study was the large data set covering all suicides that happened in Dutch residents in 1995–2015, including the demographics gender, age, and province. Since there were no exclusion criteria and drop out was not applicable, this study had no missing data, which is a strength. A limitation of this study is that no daily data were available for age groups; these data were not available to prevent loss of anonymity.

Implications for Suicide Prevention

Several suicide prevention strategies exist; in creating awareness and education for the general public and professionals, screening tools for at risk individuals, treatment of psychiatric disorders, restricted access to lethal means and responsible media reporting of suicide (1). This study contributes to the first strategy: creating knowledge and awareness about high-risk time frames. The high-risk time frames identified take place in the spring-season and in the beginning of the new year. Although we found a decline in December, and specifically at Christmas, this does not mean that one should be less aware for signals at low-incidence periods, such as Christmas. Suicides do happen at Christmas. Therefore, there must always be awareness for signals. However, we would recommend planning (mental) health care services to be available especially at high-risk moments, which is in spring and in January.

Implications for Scientific Research

This study has contributed to scientific research by updating and deepening knowledge on time trends in suicide incidence. It also makes corrections possible for naturally occurring time trends in suicide incidence over the year, which is useful when examining the effect of a suicide prevention intervention. In this study, evidence is found that time trends (still) exist in the Netherlands. More research is needed to better understand the underlying mechanisms of time trends in suicide incidence. For example, more research is needed to examine religiousness, urbanization, and method of suicide in relation to time trends. In addition, research is needed to better understand why the effect of Christmas is greater in some provinces and which combination of factors may be more or less favorable in relation to suicide rates. Moreover, we would recommend to examine the effectiveness of certain suicide prevention strategies at these high-risk moments. Multilevel suicide prevention intervention in particular seems to be promising in suicide prevention (71); however, further study on their effectiveness at these specific high-risk moments is needed.

AUTHOR CONTRIBUTIONS

EH, IE, MB, JdJ, CN, and CF-C contributed to the conception and design of this paper. EH and MB undertook the statistical analysis. EH wrote the first draft of the paper, and IE, MB, JdJ, CN, and CF-C contributed in the process of drafting and revising. CF-C supervised the procedure and the paper. All authors gave their agreement and approval for all aspects of the final version of the paper.

REFERENCES

1. Mann JJ, Apter A, Bertolote J, Beautrais A, Currier D, Haas A, et al. Suicide prevention strategies: a systematic review. *JAMA* (2005) 294(16):2064–74. doi:10.1001/jama.294.16.2064
2. WHO. *Preventing Suicide: A Global Imperative*. Geneva: World Health Organization (2014).
3. WHO. *Age-Standardized Suicide Rates (per 100 000 Population)*. (2015). Available from: http://www.who.int/gho/mental_health/suicide_rates/en/
4. Blum RW, Nelson-Mmari K. The health of young people in a global context. *J Adolesc Health* (2004) 35(5):402–18. doi:10.1016/S1054-139X(03)00537-8
5. Wasserman D, Cheng Q, Jiang G-X. Global suicide rates among young people aged 15–19. *World Psychiatry* (2005) 4(2):114–20.
6. Gvion Y, Apter A. Suicide and suicidal behavior. *Public Health Rev* (2012) 34(2):9. doi:10.1007/BF03391677
7. CBS. *Overledenen; belangrijke doodsoorzaken (korte lijst), regio*. (2016). Available from: http://statline.cbs.nl/Statweb/publication/?DM=SLNL&PA=80202NED&D1=88&D2=0&D3=0&D4=0&D5=11-19&HDR=T,G2,G1,G4&STB=G3&VW=T
8. Theorell T, Leymann H, Jodko M, Konarski K, Norbeck HE. 'Person under train' incidents from the subway driver's point of view – a prospective 1-year follow-up study: the design, and medical and psychiatric data. *Soc Sci Med* (1994) 38(3):471–5. doi:10.1016/0277-9536(94)90449-9
9. Tranah T, Farmer RD. Psychological reactions of drivers to railway suicide. *Soc Sci Med* (1994) 38(3):459–69. doi:10.1016/0277-9536(94)90448-0
10. Ajdacic-Gross V, Lauber C, Baumgartner M, Malti T, Rössler W. In-patient suicide – a 13-year assessment. *Acta Psychiatr Scand* (2009) 120(1):71–5. doi:10.1111/j.1600-0447.2009.01380.x
11. Sansone RA, Sansone LA. The Christmas effect on psychopathology. *Innov Clin Neurosci* (2011) 8(12):10.
12. Christodoulou C, Douzenis A, Papadopoulos FC, Papadopoulou A, Bouras G, Gournellis R, et al. Suicide and seasonality. *Acta Psychiatr Scand* (2012) 125(2):127–46. doi:10.1111/j.1600-0447.2011.01750.x
13. Van Houwelingen CA, Beersma DG. Seasonal changes in 24-h patterns of suicide rates: a study on train suicides in the Netherlands. *J Affect Disord* (2001) 66(2):215–23. doi:10.1016/S0165-0327(00)00308-6
14. Preti A, Miotto P. Diurnal variations in suicide by age and gender in Italy. *J Affect Disord* (2001) 65(3):253–61. doi:10.1016/S0165-0327(00)00232-9
15. Lukaschek K, Baumert J, Erazo N, Ladwig K-H. Stable time patterns of railway suicides in Germany: comparative analysis of 7,187 cases across two observation periods (1995–1998; 2005–2008). *BMC Public Health* (2014) 14(1):124. doi:10.1186/1471-2458-14-124
16. Erazo N, Baumert J, Ladwig K-H. Sex-specific time patterns of suicidal acts on the German railway system. An analysis of 4003 cases. *J Affect Disord* (2004) 83(1):1–9. doi:10.1016/j.jad.2004.04.012
17. Rådbo H, Svedung I, Andersson R. Suicides and other fatalities from train-person collisions on Swedish railroads: a descriptive epidemiologic analysis as a basis for systems-oriented prevention. *J Safety Res* (2005) 36(5):423–8. doi:10.1016/j.jsr.2005.08.003
18. Beauchamp GA, Ho ML, Yin S. Variation in suicide occurrence by day and during major American holidays. *J Emerg Med* (2014) 46(6):776–81. doi:10.1016/j.jemermed.2013.09.023
19. Zonda T, Bozsonyi K, Veres E, Lester D, Frank M. The impact of holidays on suicide in Hungary. *Omega (Westport)* (2009) 58(2):153–62. doi:10.2190/OM.58.2.e
20. Durkheim E. In: Spaulding JA, Simpson G, editors. *Suicide: A Study in Sociology*. Glencoe, IL: Free Press (1897). 1951 p.
21. Postolache TT, Mortensen PB, Tonelli LH, Jiao X, Frangakis C, Soriano JJ, et al. Seasonal spring peaks of suicide in victims with and without prior history of hospitalization for mood disorders. *J Affect Disord* (2010) 121(1):88–93. doi:10.1016/j.jad.2009.05.015
22. Zonda T, Bozsonyi K, Veres E. Seasonal fluctuation of suicide in Hungary between 1970–2000. *Arch Suicide Res* (2005) 9(1):77–85. doi:10.1080/13811110590512967
23. Flisher AJ, Parry CD, Bradshaw D, Juritz JM. Seasonal variation of suicide in South Africa. *Psychiatry Res* (1997) 66(1):13–22. doi:10.1016/S0165-1781(96)02974-5
24. Preti A, Miotto P. Seasonality in suicides: the influence of suicide method, gender and age on suicide distribution in Italy. *Psychiatry Res* (1998) 81(2):219–31. doi:10.1016/S0165-1781(98)00099-7
25. Sun J, Guo X, Ma J, Zhang J, Jia C, Xu A. Seasonality of suicide in Shandong China, 1991–2009: associations with gender, age, area and methods of suicide. *J Affect Disord* (2011) 135(1):258–66. doi:10.1016/j.jad.2011.08.008
26. Ho TP, Chao A, Yip P. Seasonal variation in suicides re-examined: no sex difference in Hong Kong and Taiwan. *Acta Psychiatr Scand* (1997) 95(1):26–31. doi:10.1111/j.1600-0447.1997.tb00369.x
27. Preti A. The influence of seasonal change on suicidal behaviour in Italy. *J Affect Disord* (1997) 44(2):123–30. doi:10.1016/S0165-0327(97)00035-9
28. Kevan SM. Perspectives on season of suicide: a review. *Soc Sci Med Med Geogr* (1980) 14(4):369–78.
29. Rihmer Z, Rutz W, Pihlgren H, Pestality P. Decreasing tendency of seasonality in suicide may indicate lowering rate of depressive suicides in the population. *Psychiatry Res* (1998) 81(2):233–40. doi:10.1016/S0165-1781(98)00106-1
30. Preti A, Miotto P, Coppi MD. Season and suicide: recent findings from Italy. *Crisis* (2000) 21(2):59. doi:10.1027//0227-5910.21.2.59
31. Ajdacic-Gross V, Bopp M, Sansossio R, Lauber C, Gostynski M, Eich D, et al. Diversity and change in suicide seasonality over 125 years. *J Epidemiol Community Health* (2005) 59(11):967–72. doi:10.1136/jech.2004.030981

32. Mackenbach J, Kunst A, Looman C. Seasonal variation in mortality in the Netherlands. *J Epidemiol Community Health* (1992) 46(3):261–5. doi:10.1136/jech.46.3.261
33. Chew KS, McCleary R. The spring peak in suicides: a cross-national analysis. *Soc Sci Med* (1995) 40(2):223–30. doi:10.1016/0277-9536(94)E0070-9
34. APP. *Nearly Half of News Stories Still Making the False Holiday-Suicide Connection.* (2016).
35. Melrose S. Seasonal affective disorder: an overview of assessment and treatment approaches. *Depress Res Treat* (2015) 2015:178564. doi:10.1155/2015/178564
36. Lam RW, Levitan RD. Pathophysiology of seasonal affective disorder: a review. *J Psychiatry Neurosci* (2000) 25(5):469–80.
37. Vreeman RC, Carroll AE. Festive medical myths. *BMJ* (2008) 337:a2769. doi:10.1136/bmj.a2769
38. Carley S, Hamilton M. Suicide at Christmas. *Emerg Med J* (2004) 21(6): 716–7. doi:10.1136/emj.2004.019703
39. Ajdacic-Gross V, Wang J, Bopp M, Eich D, Rössler W, Gutzwiller F. Are seasonalities in suicide dependent on suicide methods? A reappraisal. *Soc Sci Med* (2003) 57(7):1173–81. doi:10.1016/S0277-9536(02)00493-8
40. Jessen G, Jensen BF. Postponed suicide death? Suicides around birthdays and major public holidays. *Suicide Life Threat Behav* (1999) 29(3):272–83.
41. Bridges FS. Rates of homicide and suicide on major national holidays. *Psychol Rep* (2004) 94(2):723–4. doi:10.2466/pr0.94.2.723-724
42. Plöderl M, Fartacek C, Kunrath S, Pichler E-M, Fartacek R, Datz C, et al. Nothing like Christmas – suicides during Christmas and other holidays in Austria. *Eur J Public Health* (2014) 25(3):410–3. doi:10.1093/eurpub/cku169
43. Cavanagh B, Ibrahim S, Roscoe A, Bickley H, While D, Windfuhr K, et al. The timing of general population and patient suicide in England, 1997–2012. *J Affect Disord* (2016) 197:175–81. doi:10.1016/j.jad.2016.02.055
44. Demirci S, Dogan KH, Koc S. Evaluation of forensic deaths during the month of Ramadan in Konya, Turkey, between 2000 and 2009. *Am J Forensic Med Pathol* (2013) 34(3):267–70. doi:10.1097/PAF.0b013e3182a0a430
45. Knippenberg H. Secularisation and the rise of immigrant religions: the case of the Netherlands. *Acta Univ Carol Geogr* (2010) 44(1–2):63–82.
46. Micciolo R, Williams P, Zimmermann-Tansella C, Tansella M. Geographical and urban – rural variation in the seasonality of suicide: some further evidence. *J Affect Disord* (1991) 21(1):39–43. doi:10.1016/0165-0327(91)90017-M
47. Yip PS, Chao A, Ho T. A re-examination of seasonal variation in suicides in Australia and New Zealand. *J Affect Disord* (1998) 47(1):141–50. doi:10.1016/S0165-0327(97)00135-3
48. CBS. *Niet-natuurlijk overlijden.* Available from: https://www.cbs.nl/nl-nl/onze-diensten/methoden/onderzoeksomschrijvingen/korte-onderzoeksbeschrijvingen/niet-natuurlijk-overlijden
49. Värnik P, Sisask M, Värnik A, Laido Z, Meise U, Ibelshäuser A, et al. Suicide registration in eight European countries: a qualitative analysis of procedures and practices. *Forensic Sci Int* (2010) 202(1):86–92. doi:10.1016/j.forsciint.2010.04.032
50. World Health Organization. *International Statistical Classification of Diseases and Related Health Problems.* 10th Revision (ICD-10). Geneva: World Health Organization (2011).
51. Linsley KR, Schapira K, Kelly T. Open verdict v. suicide – importance to research. *Br J Psychiatry* (2001) 178(5):465–8. doi:10.1192/bjp.178.5.465
52. Birt C, Bille-Brahe U, Cabecadas M, Chishti P, Corcoran P, Elgie R, et al. Suicide mortality in the European Union. *Eur J Public Health* (2003) 13(2):108–14. doi:10.1093/eurpub/13.2.108
53. Bertolote JM, Fleischmann A. A global perspective in the epidemiology of suicide. *Suicidologi* (2015) 7(2):6–8. doi:10.5617/suicidologi.2330
54. Breiding MJ, Wiersema B. Variability of undetermined manner of death classification in the US. *Inj Prev* (2006) 12(Suppl 2):ii49–54. doi:10.1136/ip.2006.012591
55. Von Elm E, Altman DG, Egger M, Pocock SJ, Gøtzsche PC, Vandenbroucke JP, et al. The strengthening the reporting of observational studies in epidemiology (STROBE) statement: guidelines for reporting observational studies. *Int J Surg* (2014) 12(12):1495–9. doi:10.1016/j.ijsu.2014.07.013
56. Martin-Carrasco M, Evans-Lacko S, Dom G, Christodoulou N, Samochowiec J, Gonzalez-Fraile E, et al. EPA guidance on mental health and economic crises in Europe. *Eur Arch Psychiatry Clin Neurosci* (2016) 266(2):89–124. doi:10.1007/s00406-016-0681-x
57. Chang S-S, Stuckler D, Yip P, Gunnell D. Impact of 2008 global economic crisis on suicide: time trend study in 54 countries. *BMJ* (2013) 347:f5239. doi:10.1136/bmj.f5239
58. Stuckler D, Basu S, Suhrcke M, Coutts A, McKee M. The public health effect of economic crises and alternative policy responses in Europe: an empirical analysis. *Lancet* (2009) 374(9686):315–23. doi:10.1016/S0140-6736(09)61124-7
59. Economou M, Angelopoulos E, Peppou LE, Souliotis K, Stefanis C. Suicidal ideation and suicide attempts in Greece during the economic crisis: an update. *World Psychiatry* (2016) 15(1):83–4. doi:10.1002/wps.20296
60. Gabennesch H. When promises fail: a theory of temporal fluctuations in suicide. *Soc Forces* (1988) 67:129–45. doi:10.1093/sf/67.1.129
61. Woo J-M, Okusaga O, Postolache TT. Seasonality of suicidal behavior. *Int J Environ Res Public Health* (2012) 9(2):531–47. doi:10.3390/ijerph9020531
62. Hakko H, Räsänen P, Tiihonen J. Seasonal variation in suicide occurrence in Finland. *Acta Psychiatr Scand* (1998) 98(2):92–7. doi:10.1111/j.1600-0447.1998.tb10048.x
63. Mutz M. Christmas and subjective well-being: a research note. *Appl Res Qual Life* (2016) 11(4):1341–56. doi:10.1007/s11482-015-9441-8
64. Griffin E, Dillon CB, O'Regan G, Corcoran P, Perry IJ, Arensman E. The paradox of public holidays: hospital-treated self-harm and associated factors. *J Affect Disord* (2017) 218:30–4. doi:10.1016/j.jad.2017.04.058
65. Hawton K. Sex and suicide. Gender differences in suicidal behavior. *Br J Psychiatry* (2000) 177(6):484–5. doi:10.1192/bjp.177.6.484
66. O'Connell H, Chin A-V, Cunningham C, Lawlor BA. Recent developments: suicide in older people. *BMJ* (2004) 329(7471):895. doi:10.1136/bmj.329.7471.895
67. Juurlink DN, Herrmann N, Szalai JP, Kopp A, Redelmeier DA. Medical illness and the risk of suicide in the elderly. *Arch Intern Med* (2004) 164(11): 1179–84. doi:10.1001/archinte.164.11.1179
68. de Beurs DP, Hooiveld M, Kerkhof AJ, Korevaar JC, Donker GA. Trends in suicidal behaviour in Dutch general practice 1983–2013: a retrospective observational study. *BMJ Open* (2016) 6(5):e010868. doi:10.1136/bmjopen-2015-010868
69. CBS. *Bevolking; Kerncijfers.* (2017). Available from: http://statline.cbs.nl/Statweb/publication/?DM=SLNL&PA=37296ned&D1=14-18&D2=45-65&HDR=G1&STB=T&VW=T
70. CBS. *Arbeidsdeelname; Provincie.* (2015). Available from: http://statline.cbs.nl/Statweb/publication/?DM=SLNL&PA=83523ned&D1=12&D2=0,5-16&D3=64,l&HDR=G2,T&STB=G1&VW=T
71. Van der Feltz-Cornelis CM, Sarchiapone M, Postuvan V, Volker D, Roskar S, Grum AT, et al. Best practice elements of multilevel suicide prevention strategies. *Crisis* (2011) 23(6):319–33. doi:10.1027/0227-5910/a000109

4

Developing a Hypothetical Model for Suicide Progression in Older Adults with Universal, Selective and Indicated Prevention Strategies

*Tomoe Sakashita and Hirofumi Oyama**

Department of Social Welfare, Faculty of Health Sciences, Aomori University of Health and Welfare, Aomori, Japan

Correspondence:
Hirofumi Oyama
h_oyama@auhw.ac.jp

Suicide prevention is an increasingly important issue, especially among older people. Recent work on improving its effectiveness has focused on developing a framework aligning interventions with key risk factors and stages of the suicide process. We have developed this further, by integrating psycho-behavioral components associated with suicide, existing guidelines for identifying critical points of intervention, and the previous preventive strategies framework. Our schematic diagram shows the relationship between the suicide process and prevention strategies, combined with initiatives for linking different types of strategies, from universal strategies at population level, through selective strategies focusing on groups at risk, to indicated strategies, aimed at specific high-risk individuals. We tested our framework using previous studies assessing the impact of suicide prevention interventions on suicide rates in older adults. It was possible to place all identified interventions within the framework. Examining effectiveness within the framework suggests that some interventions may be more successful in reducing suicide rates because they developed systematic linkages between universal, selective, and indicated prevention interventions. Other studies, however, show that interventions can be successful without these linkages, so other factors may also be important. The main weakness of our framework is a lack of evidence about critical intervention points within the suicide process, which may limit its practical application. However, the framework may help to improve the linkages between types of interventions, and support practitioners in developing a wide range of strategies across different areas and stages of the suicide process.

Keywords: suicide, suicide prevention, suicide rate, older adults, Japan, hypothetical model

INTRODUCTION

Suicide is an important public health issue around the world, particularly among older people (those aged over 60) (1). Both suicide rates (2, 3) and the lethality of suicidal behavior (4, 5) are higher in this age group. Older people are more likely to have serious intent to commit suicide, with less warning, than younger people (6, 7).

Several risk factors are associated with suicide among older adults. At least one major psychiatric diagnosis is found in over 70% of suicides in this age group (8). Depression is particularly associated (8), and has a population-attributed risk of more than 40% for suicide, attempted suicide, and suicidal ideation (9–11). Several physical and psychosocial risk factors are also associated, including physical illness and functional impairment (12, 13), and age-related psychosocial stressors, such as lack of supportive social networks (14), loneliness (15), and loss of an important intimate relationship or social role (16).

There are several models of suicidal behavior (17–20). For example, the stress-diathesis theory (17) proposes that longitudinal factors predisposing individuals toward suicidal behavior are influenced by particular stressors. The psychological mechanisms underlying this model remain unclear, however, so it cannot distinguish those at imminent risk of suicidal behavior.

Suicide prevention work has used two basic approaches. The traditional approach is staged: primary, secondary, and tertiary prevention. Primary prevention aims to prevent onset of mental illness, secondary to detect and treat illness, and tertiary to reduce relapses and deterioration (21). The second approach focuses on effectiveness of interventions (2, 17, 22–24). A framework has been created to identify effective interventions, align them with suicidal risk factors, and classify them into three types of prevention strategies, universal, selective, and indicated (25, 26). Universal prevention strategies are applied across populations and individuals not necessarily identified as at particular risk of suicide (25). Selective prevention strategies are aimed at groups at risk of suicide, but not necessarily showing suicidal behavior. Indicated prevention strategies focus on high-risk individuals, such as those who have previously attempted suicide.

Suicide risk at individual level fluctuates over time (18), so efforts to reduce mortality from suicide among older adults in the community need to work with those at various levels of risk. The use of universal, selective and indicated strategies can both address stage of illness, and consider target populations (21), making it more suitable than the staged approach. Research suggests that the risk of suicidal acts could be reduced through a multilevel approach, linking different types of prevention strategies (27). However, no studies have explicitly examined the connections between levels or types of strategy. Another promising model (28) links the suicide process in older adults with the prevention framework (25, 26). It shows that indicated strategies are suitable for individuals with proximal risk factors for suicide (such as depression), selective strategies for those with distal risk factors (e.g., stress or illness), and universal strategies for the entire population, irrespective of risk status. The authors did not, however, show precisely how interventions addressed particular risk factors. This paper therefore aimed to further develop the framework to bring together the suicide process and prevention strategies at different levels.

It is important to ensure that individuals at higher risk of suicide participate in universal or selective interventions, so that they can be identified and supported appropriately. Making better, more systematic linkages between different types of prevention strategies may help with this. However, multilevel interventions and the linkages between them may have different effects (29). The effects may also vary in different age and population groups (30). This paper therefore draws on studies assessing the impact of suicide prevention interventions on suicide outcomes in older adults. It examines whether there were systematic linkages between universal, selective and indicated prevention interventions in studies evaluating the impact of interventions on suicide risk.

METHODS

Hypothetical Schema of Suicide Progression With Universal, Selective, and Indicated Prevention Strategies

This study built on previous work to develop a framework for suicide prevention, including the steps of the suicide process and time points for specific interventions (31). We combined this with the universal, selective, and indicated preventive strategies framework (25, 26), and models of suicidal behavior (28, 32) to generate a schematic diagram of the suicide process and classify prevention activity by stage.

Figure 1 shows the schema for suicide prevention (29). The left shows the four sequential steps of the suicide process: a non-suicidal state, suicidal ideation, suicidal plans, and suicidal acts. The right shows preventive strategies classified by suicide process stage and type of intervention (2, 23).

The second column integrates the stress-diathesis model for suicidal behavior (32). This model identifies particular psycho-behavioral components that may lead to progression to the next step. For example, depression, hopelessness, suicidal ideation, and impulsivity are suicide risk factors for all age groups, although acute deterioration and acute psychosocial crises are the most important predictors of suicidal ideation. Similarly, hopelessness and pessimism can lead to suicidal thoughts and plans. Emulation and access to means are also important factors in suicide (33, 34). Certain interventions may act on particular psycho-behavioral components, so can minimize progression to the next stage (31). Conwell et al.'s (28) risk factors overlap significantly with the stress-diathesis model. It is therefore helpful to link the elements of the stress-diathesis model to universal, selective, and indicated prevention strategies.

Testing the Framework Against Evidence on Suicide Prevention Programs

We wanted to know whether the schematic diagram explained findings about suicide prevention interventions. We used a literature search to identify systematic reviews and reports of systematic reviews as reliable sources of articles on intervention types and linkages (see **Appendix 1**). We included studies assessing the impact of suicide prevention interventions on suicide rates in older adults, particularly initiatives linking different types of prevention strategies.

We examined all the interventions against the diagram. We used previous studies (2, 17, 24) to categorize interventions within universal, selected and indicated strategies.

RESULTS

Identifying Studies to Test the Diagram

We identified 53 review articles, and excluded 46 because they did not meet the criteria (**Appendix 1**). One article (23) was added

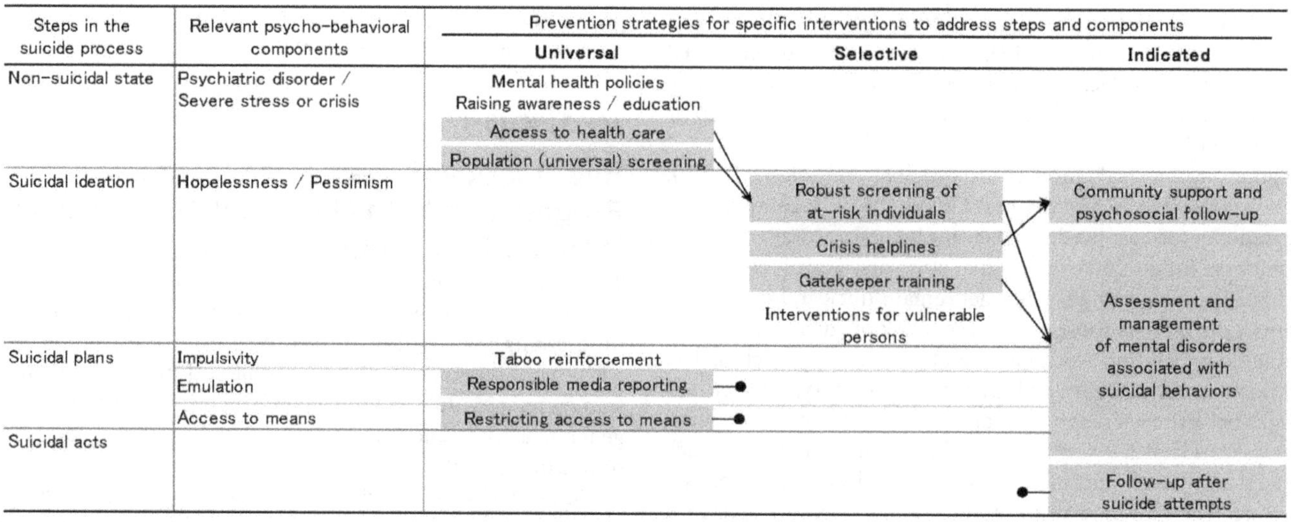

FIGURE 1 | Schematic diagram of suicide process and prevention strategies (29). Interventions highlighted in gray are supported by evidence of their efficacy in reducing suicide risk. A black arrow indicates a clear link to another intervention. A black circle indicates no known link to other interventions. The interventions at each point in the suicide process are expected to involve people at stages closer to suicide.

following cross-referencing. One report (2) was substituted for an overview (35). We found four systematic reviews (24, 36–38), two overviews (29, 39) and two reports of systematic reviews (2, 23), and their reference lists gave 17 suitable studies to test the hypothetical schema and six to examine the effect of linkages between levels of intervention on suicide rate at the population level.

Universal Prevention Strategies

Universal prevention strategies included mental health policies, awareness-raising and education, improving access to health care, and population or universal screening.

Mental Health Policies, Raising Awareness, and Education

Combining these interventions may prevent individuals from developing suicidal ideation (31). However, several systematic reviews have indicated that these interventions alone do not reduce suicidal activities among adults (40, 41). They may facilitate other preventive interventions that address acute deteriorations and psychosocial crises (42, 43), but there is no evidence that they are usually designed to be integrated directly with these strategies.

Population Screening for Mental Illness

Access to healthcare (2) and universal screening (29) have both been linked to selective preventive strategies, often because they involve the same systems and staff. One study found that community-based interventions, involving universal, in-depth screening and general care for all older people in a region with a high suicide rate, resulted in a lower suicide rate (44). These community-based interventions used a self-report instrument to assess the risk of depression among older people, and therefore identify those who may otherwise not seek help. This first stage was linked to a selective intervention involving in-depth screening of those identified as at risk, for example, because they were depressed, which is a known suicide risk factor (9–11). This provided a systematic link from universal to selective prevention. Improving education and awareness, and incorporating interventions locally, might improve uptake of screening.

Responsible Media Reporting and Restricting Access to Means of Suicide

Other universal prevention strategies include taboo reinforcement to minimize impulsivity, responsible media reporting to minimize emulation, and restricting access to means of suicide. There is evidence that some of these interventions can reduce suicide rates (2, 23, 24, 36), but no proof for others, notably taboo reinforcement. Responsible media reporting and restricting access to means are both supported by evidence, in one case of short-term benefits and in the other of benefits limited to the specific means of suicide (17). These interventions may reduce the frequency of progression toward suicidal acts (31), but are hard to integrate with selective or indicated strategies because they do not allow selection or identification of individuals to target further intervention.

Selective Prevention Strategies

Selective prevention interventions included gatekeeper training for physicians, robust screening, and counseling of at-risk individuals, the availability of crisis helplines, and interventions for vulnerable people (e.g., those experiencing severe stress).

Identifying and Referring At-Risk Individuals

Studies have found that gatekeeper training for physicians to enable them to detect and treat depression can reduce suicide rates (45, 46), probably because depression is such a common risk factor for suicide in this age group (9–11). This, like robust screening and counseling, integrates universal, and selective strategies. Previous community-based interventions using this combination resulted in lower suicide rates. These interventions involved universal, in-depth screening of older people in a region with a high suicide rate. Those who were depressed or suffering from depressive episodes were referred for semi-structured clinical interviews (44). These interventions may help to minimize hopelessness and pessimism, and therefore stop progression toward suicidal plans and acts (29, 31). The model suggests that interventions at particular time points might reasonably target people at stages closer to suicide.

Crisis Helplines and Telephone Counseling

Crisis helplines and emergency response services also reduce suicide. One study (47) provided regular telephone support for at-risk individuals and an emergency response when required. This resulted in a lower suicide rate among older women. A community agency that provided telephone counseling with emotional support, crisis intervention, referral services, and home visits reduced hopelessness, but not depressive symptoms (48). Crisis helplines, even without subsequent support, can reduce suicide risk among callers during the call itself and over subsequent weeks (49).

These selective strategies are usually closely linked to indicated strategies, often follow-up with specific individuals, but few rigorous studies have evaluated the efficacy of interventions targeted at specific vulnerable groups.

Indicated Prevention Strategies

These interventions included assessment and management of mental disorders associated with suicidal behaviors, community support, and psychosocial follow-up.

Management of Mental Disorders Associated With Suicidal Outcomes

The appropriate management of mental illness can minimize hopelessness, pessimism, and impulsivity, reducing the likelihood of individuals developing suicidal thoughts or taking action (31, 32). Antidepressants (50, 51) and collaborative care (52, 53) of older people with depression have been associated with reduced risk of suicidal ideation in institutional settings. A secondary analysis (50) of data from three studies on late-life major depression found that antidepressants and interpersonal psychotherapy reduced suicidal ideation. Other studies investigated the effect of antidepressants on suicidal ideation and behavior in patients with late-life major depression (51) and the 2-year effect of collaborative primary care interventions on suicidal ideation and depressive symptoms among older people (52). Interventions included antidepressant treatment, patient education, interpersonal psychotherapy, and care management. Both studies (51, 52) found reduced suicidal ideation among the target group. Collaborative depression care can also reduce suicidal ideation among older people (53). The sample size of treatment studies in institutional settings is usually too small to detect changes in suicide rates, but the link to risk factors such as depression (9–11) suggests that these interventions may be clinically useful to reduce suicidal acts.

These studies suggest that appropriate management of mental illness is an important part of suicide prevention, and can reduce the risk of progression toward suicide ideation, planning, and attempts. However, it may be possible to make a more direct link. One previous study in northern Japan detected individuals with depression via screening interventions (44) and successfully treated them for depression via psychiatric or primary care. This linked the management of mental illness directly with selective preventive strategies, and fits with our model's suggestion that these interventions may become more effective by linking different levels.

Community Support and Psychosocial Follow-Up

Follow-up care after attempted suicide is associated with positive outcomes, such as reduced risk of re-attempting (54–56). Follow-up care among recently discharged patients was effective in reducing suicide attempts and deaths in all age groups (54), especially those discharged from emergency departments (35, 55). This intervention may work by reducing the risk of re-attempting (56) and therefore of death by suicide, but the small numbers mean that population suicide rates are not affected. This care is also not usually designed to be integrated with other prevention strategies (37, 54), which might limit its benefits.

Linkages Between Types of Intervention

Table 1 shows the main characteristics of recent studies evaluating multilevel programs to reduce suicide rate among older adults, and shows specific linkages between types of intervention. For example, two studies linked selective and indicated interventions by emergency calls for help (47) and treatment and referrals (46). They found lower suicide rates among older women in the intervention group (47) and in the population of the intervention area (46). One study evaluated systematic linkages across types of interventions, such as recommendations to move from universal to selective interventions (44), and found reduced suicide rates in both older men and women.

Three other recent multilevel approaches (57–59) had partial linkages of primary care features (for instance, improved management of depression by physicians) between selective and indicated prevention elements, but no reported linkages between universal and selective elements. These studies reported clear reductions in attempted suicide and death by suicide, but the changes in suicide rate with large sample sizes were less clear.

This suggests that selective and indicated interventions, and close linkages between the two, are more likely to affect suicide among older people. It also suggests that multilevel approaches with systematic linkages between levels of intervention are more likely to affect the suicide rate at the population level than those with partial or subtle linkages between universal and selective interventions, in particular.

TABLE 1 | The main characteristics of recent studies evaluating multilevel programs to reduce suicide rate among older adults.

Study	Design	Target population	Intervention type and linkage					Outcome
			Universal	Linkage	Selective	Linkage	Indicated	
De Leo et al. (47)	Large cohort study comparing with the general population	Older users of service			Regular phone call for assessment and emotional support	Emergency call for help	Contacts with trained staff	Lower suicide rate among users. Significantly fewer suicides in women. No difference in male suicide rate.
Szénto et al. (46)	Large quasi-experimental	Adults of all ages in the community			Improved detection of depression following physician education	Recommendation for treatment and referral	Treatment by physician or psychiatrist	Significant reduction in suicide rate compared with control and trend.
Oyama et al. (44)	Meta-analysis of quasi-experimental studies	Older adults living in the community	Universal screening for depression Public campaign	Recommendation to participate further if screening positive No reported linkage	Robust screening for depression	Referral to physician and other health professionals	Treatment by physician and contact with health professionals	Significant reduction in suicide rate in women. No change in suicide rate in men.
Oyama et al. (44)	Meta-analysis of quasi-experimental studies	Older adults living in the community	Universal screening for depression Public campaign	Recommendation to participate further if screening positive No reported linkage	Robust screening for depression	Referral to psychiatrist or other health professionals	Treatment by psychiatrist or contact with health professionals	Significant reduction in suicide rate in women and men.
Hegerl et al. (57)	Large quasi-experimental	Adults of all ages in the community	Public campaign	No reported linkages but possibly increased patient visits	Improved detection of depression following physician education	Recommendation for treatment	Treatment by physician	Significant reduction in suicidal acts (completed plus attempted suicides) over control.
					Gatekeeper training for community facilitators	No reported outcome of linkage	Community support for suicide attempters with brief intervention	No change in suicide rate.
Székely et al. (58)	Large quasi-experimental	Adults of all ages living in the community	Public campaign (including information on crisis help lines)	No reported linkage but increased participation	Crisis helplines Improved detection of depression following physician education Gatekeeper training for community facilitators	No reported outcome of linkage Recommendation for treatment No reported outcome of linkage	Treatment by physician	Significant reduction in suicide rate compared with control and trend.
Ono et al. (59)	Large quasi-experimental	Adults of all ages living in the community	Public campaign	No reported linkage	Gatekeeper training for community facilitators	No reported outcome of linkage		Significant reduction in suicide attempts in a subgroup of older adults.
					Sporadic visits and screening for at-risk individuals	Referral to health professionals	Community support	No difference in overall change in suicide rates over control.

DISCUSSION

Our schematic diagram/framework integrates the stress-diathesis model (32), existing guidelines for identifying the critical time for interventions (31), and Gordon's preventive strategies framework (25). It therefore shows the relationship between the suicide process and suitable prevention strategies (29). Our model builds on that of Conwell et al. (28) by illustrating types of intervention strategy (2), possible linkages between interventions, and interventions related to risk factors from the stress-diathesis model (32). These risk factors are similar to those identified by Conwell et al. but focus on specific interventions rather than precise level of risk.

Practical Application of the Diagram

We hope that the diagram provides a framework to help practitioners and policy-makers to combine elements of intervention programs at different levels and produce more opportunities for effective intervention. This may, in particular, improve the detection of at-risk individuals, altering their progress through the suicide process, and resulting in fewer suicides.

Linking Interventions Across Preventive Levels

The model suggests that one reason why particular interventions may affect suicide rates may be whether the intervention is linked to others at different preventive levels. Linking interventions and levels may mean that preventive action can follow individual trajectories toward suicide more closely than separate interventions, and therefore alter these trajectories more effectively (29). For example, population-based studies of depression screening strategies and intervention among older individuals made a systematic link between universal, selective, and indicated prevention strategies (44). Rigorous community-based studies of interventions promoting regular telephone support and emergency response services among older clients (47), and encouraging physicians to attend gatekeeper training (46), linked selective and indicated strategies. These studies suggest that interventions involving assessment and management of mental illnesses associated with suicidal behaviors may be more effective if integrated with selective strategies targeting at-risk groups.

Other Effective Interventions

A number of studies, however, have identified effective interventions that were not linked to other types of prevention strategy. For example, meticulous population-based studies of universal interventions to encourage responsible media reporting and restricting access to suicidal means (17, 24) show that these interventions were not designed to be integrated with other strategies. Hospital-based studies of indicated prevention interventions, including follow-up care after suicide attempts (37, 54), suggest these interventions were also not integrated with other prevention strategies. Both these interventions were apparently effective, however, suggesting that other factors are also important in preventing suicide, such as individual risk factors.

Limitations and Suggestions for Future Research

The diagram's main weakness is the lack of evidence for the precise critical points in the suicide process. Interventions are probably more effective when targeted at particular risk factors in the stress-diathesis model (32), minimizing progression between stages. However, our model does not identify these precise risk factors, which may limit its practical use. Other weaknesses include the small number of studies used in testing. Using literature reviews to identify studies was convenient, and ensured that only validated studies were examined, but may have limited the number of studies available. Future researchers may wish to use a wider search strategy and include more studies.

CONCLUSIONS

Studies suggest that community interventions are important in reducing suicide in older adults, and that integrating universal, selective, and indicated prevention strategies may be crucial in this process. The most important relationship is probably between selective and indicated prevention interventions. These interventions are tailored to individual risk profiles, targeting those most at risk—for example, because they show signs of depression (9–11). They therefore make best use of scarce resources. Our diagram visualizes the relationships, and can help to ensure that strategies and resources are appropriately targeted and interlinked. We hope that the framework may help to improve the linkages between types of interventions, and support practitioners in developing a wide range of strategies across different areas and stages of the suicide process. It may also help policy-makers to take a more strategic approach to suicide prevention at a population level.

AUTHOR CONTRIBUTIONS

TS and HO contributed equally to the literature review and manuscript preparation, including discussion.

ACKNOWLEDGMENTS

We thank Melissa Leffler, MBA, for editing a draft of this manuscript.

REFERENCES

1. Snowdon J, Phillips J, Zhong B, Yamauchi T, Chiu HF, Conwell Y. Changes in age patterns of suicide in Australia, the United States, Japan and Hong Kong. *J Affect Disord.* (2017) 211:12–9. doi: 10.1016/j.jad.2017.01.007
2. World Health Organization. *Preventing Suicide: A Global Imperative.* Geneva: World Health Organization (2014).
3. Hawton K, van Heeringen K. Suicide. *Lancet.* (2009) 373:1372–81. doi: 10.1016/S0140-6736(09)60372-X
4. Dombrovski AY, Szanto K, Duberstein P, Conner KR, Houck PR, Conwell Y. Sex differences in correlates of suicide attempt lethality in late life. *Am J Geriatr Psychiatry.* (2008) 16:905–13. doi: 10.1097/JGP.0b013e3181860034
5. Harwood DM, Hawton K, Hope T, Jacoby R. Suicide in older people: mode of death, demographic factors, and medical contact before death. *Int J Geriatr Psychiatry.* (2000) 15:736–43. doi: 10.1002/1099-1166(200008)15:8<736::AID-GPS214>3.0.CO;2-K
6. Salib E, Rahim S, El-Nimr G, Habeeb B. Elderly suicide: an analysis of coroner's inquests into two hundred cases in Cheshire 1989–2001. *Med Sci Law.* (2005) 45:71–80.
7. Conwell Y, Duberstein PR, Cox C, Herrmann J, Forbes N, Caine ED. Age differences in behaviors leading to completed suicide. *Am J Geriatr Psychiatry.* (1998) 6:122–6. doi: 10.1097/00019442-199805000-00005
8. Conwell Y, Thompson C. Suicidal behavior in elders. *Psychiatr Clin North Am.* (2008) 31:333–56. doi: 10.1016/j.psc.2008.01.004
9. Conwell Y. Suicide later in life: challenges and priorities for prevention. *Am J Prev Med.* (2014) 47: S244-50. doi: 10.1016/j.amepre.2014.05.040
10. Goldney RD, Dal Grande E, Fisher LJ, Wilson D. Population attributable risk of major depression for suicidal ideation in a random and representative community sample. *J Affect Disord.* (2003) 74:267–72. doi: 10.1016/S0165-0327(02)00017-4
11. Beautrais AL. A case control study of suicide and attempted suicide in older adults. *Suicide Life Threat Behav.* (2002) 32:1–9. doi: 10.1521/suli.32.1.1.22184
12. Kaplan MS, McFarland BH, Huguet N, Newsom JT. Physical illness, functional limitations, and suicide risk: a population-based study. *Am J Orthopsychiatry.* (2007) 77:56–60. doi: 10.1037/0002-9432.77.1.56
13. Waern M, Rubenowitz E, Runeson B, Skoog I, Wilhelmson K, Allebeck P. Burden of illness and suicide in elderly people: case-control study. *Brit Med J.* (2002) 324:1355. doi: 10.1136/bmj.324.7350.1355
14. Turvey CL, Conwell Y, Jones MP, Phillips C, Simonsick E, Pearson JL, Wallace R. Risk factors for late-life suicide: a prospective, community-based study. *Am J Geriatr Psychiatry.* (2002) 10:398–406. doi: 10.1097/00019442-200207000-00006
15. Rubenowitz E, Waern M, Wilhelmson K, Allebeck P. Life events and psychosocial factors in elderly suicides–a case-control study. *Psychol Med.* (2001) 31:1193–202. doi: 10.1017/S0033291701004457
16. Erlangsen A, Jeune B, Bille-Brahe U, Vaupel JW. Loss of partner and suicide risks among oldest old: a population-based register study. *Age Ageing.* (2004) 33:378–83. doi: 10.1093/ageing/afh128
17. Mann JJ, Apter A, Bertolote J, Beautrais A, Currier D, Haas A, et al. Suicide prevention strategies: a systematic review. *JAMA.* (2005) 294:2064–74. doi: 10.1001/jama.294.16.2064
18. Wasserman D. *Suicide: An Unnecessary Death.* London: Martin Dunitz (2001).
19. Van Orden KA, Witte TK, Cukrowicz KC, Braithwaite SR, Selby EA, Joiner TE Jr. The interpersonal theory of suicide. *Psychol Rev.* (2010) 117:575–600. doi: 10.1037/a0018697
20. O'Conner R. Towards an integrated motivational-volitional model of suicidal behavior. In: O'Conner R, Platt S, Gordon J, editors, *International Handbook of Suicide Prevention: Research, Policy and Practice.* Chichester: John Wiley & Sons Ltd. (2011). p. 181–98.
21. Dwight EL, Foa EB, Gur RE, Hendin H, O'Brein CP, Seligman MEP, et al. Prevention of schizophrenia. In: Dwight EL, Foa EB, Gur RE, Hendin H, O'Brein CP, Romer D, Seligman MEP, Walsh BT, editors, *Treating and Preventing Adolescent Mental Health Disorders. What We Know and What We Don't Know. A Research Agenda for Improving the Mental Health for our Youth.* New York, NY: Oxford University Press USA (2005). p. 133–56.
22. Wasserman D, Wasserman C. *Oxford Textbook of Suicidology and Suicide Prevention: A Global Perspective.* New York, NY: Oxford University Press (2009). doi: 10.1093/med/9780198570059.001.0001
23. Pompili M, Tatarelli R. *Evidence-Based Practice in Suicidology: A Source Book.* Göttingen: Hogrefe Publishing (2011).
24. Zalsman G, Hawton K, Wasserman D, van Heeringen K, Arensman E, Sarchiapone M, et al. Suicide prevention strategies revisited: 10-year systematic review. *Lancet Psychiatry.* (2016) 3:646–59. doi: 10.1016/S2215-0366(16)30030-X
25. Gordon RS Jr. An operational classification of disease prevention. *Public Health Rep.* (1983) 98:107–9.
26. Mrazek PJ, Haggerty RJ. *Reducing Risks from Mental Disorders: Frontiers for Preventive Intervention Research.* Washington, DC: National Academy Press (1994).
27. Hegerl U, Rummel-Kluge C, Värnik A, Arensman E, Koburger N. Alliances against depression–a community based approach to target depression and to prevent suicidal behaviour. *Neurosci Biobehav Rev.* (2013) 37:2404–9. doi: 10.1016/j.neubiorev.2013.02.009
28. Conwell Y, Van Orden K, Caine ED. Suicide in older adults. *Psychiatr Clin North Am.* (2011) 34:451–68. doi: 10.1016/j.psc.2011.02.002
29. Sakashita T, Oyama H. Overview of community-based studies of depression screening interventions among the elderly population in Japan. *Aging Ment Health.* (2016) 20:231–9. doi: 10.1080/13607863.2015.1068740
30. Van Orden K, Deming C. Late-life suicide prevention strategies: current status and future directions. *Curr Opin Psychol.* (2017) 22:79–83. doi: 10.1016/j.copsyc.2017.08.033
31. Jenkins S, Singh B. General population strategies of suicide prevention. In Hawton K, van Heeringen K, editors. *The International Handbook of Suicide and Attempted Suicide.* New York, NY: Wiley. (2000). p 579–615.
32. Mann JJ. Neurobiology of suicidal behaviour. *Nat Rev Neurosci.* (2003) 4:819–28. doi: 10.1038/nrn1220
33. Sudak HS, Sudak DM. The media and suicide. *Acad Psychiatry.* (2005) 29:495–9. doi: 10.1176/appi.ap.29.5.495
34. Yip PS, Caine E, Yousuf S, Chang SS, Wu KC, Chen YY. Means restriction for suicide prevention. *Lancet.* (2012) 379:2393–9. doi: 10.1016/S0140-6736(12)60521-2
35. Fleischmann A, Arensman E, Berman A, Carli V, De Leo D, Hadlaczky G, et al. Overview evidence on interventions for population suicide with an eye to identifying best-supported strategies for LMICs. *Glob Ment Health.* (2016) 3:e5. doi: 10.1017/gmh.2015.27
36. Pirkis J, Too LS, Spittal MJ, Krysinska K, Robinson J, Cheung YT. Interventions to reduce suicides at suicide hotspots: a systematic review and meta-analysis. *Lancet Psychiatry.* (2015) 2:994–1001. doi: 10.1016/S2215-0366(15)00266-7
37. Milner AJ, Carter G, Pirkis J, Robinson J, Spittal MJ. Letters, green cards, telephone calls and postcards: systematic and meta-analytic review of brief contact interventions for reducing self-harm, suicide attempts and suicide. *Br J Psychiatry.* (2015) 206:184–90. doi: 10.1192/bjp.bp.114.147819
38. Lapierre S, Erlangsen A, Waern M, De Leo D, Oyama H, Scocco P, et al. A systematic review of elderly suicide prevention programs. *Crisis.* (2011) 32:88–98. doi: 10.1027/0227-5910/a000076
39. Chen YY, Wu KC, Yousuf S, Yip PS. Suicide in Asia: opportunities and challenges. *Epidemiol Rev.* (2012) 34:129–44. doi: 10.1093/epirev/mxr025
40. Dumesnil H, Verger P. Public awareness campaigns about depression and suicide: A review. *Psychiatr Serv.* (2009) 60:1203–13. doi: 10.1176/ps.2009.60.9.1203
41. Fountoulakis KN, Gonda X, Rihmer Z. Suicide prevention programs through community intervention. *J Affect Disord.* (2011) 130:10–6. doi: 10.1016/j.jad.2010.06.009
42. Matsubayashi T, Ueda M, Sawada Y. The effect of public awareness campaigns on suicides: evidence from Nagoya, Japan. *J Affect Disord.* (2014) 152-154:526–9. doi: 10.1016/j.jad.2013.09.007
43. Reynders A, Kerkhof AJ, Molenberghs G, Van Audenhove C. Attitudes and stigma in relation to help-seeking intentions for psychological problems in low and high suicide rate regions. *Soc Psychiatry Psychiatr Epidemiol.* (2014) 49:231–9. doi: 10.1007/s00127-013-0745-4
44. Oyama H, Sakashita T, Ono Y, Goto M, Fujita M, Koida J. Effect of community-based intervention using depression screening on elderly suicide risk: a meta-analysis of the evidence from Japan. *Community Ment Health J.* (2008) 44:311–20. doi: 10.1007/s10597-008-9132-0

45. Rutz W, von Knorring L, Walinder J. Long-term effects of an educational program for general practitioners given by the Swedish committee for the prevention and treatment of depression. *Acta Psychiatr Scand.* (1992) 85:83–8. doi: 10.1111/j.1600-0447.1992.tb01448.x
46. Szanto K, Kalmar S, Hendin H, Rihmer Z, Mann JJ. A suicide prevention program in a region with a very high suicide rate. *Arch Gen Psychiatry.* (2007) 64:914–20. doi: 10.1001/archpsyc.64.8.914
47. De Leo D, Dello Buono M, Dwyer J. Suicide among the elderly: the long-term impact of a telephone support and assessment intervention in northern Italy. *Br J Psychiatry.* (2002) 181:226–9. doi: 10.1192/bjp.181.3.226
48. Fiske A, Arbore P. Future directions in late life suicide prevention. *Omega-J Death Dying.* (2000) 42:37–53. doi: 10.2190/3T4G-T5U2-Q724-E0K8
49. Gould MS, Kalafat J, Harrismunfakh JL, Kleinman M. An evaluation of crisis hotline outcomes. Part 2: suicidal callers. *Suicide Life Threat Behav.* (2007) 37:338–52. doi: 10.1521/suli.2007.37.3.338
50. Szanto K, Mulsant BH, Houck P, Dew MA, Reynolds CF 3rd. Occurrence and course of suicidality during short-term treatment of late-life depression. *Arch Gen Psychiatry.* (2003) 60:610–7. doi: 10.1001/archpsyc.60.6.610
51. Nelson JC, Delucchi K, Schneider L. Suicidal thinking and behavior during treatment with sertraline in late-life depression. *Am J Geriatr Psychiatry.* (2007) 15:573–80. doi: 10.1097/JGP.0b013e318050c9c2
52. Bruce ML, Ten Have TR, Reynolds CF III, Katz II, Schulberg HC, Mulsant BH, et al. Reducing suicidal ideation and depressive symptoms in depressed older primary care patients: a randomized controlled trial. *JAMA.* (2004) 291:1081–91. doi: 10.1001/jama.291.9.1081
53. Unützer J, Tang L, Oishi S, Katon W, Williams JW Jr, Hunkeler E, et al. Reducing suicidal ideation in depressed older primary care patients. *J Am Geriatr Soc.* (2006) 54:1550–6. doi: 10.1111/j.1532-5415.2006.00882.x
54. Luxton DD, June JD, Comtois KA. Can postdischarge follow-up contacts prevent suicide and suicidal behavior? A review of the evidence. *Crisis.* (2013) 34:32–41. doi: 10.1027/0227-5910/a000158
55. Kawanishi C, Aruga T, Ishizuka N, Yonemoto N, Otsuka K, Kamijo Y, et al. Assertive case management versus enhanced usual care for people with mental health problems who had attempted suicide and were admitted to hospital emergency departments in Japan. (ACTION-J): a multicentre, randomised controlled trial. *Lancet Psychiatry.* (2014) 1:193–201. doi: 10.1016/S2215-0366(14)70259-7
56. Hepp U, Wittmann L, Schnyder U, Michel K. Psychological and psychosocial interventions after attempted suicide: an overview of treatment studies. *Crisis.* (2004) 25:108–17. doi: 10.1027/0227-5910.25.3.108
57. Hegerl U, Althaus D, Schmidtke A, Niklewski G. The alliance against depression: 2-year evaluation of a community-based intervention to reduce suicidality. *Psychol Med.* (2006) 36:1225–33. doi: 10.1017/S003329170600780X
58. Székely A, Konkolÿ Thege B, Mergl R, Birkás E, Rózsa S, et al. How to decrease suicide rates in both genders? An effectiveness study of a community-based intervention. (EAAD). *PLoS ONE.* (2013) 8:e75081. doi: 10.1371/journal.pone.0075081
59. Ono Y, Sakai A, Otsuka K, Uda H, Oyama H, Ishizuka N, et al. Effectiveness of a multimodal community intervention program to prevent suicide and suicide attempts: a quasi-experimental study. *PLoS ONE.* (2013) 8:e74902. doi: 10.1371/journal.pone.0074902

5

The Relationship Between Regulatory Emotional Self-Efficacy and Core Self-Evaluation of College Students: The Mediation Effects of Suicidal Attitude

Xiaojun Zhao[1†] and Changxiu Shi[2†]*

[1] School of Education, Hebei University, Baoding, China, [2] School of Criminal Justice, China University of Political Science and Law, Beijing, China

Correspondence:
Changxiu Shi
270729292@qq.com

† These authors have contributed equally to this work and first authors.

This study analyzed the mediation effect of a suicidal attitude from regulatory emotional self-efficacy to core self-evaluation. A measurement study was conducted among 438 college students using the Regulatory Emotional Self-Efficacy Scale, the Core Self-Evaluation Scale, and the Suicide Attitude Questionnaire. Results from the plug-in process in SPSS and the bootstrap method showed that the attitude toward suicidal behavior and the attitude toward family members of an individual who has committed suicide played a double-mediation role, from perceived self-efficacy in managing happiness to core self-evaluation. The results also showed that the attitude toward a person who committed suicide or attempted suicide played a mediation effect from perceived self-efficacy in managing curiousness to core self-evaluation. This research has great significance for improving the understanding of college students' sense of happiness and prevention for self-evaluation.

Keywords: regulatory emotional self-efficacy, suicidal attitude, core self-evaluation, mediation effect, sense of happiness

INTRODUCTION

Suicide College Students

Suicide in college students is one of the most important aspects of mental health education for college students. Suicidal ideation in college students can be discussed with respect to the following two aspects: college students' suicide behavior and suicidal attitude. However, suicidal attitude is a more important psychological factor. On the one hand, in social environments, each individual may have suicidal attitude under the influence of various negative stimulations and frustrations. Suicidal ideation occurs primarily at the cognitive level for most people and is not the leading cause of suicidal behavior. On the other hand, suicidal attitude may include the attitude of an individual that is inclined to commit suicide or the attitude of an individual that is not inclined to commit suicide. However, suicidal attitude also includes attitudes toward people who commit suicide, people who are in the environment around the individual, and related social attributes Because family and friends are also important factors affecting a suicide attempt (Frey et al., 2016).

Suicide in college students is due to academic anxiety, interpersonal difficulties, physical health, and other factors (Seiden, 1966). Body image can predict depression, depression can predict alcohol use, and alcohol use can predict proneness to suicide (Lamis et al., 2010). The Anderson–Darling test is an effective tool to identify suicide clustering (MacKenzie, 2013). However, we are more concerned about the significance of college students' suicidal attitude, rather than the suicide itself. Compared with the intervention of college students' suicidal behavior, the improvement of college students' suicide attitude has a more positive, early preventive effect. The studies on college students' suicidal attitude are important not only for suicide but also for healthy college students.

College students have permissive attitudes about suicidal behavior (Li and Phillips, 2010). After adjusting for reflection and hopelessness, brooding and suicidal ideation are closely linked (Cheref et al., 2015). An ideator with poor problem solving holds a certain attitude about suicide behavior (McAuliffe et al., 2003).

Perceived Self-Efficacy in Managing Happiness, Suicidal Attitude, and Core Self-Evaluation

Perceived self-efficacy in managing happiness refers to individual efficiency in coping with success or positive events embodied in positive emotions (Zhao et al., 2013). Related studies found that psychological elastic impact core self-evaluation (Zeng et al., 2014). Studies have found that core self-evaluation at a high level and emotion regulation ability at a high level were closely related (Kacmar et al., 2009). In addition, Judge thinks that self-efficacy affects core self-evaluation (Judge and Hurst, 2007). As mentioned earlier, perceived self-efficacy in managing happiness was a combination of the effects of self-efficacy and optimism. Therefore, perceived self-efficacy in managing happiness may affect core self-evaluation. The study put forward H1 as follows: the perceived self-efficacy in managing the happiness of college students has a significant effect on core self-evaluation.

Do suicidal attitudes, which are important in relation to people's outlook on life, play an indirect role for perceived self-efficacy in managing happiness? Suicide is the third largest factor of death for college students. Fear/anxiety and suicide attempts or self-injury are closely related (Mitchell et al., 2014). Depression significantly affects suicidal ideation (Westefeld and Furr, 1987; Furr et al., 2001; Mackenzie et al., 2011). At the same time, perceived burdensomeness can predict suicidal ideation (Wong et al., 2011). Fear/anxiety, depression, and burdensomeness belong to the category of mood. However, self-efficacy indirectly influences suicidal ideation through optimism (You and Chen, 2012). Optimism leads to low depressive symptoms or hopelessness and suicidal ideation (Bryan et al., 2013; Chang et al., 2017). In addition, there are studies that make it clear that optimism can reduce suicide risk for college students (Hirsch et al., 2007). From the perspective of psychological experience, does perceived self-efficacy in managing happiness with a combination of self-efficacy and optimism affect suicidal attitude? Suicidal ideation is partly affected by individual emotional distress, and regulatory emotional self-efficacy serves as an important aspect of emotional control related to the effects of individual suicide or attitude. Normally, the mental flexibility of an individual with a suicide identity is poor.

As a carrier of the characteristics, suicidal attitude may affect a person's overall core self-evaluation. The suicide attitude connected with one's life outlook is involved in the philosophy of life. The suicide attitude has an important influence on one's overall self-analysis. In a study of suicidal attitude, the researchers focused on attitudes toward suicide. At the same time, the family caregivers (such as family members of suicide) are an important link to reduce the number of suicides (Chiang et al., 2015). The study put forward H2 and H3 as follows. H2: the perceived self-efficacy in managing the happiness of college students indirectly affects core self-evaluation through the attitude for suicidal behavior; H3: the perceived self-efficacy in managing the happiness of college students indirectly affects core self-evaluation through attitude to family members of suicide.

Perceived Self-Efficacy in Managing Curiousness and Suicidal Attitude

Curiosity and anxiety can be regarded as two kinds of reverse drive and emotional state. The interaction of curiosity and anxiety affect the individual's attitude and behavior (Spielberger and Starr, 1994). Particularly, interpersonal curiosity is better. For an individual of high interpersonal curiosity, it is easier to understand social behavior. In social activities, an individual showing quality curiosity has more positive emotions, creating a more positive and close social experience (Kashdan et al., 2011). An individual with poor control over interpersonal curiosity may eventually exhibit deviant behavior. So, from the perspective of interpersonal environment, perceived self-efficacy in managing curiousness may affect suicidal attitude, particularly the suicidal attitude toward the person who committed suicide or attempted suicide. The study put forward H4 as follows: the perceived self-efficacy in managing the curiosity of college students indirectly affects core self-evaluation through the suicidal attitude toward a person who committed suicide or attempted suicide.

Some people have affirmatory suicidal attitude, but few people display suicidal behavior. An attitude toward suicide might affect the person's overall perception and self-evaluation. Happiness is one of the important indicators of modern social development. This study has important significance for improving the understanding of college students' sense of happiness and prevention for self-evaluation.

MATERIALS AND METHODS

Participants

The participants included 450 university students from Anhui province and Hebei province. All participating universities had cases of suicide or attempted suicide in the past year. The participants completed the informed consent form and the basic information form. The study was approved by the academic and ethics committee of school of education in Hebei University. The number of students who completed the recycling questionnaire was 441, and the recovery rate was 97.33%. After excluding invalid questionnaires, the number of participants was 438, and the effective rate was 99.32%. The participants included 128 boys and 310 girls, and 124 student cadres and 314 non-student cadres.

Measures

Regulatory Emotional Self-Efficacy (RESE) Scale

We used the RESE Scale of Chinese college students (Zhao et al., 2013). This scale included 42 items, using a 5-point scoring method. The RESE scale of Chinese university students consists of seven factors, including perceived self-efficacy in managing inferiority, happiness, jealousy, horror/fear, confidence, curiosity, and reliance. The total internal consistency coefficient is 0.913 in this test.

Suicide Attitude Questionnaire

This study uses the Suicide Attitude Questionnaire (Xiao et al., 1999). This scale includes 29 items and uses a 5-point scoring method. The scale is divided into four factors, namely, attitude toward suicide behavior (F1), attitude toward a person who committed suicide or attempted suicide (F2), attitude toward family members of an individual who has committed suicide (F3), and attitude toward euthanasia (F4). The total internal consistency coefficient is 0.647 in this test.

Core Self-Evaluation Scale

This study used the Chinese version of the Revised Core Self-Evaluation Scale (Du et al., 2012). This scale included 10 items and used a 5-point scoring method. The scale is only one factor. The internal consistency coefficient is 0.719 for this scale.

Process

The study used paper and pencil tests. The experimenters were psychology teachers with Master's or Doctorate degrees. The participants (college students) took part in psychological tests with unified instructions. The psychological tests included the following: the RESE Scale, the Suicide Attitude Questionnaire, and the Core Self-Evaluation Scale. During the self-study period of the college students', college students filled out these questionnaires. Then, the completed questionnaires were scored and analyzed.

Data Management and Analysis

The study conducted data management and analysis using the PROCESS plug-in of the SPSS 17.0 software (Hayes, 2013). The study carried out a correlation analysis and mediation effects analysis.

RESULTS AND ANALYSIS

Correlation Analysis

According to the results of the correlation coefficient (Pearson) among perceived self-efficacy in managing happiness, perceived self-efficacy in managing curiousness, attitude toward suicidal behavior, attitude toward family members of suicide, attitude toward a person who committed suicide or attempted suicide and core self-evaluation (see **Table 1**), there were two significant correlations among perceived self-efficacy in managing happiness, attitude toward suicidal behavior and core self-evaluation. There were two significant correlations among self-efficacy in managing happiness, attitude toward family members of an individual who has committed suicide and core self-evaluation. The correlation between perceived self-efficacy in managing curiousness and attitude toward a person who committed suicide or attempted suicide was significant ($p < 0.01$). The correlation between the attitude toward a person who committed suicide or attempted suicide and core self-evaluation was significant ($p < 0.001$). The variables involved in the study are significantly correlated. To further verify the hypothesis, the study conducted the corresponding mediation effect analysis.

Double Mediation Effect Analysis Based on Perceived Self-Efficacy in Managing Happiness

To further analyze the relations among perceived self-efficacy in managing happiness, attitude for suicidal behavior, attitude toward family members of an individual who has committed suicide and core self-evaluation, the study conducted a mediation effect analysis. The analysis diagram of the mediation effect is shown in **Figure 1**.

The study conducted a mediation effect analysis using the process proposed by Zhao et al. (2010), which utilized the Bootstrap method proposed by Preacher and Hayes (2004) and Hayes (2013). Data analysis was done using the PROCESS plug-in of SPSS (Hayes, 2013). The sample size of the Bootstrap analysis was 5000. Under the 95% confidence interval, the mediation effect test results do not contain 0. The direct effect of A on B was 0.116 (LLCI = 0.018, ULCI = 0.213). The indirect effect of A on B was 0.085 (LLCI = 0.038, ULCI = 0.137). Based on F1, the indirect effect of A on B was 0.054 (LLCI = 0.015, ULCI = 0.100). Based on F3, the indirect effect of A on B was 0.030 (LLCI = 0.007, ULCI = 0.066). There was a partial mediation effect found. The results showed that the double mediation effects of attitude toward suicide behavior and attitude toward family members of an individual who has committed suicide were significant. However, the mediating effect is a complementary mediating effect. Therefore, future research should consider whether there are other intermediary variables. The process from perceived self-efficacy in managing happiness to core self-evaluation included the direct and indirect effects of attitude toward suicide behavior and attitude toward family members of an individual who has committed suicide as double mediation.

Mediation Effect Analysis Based on Perceived Self-Efficacy in Managing Curiousness

To further analyze the relations among perceived self-efficacy in managing curiousness, attitude toward a person who committed suicide or attempted suicide and core self-evaluation, the study conducted a mediation effect analysis. The analysis diagram of the mediation effect is shown in **Figure 2**.

The study conducted a mediation effect analysis program. The data analysis used the PROCESS plug-in of SPSS (Hayes, 2013). The sample size of the Bootstrap analysis was 5000. Under the 95% confidence interval, the mediation effect test results do not contain 0. The indirect effect of C on D was −0.019

TABLE 1 | The correlation based on perceived self-efficacy in managing happiness and curiousness.

	$M \pm SD$	1	2	3	4	5	6
(1) Perceived self-efficacy in managing happiness	4.230 ± 0.466	1					
(2) Perceived self-efficacy in managing happiness	3.290 ± 0.763	0.295***	1				
(3) Attitude for suicidal behavior	3.070 ± 0.570	−0.134**	0.029	1			
(4) Attitude toward a person who committed suicide or attempted suicide	2.700 ± 0.424	−0.070	0.128**	0.072	1		
(5) Attitude toward family members of an individual who has committed suicide	2.504 ± 0.450	−0.236***	0.018	−0.039	0.404***	1	
(6) Core self-evaluation	3.256 ± 0.512	0.182***	0.000	0.390***	−0.222***	0.156***	1

*$p < 0.05$, **$p < 0.01$, ***$p < 0.001$.

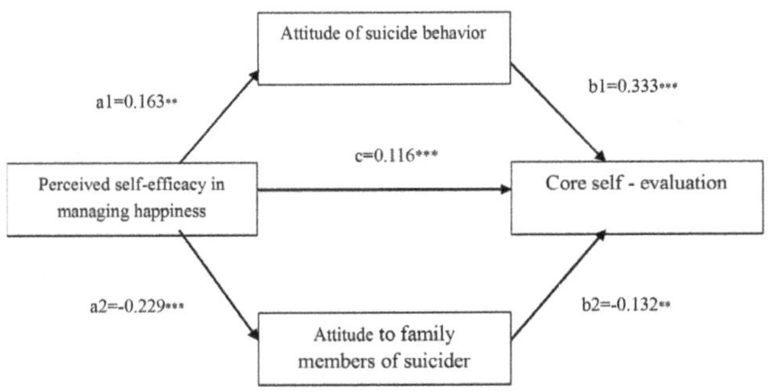

FIGURE 1 | Mediation effect diagram for attitude of suicide behavior and attitude toward family members of an individual who has committed suicide.

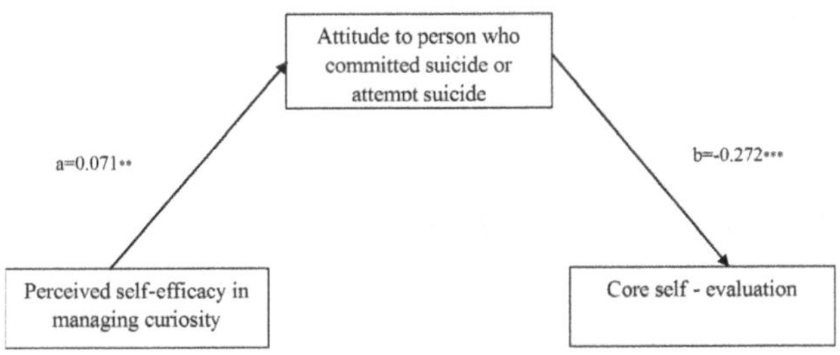

FIGURE 2 | Mediation effect diagram for attitude toward a person who committed suicide or attempted suicide.

(LLCI = −0.042, ULCI = −0.006). The direct effect of C on D was 0.019 (LLCI = −0.043, ULCI = 0.081); therefore, a complete mediation effect was found. The results showed a significant mediation effect of the attitude toward a person who committed suicide or attempted suicide.

DISCUSSION

Perceived Self-Efficacy in Managing Happiness Impact on Core Self-Evaluation

The study confirms H1, and the results are in line with previous studies (Judge and Hurst, 2007; Kacmar et al., 2009; Zeng et al., 2014; Zang et al., 2015). Psychological elastic, emotion regulation ability, and self-efficacy affect core self-evaluation. In this study, perceived self-efficacy in managing happiness refers to individual efficiency in coping with success or positive events embodied in positive emotions (Zhao et al., 2013). The core self-evaluation is a basic evaluation for their ability and value (Judge et al., 1997). Emotional elasticity is a type of regulation ability of negative emotion, and perceived self-efficacy in managing happiness reflects your perceptive ability to adjust to a happy mood in a controlled manner. These two aspects are associated in that perceived self-efficacy in managing happiness is a factor of regulatory emotional self-efficacy, as well as a type of special self-efficacy. This special self-efficacy is also likely to affect the general integrity of self-evaluation. Perceived self-efficacy in managing happiness with a nature of optimism is a type of positive individual ability. This ability will become a personality trait if it is positively exercised for a long time. This trait ultimately leads to increased ability and value.

Intermediary Effect Analysis of the Suicidal Attitude

Perceived self-efficacy in managing happiness is a reflection of positive psychology. Perceived self-efficacy in managing happiness of the optimistic nature is bound to influence one's perceptions (negative or positive) of suicide. Due to differences in cognitive nature, attitude led to the observed differentiation of the college students' self-evaluation.

Previous studies have found that self-efficacy indirectly influences suicidal ideation through optimism (You and Chen, 2012). Optimism reduces depressive symptoms (Hirsch et al., 2014), depression significantly affects suicidal ideation (Westefeld and Furr, 1987; Furr et al., 2001; Mackenzie et al., 2011). Depression belongs to the category of emotional symptoms, but optimism is a rather positive psychology. If the individuals have the ability to adjust the level and perception of their happiness, then the suicidal attitude may be improved. Once one has the ability to control environmental factors, the individual will reduce negative thoughts and actions. In contrast, individual feelings that are passively controlled by the environment will produce more negative thoughts and actions. A suicidal attitude also includes attitudes toward suicidal behavior, people who commit suicide, people who are in the environment around them, and related social attributes, since family and friends are also important factors affecting a suicide attempt (Frey et al., 2016). The study found that attitudes toward suicidal behavior and attitudes toward family members of a suicide were mediated. The perceived self-efficacy in managing happiness with a combination of self-efficacy and optimism affects suicidal ideation.

The perceived self-efficacy in managing curiousness reflects the adjustment ability of interpersonal curiosity. For an individual of high interpersonal curiosity, it is easier to understand social behavior. In social activities, an individual with quality curiosity has more positive emotions, thus creating a more positive and close social experience (Kashdan et al., 2011). A suicidal attitude is a mixture of emotion and social experience. Negative emotion and negative social experience a prompted more negative suicidal attitude. A college student with poor control over interpersonal curiosity may eventually exhibit deviant behavior. These deviant behaviors include suicide behavior and internal fighting behavior.

Related research showed that the core self-evaluation influenced suicidal ideation (Ma et al., 2013). However, this study considered that a suicidal attitude affects the core self-evaluation for the following reasons: (1) suicidal ideation and attitude for suicidal behavior are different. Suicidal ideation refers to oneself, and attitude for suicidal behavior refers to oneself or others; (2) whether related to oneself suicide or suicide involved with others, the individual's outlook on life is severely affected if one has a positive attitude toward suicide. The individual's view of life promotes a change in the self-assessment.

Prevention for Core Self-Evaluation Based on Perceived Self-Efficacy in Managing Happiness and Suicidal Attitude

The traditional intervention of core self-evaluation rarely considers the perceived self-efficacy in managing happiness and suicidal attitude. Positive psychological constructs should be an important factor in suicide intervention (Celano et al., 2017). Intervention for suicidal attitudes may be more likely to lead to a deeper variation in self-evaluation. Because suicide does not occur in a majority of people, most healthy people have a stable attitude toward suicide. A stable attitude toward suicide may have a stronger effect on one's outlook on life. The intervention plan with some techniques for building scenarios (such as virtual reality and augmented reality) may have profound implications for the ascension of self-evaluation. In addition, perceived self-efficacy in managing happiness was a combination of self-efficacy and optimism. Perceived self-efficacy in managing happiness directly affects one's attitude toward suicide and directly influences core self-evaluation. It is a reliable method to improve one's perceived self-efficacy in managing happiness through behavioral training techniques.

Limitations and Future Directions

Although this study confirmed the mediation effect of a suicidal attitude on perceived self-efficacy in managing happiness/curiousness to core self-evaluation, the following limitations were present: (1) the sample size could be larger; (2) only a single research method is used; (3) because the double-mediation effect in this study is a complementary mediating effect, there may not be any other intermediary variables. Future studies should aim to do the following: (1) analyze the mediation effects among core self-evaluation, attitude for suicidal behavior, and suicidal behavior by confirming whether there is a chain mediation effect; (2) confirm the related mechanism of sense of happiness using susceptibility theory; determining whether there is a susceptibility factor for sense of happiness would be of great value.

AUTHOR CONTRIBUTIONS

XZ and CS conceived and designed the study, performed the study, analyzed the data, and wrote the paper.

REFERENCES

1. Bryan, C. J., Ray-Sannerud, B. N., Morrow, C. E., and Etienne, N. (2013). Optimism reduces suicidal ideation and weakens the effect of hopelessness among military personnel. *Cogn. Ther. Res.* 37, 996–1003. doi: 10.1007/s10608-013- 9536-1
2. Celano, C. M., Beale, E. E., Mastromauro, C. A., Stewart, J. G., and Millstein, R. A. (2017). Psychological interventions to reduce suicidality in high-risk patients with major depression: a randomized controlled trial. *Psychol. Med.* 47, 810–821. doi: 10.1017/S0033291716002798
3. Chang, E. C., Martos, T., Sallay, V., Chang, O. D., and Wright, K. M. (2017). Examining optimism and hope as protective factors of suicide risk in hungarian college students: is risk highest among those lacking positive psychological protection. *Cogn. Ther. Res.* 41, 278–288. doi: 10.1007/s10608-016-9810-0
4. Cheref, S., Lane, R., Polanco-Roman, L., Gadol, E., and Miranda, R. (2015). Suicidal ideation among racial/ethnic minorities: moderating effects of rumination and depressive symptoms. *Cultur. Divers. Ethnic Minor. Psychol.* 21, 31–40. doi: 10.1037/a0037139
5. Chiang, C. Y., Lu, C. Y., Lin, Y. H., Lin, H. Y., and Sun, F. K. (2015). Caring stress, suicidal attitude and suicide care ability among family caregivers of suicidal individuals: a path analysis. *J. Psychiatr. Ment. Health Nurs.* 22, 792–800. doi: 10.1111/jpm.12267
6. Du, J. Z., Zhang, X., and Zhao, Y. (2012). Reliability, validation and construct confirmatory of core self-evaluations scale. *Chin. J. Psychol. Res.* 5, 54–60. doi: 10.1007/s11136-010-9833-z
7. Frey, L. M., Hans, J. D., and Cerel, J. (2016). An interpretive phenomenological inquiry of family and friend reactions to suicide disclosure. *J. Marital Fam. Ther.* 43, 159–172. doi: 10.1111/jmft.12180
8. Furr, S. R., Westefeld, J. S., McConnell, G. N., and Jenkins, J. M. (2001). Suicide and depression among college students: a decade later. *Prof. Psychol.* 32, 97–100. doi: 10.1037/0735-7028.32.1.97
9. Hayes, A. F. (2013). *Introduction to Mediation, Moderation, and Conditional Process Analysis: A Regression-Based Approach.* New York, NY: Guilford Press. Hirsch, J. K., Conner, K. R., and Duberstein, P. R. (2007). Optimism and suicide ideation among young adult college students. *Arch. Suicide Res.* 11, 177–185. doi: 10.1080/13811110701249988
10. Hirsch, J. K., Nsamenang, S. A., Chang, E. C., and Kaslow, N. J. (2014).

Spiritual well-being and depressive symptoms in female African American suicide attempters: mediating effects of optimism and pessimism. *Psychol. Relig. Spiritual.* 6, 276–283. doi: 10.1037/a0036723
11. Judge, T. A., and Hurst, C. (2007). Capitalizing on one's advantages: role of core self-evaluations. *J. Appl. Psychol.* 92, 1212–1227. doi: 10.1037/0021-9010.92.5. 1212
12. Judge, T. A., Locke, E. A., and Durham, C. C. (1997). The dispositional causes of job satisfaction: a core evaluations approach. *Res. Organ. Behav.* 19, 151–188. Kacmar, K. M., Collins, B. J., Harris, K. J., and Judge, T. A. (2009). Core self-evaluations and job performance: the role of the perceived work environment. *J. Appl. Psychol.* 94, 1572–1580. doi: 10.1037/a0017498
13. Kashdan, T. B., Mcknight, P. E., Fincham, F. D., and Rose, P. (2011). When curiosity breeds intimacy: taking advantage of intimacy opportunities and transforming boring conversations. *J. Pers.* 79, 1369–1402. doi: 10.1111/j.1467- 6494.2010.00697.x
14. Lamis, D. A., Malone, P. S., Langhinrichsen-Rohling, J., and Ellis, T. E. (2010). Body investment, depression, and alcohol use as risk factors for suicide proneness in college students. *Crisis* 31, 118–127. doi: 10.1027/0227-5910/a000012
15. Li, X., and Phillips, M. R. (2010). The acceptability of suicide among rural residents, urban residents, and college students from three locations in china: a cross- sectional survey. *Crisis* 31, 183–193. doi: 10.1027/0027-5910/a000024
16. Ma, Y. J., Li, Q. L., Wang, L. L., and Dai, X. Y. (2013). The relationships among suicidal ideation, core self-evaluation and social support for medical students. *J. Chin. Ningxia Med. Univ.* 35, 1372–1374.
17. MacKenzie, D. W. (2013). Applying the anderson-darling test to suicide clusters: evidence of contagion at U.S. universities? *Crisis* 34, 434–437. doi: 10.1027/ 0227-5910/a000197
18. Mackenzie, S., Wiegel, J. R., Mundt, M., Brown, D., Saewyc, E., Heiligenstein, E., et al. (2011). Depression and suicide ideation among students accessing campus health care. *Am. J. Orthopsychiatry* 81, 101–107. doi: 10.1111/j.1939-0025.2010. 01077.x
19. McAuliffe, C., Corcoran, P., Keeley, H. S., and Perry, I. J. (2003). Risk of suicide ideation associated with problem-solving ability and attitudes toward suicidal behavior in university students. *Crisis* 24, 160–167. doi: 10.1027//0227-5910.24. 4.160
20. Mitchell, S. M., Jahn, D. R., and Cukrowicz, K. C. (2014). The relation between illegal risk behaviors and the acquired capability for suicide. *Crisis* 35, 368–377. doi: 10.1027/0227-5910/a000274
21. Preacher, K. J., and Hayes, A. F. (2004). SPSS and SAS procedures for estimating indirect effects in simple mediation models. *Behav. Res. Methods Instrum. Comput.* 36, 717–731. doi: 10.3758/BF03206553
22. Seiden, R. H. (1966). Campus tragedy: a study of student suicide. *J. Abnorm. Psychol.* 71, 389–399. doi: 10.1037/h0023970
23. Spielberger, C. D., and Starr, L. M. (1994). "Curiosity and exploratory behavior," in *Motivation: Theory and Research*, eds H. F. O'Neil Jr and M. Drillings (Hillsdale, NJ: Lawrence Erlbaum Associates), 221–243.
24. Westefeld, J. S., and Furr, S. R. (1987). Suicide and depression among college students. *Prof. Psychol.* 18, 119–123. doi: 10.1037/0735-7028.18. 2.119
25. Wong, Y. J., Koo, K., Tran, K. K., Chiu, Y., and Mok, Y. (2011). Asian American college students' suicide ideation: a mixed-methods study. *J. Counsel. Psychol.* 58, 197–209. doi: 10.1037/a0023040
26. Xiao, S. Y., Yang, H., Dong, Q. H., and Yang, D. S. (1999). The Development, reliability and validity of suicide attitude inventory. *Chin. Ment. Health J.* 13, 250–251.
27. You, F. H., and Chen, Z. J. (2012). Impacts of academic stress, self-efficacy and optimism on suicide ideation of doctoral students. *Chin. J. Clin. Psychol.* 20, 662–665.
28. Zang, S., Liu, F. Q., Li, Y., and Lin, Y. (2015). Mediate effects of psychological capital appreciation between emotional elasticity and core self - evaluation among the ethnic minority medical students. *Chin. Gen. Pract.* 18, 1436–1440.
29. Zeng, X. J., Jiang, H., and Li, Y. X. (2014). Mental health, resilience and core self- evaluation in left-behind rural middle school students. *Chin. Ment. Health J.* 28, 947–950.
30. Zhao, X., Lynch, J. G. Jr., and Chen, Q. (2010). Reconsidering baron and kenny: myths and truths about mediation analysis. *J. Consum. Res.* 37, 197–206. doi: 10.1086/651257
31. Zhao, X. J., You, X. Q., Shi, C. X., Yang, X. F., Chu, K. W., and Peng, Z. M. (2013). Factor analysis of the regulatory emotional self-efficacy scale of Chinese college students. *Soc. Behav. Pers.* 41, 751–760. doi: 10.2224/sbp.2013.41. 5.751

6

Event-Related Potential Measures of Attention Capture in Adolescent Inpatients with Acute Suicidel Behavior

Paniz Tavakoli[1], Addo Boafo[2,3], Allyson Dale[4], Rebecca Robillard[4,5], Stephanie L. Greenham[1,3,4] and Kenneth Campbell[4]*

[1] Children's Hospital of Eastern Ontario Research Institute, Ottawa, ON, Canada, [2] Department of Psychiatry, University of Ottawa, Ottawa, ON, Canada, [3] Children's Hospital of Eastern Ontario, Ottawa, ON, Canada, [4] School of Psychology, University of Ottawa, Ottawa, ON, Canada, [5] University of Ottawa Institute of Mental Health Research, Ottawa, ON, Canada

***Correspondence:**
Paniz Tavakoli
ptava069@uottawa.ca

Impaired executive functions, modulated by the frontal lobes, have been suggested to be associated with suicidal behavior. The present study examines one of these executive functions, attentional control, maintaining attention to the task-at-hand. A group of inpatient adolescents with acute suicidal behavior and healthy controls were studied using a passively presented auditory optimal paradigm. This "optimal" paradigm consisted of a series of frequently presented homogenous pure tone "standards" and different "deviants," constructed by changing one or more features of the standard. The optimal paradigm has been shown to be a more time-efficient replacement to the traditional oddball paradigm, which makes it suitable for use in clinical populations. The extent of processing of these "to-be-ignored" auditory stimuli was measured by recording event-related potentials (ERPs). The P3a ERP component is thought to reflect processes associated with the capturing of attention. Rare and novel stimuli may result in an executive decision to switch attention away from the current cognitive task and toward a probe of the potentially more relevant "interrupting" auditory input. On the other hand, stimuli that are quite similar to the standard should not elicit P3a. The P3a has been shown to be larger in immature brains in early compared to later adolescence. An overall enhanced P3a was observed in the suicidal group. The P3a was larger in this group for both the environmental sound and white noise deviants, although only the environmental sound P3a attained significance. Other deviants representing only a small change from the standard did not elicit a P3a in healthy controls. They did elicit a small P3a in the suicidal group. These findings suggest a lowered threshold for the triggering of the involuntary switch of attention in these patients, which may play a role in their reported distractibility. The enhanced P3a is also suggestive of an immature frontal central executive and may provide a promising marker for early identification of some of the risk factors for some of the cognitive difficulties linked to suicidality.

Keywords: suicidality, executive functions, attention capture, event-related potentials, P3a

INTRODUCTION

Adolescence is a phase of life associated with possible increased risks for dangerous behaviors. The World Health Organization indicates that suicide is the fifteenth leading cause of death worldwide but represents the second leading cause of death among 10–24 years old (1). Mood disorders are among the top mental health illnesses that increase the risk of suicidal behavior (2). Research has shown that internal conflicts as well as feelings of depression and anxiety can result in suicidal behavior (3, 4).

Attempted suicide may be a different phenomenon in adolescents than in adults. This is particularly true considering that adolescence is a critical time for brain maturation and the development of cognitive and emotional personalities. Adolescents with suicidal behavior often exhibit concentration deficits that can be displayed as increased distractibility (5–7). These deficits are often increased with the presence of suicide attempts. Furthermore, distractibility in these individuals may be caused by their high emotional sensitivity to external stimuli, particularly negative emotional cues [for reviews, see Ref. (8, 9)]. This emotional sensitivity may in turn predispose these individuals to self-harming and suicidal behavior (10, 11). The present study aims to determine whether information processing commonly associated with distractibility and attention shifts are affected in adolescents with an acute risk of suicidal behavior.

Imaging studies have provided evidence that a number of regions of the frontal lobe are implicated in suicidal behavior (12–18). Marzuk et al. (19) was among one of the first to suggest that impaired executive functions, modulated by the frontal lobes, may be associated with suicidal ideation, regardless of a history of suicide attempts. A number of neuropsychological and cognitive studies have now provided support for this claim [see Ref. (20–22) for reviews]. There is much debate whether the frontal lobes modulate a single unitary or "central" executive function or whether there are many interrelated and fragmented functions (23, 24). Stuss et al. (25) have identified different subregions within the frontal lobes that reflect these separate, fragmented functions. In this regard, research has shown that suicidal ideation and actual suicide attempt are associated with many different deficits in executive functions (21, 26–31). The deficits in executive tasks that have been identified vary among studies and have not always been replicated. Part of this inconsistency can be explained by factors such as the diversity in patient samples (suicide ideation versus attempt), the nature and time (acute, recent, remote) of the attempts, comorbid disorders and medications (21). Keilp et al. (29, 32) however emphasize that common to many studies is a specific executive deficit, attentional control. This may be observed in an inability to sustain attention for long periods of time.

The need to sustain active attention is critically important to many higher aspects of cognition. Almost all neuropsychological and cognitive tasks do require attention to be maintained for the duration of the task. It is, thus, possible that reports of a dysfunction on a wide number of executive functions may be confounded by this underlying inability to sustain sufficient attention to maintain optimal performance. The present study examines an executive function that operates passively, independent of active attention. While an individual is actively engaged in a cognitive task, certain potentially highly relevant auditory events occurring outside of the current focus attention may result in a switch of attention away from the cognitive task and toward the auditory stimulation. Such control of attentional resources is called passive attention (33). In this regard, Keilp et al. (28) note that deficits in attentional control do not involve all aspects of attention but rather are more specific to this interference processing. A critical executive function is indeed to allocate attentional resources and to maintain attention to highly relevant tasks. Nevertheless, the system is fluid and flexible. For survival purposes, we must be able to detect, and act upon, potentially highly relevant information occurring outside of the current focus of attention. Nevertheless, most stimulus input that bombards the sensory receptors does in fact turn out to be irrelevant. A consequence of these interruptions is deterioration in performance of the current cognitive tasks as a result of attention being switched away. This is called "distraction." A delicate balance must thus be established that limits interruption of current cognitive demands to only very rare and highly relevant stimulus input. The Keilp et al. (28) interference hypothesis suggests that suicidal behavior may be marked by a too frequent interruption of the central executive.

It is, of course, difficult to design experimental studies to measure the extent of processing of information occurring outside the current focus of attention. The participant could be asked to detect, by button pressing, certain stimuli occurring in an unattended sensory modality. However, active attention is then being directed to that modality, bringing it into the focus of attention. Auditory event-related potentials (ERPs) allow researchers to monitor the extent of information processing of stimulus input occurring outside the focus of attention. ERPs are the minute changes in the ongoing electrical activity of the brain (the "EEG") that are elicited by external stimuli or internal psychological events. ERPs consist of a series of negative-voltage and positive-voltage "components," reflecting different aspects of information processing. Auditory stimuli are often used in the study of attention capture. This is because we hear over 360° and all auditory stimuli, whether attended or ignored, are processed to a certain extent. Visual stimuli that are not presented within the participant's visual field, on the other hand, do not activate retinal cells and are thus not processed in the visual system.

Many auditory ERP studies of attention capture employ a so-called auditory "oddball" paradigm. The participant is presented with a rapid presentation of a frequently occurring homogenous "standard" stimulus. Occasionally, a feature of the standard stimulus is changed to form a rarely occurring "deviant" stimulus. The participant is often asked to ignore the auditory sequence of stimuli while attending to another, often visual, task. The auditory ERPs are thus elicited passively, independent of active attention. Such processing is thus said to be preattentive, or preconscious. The standard stimulus elicits an obligatory negative-going component, "N1," peaking at about 100 ms after stimulus onset. This is followed by a positivity known as the "P2," occurring at about 180–200 ms. Deviant stimuli also elicit the same N1-P2. In addition, it also elicits another negative ERP component, the mismatch negativity [MMN; (34, 35)]. The MMN occurs at about 100–200 ms following the onset of the stimulus depending on the extent of change from the standard stimulus. The MMN's voltage is largest over frontocentral areas of the scalp, and it inverts in polarity (recorded as a positive potential) at the mastoids. The MMN is associated with a preconscious memory-based change detection system in which the features of the incoming auditory stimulus are compared against the features of the preceding stimuli stored in sensory memory. If a standard is now presented, the features of the incoming stimulus match those stored in a sensory memory; memory is then improved, but further processing ceases. The individual would thus not be conscious of this input. If the features do not match those stored in sensory memory, change is detected. A more recent model suggests that the MMN is elicited by the detection of deviance whenever an external auditory event does not match the brain's prediction of environmental regularities (36–39), the frequently presented standard stimulus, in this case, representing a pattern of regularity. Importantly, the change detection system operates automatically and independently of attention. Thus, the MMN is elicited even if the participant is not attending to the auditory channel in which the deviant occurs and regardless of task demands in which the participants is engaged (40–42). Highly novel deviants might elicit both a larger N1 than the standard stimuli, but also an MMN. This observed is often referred to as a deviant-related negativity (DRN) as it is not a true MMN. It represents a combined negative potential, both spatially and temporally, of the N1 and MMN. In this article, for consistency, the negativity following deviants will be described as a DRN.

The output of the change detector system is proportional to the extent of change between standard and deviant. If this output is large enough, it will send a trigger to the central executive, resulting in a passive switch of attention away from current cognitive demands and toward a probing of the "interrupting" auditory modality. The content of the auditory modality then becomes available to consciousness. This process has been associated with a later 200–250 ms positivity, maximum over centrofrontal areas of the scalp, the P3a (43). There is currently some debate about whether the P3a reflects the actual switch of attention toward incoming auditory stimuli or is a precursor process that may lead to conscious awareness [for reviews, see Ref. (44, 45)]. The current understanding is that the presence of the P3a at least reflects higher-level processing, such as the evaluation of events as being significant (46–48). Several studies have reliably shown that the presentation of certain irrelevant auditory deviants that elicit a P3a will cause a distraction away from other primary tasks as evidenced by increased reaction times and/or decreased accuracy of detection (49–52). It is important to note that while almost any perceptible acoustic change will elicit an MMN, only a few of these auditory stimuli will also elicit a P3a. The P3a is elicited by only those stimuli that signal a large extent of change. In the Näätänen model (34, 35), the threshold at which the central executive is interrupted is thought to be flexible. In certain disorders, it may be very low, resulting in abnormally frequent interruption while in other disorders, very high, resulting in an inability to detect potentially relevant events occurring outside of the focus of attention.

It has long been known that prefrontal cortical regions play an important role in the orienting of attention (53). The prefrontal cortex is however not fully mature until late adolescence [see (54, 55) for reviews]. It has been suggested that the P3a is associated with a complex network of brain regions involved in processing and evaluating novel information. These regions include the prefrontal cortex, anterior cingulate cortex, and the hippocampus (56–58). A limited number of studies have examined attention capture and the involuntary switching of attention, as measured by the P3a, in adolescents. There is evidence of an increased susceptibility to task-irrelevant information in children and younger adolescents compared to older adolescents and adults (45, 52, 59–65). It is thus possible that the threshold for interruption of the central executive is lower in younger participants.

Few studies have examined the P3a in association with suicidal behavior. Similarly, a limited number of studies have been carried out in patients with major depressive disorder (MDD), and the results are inconsistent (66–70). In adults, the amplitude of the P3a appears to be reduced in patients with MDD compared to healthy controls (66–68, 70). On the other hand, Lepistö et al. (71) examined the P3a in 10- to 13-year-old children with MDD and observed an enhanced P3a in response to the rarely occurring deviant stimuli, in contrast to the studies showing a reduced P3a in adults. Additionally, although Jandl et al. (69) did not directly compare P3a amplitudes between adult depressed suicide attempters and healthy controls, their figures show a slight enhancement of the P3a in the suicidal patients [**Figure 2** in Ref. (69)]. These limited findings thus suggest a very different pattern of processing from adolescent to adult MDD. Of course, differences in methodology and choice of types of deviant stimuli limit this conclusion. It is possible that the type of deviant stimuli used can differentially affect the interruption of the central executive in depressed/suicidal adolescents and healthy controls. Adolescents with suicidal behavior may exhibit a frequent occurrence of a P3a to deviant stimuli that do not elicit a P3a in controls. To determine whether this is the case requires the presentation of several different deviants, varying in extent of change from the standard.

A problem with ERP methodology is that the "signal" of interest (the P3a in this case) is embedded within the much larger ongoing background EEG "noise." The amplitude of the background EEG can be reduced through repeated presentation of the same stimulus and the averaging of these trials. The amplitude of the background EEG will decrease with the averaging procedure while the ERP signal should remain constant from one trial to the next. This procedure will decrease the signal-to-noise ratio. Nonetheless, in order for the ERP signal to emerge from the background EEG noise, numerous stimulus repetitions must be presented. An oddball sequence will often last from 10 to 15 min to permit a sufficiently large number of stimuli to be presented. Researchers often replicate their data, in which case the sequence will need to be repeated a second time. Furthermore, if several oddball sequences are to be presented to examine the P3a to numerous deviants, testing times could be very long indeed, exceeding 2 h. Such a long testing time may not be feasible in clinical populations.

A newer multifeature optimal paradigm (72) reduces testing time dramatically because several different deviants are presented within a single sequence. In this paradigm, standard and deviant stimuli alternate. Thus, the overall probability of occurrence of each is 0.50. However, several different types of deviants are presented. In the original multifeature paradigm, each deviant represented a change in a different feature from the standard (for example, its frequency, duration, intensity, etc.). Thus, if five different deviants are presented, even though the overall probability of occurrence of deviance was quite high (0.50), the probability of occurrence of a specific deviant was low (0.10). While a single feature of the deviant does differ from that of the standard, all other features are shared. The optimal paradigm was created with the assumption that the deviant stimuli will strengthen the memory trace of the standard in regards to the stimulus features they share. The MMNs that were elicited when an optimal paradigm was run were very similar to the MMNs elicited when separate oddball paradigms were run for each deviant (72). Recently, Tavakoli and Campbell (73) studied whether an optimal paradigm could also be used for the study of the P3a in young healthy adults. They noted that only certain deviants, white noise and novel environmental sounds, could elicit a P3a within an oddball paradigm. Other types of deviants did not. Very similar findings were found when the same deviants were used within a single optimal sequence. The advantage the multifeature optimal paradigm is that it of course significantly reduces testing times and is thus particularly suited for use with clinical populations.

Very few ERP studies have been run with suicidal populations. The present study examines processing related to a critical executive function, the capturing of attention. Most tests of executive function require the maintenance of attention for relatively long periods of time. The capture of attention is, however, a relatively passive process not requiring active attention. There is evidence that frequent interruptions of the central executive by irrelevant input are a risk factor for suicidal behavior. The present study will record ERPs during the presentation of a multifeature optimal paradigm to determine whether adolescents with suicidal behavior are more likely to show a P3a, reflecting attention capture processing.

MATERIALS AND METHODS

Participants

The study participants were 12 (10 females) adolescent psychiatric in-patients admitted for acute risk of suicide and 12 (10 females) age and gender matched healthy controls. Adolescents ranged in age from 13 to 17 years (mean = 14.9; SD = 1.2). Patients were recruited after coming to the Emergency Unit and then being admitted to the inpatient psychiatric unit at the Children's Hospital of Eastern Ontario. None of participants had any reported a history of hearing or neurological disorders. Written informed consent was obtained from all participants, and parents when necessary, prior to the start of the study. Participants received an honorarium for their participation. The study was approved by both the University of Ottawa's Health Sciences and Science Research Ethics Board and the Children's Hospital of Eastern Ontario's Research Ethics Board. The study was conducted according to the Canadian Tri-Council guidelines (Medical, Natural, and Social Sciences) on ethical conduct involving human subjects. These guidelines are similar to those used conducted with the Declaration of Helsinki.

Medications

A requirement was that potential in-patient participants were not being treated using benzodiazepines prior to the start of the study. All patients were treated with medication, including antidepressants [selective serotonin reuptake inhibitors (SSRIs) and selective serotonin and norepinephrine reuptake inhibitors] and/or atypical antipsychotics. Three patients reported sleep disturbances and were treated using melatonin. Studies have shown that the MMN is not significantly modulated by antidepressant (74, 75) or atypical antipsychotic (74, 76–80) medications. Very few studies have directly examined the effects of these medications on the amplitude of the P3a. Rydkjaer et al. (74) found no significant differences in the amplitude of the MMN and P3a among those with and without SSRI antidepressant use and also among those with and without antipsychotic use.

Psychological Assessment

The severity of depression symptoms was assessed using the Children's Depression Inventory-2 [CDI-2; (81)], a commonly used self-report rating inventory that includes 27 items. The 27 items are grouped into two major factor, each comprised of two subscales assessing emotional problems (including negative mood/physical symptoms and negative self-esteem) and functional problems (including ineffectiveness and interpersonal problems). Patients had a mean CDI-2 total score of 24.88 (SD = 9.49). Controls had a mean CDI-2 total score of 4.1 (SD = 2.93). The presence and severity of suicidal symptoms were assessed using the Suicidal Behaviors Questionnaire-Revised [SBQ-R; (82)], a brief 4-item, self-report questionnaire measuring different dimensions of suicidality: (1) lifetime suicide ideation and suicide attempt, (2) frequency of suicide ideation over the past 12 months, (3) threat of suicidal behavior, and (4) the likelihood of suicidal behavior. Patients had a mean SBQ-R score of 13.75 (SD = 2.37). Controls had a mean score of 3.5 (SD = 0.71). The CDI-2 and SBQ-R scores did significantly differ between patients and controls ($p < 0.05$ in both cases).

Neurophysiological Recording

EEG and electrooculography (EOG) activity were recorded using Grass gold-cup electrodes, filled with electrolytic paste, and affixed to the skin by surgical tape and to the scalp by gauze. Brain Products BrainAmp amplifiers and Recorder software were used for the recording of the physiological signals. The EEG was recorded from 11 electrodes across frontal, central, parietal, and occipital sites (F3, Fz, F4, C3, Cz, C4, P3, Pz, P4, O1, O2) according to the 10/20 system of electrode placement. Two additional electrodes were placed on the left and right mastoids (M1 and M2). Vertical EOG was recorded from electrodes placed at the supra-orbital and infra-orbital ridges of the left eye. A horizontal EOG was recorded from electrodes placed at the outer canthus of each eye. The nose served as a reference for all channels, including the EOG channels. Inter-electrode impedances were kept below 5 kΩ. The high-frequency filter was set at 75 Hz and the time constant was set at 2 s. The physiological data were digitized continuously at a 500 Hz sampling rate and stored on hard disk for later analyses.

Procedure and Stimuli

Auditory stimuli were presented monaurally to the right ear using EAR 3A insert earphones while participants watched a silent, subtitled movie of their choice. The auditory stimuli were thus irrelevant and participants were asked to ignore them. A multifeature auditory optimal paradigm was presented. This permitted the presentation of six different deviant stimuli within a singe sequence. The participants was presented with a sequence constructed such that every other stimulus was a 80 dB SPL 1,000 Hz "standard" pure tone ($p = 0.5$) and every other was one of six deviants (each with a $p = 0.08$). Deviants in the optimal sequence included (a) a 90 dB SPL increment pure tone, (b) a 60 dB SPL decrement pure tone, (c) an 80 dB peak SPL white noise burst, (d) different environmental sounds (with an average intensity of 80 dB SPL), (e) a higher frequency, 1,100 Hz, pure tone, and (f) a shorter duration, 100 ms, pure tone. All stimuli had a duration of 200 ms and a rise-and-fall time of 5 ms, with the exception of the duration deviant. **Table 1** lists the properties of the various auditory stimuli. The deviants were pseudorandomized so that in an array of six deviants, each deviant was presented once and the same deviant was never presented twice in a row. Thus, while every other stimulus was a deviant, the participants could not predict which specific deviant would be presented. A different environmental sound was presented on each trial so that none of the environmental sounds were repeated. The environmental sounds were downloaded from the New York Psychiatric Institute [described in Ref. (83)]. Their duration was however manipulated to be the same 200 ms as the other stimuli. The environmental sounds consisted of six different categories of stimuli including, animal sounds (e.g., dog, cat, frog), bird sounds, human-produced sounds (e.g., laughter, coughing, sneezing, hiccup), musical instruments (e.g., piano, violin, guitar), sounds within daily environments (e.g., water dripping, drilling, car, video games), and mechanically produced sounds. The first 10 tones in the sequence consisted of only standards in order to establish a memory trace for the standard stimulus. The stimulus onset asynchrony (onset-to-onset) was 600 ms. A total of 932 stimuli were presented in a single sequence, consisting of 472 trials of standards and 77 trials of each deviant. A sequence thus lasted about 9.5 min. Two blocks of auditory stimuli were presented to both patients and controls. A brief 5-min rest period was given between blocks.

TABLE 1 | The intensity, frequency, duration, and probability of the standard stimulus and the six deviant stimuli in the optimal paradigm.

Stimulus type	Intensity	Frequency	Duration	Probability
Standard	80 dB SPL	1,000 Hz	200 ms	0.50
Deviants				
Frequency	80 dB SPL	*1,100 Hz*	200 ms	0.08
Increment	*90 dB SPL*	1,000 Hz	200 ms	0.08
Decrement	*60 dB SPL*	1,000 Hz	200 ms	0.08
Duration	80 dB SPL	1,000 Hz	*100 ms*	0.08
White noise	*~80 dB SPL*	*Random*	200 ms	0.08
Environmental sounds	*~80 dB SPL*	*Mixed*	200 ms	0.08

Information in italics represents the feature of the deviant that has been changed.

ERP Analysis

The data were reconstructed using Brain Products' Analyzer2 software. The continuous EEG data was band-pass filtered between 0.5 and 20 Hz (24 dB/octave slope). A vertical EOG channel was computed by subtracting activity recorded at supraorbital and infraorbital ridges of the left eye. A horizontal EOG channel was computed by subtracting activity recorded at the outer canthus of each eye. Independent Component Analysis (84, 85) was used to identify eye movement and blink artifacts that were statistically independent of the EEG activity. These were then partialed out from the EEG trace. The continuous data were subsequently reconstructed into discrete single trial 700 ms segments, beginning 100 ms before stimulus onset and then baseline corrected. The prestimulus period for the environmental sound deviants was not stable and varied between the two groups therefore a −50 to 50 ms parastimulus baseline was applied. Segments in which EEG activity exceeded ±100 μV relative to the baseline were excluded from further analyses. No more than 5% of total trials were rejected from further analyses per participant. There was no variation in the rejection of trials across deviants. The single trials were then sorted and averaged on the basis of stimulus type (standard and six deviants) and electrode site.

Quantification and Statistical Analyses

The ERP waveform time-locked to the deviant stimuli elicited a series of positive- and negative-going components that were not apparent in the waveform following the standard stimulus. These components are best observed in a difference wave computed by subtracting, point-by-point, the standard from the deviant waveforms at each electrode site. This process removes the commonalities in processing between the standard and the deviant, leaving only processing unique to the deviant. The subtraction process is illustrated in **Figure 1**. From this difference wave, the DRN and P3a were initially identified using the grand averaged data (the average of all subjects' averages) separately for patients and controls. The DRN and P3a were measured with respect to the prestimulus zero voltage baseline. They were quantified for each individual participant using the mean of all the data points that were within ±25 ms of the peak in amplitude that was identified in the grand average.

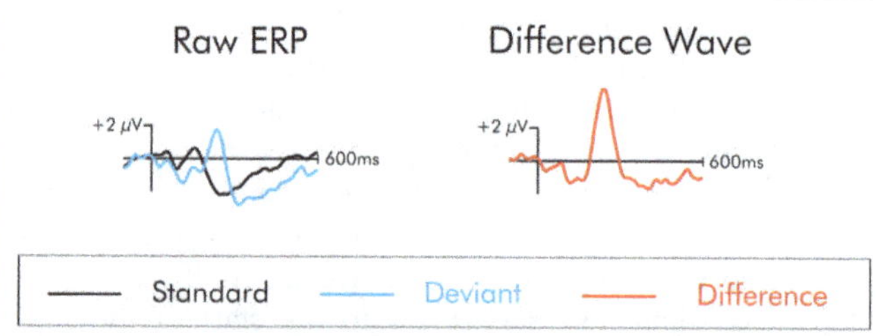

FIGURE 1 | The "raw" event-related potentials (ERPs) following the presentation of the standard and deviant are traced on the left. The difference wave on the right is constructed by subtracting the raw standard from the deviant waveforms. The subtraction process removes the commonalities in processing between the standard and the deviant leaving only processing unique to the deviant. In the difference wave, a small negativity is apparent at about 100 ms. This is the mismatch negativity/deviant-related negativity. This deviant also elicits a large positivity at about 225 ms. This is the P3a.

Previous studies have indicated that not all deviants will elicit a P3a. The statistical analysis of absent ERP components with the usual analyses of variance (ANOVA) procedure is problematic. This is because the observation of a significant amplitude difference with, for example, the P3a between participant groups cannot be used as evidence that a specific deviant did in fact elicit this component for a given group. It must be first demonstrated that the deviants elicited significant ERP components. Thus, confidence intervals were computed for the P3a. When the lower limit of the interval was significantly greater than 0 μV (i.e., in a positive direction), it was considered to be a significant positivity. The procedure was run at Cz where the P3a tends to be at maximum amplitude. Because a positive directionality was predicted, one-tailed tests of significance ($p < 0.05$) were applied to the confidence intervals. To restrict the likelihood of chance findings, the positivity had to conform to the usual latency (180–350 ms) and scalp distribution (centrofrontal maximum) of the P3a.

Electrode sites were grouped into regions of interest (ROIs), to include nine electrode sites where the ERP components have been quantified in previous studies. The ROIs allowed for an analysis of an anterior–posterior and an interhemisphere factor. Specifically for the anterior–posterior electrode factor, three electrodes for frontal (F3, Fz, F4), central (C3, Cz, C4), and parietal (P3, Pz, P4) sites were chosen for separate analysis. The DRN and P3a components were thus quantified at each of these sites within the latency range identified at Fz, and Cz, where their amplitude is largest. For the interhemisphere factor, three electrodes for left (e.g., F3), midline (e.g., Fz), and right (e.g., F4) sites were chosen for analysis.

The between-group differences in the amplitudes of the ERP components were tested using ANOVA. Specific details about the exact nature of each statistical analysis are reported in the "Results" section. Separate ANOVAs were conducted for the DRN and P3a. Significant main effects and interactions were followed up with least significant difference *post hoc* testing. For all statistical analyses, a Geisser-Greenhouse correction was used when appropriate (86).

RESULTS

Standard ERP

The DRN and P3a waveforms were calculated in the deviant-standard difference wave. As a result, an assumption is made that processing of the standard is similar for both groups and thus, whatever differences emerged were a result of differential processing of the deviant. The ERP waveform to the standard stimulus for both patients and controls in presented in **Figure 2**. This assumption was tested. The N1 and N2 were measured at Cz in the standard waveform as the mean of all data points within ±25 ms of the peak identified in the grand average. A *t*-test was run separately on the amplitude of the N1occurring at about 100 ms and P2 occurring t about 180 ms, between patients and controls. There was no significant difference in the amplitude of the N1 ($t < 1$) or P2, $t(22) = 1.88$, $p > 0.05$ between the two groups. An additional negativity at about 220 ms was also observed in the ERPs following the standard stimulus. There was no significant difference in the amplitude of this negativity between patients and controls ($t < 1$).

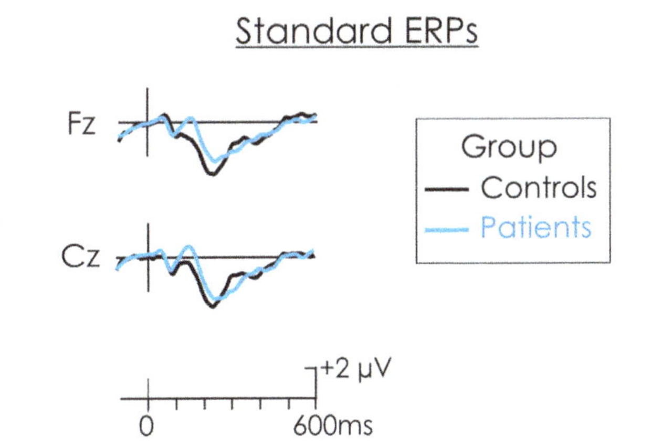

FIGURE 2 | The event-related potential (ERP) waveform to the standard stimulus for both patients (blue) and controls (black). There were no significant differences in the amplitude of the N1 or P2 between patients and controls.

Deviant-Related Negativity

A negativity, peaking at about 150 ms, was observed in the difference waveforms (**Figure 3**). In some cases, this probably reflected a larger N1 component to the deviant than to the standard. In cases in which the intensity of the deviant increased relative to the standard (i.e., increment, white noise, environmental sounds) this negativity probably reflected a composite N1 and MMN (i.e., the DRN). In the cases of the frequency, duration, and decrement deviants, the negativity probably reflects a true MMN, although for consistency will be labeled as a DRN. It was largest over frontocentral areas of the scalp and inverted in polarity at the mastoids.

A region of interest (ROI) analysis was applied to the DRN. Thus, a separate ANOVA was run on a frontal electrode (F3, Fz, F4) cluster and also on a central electrode (C3, Cz, C4) cluster where the DRN is largest. A three-way ANOVA with one between factor, group (patients vs. controls), and two within factors, deviant type (frequency, duration, decrement, increment, white noise, environmental sounds), and laterality (left, midline, right) was run. There was no significant difference in the amplitude of the DRN between patient and control groups at either the frontal or central ROIs ($F < 1$ in both cases). Similarly, there were no overall differences in the amplitude of the DRN across the deviants at frontal and central sites ($F < 1$ in both cases). The group × deviant interaction was significant for the frontal ROIs, $F(5, 110) = 2.62$, MSE = 5.22, $p < 0.05$, $\eta_p^2 = 0.11$. This was due to a larger DRN to the decrement deviant in patients compared to controls. The DRN did not differ as a function of hemisphere and interactions involving electrode site were not significant ($F < 1$ in all cases).

P3a

Not all of the deviants elicited a significant P3a. In the difference waves, a large amplitude centrofrontal maximum P3a, was observed following the white noise and environmental sound deviants, peaking at about 225 and 240 ms, respectively, for both patients and controls. For the controls, confidence interval testing

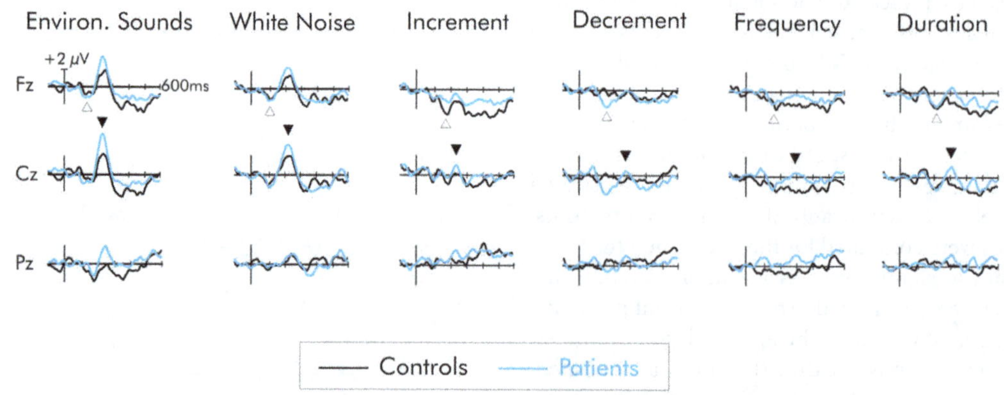

FIGURE 3 | Difference waves for the six deviant stimuli for patients (blue) and controls (black). The deviant-related negativity (DRN) is indicated by an open upward arrow and the P3a by a closed downward arrow. All deviants elicited a DRN but in general, its amplitude did not differ between groups. Only the environmental sounds and white noise elicited a large P3a. The P3a for these deviants was larger in amplitude for the patient group. The deviants representing a smaller extent of change did not elicit a P3a in the control group. A small P3a was however elicited in the patients but its amplitude did not significantly differ from that of the controls.

TABLE 2 | Mean amplitudes (SD in parentheses) at the Cz electrode site for the difference waves at the time interval of the P3a.

	Environmental sounds	White noise	Increment	Decrement	Frequency	Duration
Controls	1.54 (1.51)	1.82 (2.20)	−0.45 (3.22)	−0.55 (1.59)	−1.34 (2.45)	−0.35 (2.53)
Patients	4.04 (2.26)	3.32 (2.91)	0.02 (1.49)	0.07 (1.88)	0.18 (1.14)	0.88 (1.56)

revealed that the P3a elicited by white noise and environmental sound deviants was significantly different from the zero amplitude baseline ($p < 0.01$ in both cases). All other deviants failed to reach significance. Similarly for the patients, only the white noise and the environmental sounds elicited a significant P3a ($p < 0.001$, in both cases). All other deviants failed to reach significance. The mean amplitudes of the P3a for both groups and all deviants are presented in **Table 2**.

An initial analysis of the data for all deviants was run at Cz where the P3a was largest. A two-way omnibus ANOVA with one between factor (groups) and one within factor (six deviants) was computed. As is apparent in **Figure 3**, the overall main effect of deviant was significant, $F(5, 110) = 16.02$, MSE = 3.43, $p < 0.0001$, $\eta_p^2 = 0.42$. Significant group differences were also found, $F(1, 22) = 5.76$, MSE = 10.72, $p < 0.05$, $\eta_p^2 = 0.21$. Overall, the P3a was significantly larger for the patients than the controls. The group x deviant interaction was not significant ($F < 1$).

A large P3a was only elicited by the white noise and environmental sound deviants. For this reason, a more extensive ROI analysis was carried out separately for these deviants. While the P3a tends to be largest over central regions of the scalp, its amplitude is also large at both anterior and posterior sites. Analyses were therefore run separately at frontal (F3, Fz, F4), central (C3, Cz, C4), and parietal (P3, Pz, P4) clusters. A two-way ANOVA consisting of a between factor (group), and a within factor (laterality: left, midline, right) was separately run at each cluster.

The P3a following presentation of the white noise deviant is presented in **Figure 4**. While the amplitude of the P3a was larger in the patients than the controls, the difference was not significant at frontal, $F(1, 22) = 1.84$, MSE = 14.06, $p > 0.05$, $\eta_p^2 = 0.07$,

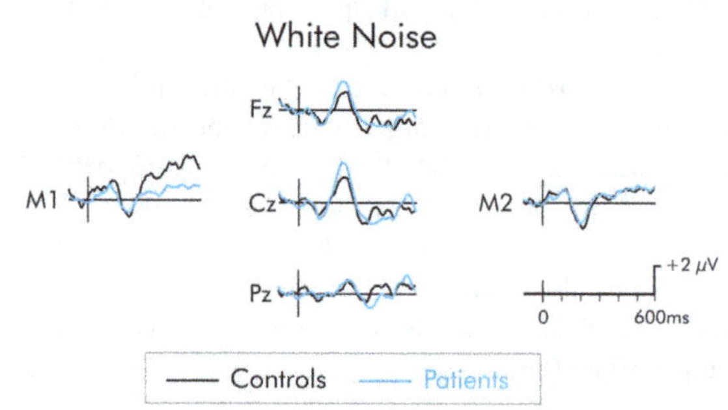

FIGURE 4 | P3a following presentation of the white noise for patients (blue) and controls (black). Although, the P3a was larger in the patient group, the between group difference was not significant.

central, $F(1, 22) = 1.94$, MSE = 16, $p > 0.05$, $\eta_p^2 = 0.08$, or parietal $F(1, 22) = 0.88$, MSE = 11.46, $p > 0.05$, $\eta_p^2 = 0.03$, ROIs. The P3a did not differ as a function of hemisphere and interactions involving electrode site were not significant ($F < 1$ in all cases).

The P3a following presentation of the environmental sound deviants is presented in **Figure 5**. The P3a was significantly larger in the patient group across frontal, $F(1, 22) = 8.14$, MSE = 7.51, $p < 0.01$, $\eta_p^2 = 0.27$, central, $F(1, 22) = 11.32$, MSE = 10.19, $p < 0.01$, $\eta_p^2 = 0.34$, and parietal, $F(1, 22) = 6.29$, MSE = 17.36, $p < 0.05$, $\eta_p^2 = 0.22$, ROIs. The P3a did not differ as a function of hemisphere and interactions involving electrode site were not significant ($F < 1$ in all cases).

The omnibus ANOVA showed the P3a was significantly larger for patients for all deviants. As is apparent in **Figure 2**, only a small

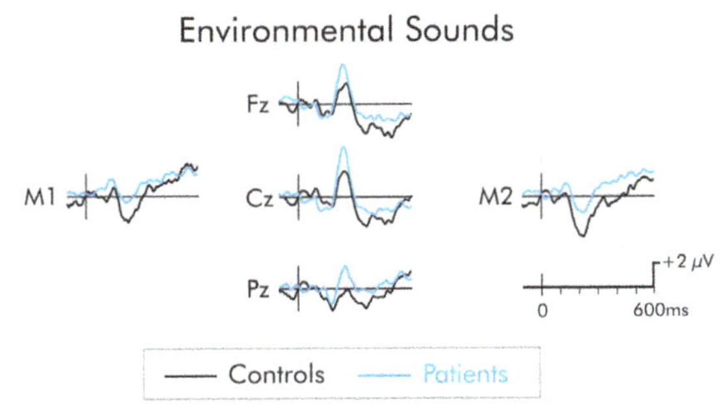

FIGURE 5 | P3a following presentation of the environmental sounds for patients (blue) and controls (black). The P3a was significantly larger in patients compared to controls. The prestimulus period for the environmental sounds was not stable and varied between the two groups. As a result, a −50 to 50 ms parastimulus baseline was used.

amplitude P3a was elicited for the patients following presentation of the frequency, duration, decrement, and increment deviants. A P3a was, however, absent for the controls for these deviants. A separate group × deviant ANOVA was run only for these deviants. To maximize likelihood of finding group differences, the ANOVA was run only at Cz where the P3a was largest. The amplitude of the P3a did not significantly vary as a result of type of deviant, $F(3, 66) = 1.00$, MSE = 2.87, $p > 0.05$, $\eta_p^2 = 0.05$. Importantly, while the amplitude of the small P3a was largest for the patient group, the difference compared to the control group was not significant, $F(1, 22) = 2.51$, MSE = 8.90, $p < 0.12$, $\eta_p^2 = 0.10$.

Correlations were also conducted on the individual participants' P3a amplitudes for the white noise and environmental sound deviants, and the scores on the CDI-2 and SBQ-R. Initially, these correlations were computed on all participants (patients and controls). These correlations were computed at the Cz electrode site where the P3a was largest. Correlations involving the white noise P3a were very small ($r = -0.08$ with the CDI-2 and $r = -0.06$ with the SBQ-R) and not significant. For the environmental sound P3a, the correlations were $r = 0.48$ with the CDI-2 and $r = 0.41$ for the SBQ-R, $p < 0.05$ and $p < 0.09$, respectively. Correlations with the CDI-2 subscales were also computed. The negative self-esteem, functional problems, ineffectiveness, and interpersonal problems subscales were significantly correlated with the environmental sound-P3a ($r = 0.49$, $r = 0.57$, $r = 0.46$, and $r = 0.64$, respectively). When only the patients were considered, the correlations between the amplitude of the P3a and CDI-2 and SBQ-R were much lower. The correlations between the environmental sound P3a and the overall CDI-2 and the SBQ-R were $r = 0.05$ and $r = -0.54$, respectively, and were not significant. Similarly, the correlations between the white noise P3a and each of the six subscales of the CDI-2 were also small and not significant ($p > 0.05$ in all cases).

DISCUSSION

A recent report by the American Centers for Disease Control and Prevention (87) has indicated that the rates for suicide have not decreased over the past several decades. This is in spite of considerably increasing mental health treatment efforts. Clearly, additional research is required to understand the factors that contribute to an increased risk of suicidal behavior.

One of these factors appears to be a dysfunction of the frontal executive functions. The present study is one of a few that have investigated an adolescent sample. This has important implications. Most previous studies have examined executive functions in adult populations. The causes and behavior associated with adolescent and adult suicide behavior may be very different. Moreover, the present study was carried out in adolescent inpatients, only days after being admitted to a local children's hospital because of an acute risk of suicide. Most previous studies have examined non-acute suicidal ideation or those with a history of previous suicide attempts. Very few studies have studied acute suicide risk with an in-patient population. It should also be noted that several features might distinguish individuals with suicidal behavior from those who only think about suicide [e.g., suicidal ideation; (88), see also, Ref. (89)]. In their review, Bredemeier and Miller (20) indicate that a majority of studies have identified executive function deficits as a risk of suicidality, especially when associated with mood disorders. The authors emphasize individual differences. Those who have actually attempted suicide appear to show the largest executive function disorders. It is not known whether these would also differ with those manifesting an acute at risk of suicide. It is quite possible that the executive function disorders would be even larger.

Many studies have identified poorer scores in suicidal groups on a number of cognitive tasks and traditional neuropsychological tests. These however require active participation and cooperation of the individual for relatively long periods to achieve successful performance. An inability to control attention has been identified as a marker of suicide behavior (29, 32). The present study thus examined executive processes involved in the capturing of attention by a rarely occurring and potentially highly relevant but unattended stimulus input. These processes are assumed to be involuntary and operate passively, and therefore do not require active attention The frontal lobe's central executive must make a decision regarding whether current cognitive demands or the potentially more relevant, intruding input has priority. If the rare stimulus event is given priority, then attention is switched to its processing and performance on cognitive tasks-at hand will deteriorate. There is evidence that suicidal behavior is associated with an inability to inhibit irrelevant processing. For example, individuals with previous suicide attempts have performed worse on the Stroop task, thought to reflect the ability to inhibit a dominant but inappropriate response, compared to individuals with suicidal ideation (90).

In the present study, participants were asked to watch a silent, subtitled video while ignoring the auditory stimuli. Several ERP studies have now indicated that the nature of the "diversion" task (watching the video in this case) is, in fact, relatively incidental. What the participant "is doing" should not affect the processing of the unattended auditory stimuli. These auditory stimuli consisted of a frequently occurring standard stimulus and six different rarely occurring deviant stimuli. The deviant stimuli varied in the extent to which they represented change from the standard. A series of well-studied ERP components were elicited by the deviant stimuli.

Deviant-Related Negativity

As expected, all deviant stimuli elicited a frontocentral maximum DRN, peaking from 100 to 150 ms after stimulus onset. The amplitude of the DRN to all but the decrement deviants did not significantly differ between adolescents with suicidal behavior and healthy controls. The amplitude of the DRN was significantly larger for this decrement deviant for the patient group. It is difficult to explain why the processing of only the decrement deviant would differ. It is possible that this is a chance finding, given the large number of comparisons that were made. The decrement deviant does represent a decrease in intensity of the standard and it would be difficult to perceive. Given the fact that the patient group did display a larger P3a amplitude to all deviants, it is possible that they were able to perceive the decrease in intensity better than the controls. The general failure to find a DRN difference between the groups suggests that the automatic auditory deviance detection is well preserved in adolescents with suicidal behavior. Thus, whatever group differences were found in the amplitude of the P3a cannot be attributed to the initial detection of change. Only a limited number of studies have examined the effects of suicidality on the MMN. These studies have only used a single deviant and have focused on adult populations (91, 92). Both Zaifu et al. (91) and Zhen et al. (92) observed decreased amplitudes of the MMN in depressed adults with suicidal behavior. Studies looking at the MMN in adults with presumably only depression, also have reported a diminished MMN amplitude (93–96). The differences between these and the present study may be because of the use of different paradigms. The present study employed an optimal sequence while the others employed an oddball sequence. This is an unlikely explanation, however. Studies of the MMN have failed to find differences when it is elicited in oddball compared to optimal sequences (72, 73, 97). Importantly task demands also differed between the present study and those studying depressed adults. In the present study, the auditory MMN was elicited passively while participants watched a video. In the adult studies, participants were asked to actively attend to the auditory sequence and detect the change in the auditory stimulus. Several studies have indicated that suicidal behavioral and depression are associated with an inability to sustain attention. Differences between healthy controls and the patient group might thus be explained by this inability to sustain attention. Attention to the auditory sequence will cause other auditory ERPs to be elicited that are not observed when the auditory sequence is ignored. These attention-related ERPs may overlap and summate with the MMN. It is these attention-related ERPs rather than the MMN that might differentiate the groups. Also, processing in adult and adolescent groups may well differ. Lepistö et al. (71) studied depressed children and similar to our results, found no difference in the MMN amplitude compared to controls.

P3a

The amplitude of the P3a was crucial to the understanding of which unattended deviant stimuli are extensively processed and interrupt executive functions maintaining attention to the task-at-hand. There is some evidence that suicidal behavior is associated with an inability to inhibit the processing of irrelevant input. In healthy young adults, a number of studies have indicated that when a pure tone is used as a standard stimulus, white noise and environmental sounds acting as deviants will be especially likely to elicit a P3a (48, 73, 98–100). So powerful are the effects of these particular deviants that they continue to elicit a P3a during the sleep onset period where conscious awareness of the external environment is gradually diminished (101). The environmental sounds even elicit a P3a during definitive stage N2 sleep (101). On the other hand, the frequency, duration, decrement, and increment deviants do not elicit a P3a in young adults during the waking state suggesting these are determined to be less relevant and thus less likely to interrupt current cognitive priorities. These results were essentially replicated in the healthy adolescent controls. A large and significant P3a was also elicited by the white noise and environmental sound deviants. No P3a was apparent to the other deviants.

To our knowledge, this is the first study to examine the P3a in suicidal adolescents. The manner in which those with an acute risk of suicide processed the different deviants was generally similar to that of the healthy controls. Thus, a large and significant P3a was observed following presentation of the white noise and environmental sound deviants. Jandl et al. (69) recorded the P3a to environmental sound deviants in depressed adults with a lifetime history of suicidal behavior. They attempted to determine whether this P3a would become attenuated over the course their study. They did not however directly present P3a amplitude differences between healthy controls and those with a history of suicidal behavior, but their **Figure 2** indicates a slight enhancement of the P3a in the suicidal group. The principle finding of the present study was that the amplitude of the P3a was also enhanced in the suicidal group. When an overall ANOVA was applied to the P3a for all deviant data, a "main effect" of group was found. Thus, the P3a for all deviants was larger for those with an acute risk of suicide compared to healthy controls. The P3a was calculated in a deviant-standard difference wave. The significant differences might therefore be a result of differential processing of either the deviant or the standard. In actual fact, ERPs to the standard stimulus were not significantly different between the two groups. Thus, the enhanced P3a in the suicidal group appears to be largely due to unusual "hyper-responsivity" to the deviant. This result does need to be interpreted with caution. Even though the group x deviant interaction was not significant, follow-up testing was nevertheless deemed to be warranted. It indicated that the group P3a difference was significant for only one deviant. The P3a following presentation of the environmental sound deviant was significantly larger for the group with acute risk of suicide. The P3a to the white noise deviant did appear larger for the suicidal adolescents; however, its amplitude was not significantly different from that of controls. An intriguing finding was that a small amplitude P3a was elicited in those at risk of suicide for the frequency, duration, increment and decrement deviants while in healthy controls, a P3a to the same deviants was absent. When an ANOVA was run only on these deviants, a tendency for a larger P3a in the suicide group was apparent, although the difference again did not reach significance.

These results do therefore provide strong support for the notion that suicidal behavior is associated with deficits in attentional control and more specifically in an inability to inhibit processing of what might be irrelevant stimulus input (28). An important executive function is to determine which of the many stimulus inputs is potentially so critical to warrant an interruption of ongoing cognitive demands. A threshold set too high will result in a failure to detect truly highly relevant events, possibly critical for survival. On the other hand, a threshold set too low will result in recurrent interruption of executive functions by what turns out to be irrelevant events, resulting in frequent distraction. The later appears to be the processing option observed with suicidal behavior. Such interruptions might also explain the reported inability to maintain and sustain attention in this group. The P3a also appears to provide a measure of maturity of the frontal lobes executive function. Mahajan and McArthur (64) and Oades et al. (65) have indicated it is larger in younger than older adolescents. The finding of an enhanced P3a in the adolescents with acute risk of suicide might thus be a reflection of immature frontal executive functions. It is also tempting to generalize beyond the present findings. Suicidality has also been associated with difficulty in inhibiting negative thoughts about oneself and a tendency for mind wandering and rumination (102). In the case of the group we studied, adolescents with an acute risk of suicide, the immature frontal central executive may also have difficulty in inhibiting the urge to act on suicidal thoughts, thus the need to urgently seek help.

Limitations

There are some limitations in the present study. The sample size is relatively small (although comparable to other ERP studies). This small sample size did not allow for a study of individual differences of other factors known to be associated with suicidality. Depression is correlated with suicidal thoughts and behavior and indeed scores on our depression index were much higher for the group at risk of suicide compared to healthy controls. Lepistö et al. (71) also reported an enhanced P3a to environmental sounds in depressed children compared to healthy controls. In our study, when the extent of depression was measured in both patients and healthy controls, a significant positive correlation was also found between this index of depression and the amplitude of the P3a to environmental sound deviants. It is therefore possible that the group differences we observed in the P3a amplitude may reflect effects of depression rather than suicidality. Keilp et al. (28, 32) noted larger impairments in executive functioning related to attention and memory in patients with high-lethality suicide attempters beyond that typically found in major depression. In the present study, when only the patients were considered, the correlation between the amplitude of P3a and depression was much lower. The extent of depression within the suicide group was thus a poor predictor of P3a amplitude and presumably its reflection of executive control of where attention is directed.

The types and dosages of various medications might also account for some of the group differences. Ideally, a non-medicated sample should also be studied. This may not be ethically or morally justifiable in those seeking emergency intervention for acute risk of suicide and deemed to require pharmaceutical treatment. Still, the types of medication used in treatment are generally considered to dampen rather than heighten the extent of information processing. It therefore seems unlikely that these medications would increase the likelihood of interruption of executive functions.

While the present study did employ an objective neurophysiological measure, the P3a, as an index of the interruption of ongoing cognitive tasks and switching of attention, it is important to note that an independent measure of this process was not available. This independent evidence of the switch of attention is generally provided by a behavioral measure, a deterioration in performance on the cognitive task in which the participant is actively engaged following presentation of the deviant. In a classic Schröger and Wolff (64) study, participants were presented with a modified oddball task consisting of short and long duration pure tones occurring with equal probability. Participants were asked to press a button corresponding to which tone had been presented. At odd times, the frequency of one of the tones was changed to form a deviant stimulus. This frequency deviation was, however, irrelevant to the primary task of duration detection and was thus to-be-ignored. The frequency deviant did, nevertheless, elicited a large P3a. Following its presentation, a prolongation of reaction times and decrease in accuracy on the duration detection task was observed. The processing of the deviant stimulus did indeed result in a switch of attention from the duration detection task resulting in the deterioration in performance. Such an active task could be modified for use with younger participants. Still, it would require the participant to remain vigilant and sustain attention for a relatively long period of time to this very difficult task. Again, attentional control appears to be highly problematic in such clinical groups.

CONCLUSION

There was little evidence of a deficit in processes related to the automatic detection of acoustic change in adolescents with an acute risk of suicide. The amplitude of the DRN following presentation of the different deviants did not differ between patients and controls. Some of the deviants, particularly the white noise and the environmental sounds, were expected to interrupt executive functions that maintain attention to an ongoing cognitive task. A later positivity, the P3a, is thought to reflect processes associated with this interruption. These deviants did in fact elicit a large P3a in both groups. However, an enhanced P3a was evident in the patient group, particularly for the environmental sound deviants. For the control group, a P3a was absent following presentation of the frequency, duration, decrement, and increment deviants. These deviants did however elicit a small P3a in the group at acute risk of suicide, although the differences were not statistically significant. These findings suggest that the threshold for triggering the involuntary switch of attention might be lower in these patients and may explain their reported enhanced distractibility. This is likely to cause difficulties in concentration and may cause deterioration in academic performance, because of an inability to sustain attention. The group differences in the P3a are suggestive of an immature frontal central executive, and perhaps may provide a promising marker for the identification of those with an increased risk of suicide. This could result in an earlier recognition and, importantly, earlier intervention of suicide in adolescence.

ETHICS STATEMENT

Written informed consent was obtained from all participants, and parents when necessary, prior to the start of the study. Participants received an honorarium for their participation. The study was approved by both the University of Ottawa's Health Sciences and Science Research Ethics Board and the Children's Hospital of Eastern Ontario's Research Ethics Board. The study was conducted according to the Canadian Tri-Council guidelines (Medical, Natural, and Social Sciences) on ethical conduct involving human subjects. These guidelines are similar to those used conducted with the Declaration of Helsinki.

AUTHOR CONTRIBUTIONS

PT, KC, AB, AD, RR, and SG contributed to the rationale and the design of the study, and read and approved the final manuscript. The manuscript was written by PT. AB carried out the psychiatric assessment and evaluation of the patient population. RR, SG, and AB assisted with the selection of the depression and suicidal inventories. PT and AD assisted with the collection and analysis of the EEG data.

ACKNOWLEDGMENTS

Financial support for this research was provided by an operating grant (8242) to KC by the Natural Sciences and Engineering Research Council (NSERC) of Canada and from funds from the Psychiatry Associates at the Children's Hospital of Eastern Ontario and from the Institute of Mental Health Research University of Ottawa. A doctoral scholarship was provided to PT from NSERC and to AD from the Social Sciences and Humanities Research Council (SSHRC) of Canada. Thank you to Joseph De Koninck for his consultations throughout the process of this study. Ashley Nixon and Alexandre Lafrenière assisted with the collection of the data.

REFERENCES

1. World Health Organization. *Preventing Suicide: A Global Imperative.* World Health Organization (2014).
2. Qin P, Nordentoft M. Suicide risk in relation to psychiatric hospitalization: evidence based on longitudinal registers. *Arch Gen Psychiatry* (2005) 62:427–32. doi:10.1001/archpsyc.62.4.427
3. McManama O'Brien KH, Becker SJ, Spirito A, Simon V, Prinstein MJ. Differentiating adolescent suicide attempters from ideators: examining the interaction between depression severity and alcohol use. *Suicide Life Threat Behav* (2014) 44:23–33. doi:10.1111/sltb.12050
4. Taliaferro LA, Muehlenkamp JJ. Risk and protective factors that distinguish adolescents who attempt suicide from those who only consider suicide in the past year. *Suicide Life Threat Behav* (2014) 44:6–22. doi:10.1111/sltb.12046
5. American Psychiatric Association. *Diagnostic and Statistical Manual of Mental Disorders.* 4th ed. Washington, DC: American Psychiatric Association (1994).
6. Burke TA, Connolly SL, Hamilton JL, Stange JP, Abramson LY, Alloy LB. Cognitive risk and protective factors for suicidal ideation: a two year longitudinal study in adolescence. *J Abnorm Child Psychol* (2016) 44:1145–60. doi:10.1007/s10802-015-0104-x
7. Polanco-Roman L, Jurska J, Quiñones V, Miranda R. Brooding, reflection, and distraction: relation to non-suicidal self-injury versus suicide attempts. *Arch Suicide Res* (2015) 19:350–65. doi:10.1080/13811118.2014.981623
8. Drevets WC. Neuroimaging and neuropathological studies of depression: implications for the cognitive-emotional features of mood disorders. *Curr Opin Neurobiol* (2001) 11:240–9. doi:10.1016/S0959-4388(00)00203-8
9. Leppänen JM. Emotional information processing in mood disorders: a review of behavioral and neuroimaging findings. *Curr Opin Psychiatry* (2006) 19:34–9. doi:10.1097/01.yco.0000191500.46411.00
10. Gratz KL. Risk factors for deliberate self-harm among female college students: the role and interaction of childhood maltreatment, emotional inexpressivity, and affect intensity/reactivity. *Am J Orthopsychiatry* (2006) 76:238. doi:10.1037/0002-9432.76.2.238
11. Nock MK, Wedig MM, Holmberg EB, Hooley JM. The emotion reactivity scale: development, evaluation, and relation to self-injurious thoughts and behaviors. *Behav Ther* (2008) 39:107–16. doi:10.1016/j.beth.2007.05.005
12. Ding Y, Lawrence N, Olie E, Cyprien F, le Bars E, Bonafe A, et al. Prefrontal cortex markers of suicidal vulnerability in mood disorders: a model-based structural neuroimaging study with a translational perspective. *Transl Psychiatry* (2015) 5:e516. doi:10.1038/tp.2015.1
13. Oquendo MA, Placidi GP, Malone KM, Campbell C, Keilp J, Brodsky B, et al. Positron emission tomography of regional brain metabolic responses to a serotonergic challenge and lethality of suicide attempts in major depression. *Arch Gen Psychiatry* (2003) 60:14–22. doi:10.1001/archpsyc.60.1.14
14. Reisch T, Seifritz E, Esposito F, Wiest R, Valach L, Michel K. An fMRI study on mental pain and suicidal behavior. *J Affect Disord* (2010) 126:321–5. doi:10.1016/j.jad.2010.03.005
15. Willeumier K, Taylor DV, Amen DG. Decreased cerebral blood flow in the limbic and prefrontal cortex using SPECT imaging in a cohort of completed suicides. *Transl Psychiatry* (2011) 1:e28. doi:10.1038/tp.2011.28
16. Wagner G, Schultz CC, Koch K, Schachtzabel C, Sauer H, Schlosser RG. Prefrontal cortical thickness in depressed patients with high-risk for suicidal behavior. *J Psychiatr Res* (2012) 46:1449–55. doi:10.1016/j.jpsychires.2012.07.013
17. Tsujii N, Mikawa W, Tsujimoto E, Adachi T, Niwa A, Ono H, et al. Reduced left precentral regional responses in patients with major depressive disorder and history of suicide attempts. *PLoS One* (2017) 12:e0175249. doi:10.1371/journal.pone.0175249
18. Van Heeringen C, Bijttebier S, Godfrin K. Suicidal brains: a review of functional and structural brain studies in association with suicidal behaviour. *Neurosci Biobehav Rev* (2010) 35:688. doi:10.1016/j.neubiorev.2010.08.007
19. Marzuk PM, Hartwell N, Leon AC, Portera L. Executive functioning in depressed patients with suicidal ideation. *Acta Psychiatr Scand* (2005) 112:294–301. doi:10.1111/j.1600-0447.2005.00585.x
20. Bredemeier K, Miller IW. Executive function and suicidality: a systematic qualitative review. *Clin Psychol Rev* (2015) 40:170–83. doi:10.1016/j.cpr.2015.06.005
21. Jollant F, Lawrence NL, Olie E, Guillaume S, Courtet P. The suicidal mind and brain: a review of neuropsychological and neuroimaging studies. *World J Biol Psychiatry* (2011) 12:319–39. doi:10.3109/15622975.2011.556200
22. Richard-Devantoy S, Berlim MT, Jollant F. A meta-analysis of neuropsychological markers of vulnerability to suicidal behavior in mood disorders. *Psychol Med* (2014) 44:1663–73. doi:10.1017/S0033291713002304
23. Miyake A, Friedman NP. The nature and organization of individual differences in executive functions: four general conclusions. *Curr Dir Psychol Sci* (2012) 21:8–14. doi:10.1177/0963721411429458
24. Norman DA, Shallice T. Attention to action: willed and automatic control of behaviour. In: Davidson RJ, Schwartz GE, Shapiro D, editors. *Consciousness and Self-Regulation: Advances in Research and Theory.* (Vol. 4), New York: Plenum Press (1986). p. 1–18.
25. Stuss DT, Shallice T, Alexander MP, Picton TW. A multidisciplinary approach to anterior attentional functions. *Ann N Y Acad Sci* (1995) 769:191–212. doi:10.1111/j.1749-6632.1995.tb38140.x
26. Gujral S, Dombrovski AY, Butters M, Clark L, Reynolds CF III, Szanto K. Impaired executive function in contemplated and attempted suicide in late life. *Am J Geriatr Psychiatry* (2014) 22:811–9. doi:10.1016/j.jagp.2013.01.025
27. King DA, Conwell Y, Cox C, Henderson RE, Denning DG, Caine ED. A neuropsychological comparison of depressed suicide attempters and nonattempters. *J Neuropsychiatry Clin Neurosci* (2000) 12:64–70. doi:10.1176/jnp.12.1.64
28. Keilp JG, Sackeim HA, Brodsky BS, Oquendo MA, Malone KA, Mann JJ. Neuropsychological dysfunction in depressed suicide attempters. *Am J Psychiatry* (2001) 158:735–41. doi:10.1176/appi.ajp.158.5.735
29. Keilp JG, Gorlyn M, Oquendo MA, Burke AK, Mann JJ. Attention deficit in depressed suicide attempters. *Psychiatry Res* (2008) 159:7–17. doi:10.1016/j.psychres.2007.08.020

30. Pu S, Setoyama S, Noda T. Association between cognitive deficits and suicidal ideation in patients with major depressive disorder. *Sci Rep* (2017) 7:e11637. doi:10.1038/s41598-017-12142-8
31. Westheide J, Quednow BB, Kuhn K-U, Hoppe C, Cooper-Mahkorn D, Hawellek B, et al. Executive performance of depressed suicide attempters: the role of suicidal ideation. *Eur Arch Psychiatry Clin Neurosci* (2008) 258:414–21. doi:10.1007/s00406-008-0811-1
32. Keilp JG, Gorlyn M, Russell M, Oquendo MA, Burke AK, Harkavy-Friedman J, et al. Neuropsychological function and suicidal behavior: attention control, memory and executive dysfunction in suicide attempt. *Psychol Med* (2013) 43:539–51. doi:10.1017/S0033291712001419
33. James W. *The Principles of Psychology*. New York: Dover (1890).
34. Näätänen R. The role of attention in auditory information processing as revealed by event-related potentials and other brain measures of cognitive function. *Behav Brain Sci* (1990) 13:201–33. doi:10.1017/S0140525X00078407
35. Näätänen R. *Attention and Brain Function*. Hillsdale, NJ: Lawrence Erlbaum (1992).
36. Näätänen R, Kujala T, Winkler I. Auditory processing that leads to conscious perception: a unique window to central auditory processing opened by the mismatch negativity and related responses. *Psychophysiology* (2011) 48:4–22. doi:10.1111/j.1469-8986.2010.01114.x
37. Paavilainen P. The mismatch-negativity (MMN) component of the auditory event-related potential to violations of abstract regularities: a review. *Int J Psychophysiol* (2013) 88:109–23. doi:10.1016/j.ijpsycho.2013.03.015
38. Winkler I. Interpreting the mismatch negativity. *J Psychophysiol* (2007) 21:147–63. doi:10.1027/0269-8803.21.34.147
39. Winkler I, Denham SL, Nelken I. Modeling the auditory scene: predictive regularity representations and perceptual objects. *Trends Cogn Sci* (2009) 13:532–40. doi:10.1016/j.tics.2009.09.003
40. Muller-Gass A, Stelmack RM, Campbell KB. The effect of visual task difficulty and attentional direction on the detection of acoustic change as indexed by the mismatch negativity. *Brain Res* (2006) 1078:112–30. doi:10.1016/j.brainres.2005.12.125
41. Muller-Gass A, Macdonald M, Schröger E, Sculthorpe L, Campbell K. Evidence for the auditory P3a reflecting an automatic process: elicitation during highly-focused continuous visual attention. *Brain Res* (2007) 1170:71–8. doi:10.1016/j.brainres.2007.07.023
42. Sussman ES, Horváth J, Winkler I, Orr M. The role of attention in the formation of auditory streams. *Percept Psychophys* (2007) 69:136–52. doi:10.3758/BF03194460
43. Escera C, Alho K, Winkler I, Näätänen R. Neural mechanisms of involuntary attention to acoustic novelty and change. *J Cogn Neurosci* (1998) 10:590–604. doi:10.1162/089892998562997
44. Parmentier F. The cognitive determinants of behavioral distraction by deviant auditory stimuli: a review. *Psychol Res* (2014) 78:321–38. doi:10.1007/s00426-013-0534-4
45. Wetzel N, Schröger E. On the development of auditory distraction: a review. *Psych J* (2014) 3:72–91. doi:10.1002/pchj.49
46. Horváth J, Winkler I, Bendixen A. Do N1/MMN, P3a, and RON form a strongly coupled chain reflecting the three stages of auditory distraction? *Biol Psychol* (2008) 79:139–47. doi:10.1016/j.biopsycho.2008.04.001
47. Hölig C, Berti S. To switch or not to switch: brain potential indices of attentional control after task-relevant and task-irrelevant changes of stimulus features. *Brain Res* (2010) 1345:164–75. doi:10.1016/j.brainres.2010.05.047
48. Wetzel N, Schröger E, Widmann A. The dissociation between the P3a event-related potential and behavioral distraction. *Psychophysiology* (2013) 50:920–30. doi:10.1111/psyp.12072
49. Berti S, Roeber U, Schröger E. Bottom-up influences on working memory: behavioral and electrophysiological distraction varies with distractor strength. *Exp Psychol* (2004) 51:249–57. doi:10.1027/1618-3169.51.4.249
50. Rinne T, Särkkä A, Degerman A, Schröger E, Alho K. Two separate mechanisms underlie auditory change detection and involuntary control of attention. *Brain Res* (2006) 1077:135–43. doi:10.1016/j.brainres.2006.01.043
51. Schröger E, Wolff C. Attentional orienting and reorienting is indicated by human event-related brain potentials. *Neuroreport* (1998) 9:3355–8. doi:10.1097/00001756-199810260-00003
52. Wetzel N, Widmann A, Berti S, Schröger E. The development of involuntary and voluntary attention from childhood to adulthood: a combined behavioral and event-related potential study. *Neurophysiol Clin* (2006) 117:2191–203. doi:10.1016/j.clinph.2006.06.717
53. Knight RT. Decreased response to novel stimuli after prefrontal lesions in man. *Electroencephalogr Clin Neurophysiol* (1984) 59:9–20. doi:10.1016/0168-5597(84)90016-9
54. Caballero A, Granberg R, Tseng KY. Mechanisms contributing to prefrontal cortex maturation during adolescence. *Neurosci Biobehav Rev* (2016) 70:4–12. doi:10.1016/j.neubiorev.2016.05.013
55. Paus T. Mapping brain maturation and cognitive development during adolescence. *Trends Cogn Sci* (2005) 9:60–8. doi:10.1016/j.tics.2004.12.008
56. Bruder GE, Kayser J, Tenke CE. Event-related brain potentials in depression: clinical, cognitive and neurophysiologic implications. In: Luck SJ, Kappenman ES, editors. *Event-Related Potential Components: The Ups and Downs of Brainwave Recordings*. New, NY: Oxford University Press (2012). p. 563–92.
57. Friedman D, Cycowicz YM, Gaeta H. The novelty P3: an event-related brain potential (ERP) sign of the brain's evaluation of novelty. *Neurosci Biobehav Rev* (2001) 25:355–73. doi:10.1016/S0149-7634(01)00019-7
58. Volpe U, Mucci A, Bucci P, Merlotti E, Galderisi S, Maj M. The cortical generators of P3a and P3b: a LORETA study. *Brain Res Bull* (2007) 73:220–30. doi:10.1016/j.brainresbull.2007.03.003
59. Wetzel N, Berti S, Widmann A, Schröger E. Distraction and reorientation in children: a behavioral and ERP study. *Neuroreport* (2004) 15:1355–8. doi:10.1097/01.wnr.0000129858.40478.be
60. Berman S, Friedman D. The development of selective attention as reflected by event-related brain potentials. *J Exp Child Psychol* (1995) 59:1–31. doi:10.1006/jecp.1995.1001
61. Dempster FN. Resistance to interference: developmental changes in a basic processing mechanism. In: Howe ML, Pasnak R, editors. *Emerging Themes in Cognitive Development*. New York, NY: Springer (1993). p. 3–27.
62. Harnishfeger KK, Bjorklund DF. The ontogeny of inhibition mechanisms: a renewed approach to cognitive development. In: Howe ML, Pasnak R, editors. *Emerging Themes in Cognitive Development*. New York, NY: Springer (1993). p. 28–49.
63. Lane DM, Pearson DA. The development of selective attention. *Merrill Palmer Q* (1982) 28:317–37.
64. Mahajan Y, McArthur G. Maturation of mismatch negativity and P3a response across adolescence. *Neurosci Lett* (2015) 587:102–6. doi:10.1016/j.neulet.2014.12.041
65. Oades RD, Dittmann-Balcar A, Zerbin D, Grzella I. Impaired attention-dependent augmentation of MMN in nonparanoid vs paranoid schizophrenic patients: a comparison with obsessive-compulsive disorder and healthy subjects. *Biol Psychiatry* (1997) 41:1196–210. doi:10.1016/S0006-3223(96)00214-4
66. Bruder GE, Stewart JW, McGrath PJ, Ma GJ, Wexler BE, Quitkin FM. Atypical depression: enhanced right hemispheric dominance for perceiving emotional chimeric faces. *J Abnorm Psychol* (2002) 111:446. doi:10.1037/0021-843X.111.3.446
67. Bruder GE, Kroppmann CJ, Kayser J, Stewart JW, McGrath PJ, Tenke CE. Reduced brain responses to novel sounds in depression: P3 findings in a novelty oddball task. *Psychiatry Res* (2009) 170:218–23. doi:10.1016/j.psychres.2008.10.023
68. Chen J, Zhang Y, Wei D, Wu X, Fu Q, Xu F, et al. Neurophysiological handover from MMN to P3a in first-episode and recurrent major depression. *J Affect Disord* (2015) 174:173–9. doi:10.1016/j.jad.2014.11.049
69. Jandl M, Steyer J, Kaschka WP. Suicide risk markers in major depressive disorder: a study of electrodermal activity and event-related potentials. *J Affect Disord* (2010) 123:138–49. doi:10.1016/j.jad.2009.09.011
70. Tenke CE, Kayser J, Stewart JW, Bruder GE. Novelty P3 reductions in depression: characterization using principal components analysis (PCA) of current source density (CSD) waveforms. *Psychophysiology* (2010) 47:133–46. doi:10.1111/j.1469-8986.2009.00880.x
71. Lepistö T, Soininen M, Čeponien R, Almqvist F, Näätänen R, Aronen ET. Auditory event-related potential indices of increased distractibility in children with major depression. *Neurophysiol Clin* (2004) 115:620–7. doi:10.1016/j.clinph.2003.10.020

72. Näätänen R, Pakarinen S, Rinne T, Takegata R. The mismatch negativity (MMN): towards the optimal paradigm. *Neurophysiol Clin* (2004) 115:140–4. doi:10.1016/j.clinph.2003.04.001
73. Tavakoli P, Campbell K. Can an auditory multi-feature optimal paradigm be used for the study of processes associated with attention capture in passive listeners? *Brain Res* (2016) 1648:394–408. doi:10.1016/j.brainres.2016.08.003
74. Rydkjaer J, Jepsen JM, Pagsberg AK, Fagerlund B, Glenthøj BY, Oranje B. Mismatch negativity and P3a amplitude in young adolescents with first-episode psychosis: a comparison with ADHD. *Psychol Med* (2017) 47:377–88. doi:10.1017/S0033291716002518
75. Takei Y, Kumano S, Hattori S, Uehara T, Kawakubo Y, Kasai K, et al. Preattentive dysfunction in major depression: a magnetoencephalography study using auditory mismatch negativity. *Psychophysiology* (2009) 46:52–61. doi:10.1111/j.1469-8986.2008.00748.x
76. Catts SV, Shelley AM, Ward PB, Liebert B, McConaghy N, Andrews S, et al. Brain potential evidence for an auditory sensory memory deficit in schizophrenia. *Am J Psychiatry* (1995) 152:213. doi:10.1176/ajp.152.2.213
77. Korostenskaja M, Dapsys K, Siurkute A, Maciulis V, Ruksenas O, Kähkönen S. Effects of olanzapine on auditory P300 and mismatch negativity (MMN) in schizophrenia spectrum disorders. *Prog Neuropsychopharmacol Biol Psychiatry* (2005) 29:543–8. doi:10.1016/j.pnpbp.2005.01.019
78. Rissling AJ, Braff DL, Swerdlow NR, Hellemann G, Rassovsky Y, Sprock J, et al. Disentangling early sensory information processing deficits in schizophrenia. *Neurophysiol Clin* (2012) 123:1942–9. doi:10.1016/j.clinph.2012.02.079
79. Umbricht D, Javitt D, Novak G, Bates J, Pollack S, Lieberman J, et al. Effects of clozapine on auditory event-related potentials in schizophrenia. *Biol Psychiatry* (1998) 44:716–25. doi:10.1016/S0006-3223(97)00524-6
80. Umbricht D, Javitt D, Novak G, Bates J, Pollack S, Lieberman J, et al. Effects of risperidone on auditory event-related potentials in schizophrenia. *Int J Neuropsychopharmacol* (1999) 2:299–304. doi:10.1017/S1461145799001595
81. Kovacs M, Staff MHS. *Children's Depression Inventory 2nd Edition (CDI-2): Multi-Health Systems.* Incorporated (2011).
82. Osman A, Bagge CL, Gutierrez PM, Konick LC, Kopper BA, Barrios FX. The suicidal behaviors questionnaire-revised (SBQ-R): validation with clinical and nonclinical samples. *Assessment* (2001) 8:443–54. doi:10.1177/107319110100800409
83. Fabiani M, Kazmerski VA, Cycowicz YM, Friedman D. Naming norms for brief environmental sounds: effects of age and dementia. *Psychophysiology* (1996) 33(4):462–75. doi:10.1111/j.1469-8986.1996.tb01072.x
84. Chaumon M, Bishop DV, Busch NA. A practical guide to the selection of independent components of the electroencephalogram for artifact correction. *J Neurosci Methods* (2015) 250:47–63. doi:10.1016/j.jneumeth.2015.02.025
85. Makeig S, Bell AJ, Jung TP, Sejnowski TJ. Independent component analysis of electroencephalographic data. In: Touretzky D, Mozer M, Hasselmo M, editors. *Advances in Neural Information Processing Systems* (1996) 8:145–51.
86. Geisser S, Greenhouse SW. An extension of box's results on the use of the F distribution in multivariate analysis. *Ann Math Stat* (1958) 29:885–91. doi:10.1214/aoms/1177706545
87. Centers for Disease Control and Prevention. *Fatal Injury Reports and Nonfatal Injury Reports. Web-Based Injury Statistics Query and Reporting System.* Atlanta, GA: National Center for Injury Prevention and Control (2014). Available from: www.cdc.gov/injury/wisqars/index.html
88. May AM, Klonsky ED. What distinguishes suicide attempters from suicide ideators? A meta-analysis of potential factors. *Clin Psychol Sci Pract* (2016) 23:5–20. doi:10.1111/cpsp.12136
89. Nock MK, Kessler RC, Franklin JC. Risk factors for suicide ideation differ from those for the transition to suicide attempt: the importance of creativity, rigor, and urgency in suicide research. *Clin Psychol Sci Pract* (2016) 23:31–4. doi:10.1093/epirev/mxn002
90. Burton CZ, Vella L, Weller JA, Twamley EW. Differential effects of executive functioning on suicide attempts. *J Neuropsychiatry Clin Neurosci* (2011) 23:173–9. doi:10.1176/appi.neuropsych.23.2.173
91. Zaifu Z, Ruoxiao H, Zhirong Y, Weixing F, Wangqiang L, Jianwei Z, et al. Correlation study of decreased mismatch negativity latency and amplitudes accompanying suicidal behavior in patients with depression. *J Neurol Neurorehabil* (2010) 2.
92. Zhen C, Zhu W, Chen Z, Zhou D, Zhang Y, Wang H, et al. Experimental study on mismatch negativity in senile depression patients with suicide behavior. *Mod Pract Med* (2012) 5:008.
93. El Massioui F, Lesèvre N. Attention impairment and psychomotor retardation in depressed patients: an event-related potential study. *Electroencephalogr Clin Neurophysiol* (1988) 70(1):46–55. doi:10.1016/0013-4694(88)90193-9
94. El Massioui F, Everett J, Martin MT, Jouvent R, Widlöcher D. Attention deficits in depression: an electrophysiological marker. *Neuroreport* (1996) 7(15–17):2483–6. doi:10.1097/00001756-199611040-00016
95. Ogura C, Nageishi Y, Omura F, Fukao K, Ohta H, Kishimoto A, et al. N200 component of event-related potentials in depression. *Biol Psychiatry* (1993) 33:720–6. doi:10.1016/0006-3223(93)90122-T
96. Qiao Z, Yu Y, Wang L, Yang X, Qiu X, Zhang C, et al. Impaired pre-attentive change detection in major depressive disorder patients revealed by auditory mismatch negativity. *Psychiatry Res* (2013) 211:78–84. doi:10.1016/j.pscychresns.2012.07.006
97. Fisher DJ, Grant B, Smith DM, Knott VJ. Effects of deviant probability on the 'optimal' multi-feature mismatch negativity (MMN) paradigm. *Int J Psychophysiol* (2011) 79(2):311–5. doi:10.1016/j.ijpsycho.2010.11.006
98. Cahn BR, Polich J. Meditation (Vipassana) and the P3a event-related brain potential. *Int J Psychophysiol* (2009) 72(1):51–60. doi:10.1016/j.ijpsycho.2008.03.013
99. Combs LA, Polich J. P3a from auditory white noise stimuli. *Neurophysiol Clin* (2006) 117(5):1106–12. doi:10.1016/j.clinph.2006.01.023
100. Frank DW, Yee RB, Polich J. P3a from white noise. *Int J Psychophysiol* (2012) 85(2):236–41. doi:10.1016/j.ijpsycho.2012.04.005
101. Tavakoli P, Varma S, Campbell K. Highly relevant stimuli may passively elicit processes associated with consciousness during the sleep onset period. *Conscious Cogn* (2018) 58:60–74. doi:10.1016/j.concog.2017.10.012
102. Miranda R, Nolen-Hoeksema S. Brooding and reflection: rumination predicts suicidal ideation at 1-year follow-up in a community sample. *Behav Res Ther* (2007) 45:3088–95. doi:10.1016/j.brat.2007.07.015

7

Understanding the Links Between Self-Report Emotional Intelligence and Suicide Risk: Does Psychological Distress Mediate This Relationship Across Time and Samples?

Sergio Mérida-López[1], *Natalio Extremera*[1*] *and Lourdes Rey*[2]

[1] *Department of Social Psychology, University of Málaga, Málaga, Spain,* [2] *Department of Personality, Assessment and Psychological Treatment, University of Málaga, Málaga, Spain*

Correspondence:
Natalio Extremera
nextremera@uma.es

Objective: In the last decades, increasing attention has been paid to examining psychological resources that might contribute to our understanding of suicide risk. Although Emotional Intelligence (EI) is one dimension that has been linked with decreased suicidal ideation and behaviors, we detected several gaps in the literature in this area regarding the research designs and samples involved. In this research, we aimed to test a mediator model considering self-report EI, psychological distress and suicide risk across samples adopting both cross-sectional and prospective designs in two independent studies.

Method: In Study 1, our purpose was to examine the potential role of psychological distress as a mediator in the relationship between self-report EI and suicide risk in a community sample comprised of 438 adults (270 women; mean age: 33.21 years). In Study 2, we sought to examine the proposed mediator model considering a 2-month prospective design in a sample of college students (n = 330 in T1; n = 311 in T2; 264 women; mean age: 22.22 years).

Results: In Study 1, we found that psychological distress partially mediated the effect of self-report EI on suicide risk. More interestingly, findings from Study 2 showed that psychological distress fully mediated the relationship between self-report EI and suicide risk at Time 2.

Conclusion: These results point out the role of psychological distress as a mediator in the association between self-report EI and suicide risk. These findings suggest an underlying process by which self-report EI may act as a protective factor against suicidal ideation and behaviors. In line with the limitations of our work, plausible avenues for future research and interventions are discussed.

Keywords: emotional intelligence, psychological distress, suicide risk, mediator model, prospective design

INTRODUCTION

In the last decades, the literature on individual differences regarding health and well-being has been expanding rapidly, thereby leading to a large body of research on psychological resources associated with mental health outcomes [e.g., (1, 2)]. Emotional Intelligence (EI) is one dimension that has shown robust associations with health-related outcomes (3), thereby constituting a particularly relevant topic in psychiatric research (4).

Two main theoretical approaches are found to build the framework for this construct: trait EI and ability EI. These views play a major role in the assessment of EI together with its training [for a review, see e.g., (5)]. In fact, there is a growing consensus in distinguishing three main construct-method pairings considering the model of EI: self-report mixed EI tests, performance-based ability EI instruments and self-report ability EI tests (6, 7). On the one hand, models of trait EI define this construct as a personality trait regarding the person's tendency to manage his or her emotional states (8). Therefore, researchers following this approach tend to use self-report mixed EI instruments. On the other hand, ability EI is referred to as a set of abilities that allow people to effectively deal with emotions (9).

According to the ability model proposed by Mayer and Salovey (10), EI is defined as "the ability to perceive accurately, appraise, and express emotion; the ability to access and/or generate feelings when they facilitate thought; the ability to understand emotion and emotional knowledge; and the ability to regulate emotions to promote emotional and intellectual growth" (10). Thus, the ability EI approach suggests implications on EI training as emotional abilities might be more susceptible to being developed and learned (9). Following the ability model of EI, performance-based ability EI tests are often used together with instruments referred to as self-report ability EI tests. In line with previous studies (11), a widely used self-report ability EI measure (i.e., Wong and Law Emotional Intelligence Scale) was chosen because it is relatively short, reliable and easy to administer. Besides, this instrument provides unique access to emotional-affective processes given by self-report ability EI tests.

EI and Suicide Risk

While suicide is considered as a public health concern because of its alarming prevalence, suicidal thoughts and behaviors represent significant indicators of suicide risk (12). In this sense, the phenomenon of suicide has been argued as a continuum [e.g., (13)]. In addition, two populations have received particular attention in psychiatric research regarding the leading prevalence of deaths caused by suicide in both populations (12, 13). On the one hand, community samples constituted of middle-aged adults are required to deal with psychosocial events (e.g., loss of job, marriage, or relationship breakdown or financial stress) that are linked to increased suicide risk in this age group (14, 15). On the other hand, college students constitute a population at high risk of suicidal thoughts and behaviors (16). As some authors have argued, the university context represents a key transitional period often perceived as a stressful time of change, thereby influencing students' suicidal thoughts and behaviors (13).

Because the perceived ability to deal with affective information has been highlighted as a relevant factor regarding health and well-being indicators [e.g., (7, 17)], it is not surprising that findings from several studies have reported significant associations between self-report ability EI and suicide risk. For instance, Abdollahi et al. (18) found that self-report ability EI buffered the association between perceived stress and suicidal ideation among depressed adolescent inpatients. In this context, Abdollahi and Talib (19) argued the protective role of self-report ability EI against suicidal ideation because of its negative associations with rumination processes. Similar findings have been found on the relationship between self-report ability EI and suicide risk indicators among college students (20, 21) and community samples (22). With respect to performance-based ability EI tests, similar results have been reported in a study with adolescents (23). More recently, Paradiso and colleagues used a well-known performance-based ability EI test (i.e., Mayer-Salovey-Caruso Emotional Intelligence Test; MSCEIT, Version 2.0) in a study with a clinic sample of veterans (24). Findings showed that suicidal thoughts were linked to lower emotion processing. As noted above, existing literature on EI and suicide has focused on the ability model of EI using both self-report ability EI tests and performance-based instruments. In sum, there is a growing body of research suggesting that the manner in which people deal with emotional information contributes to an explanation of suicide risk.

Psychological Distress as a Potential Mediator Between EI and Suicide Risk

In identifying risk factors linked with suicidality, impaired mental health constitutes identifiable vulnerabilities that increase the likelihood of suicide [e.g., (12, 25)]. In this context, prior research has reported the predictive validity of psychological risk factors on suicide risk among college students [e.g., (16)] or community samples [e.g., (26)]. Finally, the deleterious impact over time of psychological symptomatology on suicidality has been reported (27).

A broad association between EI and psychological distress indicators suggests that the perceived ability to deal with emotions is linked to individuals' psychological adjustment and adaptation [e.g., (2, 3)]. In addition, EI has been found to be involved in psychological distress processes beyond the influence of personality traits (4, 28). According to the EI framework, emotionally intelligent individuals manage their emotions in a better way than those with lower EI (5). Consequently, people with higher EI tend to adopt more adaptive regulatory strategies that are, in turn, negatively associated with negative affect and psychological distress [e.g., (29)]. Conversely, emotion dysregulation is considered a factor contributing to affective vulnerabilities that are in the basis of suicide risk (12, 30) and nonsuicidal self-injury (31). This latter risk factor has shown robust associations with increased desire for, and capability of, suicide across samples (32).

Even though researchers have focused efforts on identifying the buffering role of emotional abilities in understanding the associations between psychological risk factors such as perceived stress or depression (18, 21) and increased suicide risk, no study has examined a mediator model beyond the direct associations between these variables. In other words, there is a need for research to delineate the mechanisms through which EI might act as a protective factor to reduce suicidal thoughts and behaviors (33).

Purpose of the Present Research

As noted above, we found several gaps in the literature on EI and suicide risk that motivate our work. First, although EI is negatively related to suicide risk, the mechanisms by which EI relates to suicidal thoughts and behaviors remain unclear. Second, most of studies examining self-report EI and suicide risk indicators relied on adolescent and college student samples [e.g., (20, 21)]. Thus, studies examining the associations between EI and health indicators in more heterogeneous samples are needed to confirm the validity of these results (17, 34). Finally, current findings in the literature on EI and suicide risk share a limitation derived from the use of cross-sectional designs. In short, previous studies have failed to capture change over time and left the question of causal direction unanswered. Therefore, the findings from prospective studies may provide clarity on causal mechanisms between EI and suicide risk (22, 33). Besides, analyzing EI at Time 1 with reported suicidal ideation and behavior at Time 2 offers a more stringent test of the impact of EI on suicide risk. Moreover, this prospective design can reveal the existence of stable relationships that might not be detected when constructs are measured at only one point in time.

To begin to fill these gaps, the objective of the present work was threefold. First, we aimed to examine the associations between self-report EI, psychological distress and suicidal thoughts and behaviors in two different populations (community sample and college students) to confirm the generalizability of our results. Second, we aimed to examine whether psychological distress would mediate the relationship between self-report EI and suicide risk. Third, we analyzed the proposed mediator model considering both cross-sectional and prospective designs in two independent samples.

We undertook two studies aiming to achieve the above-described objectives. Based on prior research, we expected that: (a) direct associations would exist between self-report EI, psychological distress and suicide risk, and (b) psychological distress would operate as a mediator of the relationship between self-report EI and suicide risk. In Study 1, we explored this proposed mediator model in a community sample. In Study 2, we aimed to verify prospectively the proposed model in a sample of college students, that is, taking a temporal mediation approach to examine the effects of self-report EI on Time 2 suicide risk over a 2-month period. Our proposed mediator model is shown in **Figure 1**.

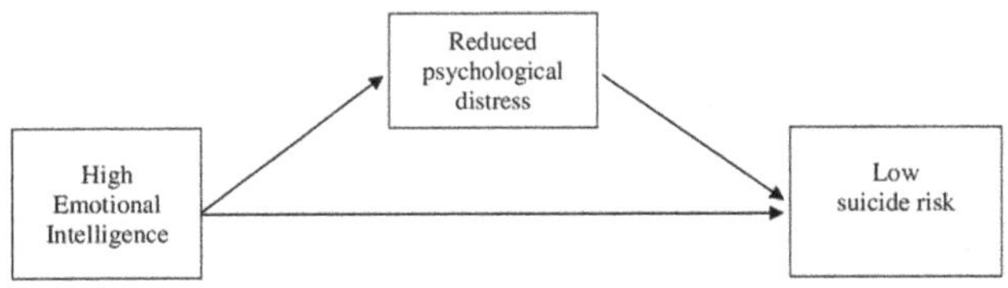

FIGURE 1 | Proposed model of the role of psychological distress in explaining the relationship between emotional intelligence to suicide risk.

STUDY 1: MATERIALS AND METHODS

Participants and Procedure

A convenience sample of 438 Spanish speaking adults (270 women; 61.60%) living in southern Spain took part in this study. The ages of participants ranged from 17 to 62 years, with a mean of 33.21 years ($SD = 11.68$). The marital status of the participants was: 57.3% single, 27.9% married, 7.5% separated/divorced, 1.8% widow/widower and 4.8% coupled. Three subjects did not indicate their marital status.

Participants were recruited with the help of psychology students at University of Malaga. In this sense, respondents were invited to participate through a snowball sampling technique via the researchers' and undergraduates' personal and professional contacts. These students were given copies of the surveys and received instructions from the teaching staff regarding how to administer the questionnaire correctly. Overall, participants were aware that by completing the questionnaires they were providing informed consent to use this data in the present research. No financial compensation was offered to the subjects for their participation. Common inclusion criteria were being aged above 18 years old at the time of this survey and willingness to participate in the research. Exclusion criteria were illiteracy in Spanish and not being interested at participating in filling in the individual, confidential and voluntary questionnaire. Participants received oral and written information about the aims of the study and were fully informed about the anonymity and the voluntary nature of the research so that potential coercion was avoided. Most importantly, it was made clear that they could stop participating in case they got distressed filling in the questionnaire. Once the participants completed the questionnaires at home, the students returned them to the teaching staff for statistical processing. The questionnaires included written information on the main purpose of the study and standard instructions on how to complete the tests. Completing the surveys lasted 15 minutes on average. In addition to sociodemographic data (age, gender and marital status), the questionnaires included well-validated scales assessing the main study variables.

Measures

To assess for self-report EI we used the Wong and Law Emotional Intelligence Scale [WLEIS; (35)]. This instrument assesses four dimensions: self-emotion appraisal, other-emotion appraisal, using of emotion, and regulation of emotion (e.g., "I am quite capable of controlling my own emotions" and "I always encourage myself to try my best"). This scale consists of 16 items rated on a 7-point Likert-type scale ranging from 1 (strongly disagree) to 7 (strongly agree). This instrument elicits a global self-report EI score, with higher scores indicating higher self-report EI levels. Therefore, we combined the subscales into a global self-report EI measure as in previous studies (22, 36). This version of WLEIS has been proven to have good validity and reliability in Spanish populations [e.g., (22)]. In this study, Cronbach's alpha for WLEIS was 0.91.

Psychological distress was assessed using the Spanish version of the short-form Depression Anxiety and Stress Scales [DASS-21; (37, 38)]. This self-report instrument assesses psychological symptoms in the past week through a Likert-type scale (e.g., "I couldn't seem to experience any positive feelings at all" and "I felt I was close to panic"). Each item is rated on a 4-point scale, with "0 = did not apply to me at all" to "3 = applied to me very much, or most of the time." We combined the subscales into a global psychological distress measure as in previous studies (39, 40). Hence, scores on the three subscales were summed, with scores coded so that higher scores showed higher psychological distress. The Spanish version of the DASS-21 has shown satisfactory psychometric properties in previous studies with community samples (34) and college students (38). Cronbach's alpha was 0.92.

Suicidal thoughts and behaviors were assessed with the Suicidal Behaviors Questionnaire-Revised [SBQ-R; (41)]. The SBQ-R consists of four items that assess different dimensions of suicidality: lifetime suicidal ideation and attempts (e.g., "Have you ever thought about or attempted to kill yourself?"), frequency of suicidal ideation in the past year (e.g., "How often have you thought about killing yourself in the past year?"), communication of suicidal behavior (e.g., "Have you ever told someone that you were going to commit suicide or that you might do it?"), and self-reported likelihood of future suicidal behavior (e.g., "How likely is it that you will attempt suicide someday?"). SBQ-R items are scored on a Likert-scale ranging from 0 or 1 (*never*) to 5 (*very often*) or 6 (*very likely*) so that higher scores indicate greater suicidal behavior. Items scores were summed to obtain a total score. For this study, the SBQ-R was professionally translated from English into Spanish using the back-translation method. The Spanish version of SBQ-R has shown adequate reliability in prior research (22). Cronbach's alpha was 0.79.

Statistical Analyses

SPSS 22.0 was used to analyze the data. First, we conducted Pearson correlation analyses to test whether self-report EI was associated with the proposed mediator (psychological distress) and outcome variable (suicide risk) in the hypothesized directions. Following Cohen (42), the correlation coefficients of 0.10, 0.30, and 0.50 represent small, medium and large effect size, respectively (42). Second, mediation analysis was conducted using the procedures recommended by Hayes (43) with total score of self-report EI as the independent variable (IV) and suicide risk as the dependent variable (DV). Psychological distress was tested as the mediator variable (MV) (43). In order to rule out the possibility that associations between self-report EI and suicide risk could be confounded by socio-demographic factors, age and gender were included as covariates.

Bootstrapping with 5,000 resamples was used in order to obtain parameter estimates for both total effect model and indirect effect model. In addition, we used the 95% bias-corrected confidence interval. If the interval does not contain a zero, then the indirect effect is considered statistically significant ($p < 0.05$). Mediation analysis was conducted with the Hayes macro PROCESS (43).

Results

Descriptive statistics and Pearson correlations are reported in **Table 1**. All of the measures were significantly associated. As predicted, self-report EI scores showed significant negative correlation with psychological distress ($r = -0.42$; $p < 0.01$). Moreover, self-report EI was found to be correlated with suicide risk in the expected direction ($r = -0.32$; $p < 0.01$). Finally, psychological distress and suicide risk were positively related ($r = 0.33$; $p < 0.01$). According to Cohen's standard (42), the effect sizes of the correlations between self-report EI, psychological distress and suicide risk were medium.

The results of the mediation analysis are summarized in **Table 2**. First, after controlling for age and gender, self-report EI was found to be significantly and negatively related to suicide risk ($B = -0.90$, $S.E. = 0.13$, $t = -7.18$, $p < 0.001$). Psychological distress was found to be significantly and positively related to suicide risk ($B = 0.08$; $S.E. = 0.02$; $t = 5.08$; $p < 0.001$). Second, inclusion of psychological distress reduced the association between self-report EI and suicide risk but this relationship remained significant ($B = -0.62$; $S.E. = 0.13$; $t = -4.59$; $p < 0.001$). Lastly, results of bootstrapping showed that psychological distress was a significant mediator of the relationship between self-report EI and suicide risk [estimate $= -0.28$; $S.E. = 0.08$, 95% CI $= (-0.46, -0.15)$].

STUDY 2: MATERIALS AND METHODS

Participants and Procedure

Participants in this prospective study were 330 undergraduate students from the University of Malaga (264 females; 80%) with a mean age of 22.22 years and ranging from 18 to 61 years ($SD = 5.53$). The marital status of the participants was: 93% single, 1.2% married, 3.9% separated/divorced and 1.5% coupled. One subject did not indicate his marital status.

Students were asked if they were willing to participate in research on "associations between emotions and well-being." Data were collected with the help of a team of research assistants. All participants completed the T1 survey and 310 participants (250 female; 80%, mean age = 22.11, $SD = 5.46$) completed the T2 survey 2 months later. Students were fully informed about the voluntary and anonymous basis of participation. It was made clear to them that their participation was voluntary and that all data would remain confidential. In this sense, participants could not be personally identified. In addition, it was made clear that they could stop participating in case they got distressed filling in the questionnaire. Participants completed the surveys as a group and received course credits for their participation in the 2-month prospective study. They were fully aware that by completing the questionnaires they were in fact providing informed consent to use this data in our research. In sum, common inclusion criteria were being aged above 18 years old, being enrolled in an industrial and organizational psychology course at the time of this survey and willingness to participate in the study. The surveys were administered in paper-and-pencil

TABLE 1 | Descriptive statistics and bivariate correlations among the study variables in Study 1.

	M	*SD*	Range	Min	Max	α	1	2	3
1. Emotional intelligence	5.11	0.92	5.44	1.56	7.00	0.91	–		
2. Psychological distress	11.44	8.10	36.00	0.00	36.00	0.92	−0.42**	–	
3. Suicide risk	4.39	2.54	16.00	3.00	19.00	0.79	−0.32**	0.33**	–

N = 438.
**$p < 0.01$.

TABLE 2 | Indirect effects of Emotional Intelligence (EI) on suicide risk through psychological distress controlling for age and gender.

	Total effect model			Indirect effect model			
Path	*B*	*SE*	*t*	*B*	*SE*	*t*	BCa 95% CI
Age[a]	0.01	0.01	1.24	0.02	0.01	1.65	
Gender[a]	0.11	0.24	0.48	0.19	0.23	0.82	
EI – distress *(a)*	−3.66	0.38	−9.56***				
distress – suicide risk *(b)*	0.08	0.02	5.08***				
EI – suicide risk *(c)*	−0.90	0.13	−7.18***				
EI – suicide risk *(c′)*	−0.62	0.13	−4.59***				
EI - distress – suicide risk *(ab)*				−0.28	0.08		[−0.46, −0.15]
R^2	0.11			0.16			
F *(df)*	17.61***	(3, 434)		20.42***	(4, 433)		

EI, Emotional Intelligence; distress, psychological distress symptoms. N = 438. a, b, c, and c′ represent unstandardized regression coefficients: a, direct association between Emotional Intelligence and suicidal behavior; b, direct association between psychological distress and suicidal behavior; c, total effect between Emotional Intelligence and suicidal behavior (not accounting for psychological distress); c′, direct effect between Emotional Intelligence and suicidal behavior (accounting for psychological distress); ab, indirect effect between Emotional Intelligence and suicidal behavior operating through psychological distress. Full mediation, c is reduced by ab to a non-significant c′; partial mediation, c is reduced by ab, but c′ remains significant; indirect only, ab, but no c and no c′ initially. BCa 95% CI, bias corrected and accelerated 95% confidence interval; 5,000 bootstrap samples. [a]Age and sex were covaried.
***$p < 0.001$.

format with writing instructions and included sociodemographic factors (e.g., age, gender and marital status) together with scales measuring our main study variables.

Measures

Self-report EI was evaluated using the Spanish version of the WLEIS (see description in Study 1). Cronbach's alpha was excellent in this study: α = 0.87 in Time 1 (T1) and α = 0.88 in Time 2 (T2). We administered the Spanish version of the DASS-21 to assess psychological distress (see description in Study 1). In this study, internal reliability was excellent (α = 0.91 in T1 and T2). Suicide risk was assessed with the Suicidal Behaviors Questionnaire-Revised (SBQ-R; see description in Study 1). In this study, Cronbach's alpha was 0.77 (in T1 and T2).

Statistical Analyses

First, we conducted Pearson correlation analyses to test the associations between self-report EI, psychological distress and suicide risk. We followed Cohen's (42) standard for estimating the correlation coefficient effect size (42). Second, we conducted a *t*-test on the outcome variable (suicide risk) assessed both at T1 and T2 in order to examine whether there were significant differences over time. In the case of significant differences in suicide risk from T1 to T2, this variable would be included as a control variable. Similarly to Study 1, mediation analysis was conducted using PROCESS (43), with a 5,000 bootstrapping sample and a 95% confidence interval to judge the statistical significance of mediation (43). SPSS 22.0 was used to analyze the data.

Results

Table 3 reports descriptive statistics and correlations among our study variables at T1 and T2. As is shown, self-report EI was negatively and significantly associated with psychological distress in both T1 ($r = -0.35$; $p < 0.01$) and T2 ($r = -0.27$; $p < 0.01$). Similarly, self-report EI was significantly and negatively related to suicide risk in both T1 ($r = -0.19$; $p < 0.01$) and T2 ($r = -0.21$; $p < 0.01$). Finally, psychological distress and suicide risk were significantly and positively related in both T1 ($r = 0.41$; $p < 0.01$) and T2 ($r = 0.29$; $p < 0.01$). Following Cohen's standard (42), the effect sizes of the correlations self-report EI-psychological distress and psychological distress-suicide risk were medium, whereas the other correlations showed small effect sizes. In *post-hoc* analyses using the Fisher r-to-z transformation, we examined the correlations between self-report EI and suicide risk in both Study 1 and Study 2 (T1). Results showed that the community sample reported significantly higher associations than the college student sample ($z = -1.90$; $p < 0.05$).

Paired samples *t*-tests found no significant differences in suicide risk between T1 and T2 [$t_{(310)} = 0.67$; $p = 0.51$], and so T1 suicide risk was not included as a control variable in the

TABLE 3 | Descriptive statistics and bivariate correlations among the study variables at Time 1 and Time 2 in Study 2.

	M	*SD*	Range	Min	Max	α	1	2	3
TIME 1									
1. Emotional intelligence	5.30	0.73	4.06	2.69	6.75	0.87	–		
2. Psychological distress	9.43	6.87	36.00	0.00	36.00	0.91	−0.35**	–	
3. Suicide risk	5.05	2.83	16.00	3.00	19.00	0.77	−0.19**	0.41**	–
TIME 2									
1. Emotional intelligence	5.31	0.73	3.88	3.06	6.94	0.88	–		
2. Psychological distress	10.26	7.41	36.00	0.00	36.00	0.91	−0.27**	–	
3. Suicide risk	4.97	2.69	13.00	3.00	16.00	0.77	−0.21**	0.29**	–

*M, Mean; SD, Standard Deviation. T1 N = 330. T2 N = 311. **p < 0.01.*

main analyses, in favor of the most parsimonious model. **Table 4** reports the results of the mediation analysis. First, we found that sociodemographic factors, age and gender were significantly related to T2 suicide risk. After controlling for age and gender, self-report EI was found to be significantly and negatively related to T2 suicide risk ($B = -0.85$; $S.E. = 0.21$; $t = -4.09$; $p < 0.001$). Likewise, psychological distress was found to be significantly and positively related to suicide risk ($B = 0.15$; $S.E. = 0.02$; $t = 7.09$; $p < 0.001$). After psychological distress was included in the model, the association between self-report EI and suicide risk decreased and it did change the significance ($B = -0.36$; $S.E. = 0.21$; $t = -1.77$; $p < 0.001$). In particular, the direct effect of self-report EI on T2 suicide risk was no longer significant after accounting for the variance predicted by psychological distress. Results of bootstrapping revealed that psychological distress totally mediated the relationship between self-report EI and T2 suicide risk (estimate = -0.49; $S.E. = 0.14$, 95% $CI = [-0.82, -0.26]$). In sum, self-report EI showed a negative effect on psychological distress, which in turn was linked to decreased suicide risk 2 months later.

DISCUSSION

The proposed research aimed to examine a mediator model involving self-report EI, psychological distress and suicide risk adopting both cross-sectional and prospective designs in two independent samples. As expected, our results showed that self-report EI was negatively related to suicidal thoughts and behaviors in both community (22) and college student samples [e.g., (20)]. Similarly, the correlations between self-report EI and psychological distress were in line with those shown by Martins et al. (3) and more recent studies on EI and health-related indicators (17, 44). In line with prior research, our results show that self-report EI facilitates positive outcomes for individuals, thereby constituting a valuable resource in preventing suicide.

Our findings in study 1 suggest that self-report EI may explain suicide risk both directly and indirectly through its influence on psychological distress. Therefore, individuals who perceive themselves more skilled in perceiving, understanding and managing their own emotions and the emotions of others seem to show decreased suicidal thoughts and behaviors via reduced psychological distress (30, 45). Study 2 helped us verifying these findings providing prospective evidence on the protective role of self-report EI on suicide risk through maintaining lower emotional distress (27).

Based upon prior research, self-report ability EI seems to be related to individuals' beliefs in their emotional skills to cope with threating events (46). Relatedly, the influence of self-report EI on lower suicide risk might occur through encouraging development of adaptive strategies that decrease the individuals' vulnerability toward negative mood states associated with the likelihood of suicidal thoughts and behaviors (22, 27). For instance, EI appears to be linked to the use of certain coping strategies such as rumination, social support seeking or emotional disclosure (47). In the same vein, a recent meta-analysis on EI and emotion regulation strategies has provided empirical evidences on the fact that higher EI individuals tend to regulate their emotions and display less emotional reactivity in response to negative emotion-eliciting events (29). In sum, individuals' beliefs in their emotional skills to deal with demanding events might reduce emotional distress symptoms that might, in turn, be key factors in determining the frequency and intensity of future suicidal thoughts and behaviors (17, 22).

LIMITATIONS AND FUTURE RESEARCH

Several limitations of this work should be considered because of its implications for future research and practice. First, a limitation of the present work may be constituted by the common method variance derived from the use of self-report measures (3). Nonetheless, the construct validity of our study variables encourage us to find this question less problematic (48). Although most of the studies in the field of EI and suicide have used self-report ability EI tests with adequate psychometric properties, future studies are advised to examine jointly both performance-based and self-report instruments of EI (2, 49). In addition, semi-structured interviews or observers' ratings of EI are advised to complement the main approaches to assess ability EI. Relatedly, although performance-based ability EI has shown incremental validity in explaining suicidal ideation above the variance accounted for by personality traits (28), further research is needed to consider the potential influence of dispositional factors on suicide risk [e.g., (50)].

TABLE 4 | Examination of the indirect effect of EI on Time 2 suicide risk through psychological distress.

	Total effect model			Indirect effect model			
Path	***B***	***SE***	***t***	***B***	***SE***	***t***	**BCa 95% CI**
Age[a]	0.05	0.03	1.86	0.06	0.03	2.17*	
Gender[a]	−0.89	0.37	−2.37*	−0.79	0.35	−2.27*	
EI – suicide risk (*c′*)	−0.36	0.21	−1.77				
EI – distress (*a*)	−3.20	0.51	−6.25***				
Distress– suicide risk (*b*)	0.15	0.02	7.09***				
EI – suicide risk (*c*)	−0.85	0.21	−4.09***				
EI - distress – suicide risk (*ab*)				−0.49	0.14		[−0.82, −0.26]
R^2	0.07			0.20			
F (*df*)	7.83***(3, 307)			19.37***(4, 306)			

EI, Emotional Intelligence; distress, psychological distress symptoms. N = 330 (T1) and 311 (T2). a, b, c, and c′ represent unstandardized regression coefficients: a, direct association between Emotional Intelligence and suicidal behavior; b, direct association between psychological distress and suicidal behavior; c, total effect between Emotional Intelligence and suicidal behavior (not accounting for psychological distress); c′, direct effect between Emotional Intelligence and suicidal behavior (accounting for psychological distress); ab, indirect effect between Emotional Intelligence and suicidal behavior operating through psychological distress. Total mediation, c is reduced by ab to a non-significant c′; partial mediation, c is reduced by ab, but c′ remains significant; indirect only, ab, but no c and no c′ initially. BCa 95% CI, bias corrected and accelerated 95% confidence interval; 5,000 bootstrap samples.
*[a]Age and sex were covaried. **$p < 0.01$; ***$p < 0.001$.*

Second, we used a self-reported measure of psychological distress rather than instruments assessing psychopathological factors. Although further research should include additional measurement methodologies, such as expert judgments or clinical diagnosis, assessment of psychological distress symptoms undoubtedly constitutes a promising line in psychiatric research (51). Although we assessed marital status as well as previous studies on EI and suicide risk did [e.g., (18, 22)], future studies are advised to examine other important sociodemographic factors such as educational level, which might function differently depending on the levels of educational attainment. Finally, although gender was controlled in our analyses, prior research has shown differences between males and females in rates of psychological symptoms [e.g., (52)], along with the prediction of suicidality (53). Therefore, gender specific moderated mediation models should be considered in future studies (54).

One of the contributions of our work is that self-report EI was found to both cross-sectionally and prospectively predict suicide risk through its influence on psychological distress. In this sense, it is noteworthy that psychological distress partially mediated this relationship in Study 1, whereas it fully mediated the association between self-report EI and T2 suicide risk in Study 2. One plausible explanation for this difference might be due to the nature of the sample. It is tentative to assume that suicide risk in the community sample may be more externally determined and depend on a higher variety of contextual and sociodemographic factors that are traditionally related to psychological distress [e.g., (14, 15, 32)]. Conversely, psychological distress symptoms might be more determinant of suicidal thoughts and behaviors in a more homogenous sample constituted by college students [e.g., (16, 55)]. Undoubtedly, future studies comparing relatively large samples are advised to replicate these findings. In addition, further research adopting longitudinal and experimental designs is needed to broaden the current understanding of the protective role of EI in suicidal thoughts and behaviors. Although sampling bias could be a potential limitation of the snowball sampling technique used in study 1 (56), the instructions on the questionnaire were brief and precise aiming at avoiding these biases to a greater extent.

Taken as a whole, our findings add support to the assumption that EI might help alleviate emotional distress, thereby decreasing the likelihood of suicidal thoughts and behaviors. These results highlight the role of EI as a promising line of intervention in preventing psychological maladjustment and suicide thoughts and behaviors (57, 58). Besides, given the literature focusing on the crucial role of negative emotional states as precursors of lower physical and mental health [e.g., (3, 17)], these findings might be valuable when designing population-based interventions (12, 57). Accordingly, interventions that target both an alleviation of psychological distress and negative mood states (59) and an increase in emotional abilities (60) may offer the most promise in working with individuals experiencing higher suicide ideation (58). In sum, our results point out the potential value of using EI-based stress reduction interventions that specifically assess and that target deficits in affective mechanisms regarding mental health-related outcomes as a potential means for reducing suicide risk (61).

With respect to practical implications derived from our findings, interventions on EI might be useful in order to increase individuals' set of adaptive emotion regulation strategies (29). The development of emotional abilities might help to increase perceived social support that, in turn, is related to lower barriers regarding help seeking behaviors (5, 62). In this context, prevention programs including EI training would be relevant for individuals in obtaining support from available services [e.g., (55)]. Given the potential value of preventive intervention programmes aiming at increasing access to mental health services (12), this line of research merits serious attention. In addition to intervention programmes targeting classic precursors of suicide such as mood dysregulation (12, 63), EI training might help individuals breaking the cycle of increasingly negative and constricted negative thinking linked to risk of suicide (19, 63). Furthermore, complementary interventions through occupational or academic training programmes might increase positive emotional states and, hence, the development of physical, social and psychological resources (58, 60). In sum, our findings open the door to future practical implications with the aim of helping individuals build a system of resiliency to sources of academic and occupational stress that might lead to impaired health risk of suicide (58).

CONCLUSION

The present work provided evidence on the mediating role of psychological distress in the association between self-report EI and suicide risk across samples (community sample and college students) using both cross-sectional and prospective designs. To the best of our knowledge, no study have been conducted to test the prospective effects of EI on suicide risk nor the explanatory mechanism by which EI may prevent suicidal thoughts and behaviors.

These findings provide preliminary evidence for the crucial role of self-report emotional abilities in reducing suicidal thoughts and behaviors via reduced psychological distress. Nonetheless, much research is needed to examine the influence of mediating and moderating factors involved in this complex association. Given the alarming prevalence of suicide as a complex public health concern, this line of research linking emotional processing with health-related outcomes requires further attention.

ETHICS STATEMENT

Since the Spanish law does not impose the requirements of ethics approval nor written informed consent in case of self-report and anonymous research carried out with healthy subjects, ethics approval was not needed in the present research. Nonetheless, participants were fully informed about the voluntary and anonymous basis of participation. In addition, they were fully aware that by completing the questionnaires they were in fact providing informed consent to use this data in the present research.

AUTHOR CONTRIBUTIONS

SM-L, NE, and LR are responsible for study conception, design and implementation, data analyses and interpretation. All the authors worked on the first draft of the work, reviewed, and approved the final manuscript.

REFERENCES

1. Cheavens JS, Cukrowicz KC, Hansen R, Mitchell SM. Incorporating resilience factors into the interpersonal theory of suicide: the role of hope and self-forgiveness in an older adult sample. *J Clin Psychol.* (2016) **72**:58–69. doi: 10.1002/jclp.22230
2. Fernández-Berrocal P, Extremera N. Ability emotional intelligence, depression, and well-being. *Emot Rev.* (2016) **8**:311–15. doi: 10.1177/1754073916650494
3. Martins A, Ramalho N, Morin E. A comprehensive meta-analysis of the relationship between emotional intelligence and health. *Pers Individ Differ.* (2010) **49**:554–64. doi: 10.1016/j.paid.2010.05.029
4. Hertel J, Schütz A, Lammers C. Emotional intelligence and mental disorder. *J Clin Psychol.* (2009) **65**:942–54. doi: 10.1002/jclp.20597
5. Mayer JD, Roberts RD, Barsade SG. Human abilities: emotional intelligence. *Annu Rev Psychol.* (2008) **59**:507–36. doi: 10.1146/annurev.psych.59.103006.093646
6. Miao C, Humphrey RH, Qian S. A meta-analysis of emotional intelligence and work attitudes. *J Occup Organ Psychol.* (2016) **90**:177–202. doi: 10.1111/joop.12167
7. Sánchez-Álvarez N, Extremera N, Fernández-Berrocal P. The relation between emotional intelligence and subjective well-being: a meta-analytic investigation. *J Posit Psychol.* (2016) **11**:276–85. doi: 10.1080/17439760.2015.1058968
8. Petrides KV, Pita R, Kokkinaki F. The location of trait emotional intelligence in personality factor space. *Br J Psychol.* (2007) **98**:273–89. doi: 10.1348/000712606X120618
9. Mayer JD, Caruso DR, Salovey P. The ability model of emotional intelligence: principles and updates. *Emot Rev.* (2016) **8**:290–300. doi: 10.1177/1754073916639667
10. Mayer JD, Salovey P. What is Emotional Intelligence? In: Salovey P, Sluyter D., editors *Emotional Development and Emotional Intelligence: Implications for Educators.* New York, NY: Basic Books (1997). p. 3–31.
11. Law KS, Wong CS, Song LJ. The construct and criterion validity of emotional intelligence and its potential utility for management studies. *J Appl Psychol.* (2004) **89**:483–96. doi: 10.1037/0021-9010.89.3.483
12. Turecki G, Brent D. Suicide and suicidal behaviour. *Lancet* (2016) **387**:1227–39. doi: 10.1016/S0140-6736(15)00234-2
13. Drum DJ, Brownson C, Burton Denmark A, Smith SE. New data on the nature of suicidal crises in college students: shifting the paradigm. *Prof Psychol-Res Pract.* (2009) **40**:213–22. doi: 10.1037/a0014465
14. Goldney RD, Wilson D, Dal Grande E, Fisher LJ, McFarlane AC. Suicidal ideation in a random community sample: attributable risk due to depression and psychosocial and traumatic events. *Aust N Z J Psych.* (2000) **34**:98–106. doi: 10.1046/j.1440-1614.2000.00646.x
15. Helson R, Soto CJ. Up and down in middle age: monotonic and nonmonotonic changes in roles, status, and personality. *J Pers Soc Psychol.* (2005) **89**:194–204. doi: 10.1037/0022-3514.89.2.194
16. Arria A, O'Grady K, Caldeira K, Vincent K, Wilcox H, Wish E. Suicide ideation among college students: a multivariate analysis. *Arch Suicide Res.* (2009) **13**:230–46. doi: 10.1080/13811110903044351
17. Mikolajczak M, Avalosse H, Vancorenland S, Verniest R, Callens M, Van Broeck N, et al. A nationally representative study of emotional competence and health. *Emotion* (2015) **15**:653–67. doi: 10.1037/emo0000034
18. Abdollahi A, Carlbring P, Khanbani M, Ghahfarokhi SA. Emotional intelligence moderates perceived stress and suicidal ideation among depressed adolescent inpatients. *Pers Individ Differ.* (2016) **102**:223–28. doi: 10.1016/j.paid.2016.07.015
19. Abdollahi A, Talib MA. Emotional intelligence as a mediator between rumination and suicidal ideation among depressed inpatients: the moderating role of suicidal history. *Psychiatry Res.* (2015) **228**:591–97. doi: 10.1016/j.psychres.2015.05.046
20. Aradilla-Herrero A, Tomás-Sábado J, Gómez-Benito J. Associations between emotional intelligence, depression and suicide risk in nursing students. *Nurse Educ Today* (2014) **34**:520–25. doi: 10.1016/j.nedt.2013.07.001
21. Ciarrochi J, Deane FP, Anderson S. Emotional intelligence moderates the relationship between stress and mental health. *Pers Individ Differ.* (2002) **32**:197–209. doi: 10.1016/S0191-8869(01)00012-5
22. Extremera N, Rey L. Attenuating the negative impact of unemployment: the interactive effects of perceived emotional intelligence and well-being on suicide risk. *PLoS ONE* (2016) **11**:e0163656. doi: 10.1371/journal.pone.0163656
23. Cha CB, Nock MK. Emotional intelligence is a protective factor for suicidal behavior. *J Am Acad Child Adolesc.* (2009) **48**:422–30. doi: 10.1097/CHI.0b013e3181984f44

24. Paradiso S, Beadle JN, Raymont V, Grafman J. Suicidal thoughts and emotion competence. *J Clin Exp Neuropsychol.* (2016) **38**:887–99. doi: 10.1080/13803395.2016.1172558
25. Verrocchio MC, Carrozzino D, Marchetti D, Andreasson K, Fulcheri M, Bech P. Mental pain and suicide: a systematic review of the literature. *Front Psychiatry* (2016) **7**:108. doi: 10.3389/fpsyt.2016.00108
26. Blüml V, Kapusta ND, Doering S, Brähler E, Wagner B, Kersting A. Personality factors and suicide risk in a representative sample of the German general population. *PLoS ONE* (2013) **8**:e76646. doi: 10.1371/journal.pone.0076646
27. Zhang Y, Law CK, Yip PSF. Psychological factors associated with the incidence and persistence of suicidal ideation. *J Affect Disord.* (2011) **133**:584–90. doi: 10.1016/j.jad.2011.05.003
28. Karim J, Shah SH. Ability emotional intelligence predicts quality of life beyond personality, affectivity, and cognitive intelligence. *Appl Res Qual Life* (2014) **9**:733–47. doi: 10.1007/s11482-013-9267-1
29. Peña-Sarrionandia A, Mikolajczak M, Gross JJ. Integrating emotion regulation and emotional intelligence traditions: A meta-analysis. *Front Psychol.* (2015) **6**:160. doi: 10.3389/fpsyg.2015.00160
30. Law KC, Khazem LR, Anestis MD. The role of emotion dysregulation in suicide as considered through the ideation to action framework. *Curr Opin Psychol.* (2015) **3**:30–5. doi: 10.1016/j.copsyc.2015.01.014
31. You J, Deng B, Lin MP, Leung F. The Interactive effects of impulsivity and negative emotions on adolescent nonsuicidal self-injury: a latent growth curve analysis. *Suicide Life-Threat Behav.* (2016) **46**:266–83. doi: 10.1111/sltb.12192
32. Klonsky ED, May AM, Glenn CR. The relationship between nonsuicidal self-injury and attempted suicide: converging evidence from four samples. *J Abnorm Psychol.* (2013) **122**:231–7. doi: 10.1037/a0030278
33. Zeidner M, Matthews G, Roberts RD. The emotional intelligence, health, and well-being nexus: what have we learned and what have we missed? *Appl Psychol -Health Well Being* (2012) **4**:1–30. doi: 10.1111/j.1758-0854.2011.01062.x
34. Extremera N, Rey L. The moderator role of emotion regulation ability in the link between stress and well-being. *Front Psychol.* (2015) **6**:1632. doi: 10.3389/fpsyg.2015.01632
35. Wong C-S, Law KS. The effects of leader and follower emotional intelligence on performance and attitude: an exploratory study. *Leadership Q.* (2002) **13**:243–74. doi: 10.1016/S1048-9843(02)00099-1
36. Wong C-S, Wong P-M, Peng KZ. Effect of middle-level leader and teacher emotional intelligence on school teachers' job satisfaction: the case of Hong Kong. *Educ Manag Adm Leadersh.* (2010) **38**:59–70. doi: 10.1177/1741143209351831
37. Lovibond SH, Lovibond PF. *Manual for the Depression Anxiety Stress Scales.* 2nd ed. Sydney, NSW: Psychology Foundation (1995).
38. Bados A, Solanas A, Andrés R. Psychometric properties of the Spanish version of depression, anxiety and stress scales (DASS). *Psicothema* (2005) **17**:679–83. Available online at: http://www.redalyc.org/html/727/72717423/
39. Henry JD, Crawford JR. The short-form version of the Depression Anxiety Stress Scales (DASS-21): construct validity and normative data in a large non-clinical sample. *Br J Clin Psychol.* (2005) **44**:227–39. doi: 10.1348/014466505X29657
40. Osman A, Wong JL, Bagge CL, Freedenthal S, Gutierrez PM, Lozano G. The depression anxiety stress scales-21 (DASS-21): further examination of dimensions, scale reliability, and correlates. *J Clin Psychol.* (2012) **68**:1322–38. doi: 10.1002/jclp.21908
41. Osman A, Bagge CL, Gutierrez PM, Konick LC, Kopper BA, Barrios FX. (2001). The suicidal behaviors questionnaire-revised (SBQ-R): validation with clinical and nonclinical samples. *Assessment* (2001) **8**:443–54. doi: 10.1177/107319110100800409
42. Cohen J. A power primer. *Psychol Bull.* (1992) **112**:155–59. doi: 10.1037/0033-2909.112.1.155
43. Hayes AF. *An Introduction to Mediation, Moderation, and Conditional Process Analysis: A Regression-Based Approach.* New York, NY: Guilford Press (2013).
44. Fernández-Abascal EG, Martín-Díaz MD. Dimensions of emotional intelligence related to physical and mental health and to health behaviors. *Front Psychol.* (2015) **6**:317. doi: 10.3389/fpsyg.2015.00317
45. Rajappa K, Gallagher M, Miranda R. Emotion dysregulation and vulnerability to suicidal ideation and attempts. *Cogn Ther Res.* (2012) **36**:833–39. doi: 10.1007/s10608-011-9419-2
46. Lazarus R. *Stress and Emotion: A New Synthesis.* New York, NY: Springer (1999).
47. Salovey P, Bedell BT, Detweiler JB, Mayer JD. Coping intelligently: emotional intelligence and the coping process. In: Snyder CR, editor. *Coping: The Psychology of what works.* New York, NY: Oxford University Press (1999). p. 141–64.
48. Conway JM, Lance CE. What reviewers should expect from authors regarding common method bias in organizational research. *J Bus Psychol.* **25**:325–34. doi: 10.1007/s10869-010-9181-6
49. Goldenberg I, Matheson K, Mantler J. The assessment of emotional intelligence: a comparison of performance-based and self-report methodologies. *J Pers Assess.* (2006) **86**:33–45. doi: 10.1207/s15327752jpa8601_05
50. Hirsch JK, Wolford K, LaLonde SM, Brunk L, Morris AP. Dispositional optimism as a moderator of the relationship between negative life events and suicide ideation and attempts. *Cogn Ther Res.* (2007) **31**:533–46. doi: 10.1007/s10608-007-9151-0
51. Cuijpers P, Smit F. Subthreshold depression as a risk indicator for major depressive disorder: a systematic review of prospective studies. *Acta Psychiatr Scand.* (2004) **109**:325–31. doi: 10.1111/j.1600-0447.2004.00301.x
52. Nolen-Hoeksema S. (2012). Emotion regulation and psychopathology: the role of gender. *Annu Rev Clin Psychol.* (2012) **8**:161–87. doi: 10.1146/annurev-clinpsy-032511-143109
53. Han K-M, Chang J, Won E, Lee M-S, Ham B-J. Precarious employment associated with depressive symptoms and suicidal ideation in adult wage workers. *J Affect Disord.* (2017) **218**:201–09. doi: 10.1016/j.jad.2017.04.049
54. Beath AP, Jones MP, Fitness J. Predicting distress via emotion regulation and coping: measurement variance in trait EI scales. *Pers Individ Differ.* (2015) **84**:45–51. doi: 10.1016/j.paid.2014.12.015
55. Farabaugh A, Bitran S, Nyer M, Holt DJ, Pedrelli P, Shyu I, et al. Depression and suicidal ideation in college students. *Psychopathology* (2012) **45**:228–34. doi: 10.1159/000331598
56. Hendricks VM, Blanken P. Snowball sampling: theoretical and practical considerations. In Hendricks VM, Blanken P, Adriaans N, editors. *Snowball Sampling: A Pilot Study on Cocaine Use.* Rotterdam:IVO (1992). p. 17–35.
57. Slaski M, Cartwright S. (2003). Emotional intelligence training and its implications for stress, health and performance. *Stress Health* (2003) **19**:233–39. doi: 10.1002/smi.979
58. Wingate LR, Burns AB, Gordon KH, Perez M, Walker RL, Williams FM, et al. Suicide and positive cognitions: positive psychology applied to the understanding and treatment of suicidal behavior. In Ellis TE, editor. *Cognition and Suicide: Theory, Research, and Therapy.* Washington, DC: American Psychological Association (2006). p. 261–83.
59. Salovey P, Rothman AJ, Detweiler JB, Steward WT. Emotional states and physical health. *Am Psychol.* (2000) **55**:110–21. doi: 10.1037/0003-066X.55.1.110
60. Hodzic S, Scharfen J, Ripoll P, Holling H, Zenasni F. How efficient are emotional intelligence trainings: a meta-analysis. *Emot Rev.* (2017). doi: 10.1177/1754073917708613. [Epub ahead of print].
61. Campo M, Laborde SJP, Weckemann S. Emotional Intelligence Training: Implications for Performance and Health. In: Columbus AM, editor. *Advances in Psychology Research.* New York, NY: Nova Science Publishers (2015). p. 75–92.
62. Aldrich RS. Suicide prevention: college students' intention to intervene. *Arch Suicide Res.* (2017) **21**:403–12. doi: 10.1080/13811118.2016.1211041
63. Catanzaro SJ. Mood regulation and suicidal behavior. In: Joiner T, Rudd MD, editors. *Suicide Science: Expanding the Boundaries.* New York, NY: Kluwer Academic Publishers (2002). p. 81–103.

8

Personality and Suicidal Behavior in Old Age

Anna Szücs[1,2], Katalin Szanto[2], Jean-Michel Aubry[1] and Alexandre Y. Dombrovski[2]*

[1] Department of Psychiatry, Faculty of Medicine, University of Geneva, Geneva, Switzerland, [2] Decision Neuroscience and Psychopathology Laboratory, Department of Psychiatry, School of Medicine, University of Pittsburgh, Pittsburgh, PA, United States

***Correspondence:**
Anna Szücs
anna.szuecs@etu.unige.ch,
szuecs.anna@gmail.com

Background: Suicide rates generally peak in the second half of life and are particularly high in older men; however, little is known about the contribution of dispositional factors to late-life suicide. Maladaptive personality traits have been strongly implicated in suicide among younger adults, but the extent to which they continue to play a role in late-life suicidal behavior is unclear. We also do not know whether specific personality profiles interact with the stressors of aging to cause suicidal behavior.

Methods: We sought to synthesize the data on personality pathology in late-life suicidal ideation and behavior *via* a systematic review using the PubMed, Google Scholar, PsycInfo, Scopus, Ovid, Web of Science, Embase, and Cochrane search engines. The included key words related to three descriptors: "personality," "suicide," and "elderly." Included articles evaluated personality based on the Five-Factor Model (FFM) or ICD/DSM diagnostic criteria in older samples with minimum age cutoffs of 50 years or older. Our original search identified 1,183 articles, of which 31 were retained.

Results: Included studies were heterogeneous in their design and personality measurements. Studies of categorical personality disorders were particularly scarce and suggested a stronger association with late-life suicidal ideation than with death by suicide. Only obsessive–compulsive and avoidant personality traits were associated with death by suicide in old age, but only in studies that did not control for depression. All personality constructs were positively linked to suicidal ideation, except for histrionic personality, which emerged as a negative predictor. Studies employing the FFM also indicated that older adults who died by suicide were less likely to display a maladaptive personality profile than elderly suicide attempters and younger suicide victims, having both lower levels of neuroticism and higher levels of conscientiousness than these comparison groups. Nevertheless, older suicide victims displayed lower levels of openness to experience than younger victims in two samples.

Conclusion: Maladaptive personality manifests in milder, subthreshold, and more heterogeneous forms in late-life vs. early-life suicide. An inability to adapt to the changes occurring in late life may help explain the association between suicide in old age and higher conscientiousness as well as obsessive–compulsive and avoidant personality disorders.

Keywords: aged, elderly, suicide, attempted suicide, suicidal ideation, personality, personality disorder, Five-Factor Model

INTRODUCTION

Rationale

There has been a continuous rise in suicide rates in the United States, increasing from 10.5 to 13 per 100,000 between 1999 and 2014 (1). Suicide rates peak after age 45 for both males and females, with the highest rates in the population found in older white men aged 85 or older, for whom rates are as high as 50.7 per 100,000 (2). The known risk factors for suicide in old age remain largely unspecific, however, giving us only a limited understanding of the psychological mechanisms involved. For example, depression, physical decline, family discord, social isolation, and financial issues are well-established risk factors for suicide (3–6), but they are also present in many older adults who never engage in suicidal behavior. According to the stress–diathesis model, suicidal individuals may possess lifelong traits of vulnerability, and it is the interaction between such traits and acute stressors that triggers suicidal behavior (7). Maladaptive personality traits are strongly implicated both with suicide among younger adults and with failure to cope with the stressors of aging (8–10). Thus, the stress–diathesis framework informs two questions. First, to what extent do the personality features implicated in suicide among younger adults confer suicide risk in old age? Second, what personality profiles are uniquely associated with late-life suicide by virtue of their interaction with the stressors of aging (e.g., physical decline)? We can even entertain the possibility of pleiotropic effects (11, 12) wherein traits that confer a reproductive advantage earlier in life could increase suicide risk in old age. To the best of our knowledge, in the existing literature, there is no consensus on these questions.

On the other hand, an association between personality disorders and suicidal behavior has been reported in most studies examining younger adults (13, 14). All personality disorders, with the exception of schizoid and histrionic, are associated with increased suicide risk in clinical or community-dwelling adult samples (14–18). Studies using dimensional models of personality also link both suicide attempts and death by suicide with high neuroticism and low extraversion, two traits that are also correlated with depression and broadly defined psychopathology (19–23). Borderline personality disorder (BPD) has been most strongly implicated in adult suicidal behavior, being linked to multiple attempts starting at an earlier age, and often mediated by impulsivity (14, 24, 25). However, externalizing aspects of BPD and impulsive traits specifically are most severe in young adulthood and tend to subside with age (26, 27). Moreover, in contrast to the high-impulsivity, lower-lethality suicidal behavior of younger age groups, the elderly tend to carry out fewer but higher-lethality suicidal acts, characterized by careful planning, and often occurring without warning signs (28, 29). These observations suggest that suicidal behavior in old age may be associated with personality profiles that are distinct from borderline and Cluster B pathology.

Objectives

This study aims to provide a comprehensive overview of the existing literature on the personality profiles of the suicidal elderly. Section "Results" first summarizes the characteristics of the studies, then reports data on personality pathology as a whole, and finally focuses separately on each DSM personality disorder and Five-Factor domain. Although the definition of personality can encompass *all individual differences in characteristic patterns of thinking, feeling, and behaving* (30), our theoretical focus on categorical personality disorders and the Big Five precluded us from reviewing studies that assessed other trait-like constructs, such as impulsivity or aggression. In this study, we considered behavior to be suicidal if it was self-injurious and enacted with intent to kill oneself, and suicidal ideation as thoughts of taking one's own life (31). These definitions do not include para-suicide or passive death wish. Even though ideation, attempt, and death by suicide are interconnected entities, they do not correspond to entirely identical clinical populations, since the majority of ideators will never attempt suicide (32), and the majority of attempters do not die by suicide (33). Supporting this view, distinct yet partially overlapping personality profiles have been found in adult suicide ideators and attempters (34–36). Thus, this review will address findings on death by suicide, attempted suicide, and suicidal ideation separately in each subsection.

Research Question

The question we sought to answer is whether elderly who engage in suicidal behavior display qualitatively different personality profiles compared to their younger counterparts. Given the abatement of externalizing behaviors with aging, including BPD symptoms, we hypothesized that the contribution of these traits to suicidal behavior will diminish in old age. Furthermore, we sought to clarify whether differences in personality profiles exist in the elderly between those with ideation exclusively, attempt, and death by suicide. Based on the findings in younger samples mentioned earlier, we expect to see an overall stronger association of dysfunctional personality with suicidal ideation than death by suicide, and moderate levels associated with attempted suicide.

METHODS

A systematic search was conducted using PubMed, Ovid, Embase, PsycInfo, Cochrane, Web of Science, Scopus, and Google Scholar by cross-referencing three descriptor fields with the following key words (**Figure 1**): personality (34 key words); suicide (5 key words); and elderly (7 key words). Key words were searched in title and abstract when possible, or else in abstract only (Ovid, PsycInfo), and finally in title only where none of the above were available (Google Scholar, Web of Science). In PubMed, where the added ability to use MeSH terms is available, we complemented our search formula with the following MeSH terms: "Personality/psychology," "Personality Disorders/psychology," "Human Characteristics," and "Impulsive Behavior" were added to the descriptor *personality*, "suicide" was added to the descriptor *suicide* and "aged" to the descriptor *elderly*. In Embase, search terms were both used as free text and mapped on Emtree terms. Reference tracking was done on all included articles to check for additional publications that met inclusion. The search encompassed all articles published through January 31, 2017, with no beginning time limit and no restrictions on publication status. Our methodology and inclusion criteria

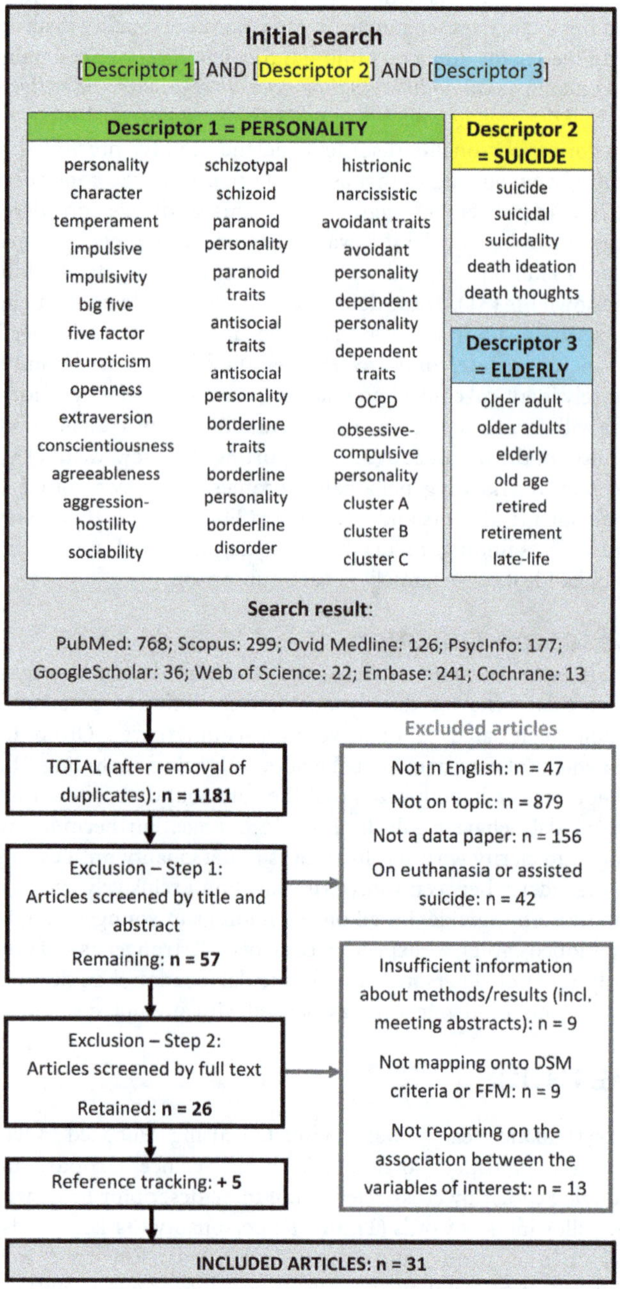

FIGURE 1 | Flow diagram of the studies retrieved for the review. The key words under each descriptor were separated by "OR" for the search. On PubMed, corresponding MeSH terms were added to each descriptor field: Personality, Personality Disorders, Human Characteristics and Impulsive Behavior to Descriptor 1; Suicide to Descriptor 2, and Aged to Descriptor 3. Abbreviation: FFM, Five-Factor Model.

were defined and documented at the beginning of the project. Publications were included if written in English and describing a research study. In addition, articles had to report an assessment of personality specifically, related to any combination of death by suicide, attempted suicide and suicidal ideation. The suicidal behavior/ideation described could not pertain to assisted suicide or euthanasia. Personality had to be assessed *via*, or map onto the Five-Factor Model (FFM) or DSM/ICD personality constructs. Studies where personality was not reported separately from other psychiatric diagnoses were excluded, as were all studies not distinguishing between older adults and other age groups, or between suicidal behavior and para-suicide. Older age was defined as equal to or above 50 years. Finally, included articles had to contain sufficient data to evaluate the quality of their findings (e.g., this was not the case for meeting abstracts). In addition to these initial criteria, we later refined the definition of research study to those having a minimum *N* of 20 to exclude case reports and small qualitative studies oversampling clinically illustrative cases with weakly generalizable data. The first author, AS, performed the initial screening and then reviewed eligibility of potentially includable articles with AD based on their full text. Of the 1,181 articles found, 1,124 were excluded during the initial screening for one of the following reasons: not written in English (47 articles), not on topic (including all articles about para-suicide/deliberate self-harm; 879 articles), not a data paper (156 articles), having a euthanasia/assisted suicide focus (42 articles). From the 57 remaining articles, further 31 were excluded based on their full text, either because they contained an insufficient amount of information about methods or results (9 articles), were not mapping onto DSM or FFM personality constructs (9 articles), or were not reporting on the association between personality and suicidal behavior/ideation in the elderly (13 articles). Twenty-six articles were retained for the review, and five more were found by reference tracking.

RESULTS

Study Characteristics

General Characteristics

Of the 31 included articles (**Tables 1–4**), one was from 1976 (37), and all others were published after 1990, with seven articles between 1990 and 2000 (38–44), 13 articles between 2001 and 2010 (45–57), and 10 articles between 2011 and 2016 (58–67). The association between personality and either death by suicide, attempted suicide or suicidal ideation was the primary outcome in 18 articles (39, 41, 43, 45, 46, 48, 50, 51, 53–56, 59, 61, 63, 65–67), while the other 13 articles reported on personality in relation to a different study focus (37, 38, 40, 42, 44, 47, 49, 52, 57, 58, 60, 62, 64). Except for one qualitative study on death by suicide (56) (displayed in **Table 2**), all studies were quantitative. Five studies followed a purely descriptive design, without control groups (40, 42, 50, 52, 56), and only nine of the remaining studies included non-suicidal psychiatric controls (39, 43, 44, 46–48, 51, 53, 57). Seventeen articles reported categorical personality disorder diagnoses (**Tables 1–3**), and 14 measured dimensional personality traits (**Tables 4** and **5**), while one article utilized both (displayed in both **Tables 2** and **4**) (59). Dimensional measures were used in an increasing fraction of articles over time: in 8/21 articles between 1976 and 2010 versus 6/10 from 2011 to 2016.

Age Cutoffs

Age cutoffs ranged from 50 to 75 years, with a majority of studies including either participants aged 60 years (11 articles) or 65 years

(12 articles) and older. Only one study had an age cutoff as high as 75 years (61). Mean age was, however, above 70 years in 17/24 articles where these data were available (several studies indicated the percentage of elderly subjects in different age subgroups without reporting a global value for mean age).

Personality Measures

Even though 17 articles reported on categorical personality disorders, findings about specific personality diagnoses remained scarce in death by suicide and attempted suicide: 6/17 studies reported only global data on personality disorders (38–40, 44, 52, 57), and two others solely specified BPD in addition to total personality disorders (42, 58) (**Table 1**). Of the remaining nine publications, findings on death by suicide were reported in three articles (37, 45, 50), two of which were based on the same study (**Table 2**). No article assessed distinct personality disorders in attempted suicide. Suicidal ideation was assessed by six studies (47, 53, 59, 65–67), of which four were based on the same population (community-dwelling older adults in Colorado, USA) (**Table 3**). One study on suicidal ideation focused exclusively on narcissistic personality disorder (53).

Of the 14 articles measuring dimensional personality traits (**Table 4**), two based their findings on the Eysenck Personality Model, assessing only Neuroticism in one case (64), and Neuroticism and Extroversion in the other (61). Based on the reasonable levels of correlation established by Costa and McCrae between Eysenck's Neuroticism and Extroversion and the Five-Factor neuroticism and extraversion domains (68), we considered these constructs equivalent when reporting results. All other studies used the FFM. Most of them exclusively included results for the five main factors, however, 6/14 articles reported findings on the facet level. Subcomponents derived from the NEO-FFI (NEO Five Factor Inventory) such as *negative emotions*, were interpreted together with the most highly correlated facets derived from the NEO-PI-R (NEO Personality Inventory Revised), in this case, *anxiety* (69). Three studies with facet-level analyses focused only on specific sets of facets (46, 54, 62). Overall, five articles provided dimensional data on death by suicide (41, 49, 55, 60, 63), seven on attempted suicide (43, 46, 48, 49, 55, 61, 62), and six others on suicidal ideation (43, 48, 51, 54, 59, 64). Four articles reported on multiple suicidal outcomes (43, 48, 49, 55). Two articles reported findings based on the same study (60, 63). Seven out of the 14 studies based on dimensional models had overlapping samples (elderly patients recruited in the teaching hospitals of the University of Rochester, NY, USA), and two others shared a recruitment source (community-dwelling older adults in Colorado, USA) (**Table 4**). The dimensional findings, however, came from at least three different sample sources for each suicidal outcome (death, attempt, and ideation).

Definition of Death by Suicide, Attempted Suicide, and Suicidal Ideation

Not surprisingly, older suicide victims were the most uniformly defined study group, with the obvious inclusion criterion being death by suicide occurring in old age. One study comparing individuals who died by suicide to older attempters also excluded suicide victims with a lifetime history of attempt (55).

While most articles did not define suicide attempt, two studies reportedly used the definition of the World Health Organization (57, 61): "Those situations in which a person has performed a life-threatening act with the intent of putting his or her life into danger or giving the appearance of such an intent" (70). Other studies defined suicide attempts as any intentional self-destructive act, without necessitating an expressed intent to die, blurring the line between suicide and para-suicide (40, 46, 48). Most studies used the presence of lifetime attempt history to define their attempters, whereas others necessitated a recent attempt, only including older individuals from either inpatient or emergency units (38, 44, 49, 57, 61, 62). In 4/6 of these cases, history of prior attempts was either controlled for statistically (49, 57) or excluded from the control group (61, 62).

Some studies included passive death wish in their definition of suicidal ideation (43, 51). Further adding to the samples' heterogeneity, studies of elderly suicide ideators neither excluded nor controlled for subjects with past history of suicide attempts. Thus, findings about suicide ideators should be interpreted with caution, since they reflect more a global suicidal risk than pure suicidal contemplation.

Correlates and Possible Mediators

Gender

An established pattern in the literature is that men are more likely to die by suicide while women are more likely to have non-fatal attempts and subsequent mental health contact (71). Thus, a selection bias cannot be excluded in the 14 studies whose suicidal sample was exclusively recruited based on previous contact with psychiatric health services (37, 39, 40, 43, 44, 46–49, 51–53, 55, 57, 61, 62) as these studies might have oversampled women. While personality pathology increased with late-life suicidal behavior in both genders in most studies, several reported a higher female to male ratio. Lawrence and colleagues found a fivefold higher rate ratio in females with personality pathology than in males for both attempted suicide and death by suicide (44). Qin, whose population study assessed psychiatric illness *via* the last hospitalization-based principal diagnosis, also reported a threefold higher prevalence of personality pathology in female versus male suicides (58). Not supporting these findings, one case–control study, with separate regression models for elderly male and female attempters, reported that neuroticism was a significant, positive predictor in men but not in women (62). In addition, the Lausanne Study indicated a 1.3 male to female ratio for the prevalence of suicide in former inpatients with personality disorders (37), and Harwood and colleagues' psychological autopsy study did not find a significant gender difference in personality disorder rates (45). The majority of case–control studies included in the review controlled for the potential effect of gender, with only four that did not, or for which this information was missing (40, 47, 65, 66).

Depressive Disorders

Depressive disorders in old age have been separately associated with both suicidal behavior (28, 72), and personality disorders (9, 73). Personality disorders co-occur in 10–30% of depressed elderly, with Cluster C disorders being the most frequent and

Cluster B disorders the rarest (9). Patients with personality disorders were found to be up to four times more likely to suffer from the persistence or the re-emergence of depressive symptoms (39, 47) and were younger at first onset (39). Morse and Lynch found that the presence and not the severity of personality pathology was correlated with poor prognosis of depressive symptoms in the elderly (47). Of the studies included in this review, only 4/12 studies of death by suicide (49, 55, 58, 60) and 7/12 of suicidal ideation (43, 47, 48, 51, 53, 54, 65) controlled for depression when evaluating the relationship between personality and suicide risk. Studies of attempted suicide were more diligent in this regard, their recruitment source most often being pools of depressed patients. Only one comparative study on attempted suicide lacked any form of adjustment for depressive disorders (44). In 143 older primary care patients, Jahn and colleagues found that depressive symptoms mediated the effect of pathological personality traits on suicidal ideation (65). While none of the studies investigated whether depressive symptoms mediate the effect of personality disorders on suicidal behavior, Nieto and colleagues found that personality disorders occurred independently of all Axis-I diagnoses in 5.2% of older adults aged 65 or above who made a medically serious suicide attempt ($N = 38$) (38).

Interpersonal Functioning

Impaired interpersonal functioning is the core feature of personality disorders and a risk factor for suicidal behavior in late-life (74). It is therefore expected to explain the effect of personality pathology on suicidal behavior and ideation. Kunik and colleagues found that depressed inpatients were more likely to be single, separated or divorced if they were diagnosed with a comorbid Axis-II disorder (39). In light of the finding that older adults most often tend to give warning signs about their suicidal intent to their next-of-kin (75), it may be particularly difficult for socially isolated elderly to reach out for help when needed. Conceptualizing the question from the perspective of the interpersonal theory of suicide, Jahn and colleagues identified perceived burdensomeness and thwarted belongingness as mediators between personality disorders and suicidal ideation in older adults aged 65 years or over ($N = 143$) (65). However, Eades found a direct relationship of pathological personality traits and suicidal ideation that was stronger than through either thwarted belongingness or perceived burdensomeness in a community sample of 102 individuals aged 60 or above (67).

Environmental Stressors

The longitudinal findings of the Lausanne Study suggest higher late-life suicide rates in psychiatric patients who displayed a "specific vulnerability to environmental stress, evident already years ago during their first admission" (37). Harwood and colleagues investigated personality traits in a subsample of individuals who died by suicide and did not have a psychiatric diagnosis ($N = 23$). Their findings indicated that personality trait accentuation was present in 44% of suicide victims, often concomitantly with recent life events that were thought to have triggered the suicidal act (50). Consistent with Mann's stress–diathesis model of suicide, these findings support the presence of an increased chronic vulnerability that is exacerbated by negative life events in older individuals with already subclinical levels of personality pathology (7).

Synthesized Findings

Prevalence of Any Personality Disorder in Late-Life Suicide

A psychological autopsy by Harwood and colleagues and a retrospective cohort study by Henriksson and colleagues estimated that respectively, 14 and 16%, of adults who died by suicide after the age of 60 had personality disorders (42, 45). These rates are somewhat higher than the 10% community prevalence of personality disorders in adults above 50 years reported by a meta-analysis (76), but the difference remains small considering possible confounding with other psychopathology. Including only principal diagnoses in their analysis, Hunt and colleagues' and Qin's population studies found a much lower prevalence of personality disorders in late-life suicide victims, namely between 1.5 and 5% (52, 58). However, these latter findings are likely less accurate since personality disorders are rarely considered principal diagnoses in this age group (42). Examining personality trait accentuation in addition to personality disorders, Harwood and colleagues' psychological autopsy study found that subthreshold accentuated personality traits were present in 28% of older adults who died by suicide ($N = 100$) (45). Thus, altogether, 44% of the suicide victims in Harwood and colleagues' sample had some level of personality pathology.

Despite these relatively high rates of pathological personality disorders and traits in late-life suicide, all studies with younger comparison groups found decreasing prevalence of personality pathology with age (42, 52, 57, 58). The prevalence of any personality disorder was reported to be 2.4 and 2.6 times lower, respectively, in elderly suicide victims aged 60 or above (42), and suicide attempters aged 55 or above (57) than in the younger comparison groups. Both Hunt and colleagues and Harwood and colleagues found that the prevalence of personality disorders further decreased between 60 and 75 years of age in elderly suicide victims (respectively, from 4.0 to 2.3% for personality disorders as primary diagnoses and from 19.7 to 10.6% at any detectable level) (45, 52).

This significant decrease in older people may be due to the attenuation of symptoms of certain commonly diagnosed personality disorders such as BPD, and/or to a survival bias related to increased premature mortality due to personality pathology. Furthermore, a detection bias is likely in old age given that personality disorders may be masked by overlapping cognitive deficits in a subset of older patients seeking psychiatric care (77). In turn, suicidal behavior may also be under-detected in old age: studies highlighted a decreased number of psychiatric hospitalizations of older adults, both before dying by suicide (58), and after a suicide attempt (44). This may be in part related to diagnostic biases. Indeed, comorbid cognitive deficits, delirium or other organic conditions often lead to medical rather than psychiatric hospitalizations in the elderly with decompensated psychopathology (78); primary health care providers have been found less likely to assess psychopathology in older adults than in younger patients (79); suicidal and death ideation are perceived as part of normal aging by many clinicians (80); and social isolation can cause low-lethality suicide attempts to go unnoticed.

Association of Personality Disorder Diagnosis With Suicidal Behavior and Ideation in the Elderly

Death by Suicide

A positive correlation between personality pathology and death by suicide was supported by most studies, although none were designed to separate unique contributions of personality disorders from those of other types of psychopathology. Harwood and colleagues found both personality disorders and traits being more frequent in a subsample of 54 elderly suicide cases compared to age- and sex-matched controls deceased from natural causes (45). Qin determined a respectively sixfold and ninefold higher prevalence of personality disorders in older females and males who died by suicide compared to general population controls (58). In a sample of psychiatric patients aged 60 years or older, Lawrence and colleagues found that personality disorders had the fifth highest suicide rate among all principal psychiatric diagnoses in the elderly, which was more than twofold higher than in the age-matched general population of Western Australia (risk ratio of 2.1, $n = 447$) (44). A single longitudinal study examined the prevalence of suicide in individuals with severe personality disorders: the Lausanne Study was conducted in Switzerland from 1963 to investigate aging in all former psychiatric inpatients of the Lausanne University Psychiatric Hospital (N = 5,661). The investigator found that personality disorders were the third

TABLE 1 | Studies with categorical measures reporting globally on personality disorders.

	Study	Sample	Age (years)	PD assessment	Summary of results
Death by suicide	Henriksson et al., 1995 (42) Finland Retrospective cohort study, descriptive	229 suicides of which 43 older suicides	≥60	Interviews with relatives and doctor (DSM-III-R)	*Prevalence of PDs in elderly*: suicide victims: 14%; younger suicides: 34%
	Hunt et al., 2006 (52) England and Wales National clinical survey, descriptive	41,959 suicides of which 597 older suicides	≥65	Retrospective diagnosis by consultant psychiatrist (ICD-10)	*Suicides with PD*: 19% (<25 years) 15.3% (25–34 years) 10.8% (35–44 years) 7.8% (45–54 years) 3.3% (55–64 years) 4.0% (65–74 years) 2.3% (≥75 years)
	Qin, 2011 (58) Denmark Population study, retrospective	1,169 suicides (4,175 older) 4,231,219 population controls (193,251 older)	>60	Coded medical records (ICD-10)	*Prevalence of PDs as principal diagnoses*: Suicides: M: 1.5%, F: 4.8% Controls: M: 0.2%, F: 0.5%
Suicide and attempt	Lawrence et al., 2000 (44) Western Australia Hospitalization-based population study, retrospective	447 suicides 1,596 attempted suicides Control values: population distribution	≥60	Medical records (ICD-9)	*PD rate ratios*: Suicide: M: 2.3, F: 12.3 Attempt: M: 2.4, F: 11.8 *Risk ratio (proportional hazards regression of PDs as risk factors)*: Suicide: 2.1 Attempt: 10.2
Attempted suicide	Nieto et al., 1992 (38) Spain, Barcelona Retrospective comparative study	257 suicide attempters with medically serious attempts of which 38 elderly	≥65	Medical records (DSM-III-R)	*PDs with no Axis-I comorbidities in attempters aged ≥65*: 5.2% *All PDs in three attempter age groups*: ≥65 years (n = 38): 6 (15.8%) 31–64 years (n = 120): 25 (21.8%) 0–30 years (n = 99): 45 (45.5%) Oldest group different from youngest group (p = 0.003)
	Kunik et al., 1993 (39) USA (PA) Case–control study, cross-sectional	143 patients with major depression of which 37 with PD	≥60	Consensus conference (DSM-III-R)	*History of attempts*: patients with PD: 35% depressed controls: 20% *Correlation (attempts-PD)*: $\chi^2(1) = 3.8, p = 0.06$
	Draper, 1994 (40) Sydney, Australia Retrospective cohort study	69 attempted suicides	≥65	Medical records (DSM-III/III-R, ICD-9)	*Any PD diagnosis*: 26% as secondary diagnosis
	Miret et al., 2010 (57) Madrid, Spain Hospitalization-based population study, cross-sectional	1,970 attempted suicides, from which 113 late-life attempts	≥55	Medical records (ICD-9)	*Prevalence of PDs as principal diagnoses*: Older attempters: n = 10 (8.8%) Younger attempters: n = 171 (22.6%)

PD, personality disorder, M, males, F, females.

most common baseline psychopathology after mood disorders and alcohol dependence among the 107 suicides that were carried out by patients between 57 and 77 years of age (37). The prevalence of suicide in the subgroup of patients with personality disorders was 6.8% in males and 5.4% in females (n = 266), respectively, more than threefold and fivefold higher than in the age- and gender-matched general population. However, the severe pathology that triggered hospitalizations in this group of patients precludes generalization of these findings to personality disorders observed in the community.

Attempted Suicide

Examining only primary diagnoses, Miret and colleagues reported a prevalence of 8.8% for personality disorders in hospitalized patients aged 50 and older who had made a recent suicide attempt (N = 113) (57). Draper found a higher prevalence (26%) considering secondary diagnoses mentioned in the hospital records of 69 attempters aged 65 or above (40). In addition, Nieto and colleagues reported that personality disorders were present without comorbid Axis-I disorders in 5.2% of 38 older adults aged 65 or above who made a medically serious suicide attempt (38). This fraction was lower than in young attempters (30 or younger) from the same study (45.5%, p = 0.003), but did not differ significantly from middle-aged attempters (31–65 years) (21.8%). Lawrence and colleagues reported a risk ratio of 10.2 for suicide attempts given a principal diagnosis of personality disorder (n = 1,596), almost five times higher than the 2.1 risk ratio for death by suicide (44). Examining psychiatric patients with personality disorders (n = 37), Kunik and colleagues found a 35% lifetime prevalence of attempted suicide. This prevalence, however, was not significantly different from the 20% seen in the clinical control group without personality disorders [$n = 117; \chi^2(1) = 3.76, p = 0.06$] (39).

Suicidal Ideation

Studies found a positive association with suicidal ideation and almost all categories of pathological personality traits in late life, with the exception of histrionic and sadistic traits (47, 59, 65–67). None of these studies, however, excluded suicide ideators with a past history of attempt. No correlation was found between the severity of pathological personality traits and the severity of suicidal ideation (47).

ICD/DSM Personality Disorders in Late-Life Suicide

Using ICD-8 personality diagnoses the abovementioned Lausanne Study found that neurotic and psychopathic (antisocial) personality disorders were the most prevalent in former

TABLE 2 | Categorical findings on separate personality disorder diagnoses in death by suicide, and qualitative findings.

	Study	Sample	Age (years)	PD assessment	Summary of results
DSM/ICD	Harwood et al., 2001 (45) England Psychological autopsy study; case–control study in a subsample	100 elderly suicides 54 included in case–control part Controls: 54 age- and gender-matched natural deaths	≥60	Informants (ICD-10)	*Prevalence of PD*: Suicides: 14.8%, controls: 3.7% *Prevalence of PD trait accentuation*: Suicides: 33.3%, controls: 13% *PDs (n = 16)*: Anankastic (n = 4); dissocial (n = 4); histrionic (n = 4); other (n = 3); mixed (n = 5) *PD trait accentuation (n = 28)*: Anankastic n = 19; anxious n = 13; dependent n = 9; histrionic n = 6; other n = 10 *Case–control part*: Correlation with suicide (Fisher's exact test): Anankastic traits: p = 0.012 Anxious traits: p = 0.015
	Harwood et al., 2006 (50) England Psychological autopsy study, descriptive	23 suicides without ante-mortem psychiatric diagnoses No controls	≥60	Informants (ICD-10)	*PD (n = 1)*: dissocial (n = 1) *PD trait accentuation (n = 10):* Anankastic (n = 8); paranoid (n = 3)
	Ciompi, 1976 (37) Switzerland Longitudinal study in psychiatric patients	1,891 deaths between age 57 and 77 years, of which 266 patients with PD (14%) Control values: average population distribution	≥57	Medical records (psychodynamic nosology of the time)	*Patients with PD who died by suicide*: Of all male deaths = 13 (6.8%) Of all female deaths = 4 (5.4%) *Control values in general population*: Suicides out of male deaths = 1.8% Suicides out of female deaths = 0.7% *Most frequent PDs in suicides:* Psychopathic and neurotic PDs
Qualitative	Kjølseth et al., 2009 (56) Norway Qualitative psychological autopsy study	23 older suicide victims No controls	≥60	Qualitative interviews	*Life history*: hard-working achievers, source of help/advice for relatives *Personality traits*: stubborn, willing to do everything by themselves *Relationships*: introverted, distant or egoistic, with strong self-control

PD, personality disorder.

psychiatric patients who died by suicide after the age of 57 (37). In the psychodynamic nosology of the time, a "neurotic personality organization" included hysterical (i.e., histrionic), depressive-masochistic (best mapping onto self-defeating personality from DSM-III), obsessive (mapping onto obsessive–compulsive), as well as avoidant personalities (81). These findings support a role of Clusters B and C in late-life suicide, which is consistent with the more recent results detailed below. As mentioned, no study reported data on specific personality disorders and attempted suicide in the elderly.

Cluster A

Paranoid Personality Disorder. In Harwood and colleagues' secondary analysis of cases without an ante-mortem psychiatric diagnosis ($N = 23$), paranoid traits were the second most frequent (13%) (50). However, in the absence of a control group, this finding remains difficult to interpret given the relatively high prevalence of paranoid personality in the general population (2–5%) (82, 83).

There was nevertheless a positive correlation of suicidal ideation with paranoid personality in all studies that investigated it (47, 59, 65, 67).

Schizoid Personality Disorder. There is no evidence linking schizoid personality disorder to late-life suicide, in spite of the documented worsening of schizoid personality with aging (84). To the best of our knowledge, this disorder is not associated with suicidal behavior earlier in life either.

A positive correlation was however found in all studies investigating schizoid traits in suicidal ideation (47, 59, 65).

Schizotypal Personality Disorder. No evidence linked schizotypal personality disorder to late-life suicide.

Three studies, with possibly overlapping community samples recruited in Colorado, found a positive correlation with suicidal ideation (59, 65, 67); however, such a relationship was not confirmed by Morse and Lynch in a depressed sample with a different recruitment source (47).

Despite the high co-occurrence of schizotypal personality disorder with BPD in the general population (85, 86), its role in suicidal behavior remains also unclear earlier in life.

Cluster B

Antisocial (and Dissocial) Personality Disorder. Studies in younger adults have linked antisocial personality to suicide attempts (17, 87, 88) and death by suicide (18). Moreover, antisocial personality traits appear to persist, or only partially remit with increasing age in most individuals (89), suggesting a possible high suicide risk throughout the lifetime, yet data so far remain inconclusive. The Lausanne Study found a high prevalence of psychopathic (antisocial) personality disorder in former patients who died by suicide after the age of 57 (37). Harwood and colleagues found dissocial personality disorder to be among the three most prevalent personality disorders in their study, with 4% of suicide victims reaching full diagnostic criteria for it (45).

TABLE 3 | Categorical findings on suicidal ideation.

	Study	Sample	Age (years)	Assessment	Summary of results
DSM-IV-TR	Segal et al., 2012 (59) USA (CA) Cross-sectional	109 community-dwelling older adults evaluated for SI	≥65	SI scale: GSIS PD scale: Coolidge Axis-II Inventory	*Positive correlation with SI*: all PDs except histrionic *Positive predictor of SI*: borderline PD *Negative predictor of SI*: histrionic PD
	Segal et al., 2015 (66) USA (CA) Cross-sectional				*Positive correlation of SI with former PDs*: depressive PD
	Jahn et al., 2015 (65) USA (CA) Cross-sectional	143 community-dwelling older adults evaluated for SI	≥65	SI scale: GSIS PD scale: SCID-II-PQ	*Positive correlation with SI (in decreasing order)*: avoidant, schizotypal, depressive, borderline, schizoid, dependent, passive-aggressive, and paranoid personality traits *No significant correlation*: obsessive-compulsive, narcissistic, histrionic, and antisocial traits
	Eades et al., 2016 (67) USA (CA) Cross-sectional	102 community-dwelling older adults evaluated for SI	≥61	SI scale: GSIS PD scale: Coolidge Axis-II inventory	*Positive correlation with SI (in decreasing order)*: Depressive, schizoid, schizotypal, passive-aggressive, avoidant, paranoid, borderline, dependent, obsessive–compulsive, and self-defeating *No significant correlation*: histrionic, antisocial, sadistic
	Morse and Lynch, 2004 (47) USA Cross-sectional	63 depressed inpatients, from which 17 with PD	≥64	SI scale: ASIQ PD scale: WISPI	*SI*: no significant correlation with total personality disorders
DSM-III & -IV	Heisel et al., 2007 (53) Canada Cross-sectional, case–control study	538 depressed elderly; 20 with narcissistic PD (n = 13)/PD traits (n = 7)	≥65	SI scale: HRSD suicide item PD diagnosis: medical records	*Narcissistic PD*: positive predictor of SI *Narcissistic PD traits*: not significant predictors

PD, personality disorder; SI, suicidal ideation; GSIS, Geriatric Suicide Ideation Scale; SCID-II-PQ, Structured Clinical Interview for DSM-IV-TR Axis II—Personality Questionnaire; ASIQ, Adult Suicide Ideation Questionnaire; WISPI, Wisconsin Personality Disorders Inventory IV; HRSD, Hamilton Rating Scale for Depression.

However, in the case–control part of their study (n = 54), the prevalence of antisocial personality did not differ between suicide victims and controls.

While one study (59) found an association between antisocial traits and suicidal ideation in old age, three others did not (47, 65, 67).

Borderline (and Emotionally Labile) Personality Disorder (BPD). In spite of its important role in suicides earlier in life, BPD showed no significant association with death by suicide in old age. Moreover, two studies found a significantly lower prevalence of BPD in both elderly suicides and controls than in younger age groups (42, 58), which is unsurprising given that most features of BPD tend to remit with age (90).

However, all studies investigating suicidal ideation found a positive correlation with borderline personality traits (47, 59, 65, 67). Segal and colleagues also identified borderline traits as the only positive predictor of suicidal ideation in a community sample of 109 adults aged 60 or above (59).

As mentioned earlier, BPD in old age may be subject to a survival bias. In a 27-year long longitudinal study in BPD patients (N = 165), Paris and Zweig-Frank reported death by suicide in as many as 10.3% of their sample with a mean age at death of 37.2 years (91). Despite persisting problems with interpersonal functioning, the surviving cohort showed significant improvement, with only five patients meeting full criteria for BPD by the end of the follow-up. Although an increase in attempts' lethality with advancing age has been reported by Soloff and colleagues (87), Pompili and colleagues' meta-analysis of suicide in BPD found a higher incidence of suicides in short-term follow-ups, suggesting lower suicidal rates during the chronic phases of BPD (92). Overall, these findings suggest that suicide risk decays, albeit incompletely, in the borderline patients who survive to old age.

Histrionic Personality Disorder. Even though histrionic personality is considered to be only mildly impairing and not linked to major emotional disability in the general population (82), Harwood and colleagues found full diagnostic criteria for histrionic personality disorder in 4 out of 100 individuals who died by suicide. Moreover, they found subthreshold histrionic traits in six others, making this personality construct the third most frequent in their sample, and the most prevalent Cluster B disorder (45). As discussed earlier, hysterical (former version of histrionic) disorder was also associated with suicides in the Lausanne Study (37).

These findings contrast with the absence of positive correlation found between suicidal ideation in old age and histrionic personality (47, 59, 65, 67). This disorder was in fact the only negative predictor of suicidal ideation in Segal and colleagues' study (59), corroborating a potential protective impact on suicide risk.

In younger adults, a protective effect of comorbid histrionic personality disorder was found in an adult sample of female attempters with BPD (93).

Narcissistic Personality Disorder. To date, no definite association has been found between narcissistic personality disorder and death by suicide in old age. However, in a qualitative psychological autopsy study conducted by Kjølseth and colleagues with the informants of 23 elderly who died between 65 and 90 years of age in Norway, the majority of suicide victims were described as self-centered over-achievers, with a need to control others, sometimes despite generating conflicts due to their authoritarianism (56).

Narcissistic personality disorder was positively correlated with late-life suicidal ideation in all studies (47, 59, 67) but one (65). In addition, it was a predictor of suicidal ideation in a retrospective database analysis specifically focusing on narcissistic personality in adults aged 65 years and older (N = 538) (53).

Narcissistic personality disorder has been identified as a risk factor for suicide in middle-aged adults by a 10-year long longitudinal study reporting a positive correlation between narcissistic personality and number of suicide attempts in a clinical sample of 431 middle-aged adults (aged 18–45 years upon enrollment) (15). In the clinical literature, Kernberg also implicated pathological narcissism in existential crises in the second half of life (94). He discussed how suicide may appeal to narcissistic patients as a means of relieving guilt over past mistakes or missed opportunities for greatness, as "external reality gradually demonstrates [that their grandiose] fantasies are no longer viable." This risk may likely persist after age 50. However, the low general prevalence of narcissistic personality disorder, estimated at 0.8% (83), suggests that higher-powered studies are needed to detect a potential association.

Cluster C

Avoidant (and Anxious) Personality Disorder. Despite an absence of subjects meeting full criteria for anxious personality disorder, Harwood and colleagues found a higher rate of anxious personality trait accentuation in suicide victims than in natural death controls, with 13% of suicide victims displaying anxious traits (45).

Furthermore, avoidant personality disorder was positively correlated with suicidal ideation in all studies (47, 59, 65, 67).

Age-related social isolation is possibly more pronounced in avoidant individuals, as the traits related to social ineptitude were found among the disorder's most stable diagnostic criteria (95). Avoidant personality disorder in the elderly is also highly prevalent in dysthymic disorder (73), an independent risk factor for suicide (96). Some evidence alternatively supports a lifelong risk between avoidant personality disorder and both suicide attempts (97) and death by suicide earlier in life (18).

Dependent Personality Disorder. Dependent personality disorder has a high prevalence in the general elderly population (76) and has been associated with suicides and suicide attempts earlier in life (18, 85). Nevertheless, this disorder showed no significant association with death by suicide in old age.

A positive correlation between dependent personality traits and suicidal ideation was found in most (59, 65, 67), but not all studies (47).

Obsessive–Compulsive (and Anankastic) Personality Disorder (OCPD). OCPD displays the strongest association with death by suicide in the existing studies, although the relationship is thin and the studies lack adequate controls. In Harwood and colleagues' psychological autopsy study ($N = 100$), out of the 44 suicide victims with personality pathology there were 23 cases (52.3%) with anankastic (obsessive–compulsive) personality disorder ($n = 4$) or trait accentuation ($n = 19$). OCPD was also associated with suicide in the case–control part of the study ($n = 54$). In a secondary analysis examining subjects without a psychiatric diagnosis, anankastic personality trait accentuation was present in 8/23 subjects (34.8%) (50). Some of the personality characteristics described by Kjølseth and colleagues' qualitative findings also map onto OCPD, such as reluctance to accept help from others, self-discipline, high professional competence, hard-work, introversion, and stubbornness ($N = 23$) (56).

Evidence of the association between OCPD and suicidal ideation remains inconsistent, with two studies reporting a positive correlation (59, 67) and two others reporting none (47, 65).

OCPD is the most common personality disorder in the general population, with a prevalence of 3–8% (98). It is also the personality disorder with the highest prevalence (17.1%) among elderly patients with dysthymic disorder (73, 99), which, as mentioned previously, is independently associated with late-life suicide (96). Along with schizoid personality disorder, OCPD is one of only two Axis-II conditions found to become accentuated in old age (84, 100), even in individuals who seemed unimpaired earlier in life (101, 102). Consistent with the qualitative findings of Kjølseth, three OCPD traits related to cognition and interpersonal functioning seem to display a stable and long-lasting pattern: preoccupation with details, rigidity and stubbornness, and reluctance to delegate (95, 103). These characteristics could cause a perception of loss of control in old age stemming from physical and cognitive decline, leaving suicide as a way to regain control. Supporting this hypothesis, two qualitative psychological autopsy reports examined elderly suicide victims who had, respectively, the conviction of having cancer ($n = 8$) or a chronic dyspnea diagnosis ($n = 14$), and both described a similar, rigid personality style in a majority of cases (5/8 and 12/14, respectively) (104, 105). In studies of decision-making, an extreme willingness to wait for delayed rewards has been found in both OCPD patients and high-lethality older attempters, indicating their common tendency to focus on long-term rewards, without considering alternate solutions (106, 107). The extent to which OCPD patients premeditate attempts, however, remains subject to controversy. Whereas some case–control studies in clinical adult samples support the notion of single attempts in OCPD (108), others report a more borderline-like pattern with impulsive suicidal behavior, multiple attempts, and lower intent to die (16). In a series of case reports on high-lethality first time suicide attempters with a double-diagnosis of OCPD and mood disorders, 6/7 cases were aged 56 or above, and all of them described transient, sudden loss of control preceding their suicidal act (109). However, this behavior may be attributed as much to impulsivity as to a general lack of perspective of alternative options.

Five-Factor Model

See **Table 5** for a summary of findings.

Neuroticism

Although high neuroticism has been linked to death by suicide in younger age groups (41), older psychiatric patients who died by suicide displayed lower levels of neuroticism than both their younger counterparts (60, 63), and those who survived their attempt (55). Interestingly, older victims were more similar to healthy controls than they were to attempters. Even though two studies found higher levels of neuroticism in older suicide victims than in healthy controls (41, 60), on the facet level, only trait depression (the tendency to feel sad) and trait self-consciousness (the tendency to be easily intimidated) were higher (41). Suicide victims and healthy controls did not significantly differ in the facets that capture negative emotional reactivity, namely vulnerability (the tendency to panic easily), trait anxiety (the tendency to worry), impulsiveness (the tendency to act impulsively), and anger–hostility (the tendency to get angry easily) (41). Anger–hostility was also the only similar facet between suicide victims and attempters (55).

Among older suicide attempters, two studies conducted in Hong Kong, China, found increased levels of neuroticism compared to healthy controls (49, 62), but this finding did not survive controlling for current major depression, past suicide attempts, physical comorbidities, demographic factors, and life events in one of them (49). Other studies observed no difference from healthy controls (61), or depressed controls (48). Again, differences emerged at the facet level, with higher levels of all facets in attempters than in depressed controls, except for trait anxiety and anger–hostility (48). Lower trait anxiety was in fact found to be a predictor of the attempter status, while lower anger–hostility was associated with fewer attempts, higher lethality of method, and higher intent to die (46). Compared to healthy controls, higher levels of anger–hostility predicted attempter status in men, but not in women, while higher impulsivity was observed in elderly attempters of both sexes (62).

Higher levels of neuroticism unequivocally differentiated elderly suicide ideators from healthy controls (59, 64). However, in depressed samples, only one (43) out of three studies found higher levels of neuroticism in ideators than in controls, with the others reporting no difference (48, 51). Higher trait depression was the only facet that correlated with the severity of suicidal ideation from the neuroticism domain in a sample of depressed elderly (48), indicating that differences may be limited to only isolated facets.

Extraversion

Lower levels of extraversion were found in older adults who died by suicide compared to healthy controls in some (49, 60), but not all studies (41). Furthermore, in Tsoh and colleagues' study, the effect disappeared in the multivariate analysis that controlled for current major depression, past suicide attempts, physical comorbidities, demographic factors, and life events (49). Extraversion did not distinguish between older adults who died by suicide and those who only attempted it (49, 55).

Findings examining elderly suicide attempters and ideators were also inconclusive. Three studies using the same recruitment source found that elderly depressed inpatients who made an attempt at age 50 or older had lower levels of extraversion than depressed controls, both globally, and for the specific facets of gregariousness (seeking company of others), warmth (making friends easily), and positive emotions (tendency to be joyful) (43, 46, 48). In addition, lower positive emotions were identified as an independent predictor of a greater number of attempts (46). However, older suicide attempters did not differ from general population controls on extraversion in two other studies controlling for age, sex, and major depression (49, 61). These inconsistent findings may be explained by sex differences, since lower levels of extraversion were present in elderly male, but not female attempters in a sex-stratified study (62). A sampling bias cannot be excluded, however. Alternatively, given the higher age cutoff in the three latter studies (65–75 years), this inconsistency might arise from a survival bias, as higher levels of extraversion have been associated with a decreased risk of death in the elderly (110).

Similarly to elderly attempters, suicide ideators aged 50 or older differed from depressed controls by reporting lower levels of both warmth and positive emotions in two studies having the same recruitment source as the three studies mentioned earlier (48, 51). They did not differ from healthy controls on extraversion

TABLE 4 | Characteristics of studies with dimensional findings (see **Table 5** for a summary of findings).

Study		Sample	Age (years)	Assessment
Suicide	Duberstein et al., 1994 (41) USA (NY, Rochester) Psychological autopsy study	52 suicides 30 healthy controls	≥50	NEO-PI
	De Leo et al., 2013 (60) Australia (QLD, NSW) Case–control study Draper et al., 2014 (63) Australia (QLD, NSW) Case–control study	261 suicides, of which 73 older 182 sudden death controls of which 79 older	≥60	NEO-FFI
Suicide, attempted suicide	Tsoh et al., 2005 (49) China (Hong Kong) Case–control study	67 suicide victims 66 suicide attempters 91 healthy controls	≥65	NEO-FFI
	Useda et al., 2007 (55) USA (NY, Rochester) Case–control study	60 depressed attempters 43 suicides	≥50	NEO-PI-R
Attempted suicide	Seidlitz et al., 2001 (46) USA (NY, Rochester) Case–control study	45 depressed attempters 36 depressed controls	≥50	NEO-PI-R (emotion facets)
	Wiktorsson et al., 2013 (61) Sweden Case–control study	72 hospitalized attempters 288 healthy controls	≥75	EPI (N and E subscales)
	Chan et al., 2014 (62) China (Hong Kong) Case–control study	77 suicide attempters 99 healthy controls	≥65	NEO-FFI NEO-PI facets
Attempted suicide, suicidal ideation	Duberstein et al., 2000 (43) USA (NY, Rochester) Case–control study	45 depressed attempters 32 patients with recent suicidal ideation (1 week) 61 patients without recent SI 36 depressed controls	≥50	SSI NEO-PI-R
	Useda et al., 2004 (48) USA (NY, Rochester) Case–control study	67 depressed attempters 43 depressed controls + Assessment of severity of SI	≥50	SSI NEO-PI-R
Suicidal ideation	Heisel et al., 2006 (51) USA (NY, Rochester) Case–control study	32 depressed suicide ideator 101 depressed controls	≥50	SSI NEO-PI-R
	Hirsch et al., 2007 (54) USA (NY, Rochester) Case–control study	462 older adults recruited from a primary care setting of which 37 suicide ideators	≥65	SCID and HRSD (SI questions) NEO-FFI
	Segal et al., 2012 (59) USA (CO, Colorado Springs) Cross-sectional	109 community-dwelling elderly	≥65	GSIS NEO-FFI
	Kim and Ahn, 2014 (64) USA (LA) Cross-sectional	220 community-dwelling elderly Korean immigrants	≥60	SSI EPQR (N subscale)

SI, suicidal ideation; NEO-PI, NEO Personality Inventory, NEO-FFI, NEO Five-Factor Inventory; EPI, Eysenck Personality Inventory; EPQR, Eysenck Personality Questionnaire; SSI, Scale for Suicide Ideation; SCID, Structured Clinical Interview; HRSD, Hamilton Rating Scale for Depression; NEO-PI, NEO Personality Inventory; NEO-PI-R, NEO Personality Inventory Revised; GSIS, Geriatric Suicide Ideation Scale.

in a community-based sample aged 60 or older ($N = 109$) (59). From the three subcomponents of extraversion derived from NEO-FFI self-reports, positive affect (being joyful), but not sociability (being outgoing and sociable) or activity (tendency to be energetic and busy), was identified as a negative predictor for suicidal ideation (54).

The fact that distinctively socially oriented facets of extraversion (namely, warmth, positive emotions, and gregariousness) differentiated elderly suicide attempters from depressed controls may suggest that a tendency toward social isolation could predispose to suicidal behavior in old age. Even though younger individuals who died by suicide were also found to have lower levels of extraversion than healthy controls (20, 41), in their case, lower levels of activity (being frequently busy) and assertiveness (tendency to take charge) were distinguishing facets in addition to lower positive emotions (41).

TABLE 5 | Summary of dimensional findings on death by suicide, attempted suicide, and suicidal ideation.

Domains; facets	Suicide victims	Suicide attempters	Suicide ideators
Neuroticism	> HC (41, 60), ≈ HC (49)[a,b] < SA (55)[a,b], ≈ SA (49)[a] < ySV (60) (63)[c]	> HC (62), ≈ HC (49)[a,b] (61)[b] ≈ DC (43)	> HC (59) (64)[a] > DC (43), ≈ DC (51)[a,b]
Depression	*> HC (41); < SA (55)[a,b]*	*≈ DC (46, 48)*	*> DC (48)*
Self-consciousness	*> HC (41); < SA (55)[a,b]*	*> DC (48), ≈ DC (46)*	*≈ DC (48)*
Impulsiveness	*≈ HC (41); < SA (55)[a,b]*	*> HC (62); > DC (48)*	*≈ DC (48)*
Vulnerability	*≈ HC (41); < SA (55)[a,b]*	*> DC (48)*	*≈ DC (48)*
Anxiety/negative affect[g]	*≈ HC (41); < SA (55)[a,b]*	*< DC (46), ≈ DC (48)*	*≈ HC (54)[a,b,g]; ≈ DC (48)*
Anger–hostility	*≈ HC (41); ≈ SA (55)[a,b]*	*> HC (62)[e], ≈ HC (62)[f] ≈ DC (46, 48) More attempts (46) Lower lethality and intent (46)*	*≈ DC (48)*
Extraversion	< HC (60), ≈ HC (41) (49)[a,b] ≈ SA (49)[a] (55)[a,b] ≈ ySV (60, 63)	< HC (62)[e], ≈ HC (49)[a,b] (61)[b] (62)[f] < DC (43) Fewer attempts (43)	≈ HC (59) ≈ DC (51)[a,b]
Positive emotions/positive affect[g]	*No data*	*< DC (46) (48)[a,b] Fewer attempts (46) (48)[a,b]*	*< HC (54)[a,b,g]; < DC (48)*
Warmth	*No data*	*≈ DC (46, 48)*	*< DC (48)[a,b]*
Gregariousness/sociability[g]	*No data*	*≈ DC (48)*	*≈ HC (54)[a,b,g]; ≈ DC (48)*
Openness to experience	< HC (41), ≈ HC (49)[a,b] (60) ≈ SA (49)[a] (55)[a,b] > ySV (41) (60) (63)[c]	≈ HC (49)[a,b] (62) ≈ DC (48)	≈ HC (59) > DC (43) (51)[a,b], ≈ DC (48)
Openness to esthetics	*< HC (41)*	*≈ DC (48)*	*No data*
Openness to action	*< HC (41); < ySV (41)*	*≈ DC (48)*	*No data*
Conscientiousness	≈ HC (41) (49)[a,b] (60) > SA (49)[a] (55)[a,b] > ySV (60) (63)[d]	< HC (49)[a] (62)[e], ≈ HC (62)[f] ≈ DC (43)	≈ HC (59) ≈ DC (48) (51)[a,b]
Dutifulness	*> SA (55)[a,b]*	*≈ DC (48)*	*No data*
Achievement-striving	*> SA (55)[a,b]*	*≈ DC (48)*	*No data*
Self-discipline	*> SA (55)[a,b]*	*≈ DC (48)*	*No data*
Deliberation	*> SA (55)[a,b]*	*≈ DC (48)*	*No data*
Agreeableness	≈ HC (41) (49)[a,b] (60) ≈ SA (49)[a] (55)[a,b] ≈ ySV (60 63)	*≈ HC (49)[a,b] (62) ≈ DC (43)*	≈ HC (59) < DC (43), ≈ DC (48) (51)[a,b]
Modesty	*No data*	*> DC (48)[a,b] More attempts (48)[c]*	*> DC (48)[a,b]*

All five domains of the Five-Factor Model and their facets with significant findings are displayed with corresponding references.

>, higher levels than; <, lower levels than; ≈, not statistically different from; HC, healthy controls; DC, depressed controls; SA, elderly suicide attempters; ySV, younger suicide victims.

[a]Result after adjusting for general health status (physical and/or cognitive).

[b]Result after adjusting for psychiatric status (any Axis-I pathology or depression).

[c]In psychiatric subgroup.

[d]In non-psychiatric subgroup.

[e]Males.

[f]Females.

[g]Subcomponents derived from the NEO-FFI.

Openness to Experience

Findings with respect to openness to experience in late-life suicide are inconsistent across studies comparing older suicide victims either to healthy controls or to older attempters. In comparison with healthy controls, Duberstein and colleagues initially found lower levels of openness to experience in older adults who died by suicide, with significant differences in the openness to esthetics (sensitivity to any form of art), and in the openness to action facets (preference of variety to routine) (41). These findings were, however, not replicated in further studies (when considering adjusted odds ratios in Tsoh and colleagues' study) (49, 60). Compared to attempters, elderly victims were found to have either lower or not significantly different levels of openness to experience (49, 55). The effect of age was more consistent, with older suicide victims displaying lower levels of openness than their younger counterparts (41, 60, 63). Duberstein and colleagues identified that the greatest difference between the two age groups was in openness to action, indicating a higher preference for routine in older versus younger suicide victims (41).

Elderly suicide attempters showed no difference in openness to experience compared to healthy as well as depressed controls (46, 48, 49, 62).

In older suicide ideators, some (43, 51) but not all studies (48) found higher openness to experience when compared to depressed controls. No difference was found between ideators and healthy controls (59).

Thus, the role of openness to experience in late-life suicide remains unclear. According to Duberstein, lower levels of openness to experience in older suicide victims (compared to younger victims and healthy controls) may arise from a reduced capability to cope with age-related changes or losses due to excessive, short-sighted, concrete thinking and a rigidly defined self-image (111). Consistent with this theory, higher levels of openness to experience have been positively associated with volunteer work and better cognition in old age (10). It is, however, also possible that the lower levels of openness to action found in older versus younger adults who died by suicide may arise from a maturational effect, since a decrease in this facet has been associated with normal aging (112).

Conscientiousness

Higher levels of conscientiousness distinguished older suicide victims from younger victims (60, 63), as well as from older attempters in clinical samples (49, 55). The difference with attempters was also apparent at the facet level, where suicide victims displayed higher dutifulness (proneness to follow the rules), achievement-striving (tendency to work-hard/overachieve), and self-discipline (capability to get things done when needed) (55). Of three studies (41, 49, 60), only Tsoh and colleagues found lower levels conscientiousness in elderly suicide victims compared to general population controls in a univariate analysis, but the finding did not survive controlling for current major depression, past suicide attempts, physical comorbidities, sociodemographic factors and life events (49).

Studies comparing elderly suicide attempters versus general population controls found either lower conscientiousness in attempters (49) or similar levels in the two groups (61). No differences were found between older suicide attempters and depressed controls (43, 48). In a sex-stratified study, lower levels of conscientiousness were present in elderly male attempters compared to healthy controls, although no such difference was found in females (62).

Elderly suicide ideators showed no difference in their levels of conscientiousness compared to healthy or depressed controls (48, 51, 59).

Overall, higher levels of conscientiousness seem to discriminate suicides from unsuccessful attempts in depressed older adults, as well as late-onset suicides from early-onset ones. These relatively higher levels of conscientiousness in older suicides appear to be consistent with ICD/DSM-findings reporting an association with OCPD (see in the corresponding subsection). In a meta-analysis, OCPD was the only Axis-II diagnosis positively correlated with conscientiousness (113). Although higher levels of conscientiousness have been linked to several facets of successful aging (10, 114), the above findings suggest that this trait could also contribute to negative outcomes in late life, especially when co-occurring with depression.

Agreeableness

Studies have found no difference in agreeableness in older suicide victims compared to younger victims, healthy controls, and elderly attempters (41, 49, 55, 60, 63). Although Tsoh and colleagues found that elderly who died by suicide had higher levels of agreeableness than elderly attempters, this effect did not hold in the multivariate model controlling for current depressive disorder, history of suicide attempt, physical comorbidities, demographic factors, and life events (49).

No study found overall differences in agreeableness between elderly suicide attempters and healthy or depressed controls, with the exception of the unadjusted effect reported by Tsoh and colleagues that indicated lower levels of agreeableness in attempters (43, 49, 61, 62).

With respect to elderly suicide ideators, most studies found no difference in agreeableness compared to both healthy and depressed controls (48, 51, 59).

Thus, agreeableness does not seem to distinguish older adults who attempt or die by suicide from the general elderly population.

DISCUSSION

Main Findings

Maladaptive personality seems to play a role in suicidal behavior in old age, although it is most often present in milder, subthreshold forms. The existing literature points toward heterogeneity in personality profiles of older adults with suicidal ideation or behavior. Suicidal ideation was predicted by narcissistic and borderline personality and was positively associated with all other personality disorders as indicated by at least one study, with the exception of histrionic personality. By contrast, only obsessive–compulsive and avoidant personality disorders were implicated in death by suicide, although this association may be confounded by depression.

Studies using the Big Five further characterized older adults who died by suicide as being more neurotic than healthy individuals, but less neurotic and more conscientious than older adults who only carried out non-fatal attempts. The limited evidence that we have links maladaptive personality with recurrent suicide attempts of largely lower severity. For example, lower anger–hostility was associated with a smaller number of attempts, higher lethality of method and higher intent to die, while lower positive emotions were identified as an independent predictor of a greater number of attempts (46).

We take these findings as evidence that a subset of aging individuals with personality disorders, BPD being the prototype, continue to display chronic suicidal ideation and repeated suicide attempts. On the other hand, the emergence of serious suicidal behavior in late life is associated with more intact personality in a majority of individuals and, possibly, obsessive–compulsive traits in a significant minority.

An important alternative hypothesis is that dysfunctional personality traits involved in late-life suicide are not well captured by existing criteria and measures, possibly reflecting effects of neurodegeneration and other aspects of brain aging. Cognitive rigidity, for instance, often appears in qualitative case descriptions and may sensitize older adults to acute stressors (56, 104, 105). It is, however, only partially captured by categorical OCPD criteria, higher conscientiousness, and lower openness to action (a facet of openness to experience), which may be overrepresented among late-life vs. early-life suicides.

Limitations

The assessment of DSM/ICD personality disorder criteria may not be best suited for the characterization of personality in the elderly. DSM personality disorders map better onto younger than older adults in whom many of the criteria become difficult to evaluate (115, 116). In addition, personality assessment in psychological autopsy studies likely under-detects internalizing traits over the life course, reflected in only moderate consistency with ante-mortem Axis-II diagnoses found in adults (kappa = 0.65) (117). Therefore, older suicide attempters with highly medically lethal attempts probably provide the best *in vivo* window into death by suicide. Unfortunately, categorical data focusing on separate personality disorders in the elderly were absent in attempters, scarce in older suicide victims, and lacking comparisons with depressed non-suicidal control groups. These limitations make it impossible to draw strong conclusions about late-life suicidal behavior in patients with specific personality disorders.

Moreover, suicidal behavior is heterogeneous in its life course, planning, method selection, and medical consequences (106, 118). The studies reviewed here did not generally consider this heterogeneity in their design and analytic approach, and the relationship between the older individual's personality profile and the life course and characteristics of his/her suicidal behavior remains largely unexplored. More work is needed, both to identify reliable predictors of any suicidal behavior in old age and, more importantly, parse the behavior's heterogeneity.

Clinical Implications

From a clinical perspective, these results suggest that older adults who are evaluated for suicidal ideation are not necessarily representative of those who die by suicide. Among the latter individuals, only a subgroup seems to display dysfunctional personality features, with a rigid vulnerability being possibly as common as an emotionally labile one. This heterogeneity highlights the challenges in assessing suicidal risk in the elderly. One needs to be cautious in drawing conclusions from the patient's personality profile, and other risk factors such as access to firearms, depression, addiction, psychosis, and pain should be given greater weight at the current state of knowledge.

Future Directions

Disorders of aging can also alter personality. Dementia brings about a progressive personality change (119), exaggeration of existing personality traits and mood disturbances being the most frequent manifestations. A longitudinal study found that, in prodromal Alzheimer's disease, increased rigidity was the most frequent alteration, occurring in 25% of the individuals subsequently converting to dementia, closely followed by apathy (24%), egocentricity (21%), and impaired emotional control (18%) (120). Other investigators reported higher levels of neuroticism, as well as lower levels of both extraversion and conscientiousness in patients with Alzheimer type dementia (121, 122). Similarly, higher levels of neuroticism, as well as lower levels of extraversion and goal orientation have been reported in either premorbid or beginning stages of Parkinson's disease (123–125). Such personality characteristics may be associated with alterations in the dopaminergic system and therefore predate motor symptoms of parkinsonism (126). Thus, the behavioral effects of neurodegeneration may in part explain the divergence in personality profiles between younger and older suicides. For example, it is possible that the accentuation of rigid personality traits contributes to suicide risk by impairing individuals' ability to cope with their progressive loss of cognitive abilities. Moreover, organic mental disorder may similarly contribute to the heterogeneity of personality profiles found in older adults at risk of suicide and has been linked to an overall under-detection of personality disorders in the elderly (77). Interestingly, new forms of impulsivity may also emerge in neurocognitive disorders, as in the case of the disruption of the indirect (no-go) and hyper-direct ("cortical brake") pathways by dopamine agonists and subthalamic nucleus stimulation in Parkinson's disease, where some studies point to treatment-emergent suicidal behavior (127, 128).

Another neurocognitive mechanism worth investigating further is executive dysfunction. This construct has already been linked to late-onset, treatment-resistant depression (129, 130) as well as to suicidal behavior (131). Moreover, there appears to be a correlation between deficits in executive functioning and certain personality disorders, such as antisocial, borderline and obsessive–compulsive (132–134).

The question of the best approach to characterize personality in older adults at increased risk of suicide remains open. Research is increasingly shifting toward dimensional measures, which have the advantages of being assessable through self-report and increasing statistical power by virtue of being parametric. Clinical constructs underlying categorical personality disorders, however, appear to possess unique explanatory and heuristic value above and beyond the Big Five in the study of suicidal behavior (135). In addition to traditional personality measures, complementary neuropsychological tools may be needed, including experimental paradigms assessing decision-making and social interactions, similarly to the way other trait-level constructs, such as impulsivity, are investigated (136).

Conclusion

Despite the scarcity of published studies, this review highlights (1) the smaller role that Cluster B personality disorders and their defining constructs play in late-life suicide compared to suicide in younger adults and (2) a possible role for Cluster C disorders, such as OCPD, in late-life suicide. Almost nothing is known about the contribution of personality change due to neurodegenerative and vascular diseases. The reasons for the generally lower prevalence of diagnosable personality disorders in older vs. younger adults who engage in suicidal behavior are likely to include actual change in the behavioral expression of personality across the lifespan, poorer fit of diagnostic instruments, and the contributions of neurodegenerative and vascular brain changes. We would be remiss not to mention the possibility, often rejected by psychiatrists, that some proportion of late-life suicidal behavior may be rational in that it is not explained by psychopathology. Future research will reveal to what extent this may be true, and to what extent suicide in characterologically unaffected older adults is motivated by concerns such as depression, psychosis, addiction, or impaired cognition and decision-making.

AUTHOR CONTRIBUTIONS

AD and KS conceived and directed the project; AS collected data, structured and drafted the article. All authors contributed to the theoretical framework, data interpretation as well as the development of the manuscript.

ACKNOWLEDGMENTS

We thank Maria Alessi, Laura Kenneally, Ariel Eytan, and George Tsimploulis for editorial and conceptual input. This work was supported by the University of Geneva (Boninchi Foundation Fellowship and Open-Access Funds to AS; Department of Psychiatry to JA), as well as the National Institute of Medical Health (NIMH R01MH048463, R01MH100095 to AD; R01MH085651 to KS).

REFERENCES

1. National Institute of Mental Health (NIMH). *Suicide [Internet]*. (2017) [cited 2018 Feb 27]. Available from: https://www.nimh.nih.gov/health/statistics/suicide.shtml#part_154969
2. American Association of Suicidology. *Elderly Suicide Fact Sheet Based on 2012 Data [Internet]*. (2014) [cited 2016 Dec 19]. Available from: http://www.suicidology.org/Portals/14/docs/Resources/FactSheets/Elderly2012.pdf
3. Waern M, Rubenowitz E, Runeson B, Skoog I, Wilhelmson K, Allebeck P. Burden of illness and suicide in elderly people: case-control study. *BMJ* (2002) 324(7350):1355. doi:10.1136/bmj.324.7350.1355
4. Waern M, Rubenowitz E, Wilhelmson K. Predictors of suicide in the old elderly. *Gerontology* (2003) 49(5):328–34. doi:10.1159/000071715
5. Juurlink DN, Herrmann N, Szalai JP, Kopp A, Redelmeier DA. Medical illness and the risk of suicide in the elderly. *Arch Intern Med* (2004) 164(11):1179–84. doi:10.1001/archinte.164.11.1179
6. Fässberg MM, Cheung G, Canetto SS, Erlangsen A, Lapierre S, Lindner R, et al. A systematic review of physical illness, functional disability, and suicidal behaviour among older adults. *Aging Ment Health* (2016) 20(2):166–94. doi:10.1080/13607863.2015.1083945
7. Mann JJ, Waternaux C, Haas GL, Malone KM. Toward a clinical model of suicidal behavior in psychiatric patients. *Am J Psychiatry* (1999) 156(2):181–9.
8. Heikkinen ME, Henriksson MM, Isometsä ET, Marttunen MJ, Na HM, LöNnqvist JK. Recent life events and suicide in personality disorders. *J Nerv Amp Ment Dis* (1997) 185(6):373–81. doi:10.1097/00005053-199706000-00003
9. Devanand D. Comorbid psychiatric disorders in late life depression. *Biol Psychiatry* (2002) 52(3):236–42. doi:10.1016/S0006-3223(02)01336-7
10. Baek Y, Martin P, Siegler IC, Davey A, Poon LW. Personality traits and successful aging: findings from the Georgia centenarian study. *Int J Aging Hum Dev* (2016) 83(3):207–27. doi:10.1177/0091415016652404
11. Medawar PB. *Uniqueness of the Individual*. London: Methuen (1957).
12. Williams GC, Williams DC. Natural selection of individually harmful social adaptations among sibs with special reference to social insects. *Evolution* (1957) 11(1):32–9. doi:10.2307/2405809
13. Giner L, Blasco-Fontecilla H, Mercedes Perez-Rodriguez M, Garcia-Nieto R, Giner J, Guija JA, et al. Personality disorders and health problems distinguish suicide attempters from completers in a direct comparison. *J Affect Disord* (2013) 151(2):474–83. doi:10.1016/j.jad.2013.06.029
14. May AM, Klonsky ED, Klein DN. Predicting future suicide attempts among depressed suicide ideators: a 10-year longitudinal study. *J Psychiatr Res* (2012) 46(7):946–52. doi:10.1016/j.jpsychires.2012.04.009
15. Ansell EB, Wright AGC, Markowitz JC, Sanislow CA, Hopwood CJ, Zanarini MC, et al. Personality disorder risk factors for suicide attempts over 10 years of follow-up. *Personal Disord* (2015) 6(2):161–7. doi:10.1037/per0000089
16. Diaconu G, Turecki G. Obsessive-compulsive personality disorder and suicidal behavior: evidence for a positive association in a sample of depressed patients. *J Clin Psychiatry* (2009) 70(11):1551–6. doi:10.4088/JCP.08m04636
17. Verona E, Sachs-Ericsson N, Joiner TE. Suicide attempts associated with externalizing psychopathology in an epidemiological sample. *Am J Psychiatry* (2004) 161(3):444–51. doi:10.1176/appi.ajp.161.3.444
18. Foster T, Gillespie K, McClelland R, Patterson C. Risk factors for suicide independent of DSM-III-R axis I disorder. Case-control psychological autopsy study in northern Ireland. *Br J Psychiatry* (1999) 175(2):175–9. doi:10.1192/bjp.175.2.175
19. Brezo J, Paris J, Turecki G. Personality traits as correlates of suicidal ideation, suicide attempts, and suicide completions: a systematic review. *Acta Psychiatr Scand* (2006) 113(3):180–206. doi:10.1111/j.1600-0447.2005.00702.x
20. Fang L, Heisel MJ, Duberstein PR, Zhang J. Combined effects of neuroticism and extraversion: findings from a matched case control study of suicide in rural China. *J Nerv Ment Dis* (2012) 200(7):598–602. doi:10.1097/NMD.0b013e31825bfb53
21. Pallis DJ, Jenkins JS. Extraversion, neuroticism, and intent in attempted suicides. *Psychol Rep* (1977) 41(1):19–22. doi:10.2466/pr0.1977.41.1.19
22. Stanković Z, Saula-Marojević B, Potrebić A. Personality profile of depressive patients with a history of suicide attempts. *Psychiatr Danub* (2006) 18(3–4):159–68.
23. Yen S, Siegler IC. Self-blame, social introversion, and male suicides: prospective data from a longitudinal study. *Arch Suicide Res* (2003) 7(1):17–27. doi:10.1080/13811110301569
24. Brodsky BS, Groves SA, Oquendo MA, Mann JJ, Stanley B. Interpersonal precipitants and suicide attempts in borderline personality disorder. *Suicide Life Threat Behav* (2006) 36(3):313–22. doi:10.1521/suli.2006.36.3.313
25. Rihmer Z, Benazzi F. Impact on suicidality of the borderline personality traits impulsivity and affective instability. *Ann Clin Psychiatry* (2010) 22(2):121–8.

26. Stone MH, Hurt SW, Stone DK. The PI 500: long-term follow-up of borderline inpatients meeting DSM-III criteria I. Global outcome. *J Personal Disord* (1987) 1(4):291–8. doi:10.1521/pedi.1987.1.4.291
27. Zanarini MC, Frankenburg FR, Reich DB, Fitzmaurice G. Time to attainment of recovery from borderline personality disorder and stability of recovery: a 10-year prospective follow-up study. *Am J Psychiatry* (2010) 167(6):663–7. doi:10.1176/appi.ajp.2009.09081130
28. Frierson RL. Suicide attempts by the old and the very old. *Arch Intern Med* (1991) 151(1):141. doi:10.1001/archinte.151.1.141
29. Conwell Y, Duberstein PR, Cox C, Herrmann J, Forbes N, Caine ED. Age differences in behaviors leading to completed suicide. *Am J Geriatr Psychiatry* (1998) 6(2):122–6. doi:10.1097/00019442-199805000-00005
30. American Psychological Association (APA). *Personality [Internet].* (2018) [cited 2018 Feb 6]. Available from: http://www.apa.org/topics/personality/index.aspx
31. O'Carroll PW, Berman AL, Maris RW, Moscicki EK, Tanney BL, Silverman MM. Beyond the tower of Babel: a nomenclature for suicidology. *Suicide Life Threat Behav* (1996) 26(3):237–52.
32. Chan LF, Shamsul AS, Maniam T. Are predictors of future suicide attempts and the transition from suicidal ideation to suicide attempts shared or distinct: a 12-month prospective study among patients with depressive disorders. *Psychiatry Res* (2014) 220(3):867–73. doi:10.1016/j.psychres.2014.08.055
33. Suominen K, Isometsä E, Suokas J, Haukka J, Achte K, Lönnqvist J. Completed suicide after a suicide attempt: a 37-year follow-up study. *Am J Psychiatry* (2004) 161(3):562–3. doi:10.1176/appi.ajp.161.3.562
34. Rudd MD, Joiner T, Rajab MH. Relationships among suicide ideators, attempters, and multiple attempters in a young-adult sample. *J Abnorm Psychol* (1996) 105(4):541–50. doi:10.1037/0021-843X.105.4.541
35. Gil S. Suicide attempters vs. ideators: are there differences in personality profiles? *Arch Suicide Res* (2005) 9(2):153–61. doi:10.1080/13811110590904007
36. Brezo J, Paris J, Tremblay R, Vitaro F, HéBert M, Turecki G. Identifying correlates of suicide attempts in suicidal ideators: a population-based study. *Psychol Med* (2007) 37(11):1551–62. doi:10.1017/S0033291707000803
37. Ciompi L. Late suicide in former mental patients. *Psychopathology* (1976) 9(1):59–63. doi:10.1159/000283665
38. Nieto E, Vieta E, Lazaro L, Gasto C, Cirera E. Serious suicide attempts in the elderly. *Psychopathology* (1992) 25(4):183–8. doi:10.1159/000284770
39. Kunik ME, Mulsant BH, Rifai AH, Sweet R, Pasternak R, Rosen J, et al. Personality disorders in elderly inpatients with major depression. *Am J Geriatr Psychiatry* (1993) 1(1):38–45. doi:10.1097/00019442-199300110-00006
40. Draper B. Suicidal behaviour in the elderly. *Int J Geriatr Psychiatry* (1994) 9(8):655–61. doi:10.1002/gps.930090810
41. Duberstein PR, Conwell Y, Caine ED. Age differences in the personality characteristics of suicide completers: preliminary findings from a psychological autopsy study. *Psychiatry* (1994) 57(3):213–24. doi:10.1080/00332747.1994.11024686
42. Henriksson MM, Marttunen MJ, Isometsä ET, Heikkinen ME, Aro HM, Kuoppasalmi KI, et al. Mental disorders in elderly suicide. *Int Psychogeriatr* (1995) 7(2):275–86. doi:10.1017/S1041610295002031
43. Duberstein PR, Conwell Y, Seidlitz L, Denning DG, Cox C, Caine ED. Personality traits and suicidal behavior and ideation in depressed inpatients 50 years of age and older. *J Gerontol B Psychol Sci Soc Sci* (2000) 55(1):18–26. doi:10.1093/geronb/55.1.P18
44. Lawrence D, Almeida OP, Hulse GK, Jablensky AV, Holman CD. Suicide and attempted suicide among older adults in Western Australia. *Psychol Med* (2000) 30(4):813–21. doi:10.1017/S0033291799002391
45. Harwood D, Hawton K, Hope T, Jacoby R. Psychiatric disorder and personality factors associated with suicide in older people: a descriptive and case-control study. *Int J Geriatr Psychiatry* (2001) 16(2):155–65. doi:10.1002/1099-1166(200102)16:2<155::AID-GPS289>3.0.CO;2-0
46. Seidlitz L, Conwell Y, Duberstein P, Cox C, Denning D. Emotion traits in older suicide attempters and non-attempters. *J Affect Disord* (2001) 66(2–3):123–31. doi:10.1016/S0165-0327(00)00300-1
47. Morse JQ, Lynch TR. A preliminary investigation of self-reported personality disorders in late life: prevalence, predictors of depressive severity, and clinical correlates. *Aging Ment Health* (2004) 8(4):307–15. doi:10.1080/13607860410001709674
48. Useda JD, Duberstein PR, Conner KR, Conwell Y. Personality and attempted suicide in depressed adults 50 years of age and older: a facet level analysis. *Compr Psychiatry* (2004) 45(5):353–61. doi:10.1016/j.comppsych.2004.06.002
49. Tsoh J, Chiu HFK, Duberstein PR, Chan SSM, Chi I, Yip PSF, et al. Attempted suicide in elderly Chinese persons: a multi-group, controlled study. *Am J Geriatr Psychiatry* (2005) 13(7):562–71. doi:10.1097/00019442-200507000-00004
50. Harwood D, Hawton K, Hope T, Jacoby R. Suicide in older people without psychiatric disorder. *Int J Geriatr Psychiatry* (2006) 21(4):363–7. doi:10.1002/gps.1473
51. Heisel MJ, Duberstein PR, Conner KR, Franus N, Beckman A, Conwell Y. Personality and reports of suicide ideation among depressed adults 50 years of age or older. *J Affect Disord* (2006) 90(2–3):175–80. doi:10.1016/j.jad.2005.11.005
52. Hunt IM, Kapur N, Robinson J, Shaw J, Flynn S, Bailey H, et al. Suicide within 12 months of mental health service contact in different age and diagnostic groups: national clinical survey. *Br J Psychiatry* (2006) 188(2):135–42. doi:10.1192/bjp.188.2.135
53. Heisel MJ, Links PS, Conn D, van Reekum R, Flett GL. Narcissistic personality and vulnerability to late-life suicidality. *Am J Geriatr Psychiatry* (2007) 15(9):734–41. doi:10.1097/01.JGP.0000260853.63533.7d
54. Hirsch JK, Duberstein PR, Chapman B, Lyness JM. Positive affect and suicide ideation in older adult primary care patients. *Psychol Aging* (2007) 22(2):380–5. doi:10.1037/0882-7974.22.2.380
55. Useda JD, Duberstein PR, Conner KR, Beckman A, Franus N, Tu X, et al. Personality differences in attempted suicide versus suicide in adults 50 years of age or older. *J Consult Clin Psychol* (2007) 75(1):126–33. doi:10.1037/0022-006X.75.1.126
56. Kjølseth I, Ekeberg O, Steihaug S. "Why do they become vulnerable when faced with the challenges of old age?" Elderly people who committed suicide, described by those who knew them. *Int Psychogeriatr* (2009) 21(5):903–12. doi:10.1017/S1041610209990342
57. Miret M, Nuevo R, Morant C, Sainz-Cortón E, Jiménez-Arriero MA, López-Ibor JJ, et al. Differences between younger and older adults in the structure of suicidal intent and its correlates. *Am J Geriatr Psychiatry* (2010) 18(9):839–47. doi:10.1097/JGP.0b013e3181d145b0
58. Qin P. The impact of psychiatric illness on suicide: differences by diagnosis of disorders and by sex and age of subjects. *J Psychiatr Res* (2011) 45(11):1445–52. doi:10.1016/j.jpsychires.2011.06.002
59. Segal DL, Marty MA, Meyer WJ, Coolidge FL. Personality, suicidal ideation, and reasons for living among older adults. *J Gerontol B Psychol Sci Soc Sci* (2012) 67(2):159–66. doi:10.1093/geronb/gbr080
60. De Leo D, Draper BM, Snowdon J, Kõlves K. Suicides in older adults: a case-control psychological autopsy study in Australia. *J Psychiatr Res* (2013) 47(7):980–8. doi:10.1016/j.jpsychires.2013.02.009
61. Wiktorsson S, Berg AI, Billstedt E, Duberstein PR, Marlow T, Skoog I, et al. Neuroticism and extroversion in suicide attempters aged 75 and above and a general population comparison group. *Aging Ment Health* (2013) 17(4):479–88. doi:10.1080/13607863.2012.749835
62. Chan SMS, Chiu FKH, Lam CWL, Wong SMC, Conwell Y. A multidimensional risk factor model for suicide attempts in later life. *Neuropsychiatr Dis Treat* (2014) 10:1807–17. doi:10.2147/NDT.S70011
63. Draper B, Kõlves K, De Leo D, Snowdon J. A controlled study of suicide in middle-aged and older people: personality traits, age, and psychiatric disorders. *Suicide Life Threat Behav* (2014) 44(2):130–8. doi:10.1111/sltb.12053
64. Kim BJ, Ahn J. Factors that influence suicidal ideation among elderly Korean immigrants: focus on diatheses and stressors. *Aging Ment Health* (2014) 18(5):619–27. doi:10.1080/13607863.2013.866631
65. Jahn DR, Poindexter EK, Cukrowicz KC. Personality disorder traits, risk factors, and suicide ideation among older adults. *Int Psychogeriatr* (2015) 27(11):1785–94. doi:10.1017/S1041610215000174
66. Segal DL, Gottschling J, Marty M, Meyer WJ, Coolidge FL. Relationships among depressive, passive-aggressive, sadistic and self-defeating personality disorder features with suicidal ideation and reasons for living among older adults. *Aging Ment Health* (2015) 19(12):1071–7. doi:10.1080/13607863.2014.1003280

67. Eades A, Segal DL, Coolidge F, Feliciano L. *Suicide Among Older Adults: An Exploration of the Effects of Personality and Self-Esteem on Thwarted Belongingness, Perceived Burdensomeness, and suicidal ideation [MA Thesis]*. Colorado Springs: University of Colorado, Department of Psychology (2016).
68. Costa PT, McCrae RR. Primary traits of Eysenck's P-E-N system: three- and five-factor solutions. *J Pers Soc Psychol* (1995) 69(2):308–17. doi:10.1037/0022-3514.69.2.308
69. Saucier G. Replicable item-cluster subcomponents in the NEO five-factor inventory. *J Pers Assess* (1998) 70(2):263–76. doi:10.1207/s15327752jpa7002_6
70. *Multisite Intervention Study on Suicidal Behaviours-SUPRE-MISS: Protocol of SUPRE-MISS*. World Health Organization – Multisite Intervention Study on Suicidal Behaviours 2002.
71. Mościcki EK. Gender differences in completed and attempted suicides. *Ann Epidemiol* (1994) 4(2):152–8. doi:10.1016/1047-2797(94)90062-0
72. Waern M, Runeson BS, Allebeck P, Beskow J, Rubenowitz E, Skoog I, et al. Mental disorder in elderly suicides: a case-control study. *Am J Psychiatry* (2002) 159(3):450–5. doi:10.1176/appi.ajp.159.3.450
73. Devanand DP, Turret N, Moody BJ, Fitzsimons L, Peyser S, Mickle K, et al. Personality disorders in elderly patients with dysthymic disorder. *Am J Geriatr Psychiatry* (2000) 8(3):188–95. doi:10.1097/00019442-200008000-00002
74. Harrison KE, Dombrovski AY, Morse JQ, Houck P, Schlernitzauer M, Reynolds CF, et al. Alone? Perceived social support and chronic interpersonal difficulties in suicidal elders. *Int Psychogeriatr* (2010) 22(03):445. doi:10.1017/S1041610209991463
75. Waern M, Beskow J, Runeson B, Skoog I. Suicidal feelings in the last year of life in elderly people who commit suicide. *The Lancet* (1999) 354 (9182):917–8. doi:10.1016/S0140-6736(99)93099-4
76. Abrams RC, Horowitz SV. Personality disorders after age 50: a meta-analysis. *J Personal Disord* (1996) 10(3):271–81. doi:10.1521/pedi.1996.10.3.271
77. Kunik ME, Mulsant BH, Rifai AH, Sweet R, Pasternak R, Zubenko GS. Diagnostic rate of comorbid personality disorder in elderly psychiatric inpatients. *Am J Psychiatry* (1994) 151(4):603–5. doi:10.1176/ajp.151.4.603
78. Koenig HG, Meador KG, Cohen HJ, Blazer DG. Detection and treatment of major depression in older medically ill hospitalized patients. *Int J Psychiatry Med* (1989) 18(1):17–31. doi:10.2190/QUP8-XL19-TKXK-CRE5
79. German PS, Shapiro S, Skinner EA, Von Korff M, Klein LE, Turner RW, et al. Detection and management of mental health problems of older patients by primary care providers. *JAMA* (1987) 257(4):489. doi:10.1001/jama.257.4.489
80. Uncapher H, Areán PA. Physicians are less willing to treat suicidal ideation in older patients. *J Am Geriatr Soc* (2000) 48(2):188–92. doi:10.1111/j.1532-5415.2000.tb03910.x
81. Magnavita JJ. *Handbook of Personality Disorders – Theory and Practice [Internet]*. New Jersey, United States: John Wiley & Sons, Inc (2004).
82. Grant BF, Hasin DS, Stinson FS, Dawson DA, Chou SP, Ruan WJ, et al. Prevalence, correlates, and disability of personality disorders in the United States: results from the national epidemiologic survey on alcohol and related conditions. *J Clin Psychiatry* (2004) 65(7):948–58. doi:10.4088/JCP.v65n0711
83. Torgersen S, Kringlen E, Cramer V. The prevalence of personality disorders in a community sample. *Arch Gen Psychiatry* (2001) 58(6):590–6. doi:10.1001/archpsyc.58.6.590
84. Engels GI, Duijsens IJ, Haringsma R, van Putten CM. Personality disorders in the elderly compared to four younger age groups: a cross-sectional study of community residents and mental health patients. *J Pers Disord* (2003) 17(5):447–59. doi:10.1521/pedi.17.5.447.22971
85. Zimmerman M, Coryell W. DSM-III personality disorder diagnoses in a nonpatient sample: demographic correlates and comorbidity. *Arch Gen Psychiatry* (1989) 46(8):682. doi:10.1001/archpsyc.1989.01810080012002
86. Lentz V, Robinson J, Bolton JM. Childhood adversity, mental disorder comorbidity, and suicidal behavior in schizotypal personality disorder. *J Nerv Ment Dis* (2010) 198(11):795–801. doi:10.1097/NMD.0b013e3181f9804c
87. Soloff PH, Lis JA, Kelly T, Cornelius J, Ulrich R. Risk factors for suicidal behavior in borderline personality disorder. *Am J Psychiatry* (1994) 151(9):1316–23. doi:10.1176/ajp.151.9.1316
88. Roth KB, Borges G, Medina-Mora M-E, Orozco R, Ouéda C, Wilcox HC. Depressed mood and antisocial behavior problems as correlates for suicide-related behaviors in Mexico. *J Psychiatr Res* (2011) 45(5):596–602. doi:10.1016/j.jpsychires.2010.10.009
89. Black DW, Baumgard CH, Bell SE. A 16- to 45-year follow-up of 71 men with antisocial personality disorder. *Compr Psychiatry* (1995) 36(2):130–40. doi:10.1016/S0010-440X(95)90108-6
90. Zanarini MC, Frankenburg FR, Reich DB, Fitzmaurice GM. Fluidity of the subsyndromal phenomenology of borderline personality disorder over 16 years of prospective follow-up. *Am J Psychiatry* (2016) 173(7):688–94. doi:10.1176/appi.ajp.2015.15081045
91. Paris J, Zweig-Frank H. A 27-year follow-up of patients with borderline personality disorder. *Compr Psychiatry* (2001) 42(6):482–7. doi:10.1053/comp.2001.26271
92. Pompili M, Girardi P, Ruberto A, Tatarelli R. Suicide in borderline personality disorder: a meta-analysis. *Nord J Psychiatry* (2005) 59(5):319–24. doi:10.1080/08039480500320025
93. Shearer SL, Peters CP, Quaytman MS, Wadman BE. Intent and lethality of suicide attempts among female borderline inpatients. *Am J Psychiatry* (1988) 145(11):1424–7. doi:10.1176/ajp.145.11.1424
94. Kernberg OF. *Internal World and External Reality*. New York, United States: Jason Aronson, Inc (1980).
95. McGlashan TH, Grilo CM, Sanislow CA, Ralevski E, Morey LC, Gunderson JG, et al. Two-year prevalence and stability of individual DSM-IV criteria for schizotypal, borderline, avoidant, and obsessive-compulsive personality disorders: toward a hybrid model of axis II disorders. *Am J Psychiatry* (2005) 162(5):883–9. doi:10.1176/appi.ajp.162.5.883
96. Alexopoulos GS. Depression in the elderly. *The Lancet* (2005) 365(9475): 1961–70. doi:10.1016/S0140-6736(05)66665-2
97. Yen S, Pagano ME, Shea MT, Grilo CM, Gunderson JG, Skodol AE, et al. Recent life events preceding suicide attempts in a personality disorder sample: findings from the collaborative longitudinal personality disorders study. *J Consult Clin Psychol* (2005) 73(1):99–105. doi:10.1037/0022-006X.73.1.99
98. Diedrich A, Voderholzer U. Obsessive–compulsive personality disorder: a current review. *Curr Psychiatry Rep* (2015) 17(2):2. doi:10.1007/s11920-014-0547-8
99. Grant JE, Mooney ME, Kushner MG. Prevalence, correlates, and comorbidity of DSM-IV obsessive-compulsive personality disorder: results from the national epidemiologic survey on alcohol and related conditions. *J Psychiatr Res* (2012) 46(4):469–75. doi:10.1016/j.jpsychires.2012.01.009
100. Ullrich S, Coid J. The age distribution of self-reported personality disorder traits in a household population. *J Pers Disord* (2009) 23(2):187–200. doi:10.1521/pedi.2009.23.2.187
101. Chen H, Cohen P, Crawford TN, Kasen S, Johnson JG, Berenson K. Relative impact of young adult personality disorders on subsequent quality of life: findings of a community-based longitudinal study. *J Pers Disord* (2006) 20(5):510–23. doi:10.1521/pedi.2006.20.5.510
102. Skodol AE, Gunderson JG, McGlashan TH, Dyck IR, Stout RL, Bender DS, et al. Functional impairment in patients with schizotypal, borderline, avoidant, or obsessive-compulsive personality disorder. *Am J Psychiatry* (2002) 159(2):276–83. doi:10.1176/appi.ajp.159.2.276
103. Grilo CM, Skodol AE, Gunderson JG, Sanislow CA, Stout RL, Shea MT, et al. Longitudinal diagnostic efficiency of DSM-IV criteria for obsessive-compulsive personality disorder: a 2-year prospective study. *Acta Psychiatr Scand* (2004) 110(1):64–8. doi:10.1046/j.0001-690X.2003.00223.x
104. Conwell Y, Caine ED, Olsen K. Suicide and cancer in late life. *Hosp Community Psychiatry* (1990) 41(12):1334–9.
105. Horton-Deutsch SL, Clark DC, Farran CJ. Chronic dyspnea and suicide in elderly men. *Hosp Community Psychiatry* (1992) 43(12):1198–203.
106. Dombrovski AY, Szanto K, Siegle GJ, Wallace ML, Forman SD, Sahakian B, et al. Lethal forethought: delayed reward discounting differentiates high- and low-lethality suicide attempts in old age. *Biol Psychiatry* (2011) 70(2):138–44. doi:10.1016/j.biopsych.2010.12.025
107. Pinto A, Steinglass JE, Greene AL, Weber EU, Simpson HB. Capacity to delay reward differentiates obsessive-compulsive disorder and obsessive-compulsive personality disorder. *Biol Psychiatry* (2014) 75(8):653–9. doi:10.1016/j.biopsych.2013.09.007
108. Dirks BL. Repetition of parasuicide – ICD-10 personality disorders and adversity. *Acta Psychiatr Scand* (1998) 98(3):208–13. doi:10.1111/j.1600-0447.1998.tb10068.x

109. Raja M, Azzoni A. The impact of obsessive-compulsive personality disorder on the suicidal risk of patients with mood disorders. *Psychopathology* (2007) 40(3):184–90. doi:10.1159/000100366
110. Wilson RS, Krueger KR, Gu L, Bienias JL, Mendes de Leon CF, Evans DA. Neuroticism, extraversion, and mortality in a defined population of older persons. *Psychosom Med* (2005) 67(6):841–5. doi:10.1097/01.psy.0000190615.20656.83
111. Duberstein PR. Openness to experience and completed suicide across the second half of life. *Int Psychogeriatr* (1995) 7(2):183–98. doi:10.1017/S1041610295001967
112. Costa PT, McCrae RR. Personality in adulthood: a six-year longitudinal study of self-reports and spouse ratings on the NEO personality inventory. *J Pers Soc Psychol* (1988) 54(5):853–63. doi:10.1037/0022-3514.54.5.853
113. Samuel D, Widiger T. A meta-analytic review of the relationships between the five-factor model and DSM-IV-TR personality disorders: a facet level analysis. *Clin Psychol Rev* (2008) 28(8):1326–42. doi:10.1016/j.cpr.2008.07.002
114. Wilson RS, Boyle PA, Yu L, Segawa E, Sytsma J, Bennett DA. Conscientiousness, dementia related pathology, and trajectories of cognitive aging. *Psychol Aging* (2015) 30(1):74–82. doi:10.1037/pag0000013
115. Casey DA, Schrodt CJ. Axis II diagnoses in geriatric inpatients. *J Geriatr Psychiatry Neurol* (1989) 2(2):87–8.
116. Fogel BS, Westlake R. Personality disorder diagnoses and age in inpatients with major depression. *J Clin Psychiatry* (1990) 51(6):232–5.
117. Kelly TM, Mann JJ. Validity of DSM-III-R diagnosis by psychological autopsy: a comparison with clinician ante-mortem diagnosis. *Acta Psychiatr Scand* (1996) 94(5):337–43. doi:10.1111/j.1600-0447.1996.tb09869.x
118. Szanto K, Galfalvy H, Vanyukov PM, Keilp JG, Dombrovski AY. Pathways to late-life suicidal behavior: cluster analysis and predictive validation of suicidal behavior. *J Clin Psychiatry* (2017) 79(2):17m11611. doi:10.4088/JCP.17m11611
119. Helmes E, Norton MC, Østbye T. Personality change in older adults with dementia: occurrence and association with severity of cognitive impairment. *Adv Aging Res* (2013) 2(1):27–36. doi:10.4236/aar.2013.21004
120. Balsis S, Carpenter BD, Storandt M. Personality change precedes clinical diagnosis of dementia of the Alzheimer type. *J Gerontol B Psychol Sci Soc Sci* (2005) 60(2):98–101. doi:10.1093/geronb/60.2.P98
121. Duchek JM, Balota DA, Storandt M, Larsen R. The power of personality in discriminating between healthy aging and early-stage Alzheimer's disease. *J Gerontol B Psychol Sci Soc Sci* (2007) 62(6):353–61. doi:10.1093/geronb/62.6.P353
122. Duberstein PR, Chapman BP, Tindle HA, Sink KM, Bamonti P, Robbins J, et al. Personality and risk for Alzheimer's disease in adults 72 years of age and older: a 6-year follow-up. *Psychol Aging* (2011) 26(2):351–62. doi:10.1037/a0023405
123. Bower JH, Grossardt BR, Maraganore DM, Ahlskog JE, Colligan RC, Geda YE, et al. Anxious personality predicts an increased risk of Parkinson's disease. *Mov Disord* (2010) 25(13):2105–13. doi:10.1002/mds.23230
124. Heberlein I, Ludin H-P, Scholz J, Vieregge P. Personality, depression, and premorbid lifestyle in twin pairs discordant for Parkinson's disease. *J Neurol Neurosurg Psychiatry* (1998) 64(2):262–6. doi:10.1136/jnnp.64.2.262
125. Glosser G, Clark C, Freundlich B, Kliner-Krenzel L, Flaherty P, Stern M. A controlled investigation of current and premorbid personality: characteristics of Parkinson's disease patients. *Mov Disord* (1995) 10(2):201–6. doi:10.1002/mds.870100211
126. Menza MA, Golbe LI, Cody RA, Forman NE. Dopamine-related personality traits in Parkinson's disease. *Neurology* (1993) 43(3 Pt 1):505–8. doi:10.1212/WNL.43.3_Part_1.505
127. Voon V, Krack P, Lang AE, Lozano AM, Dujardin K, Schüpbach M, et al. A multicentre study on suicide outcomes following subthalamic stimulation for Parkinson's disease. *Brain* (2008) 131(10):2720. doi:10.1093/brain/awn214
128. Lee T, Lee HB, Ahn MH, Kim J, Kim MS, Chung SJ, et al. Increased suicide risk and clinical correlates of suicide among patients with Parkinson's disease. *Parkinsonism Relat Disord* (2016) 32:102–7. doi:10.1016/j.parkreldis.2016.09.006
129. Lockwood KA, Alexopoulos GS, van Gorp WG. Executive dysfunction in geriatric depression. *Am J Psychiatry* (2002) 159(7):1119–26. doi:10.1176/appi.ajp.159.7.1119
130. Alexopoulos GS, Kiosses DN, Heo M, Murphy CF, Shanmugham B, Gunning-Dixon F. Executive dysfunction and the course of geriatric depression. *Biol Psychiatry* (2005) 58(3):204–10. doi:10.1016/j.biopsych.2005.04.024
131. Richard-Devantoy S, Berlim MT, Jollant F. A meta-analysis of neuropsychological markers of vulnerability to suicidal behavior in mood disorders. *Psychol Med* (2014) 44(8):1663–73. doi:10.1017/S0033291713002304
132. LeGris J, van Reekum R. The neuropsychological correlates of borderline personality disorder and suicidal behaviour. *Can J Psychiatry* (2006) 51(3):131–42. doi:10.1177/070674370605100303
133. Krakowski MI, Foxe J, de Sanctis P, Nolan K, Hoptman MJ, Shope C, et al. Aberrant response inhibition and task switching in psychopathic individuals. *Psychiatry Res* (2015) 229(3):1017–23. doi:10.1016/j.psychres.2015.06.018
134. Fineberg NA, Day GA, de Koenigswarter N, Reghunandanan S, Kolli S, Jefferies-Sewell K, et al. The neuropsychology of obsessive-compulsive personality disorder: a new analysis. *CNS Spectr* (2015) 20(5):490–9. doi:10.1017/S1092852914000662
135. Morey LC, Zanarini MC. Borderline personality: traits and disorder. *J Abnorm Psychol* (2000) 109(4):733–7. doi:10.1037/0021-843X.109.4.733
136. Sharma L, Markon KE, Clark LA. Toward a theory of distinct types of "impulsive" behaviors: a meta-analysis of self-report and behavioral measures. *Psychol Bull* (2014) 140(2):374–408. doi:10.1037/a0034418

9

Childhood Maltreatment, Pathological Personality Dimensions and Suicide Risk in Young Adults

Giorgio Falgares[1], Daniela Marchetti[2], Giovanna Manna[1], Pasquale Musso[3], Osmano Oasi[4], Daniel C. Kopala-Sibley[5,6], Sandro De Santis[7] and Maria C. Verrocchio[2]*

[1] Department of Psychological, Pedagogical and Educational Sciences, University of Palermo, Palermo, Italy, [2] Department of Psychological, Health and Territorial Sciences, University of Chieti–Pescara, Chieti, Italy, [3] Department of Languages and Educational Sciences, University of Calabria, Rende, Italy, [4] Department of Psychology, Catholic University of Sacred Heart, Milan, Italy, [5] Department of Psychiatry, Mathison Centre for Mental Health Research and Education, Hotchkiss Brain Institute, University of Calgary, Calgary, AB, Canada, [6] Alberta Children's Hospital Research Institute, University of Calgary, Calgary, AB, Canada, [7] Azienda Provinciale peri Servizi Sanitari, Provincia Autonoma di Trento, Trento, Italy

***Correspondence:**
Giovanna Manna
giovanna.manna@unipa.it

Several studies have demonstrated that child maltreatment (psychological, physical, and sexual abuse, and neglect) may be a significant factor in the development of pathological personality traits that increase the risk for suicidal ideation and behavior from adolescence to adulthood. Currently, the challenge is to understand how different forms of early negative experiences render an individual prone to develop specific personality traits and, in turn, be more vulnerable to suicide risk. To understand the relationship between childhood maltreatment and personality dimensions in suicide risk, our study aims to explore the role of self-criticism and dependency, two different pathological personality traits, as potential mediators of the link between different types of childhood maltreatment and suicide risk in young adults. For this purpose, 306 students from three Italian public universities were recruited. We used the Italian version of the Childhood Experience of Care and Abuse Questionnaire (CECA.Q) to assess experiences of lack of care by parents (i.e., antipathy and neglect) as well as psychological and physical abuse before the age of 17 years. The Depressive Experiences Questionnaire (DEQ) was used to assess the personality dimensions of self-criticism and dependency, and the Suicide History Self-Rating Screening Scale was administered to assess suicide risk. Results revealed that lack of care and psychological abuse were significantly associated with suicide risk and this association was partially mediated by the maladaptive personality dimension of self-criticism. These findings suggest that the combined effect of specific forms of dysfunctional parental behavior during childhood and the development of rigid and dysfunctional negative personality traits may increase the risk for suicidal ideation and behavior during adulthood.

Keywords: child maltreatment, personality traits, suicidal ideation, suicidal behavior, mediation effect

INTRODUCTION

Child maltreatment, such as physical and mental injury as well as sexual abuse and neglect, refers to acts of commission or omission by a parent or other caregiver that results in harm, or the threat of harm, to a child even if the harm is unintentional (Gilbert et al., 2009). These acts deprive children of the security and emotional support necessary for healthy development (Dube et al., 2003).

A large body of research has demonstrated that childhood maltreatment can lead to a range of adverse health outcomes later in life, such as depression, anxiety, substance abuse, and delinquent behavior (Bruffaerts et al., 2010; Brodsky and Biggs, 2012; Gershon et al., 2013).

Several studies have also documented that childhood maltreatment is an important risk factor for suicidal ideation and suicidal attempts (Enns et al., 2006; Brodsky and Stanley, 2008; Barbosa et al., 2014; Puzia et al., 2014; Afifi et al., 2016; Sachs-Ericsson et al., 2016). Recently, efforts have been made to understand the different impact of specific forms of maltreatment on adolescent and adult personality functioning (Witt et al., 2016) and, in turn, on risk for suicide (Dunn et al., 2013). Specifically, an important goal is to identify and understand the processes through which different forms of child maltreatment confer risk for suicidality later in life (Brent, 2011; Nock, 2012).

From this point of view, while several studies explored the mediating role of mental disorders, such as depression, anxiety, and borderline personality disorder (Anderson et al., 2002; Hahm et al., 2010; Gershon et al., 2013; Infurna et al., 2016a), relatively fewer studies have focused on the role of personality dimensions (e.g., low self-esteem and perfectionism) and how these can contribute to risk for suicidal behavior from adolescence to adulthood (Glassman et al., 2007; Campos and Holden, 2014).

Particularly, several studies have demonstrated that the pathological personality dimensions of self-criticism (Fazaa and Page, 2003; O'Connor, 2007; Campos and Mesquita, 2014; Falgares et al., 2017a) and dependency (Bornstein and O'Neill, 2000) are significant risk factors for suicide risk and are influenced by dysfunctional early relationships, such as those with parents (Blatt, 2004; Campos et al., 2013; Falgares et al., 2017a). However, to our knowledge, no study has specifically examined the links between childhood maltreatment, self-criticism and dependency, and risk for suicidality in adulthood. Accordingly, in this study we aimed to investigate the role of self-criticism and dependency as potential mediators of the relationship between different types of child maltreatment and suicide risk in young adults.

The Association Among Developmental Adversities, Self-Criticism and Dependency

In Blatt's (2008) two-configurations model, mature personality is a synergistic and balanced product of two main developmental dimensions: interpersonal relatedness, that is the capacity to be involved in intimate, mature, and mutually satisfactory relationships; and self-definition, involving the development of a realistic, integrated, and differentiated identity (see Luyten and Blatt, 2013; Kopala-Sibley and Zuroff, 2014, for reviews).

A delay or disruption in this normal developmental dialectic process could result in a rigid preoccupation with one of these two dimensions. An overemphasis on issues of relatedness is the basis of a pathological personality style that Blatt labeled *dependent/anaclitic*. In contrast, an overemphasis on issues of self-definition is the basis of the *self-critical/introjective* personality style (Blatt and Blass, 1996). According to Campos et al. (2014), a dependent personality style is characterized by intense feelings of loneliness, abandonment, helplessness, and weakness. Because of the lack of internalization of the experiences of care and affection or of the qualities of supportive and loving individuals, others are valued primarily for the care, and satisfaction they provide (Blatt, 1974, 2004). A self-critical personality style, in contrast, is characterized by feelings of unworthiness, inferiority, failure, and guilt, and involves a tendency to adopt a punitive self-stance once standards are not met (Blatt and Zuroff, 1992; Shahar and Priel, 2003).

Based on this theoretical framework, Blatt et al. (1976) developed the Depressive Experiences Questionnaire (DEQ). This self report questionnaire measures three orthogonal factors: dependency, self-criticism, and efficacy. Subsequently, Blatt et al. (1995) factor analyzed the construct of dependency and identified two facets. The first facet, dependence, involves a more immature tendency, including feelings of helplessness, fears, and apprehensions about separation and rejection. The second facet, relatedness, is characterized as more mature, and includes items that describe feelings of loneliness and loss in reaction to the end of a relationship with a particular individual. Other independent lines of research have similarly concluded that dependency has relatively more and less adaptive aspects (Rude and Burnham, 1995). It should be noted that self-criticism, dependence, and relatedness are not categorical personality types. They are conceptualized as continuous, nearly orthogonal dimensions of individual difference (Zuroff et al., 2004).

Some studies have found a connection between self-criticism and dependency and child maltreatment or poor-quality parenting. Campos et al. (2010) found that self-criticism mediated the relationship between early caretaking relationships with the mother and depressive symptoms. Neediness – a sub factor of dependency – mediated the relationship between early maternal overprotection and depressive symptoms. Some data show that emotional abuse, more than physical and sexual abuse, confers risk for the development of suicidal ideation (Puzia et al., 2014). On the contrary, other studies demonstrate that sexual and physical abuse are the strongest predictors of the initial development as well as the persistence of suicidal behavior (Bruffaerts et al., 2010). Lassri and Shahar (2012) suggested that self-criticism is an important mediator of the relationship between childhood emotional maltreatment and psychopathology in a group of undergraduate students. In the same way, but in a group of eating disorder patients, Speranza et al. (2005) found that self-criticism but not dependency is correlated with negative events or experiences in childhood. Baetens et al. (2015) highlighted that perceived parental expressed emotions have an important effect on adolescents' well-being and non-suicidal self-injury (NSSI), with self-criticism mediating this relationship. An overview of the literature about this topic indicates that self-criticism is an important predictor of suicidality (Campos et al., 2013).

The Association Among Self-Criticism, Dependency and Suicide Risk

The link among self-criticism, dependency and suicide risk has been investigated in several studies (see Falgares et al., 2017a for a summary). Fazaa and Page (2003) found that highly self-critical patients were more likely to have attempted suicide in response to a failure, and that their intent in attempting suicide was to escape from the actual events–expectations discrepancy. Dependent patients were more likely to have made their attempt in response to an interpersonal trigger which suggests that their intention in attempting suicide was to communicate their feelings of distress to others. Fazaa and Page (2009) also reported that adult participants with higher dependency showed higher rescue scores (i.e., using methods that made rescue more likely). In contrast, higher self-criticism was associated with a greater wish to die. Fehon et al. (2000) analyzed associations between dependency, self-criticism, impulsivity, and suicidal behavior in a sample of depressed hospitalized adolescents. They found that suicide risk did not significantly differ between highly self-critical and highly dependent patients. However, dependent individuals appeared generally to be more engaged in patterns of impulsive gestures and attempts, whereas self-critical individuals appeared less impulsive and more likely to plan acts of self-harm. Klomek et al. (2008), in a cross-sectional study, examined the relationship between suicidality and dependent and self-critical vulnerabilities among adolescents and found that suicidal participants have significantly higher levels of both self-criticism and dependency than non-suicidal inpatients and healthy controls. In a sample of adults, Campos et al. (2013) found that depressive symptoms mediated the association between self-critical perfectionism and suicidality. Highly self-critically perfectionistic individuals are vulnerable to intense depression, often accompanied by suicidal impulses, when confronted with stressful life events and, in particular, events that disrupt self-definition or a sense of personal achievement. Campos and Mesquita (2014) tested a model of suicidality that included dependency, self-criticism, anger-temperament, depression, and anger-in in a community of adolescents. Self-critical, dependent, and anger-in traits predicted depression, which in turn predicted suicidality directly and indirectly through anger-in. Finally, Campos and Holden (2014) in a Portuguese non-clinical sample of adults found that highly self-critical depressed individuals, were more likely to show help-seeking behaviors for emotional suffering (i.e., have visited a mental health professional) and were at greater risk for suicidal behaviors relative to less self-critical individuals.

Based on the above considerations, we aim to explore the mediating role of self-criticism and dependence/relatedness (the two factors of the dependent personality) in the relationship between different forms of child maltreatment and suicidal risk. Specifically, in line with previous studies that found that emotional maltreatment predicts negative attribution of the self (Pagura et al., 2006; Soffer et al., 2008), we hypothesized that antipathy and neglect, as well as psychological abuse, would be associated with higher levels of self-criticism. Furthermore, according to other studies (Grilo et al., 1999; Mendelson et al., 2002), we expected that physical and sexual abuse would be associated with higher levels of dependency. Finally, self-criticism is expected to be more strongly associated with suicide risk relative to dependency (Campos and Holden, 2014). It is important to note that some studies consider antipathy and neglect as one factor (Schimmenti and Bifulco, 2015). Following these studies, we chose to use the term "lack of care" to refer to these two forms of maltreatment.

MATERIALS AND METHODS

Participants

Participants were drawn from a multisite undergraduate student data set ($N = 306$) collected at public universities located in northern (Lombardy), central (Abruzzo), and southern (Sicily) Italian regions. More than 96% of these students were attending psychology courses, characterized in Italy by a high female prevalence (more than 80%, see AlmaLaurea, 2017). Only a small proportion of them (1.63%) had missing information on one or more of the study variables. These participants were excluded from the analyses, given that the p-value for Little's Missing Completely At Random test was not significant, $\chi^2(19) = 16.27$, $p = 0.64$, and because attrition analyses revealed no significant associations between demographic variables and missingness. We also excluded eight participants for having extreme outlier values after preliminary data processing. Our final sample thus consisted of 293 young adults (males = 16.72% and females = 83.28%, which closely reflects the gender distribution of the population of psychology students) aged 18–27 years ($M = 21.57$, $SD = 2.02$). Almost all of them were Caucasian Italians (95.22%), had no current occupation (92.83%), and were unmarried (97.27%). The majority came from middle-class backgrounds (80.20%), had married and cohabiting parents (81.91%) who had at least a high school education (71.33% for mothers and 64,85% for fathers). Nearly all participants indicated their birth mother (97.95%) and birth father (98.63%) as the reference figures who brought them up in childhood. About 11% had parental loss before 17 years of age (specifically, about 3.5% experienced death of mother or father and 7.5% parental separation). Only one (0.34%) had a previous hospitalization experience for psychological/psychiatric reasons, while about 16% had some psychological counseling with a psychologist or psychiatrist (including the freely accessible sessions provided by the university psychological counseling services), consisting of at least five meetings and usually for not more than 1 year.

Measures

Socio-Demographics

Respondents were asked to indicate their gender, age, ethnicity, occupation, marital status, SES level, previous hospitalization experience, previous psychological counseling and its typology, as well as their parents' marital status and education.

Childhood Experience of Care and Abuse Questionnaire

The Childhood Experience of Care and Abuse Questionnaire (CECA.Q; Bifulco et al., 2005) was used to retrospectively assess adverse childhood experiences before the age of 17. The CECA.Q was developed to mirror the corresponding interview measure (CECA; Bifulco et al., 1994) and showed good internal consistency in different contexts (e.g., Smith et al., 2002; Verrocchio et al., 2014; Infurna et al., 2016b). Accordingly, the translated Italian version of the CECA.Q used in this study was adapted by considering the validated Italian CECA interview (Giannone et al., 2011) and following the recommendations of the International Test Commission (2005). As suggested by the validation work of Bifulco et al. (2005), the Italian version of the questionnaire incorporates sections on parental loss, reference figures in childhood, and assesses parental care (antipathy and neglect), and parental psychological, physical, and sexual abuse.

Parental loss refers to either parental death or separation of 1 year or more due to a parent moving and permanently living elsewhere before age 17. These life events are important, considering, for example, that Agid et al. (1999) found that loss due to separation and loss due to death are both risk factors for mood disorders. Parental loss was assessed by asking two questions: (1) "Did either parent die before you were age 17?" and (2) "Have you ever been separated from your parent for 1 year or more before you were age 17," both rated as 0 (*no*) and 1 (*yes*) for both the mother and the father. Three successive questions asked about the age, duration, and reason for separation from the parent(s). For this section, the score could range from 0 to 4, with higher scores indicating more severe loss during childhood. However, the distribution of the score was highly skewed (>3) due to a large number of observations at 0. To ensure an adequate sufficient distribution of cases for analysis (in practice, this usually means a minimum number of 10–20 cases per cell when considering each discrete value of the distribution, e.g., Warner, 2012, and Hahs-Vaughn, 2016), the variable was dichotomized (see MacCallum et al., 2002) with a score of 0 for absence of death of parents or separation from them for 1 year or more before age 17 and a score of 1 indicating the presence of at least one death of a parent or separation from one parent for 1 year or more before age 17.

Antipathy refers to hostility, coldness or rejection as well as 'scapegoating' behavior shown toward the child by parents or surrogate parents. The related subscale consists of eight paired items for maternal and paternal figures (sample item: "At times she/he made me feel I was a nuisance"). Items were rated on a 5-point Likert scale ranging from 1 (*no, not at all*) to 5 (*yes, definitely*) and were summed to create two indicators of maternal ($\alpha = 0.84$) and paternal ($\alpha = 0.87$) antipathy. In this study, we averaged these two variables to obtain a single indicator of parental antipathy (score ranging from 8 to 40, with higher scores indicating more parental antipathy during childhood).

Neglect refers to a distinct disinterest in the child's material and physical care (e.g., food, clothing, and health), friendships, schoolwork, career prospects, and whereabouts. The related subscale consists of eight paired items for maternal and paternal figures (sample item: "She/he neglected my basic needs, e.g., food and clothes"). Items were rated on a 5-point Likert scale ranging from 1 (*no, not at all*) to 5 (*yes, definitely*) and were summed to create two indicators of maternal ($\alpha = 0.79$) and paternal ($\alpha = 0.88$) neglect. In this study, we averaged these two variables to obtain a single indicator of parental neglect (score ranging from 8 to 40, with higher scores indicating more parental neglect during childhood).

Psychological abuse refers to a highly controlling and domineering relationship of parental figures with the child, including humiliation, terrorization, cognitive disorientation, exploitation, and corruption or intentional deprivation of needs or valued objects. The range of such experiences and their frequency determine the severity of this form of abuse. The related subscale consists of 17 psychological abuse items paired with frequency items for maternal and paternal figures (sample item: "She/he liked to see me suffer" and "How Frequent?"). Items regarding the amount of psychological abuse were rated as 0 (*no*), 1 (*unsure*), or 2 (*yes*), while frequency items were rated as 0 (*never*), 1 (*once*), 2 (*rarely*), and 3 (*often*). In this study, each pair of items were multiplied, and the obtained scores were summed to create indicators of maternal ($\alpha = 0.85$) and paternal ($\alpha = 0.83$) psychological abuse. We averaged these two variables to obtain a single indicator of parental psychological abuse (score ranging from 0 to 102, with higher scores indicating more parental psychological abuse).

Physical abuse refers to violence toward the child by parents or other caregivers in the household, including attacks where implements such as belts or sticks are used, or punching or kicking occurs with the possibility of causing harm. The screening question for this section was "When you were a child or teenager, were you ever hit repeatedly with an implement (such as a belt or stick) or punched, kicked, or burnt by someone in the household?," rated as 0 (*no*) and 1 (*yes*). Severity was determined by using four dichotomous items (0 = *no*, 1 = *yes*), measuring the intensity of the attack and its frequency (example item: "Did the hitting happen on more than one occasion?"). Thus, severity could range from 0 to 4, with higher scores indicating more severe physical abuse. We multiplied the obtained scores for each participant to obtain a single indicator of psychological abuse. However, because the distribution of this comprehensive score was highly skewed (>3) and to ensure an adequate distribution of cases for analysis, this variable was dichotomized with a score of 0 for absence of any episode of physical abuse and a score of 1 for presence of one or more of such episodes.

Sexual abuse refers to age-inappropriate physical contact or approach of a sexual nature by any adult to the child. Screening questions for this section were: (1) "When you were a child or teenager, did you ever have any unwanted sexual experiences?," (2) "Did anyone force you or persuade you to have sexual intercourse against your wishes before age 17?," and (3) "Can you think of any upsetting sexual experiences before age 17 with a related adult or someone in authority, e.g., teacher?" These questions were rated as 0 (*no*) and 1 (*yes*), with score ranging from 0 to 3 and higher scores indicating more sexual abuse during childhood. Severity was determined by using seven dichotomous items (0 = *no*, 1 = *yes*), measuring the degree and intrusiveness of sexual contact, the relationship of trust with the perpetrator, and the frequency and duration of the abuse (example items: "Was the other person someone you knew?," "Did this person do it to you on more than one occasion?," and "Did it involve sexual intercourse?"). Thus, severity could range from 0 to 7, with higher scores indicating more severe sexual abuse. We multiplied the obtained scores for each participant to obtain a single indicator of sexual abuse. However, because the distribution of this comprehensive score was highly skewed (> 3) and to ensure an adequate distribution of cases for analysis, this variable was dichotomized with a score of zero for absence of any episode of sexual abuse and a score of one for presence of one or more of such episodes.

Depressive Experiences Questionnaire

The 66-item self-report Italian version of the DEQ (Blatt et al., 1976; Falgares et al., 2017b) was used to assess pathological personality traits. Despite its name, the DEQ measures stable personality traits which confer risk for the development of depression, but which do not measure acute depression (Mongrain and Zuroff, 1994; Zuroff et al., 2004). The DEQ yields factor scores for three primary factors: dependency, self-criticism, and efficacy. Within the DEQ dependency scale, it is possible to distinguish two subscales: dependence and relatedness (Blatt et al., 1995). For the purposes of this study, the third primary factor (i.e., efficacy) was not considered, while we used the two subscales of dependency, dependence (example item: "Without support from others who are close to me, I would be helpless") and relatedness (example item: "I would feel like I'd be losing an important part of myself if I lost a very close friend"), and the self-criticism scale (example item: "I tend to be very critical of myself"). Items were scored on a 7-point Likert scale, ranging from 1 (*strongly disagree*) to 7 (*strongly agree*). Self-criticism was scored using the original factor scores of Blatt et al. (1976). Dependence and relatedness were scored using the scoring method of Blatt et al. (1995) by summing the items contained in the subscales (respectively, 10 and 8 items). The Italian version of the DEQ has good internal consistency and validity, similar to those of the original DEQ (Falgares et al., 2017b). In the present study, reliability as measured with the Cronbach's α was 0.83 for self-criticism, 0.72 for dependence, and 0.79 for relatedness.

Suicidal History Self-Rating Screening Scale

The 16-item Suicidal History Self-Rating Screening Scale (SHSS; Innamorati et al., 2011) was used to assess propensity for suicide risk. Items were rated on a dichotomous scale (0 = *no*, 1 = *yes*). The SHSS assesses suicidal ideation (example item: "Have you ever thought about taking your own life?"), planning (example item: "Have you ever planned a way of taking your own life?"), or attempts (example item: "Have you ever tried to take your own life?") both in the previous year and lifetime. Despite these different facets of suicide, a one-factor solution was obtained in the validation study of the scale (with a clinical sample), having a Kuder-Richardson-20 index of 0.95 and mean inter-item correlation of 0.53 (Innamorati et al., 2011). Another study with a non-clinical sample confirmed one-factor structure of the SHSS (Pompili et al., 2016). The SHSS has demonstrated good internal consistency and validity (Innamorati et al., 2011; Pompili et al., 2016). For these reasons, as well as due to analytical issues (see section "Descriptive Statistics and Preliminary Analyses"), a unitary score was used. Thus, items were summed to provide a score ranging between 0 and 16, with higher scores indicating higher propensity to suicide. For the present sample, Cronbach alpha was 0.87.

Procedure

The local psychology department's ethics committees approved this study and all procedures were performed in accordance with the Italian Association of Psychology (2015) ethical principles for psychological research, inspired by the Declaration of Helsinki and its revisions (World Medical Association, 2001) as well as by the American Psychological Association [APA]'s (2010) ethics guidelines. Data were collected during class time at three Italian universities (in the cities of Palermo, Chieti, and Milan). After informing participants about the purpose of the research, the voluntary nature of participation and the anonymity of responses, students in each class were asked to participate in the study. More than 95% agreed to participate and written informed consent was obtained from all of them prior to collecting data in groups of 25–30 students in a large space in order to ensure anonymity. Trained Italian researchers collected the data in each university. Participants could withdraw at any time. All students were told to call the psychology departments for any further information about the research.

Statistical Analysis

We followed three main steps to conduct data analysis. First, we computed descriptive statistics for the key observed study variables including their prevalence in terms of moderate or marked levels as well as means and standard deviations, skewness and kurtosis indices, and minimum and maximum values of standardized scores. The latter descriptive analysis results allowed verification of the univariate normality of the distributions. When it was the case, non-normally distributed variables were transformed to improve normality and extreme outliers. Scores beyond | 3.29| standard deviations from the mean (Tabachnick and Fidell, 2013), were excluded from the analyses (not exceeding 5% of total participants including cases eliminated for having missing data). Furthermore, we used the Mahalanobis distance and the Mardia's multivariate kurtosis coefficient to test the multivariate normality and identify other potential multivariate outliers. Then, the final descriptive statistics for the study variables were computed.

Second, we evaluated the associations of socio-demographic with the main study variables. Particularly, we conducted a multivariate analysis of variance (MANOVA) to examine whether participants' scores for antipathy, neglect, psychological abuse, physical abuse, dependence, relatedness, self-criticism, and propensity for suicide differed based on region of university education (1 = North Italy, Lombardy; 2 = Central Italy, Abruzzo; 3 = South Italy, Sicily), gender (0 = male; 1 = female),

SES (dummy coded: 0 = low-medium; 1 = medium-high); parents' marital status (dummy coded: 0 = cohabiting; 1 = not cohabiting), parents' education (dummy coded: 0 = at most one of parents with high school diploma; 1 = both parents with at least high school diploma), parental loss (as described in the section "Measures" this variable was dichotomized with 0 = no death of parents or separation from them for 1 year or more before age 17; 1 = at least death of one parent or separation from one parent for 1 year or more before age 17), and previous psychological counseling (0 = no; 1 = yes). We computed Pearson's correlation coefficients to describe potential significant relations between age and the above-mentioned key study variables.

Third, after reporting bivariate correlations for the key study variables including the significant control demographic variables, we used structural equation modeling (SEM) to explore the mediating processes in the relation between different forms of childhood maltreatment and suicide risk in emerging adulthood. We initially presented the *a priori* model including the antecedent, mediating, outcome, and control variables as well as direct and indirect paths. Then, we carried out SEM analyses to test this model within *Mplus 7.2* (Muthén and Muthén, 2014) using the maximum likelihood estimation method. All indirect effects were tested using a Bootstrap sample of 1000 for the 95% confidence intervals. To evaluate the model fit we used multiple criteria (see Hu and Bentler, 1999; Kline, 2010; Faraci and Musso, 2013): the chi-square (χ^2) statistic, the comparative fit index (CFI; Bentler, 1990), the Tucker-Lewis index (TLI; also called the non-normed fit index or NNFI, Bentler and Bonett, 1980), the root mean square error of approximation (RMSEA; Steiger, 1990) and its 90% confidence interval (CI) (Browne and Cudeck, 1993), and standardized root mean square residual (SRMR; Bentler, 2006). Based on results from a Monte Carlo analysis, Hu and Bentler (1999) suggested that a reasonably good fit is supported when CFI and TLI values are close to or greater than 0.95, RMSEA values are close to or less than 0.06, and SRMR values are close to or less than 0.08. For the RMSEA 90% CI, values below 0.05 for the lower bound and below 0.08 for the upper bound suggest acceptable fit (MacCallum et al., 1996).

RESULTS

Descriptive Statistics and Preliminary Analyses

An initial data inspection showed that physical abuse, sexual abuse and the subscales of suicidal planning and suicidal attempts of SHSS presented a large number of observations equal to zero and were highly skewed (>3). This resulted in a not-positive definite covariance matrix. Thus, physical abuse and sexual abuse were dichotomized, while the three subscales of the SHSS were computed together to obtain a comprehensive score (for both choices, see section "Measures" for further details). **Tables 1, 2** summarize the descriptive statistics. Both the prevalence and the mean scores of the key study variables generally confirmed the non-clinical nature of the sample. Antipathy, neglect, psychological abuse, and propensity for suicide were not normally distributed (**Table 2**) with skewness and kurtosis values >|1.00| (Curran et al., 1996; Kline, 2010) as well as maximum values of standardized scores >3.29 (as dichotomous variables, physical abuse and sexual abuse were excluded from these considerations). For these reasons, a transformation was applied for non-normal variables by computing the square root for each distribution as the best solution. After re-calculating descriptive statistics for the transformed variables, eight cases presenting extreme outlier standardized scores (>|3.62| , calculated as 3.29 plus a tolerance of 10%) were excluded from the sample. The new distributions showed adequate skewness and kurtosis values (see **Table 2**). Because less than 10% of respondents indicated experiences of sexual abuse, we excluded this variable from subsequent analyses because this small number continued to preclude meaningful results. Using Mahalanobis distance with $p < 0.001$, no cases were identified as multivariate outliers. However, Mardia's multivariate kurtosis coefficient slightly exceeded the critical value. We detected five potential multivariate outliers. After performing the subsequent analyses without or with these cases, we found no effect on the pattern of results. Thus, we retained these five cases in the final sample.

We then examined the influence of the demographic variables (region of university education, gender, SES, parents' marital status, parents' education, parental loss, and previous psychological appointments) on the key study variables. The MANOVA resulted in a significant multivariate effect of gender, Wilks' $\lambda = 0.93$, $F(8,212) = 2.11$, $p = 0.036$, $\eta^2 = 0.07$. Univariate analyses of variance (ANOVAs) showed that gender had a significant effect on Dependence, $F(1,219) = 4.23$, $p = 0.041$, $\eta^2 = 0.02$, and Relatedness, $F(1,219) = 5.09$, $p = 0.025$, $\eta^2 = 0.02$. Females reported significantly higher levels of dependence and relatedness than did males. No significant multivariate effects were observed for region of university education, Wilks' $\lambda = 0.92$, $F(16,424) = 1.10$, $p = 0.35$, $\eta^2 = 0.04$, SES, Wilks' $\lambda = 0.95$, $F(8,212) = 1.46$, $p = 0.17$, $\eta^2 = 0.05$, parents' marital status, Wilks' $\lambda = 0.99$, $F(8,212) = 0.22$, $p = 0.99$, $\eta^2 = 0.01$, parents' education, Wilks' $\lambda = 0.98$, $F(8,212) = 0.60$, $p = 0.78$, $\eta^2 = 0.02$, parental loss, Wilks' $\lambda = 0.98$, $F(8,212) = 0.66$, $p = 0.72$, $\eta^2 = 0.02$, and previous psychological counseling, Wilks' $\lambda = 0.94$, $F(8,212) = 1.61$, $p = 0.12$, $\eta^2 = 0.06$. Furthermore, age was significantly and negatively related to dependence, $r = -0.14$, $p = 0.015$, and relatedness, $r = -0.16$, $p = 0.007$, but not to the other variables (see **Table 2**).

SEM Analysis of the Mediation Model

Based on the preliminary analyses, gender and age were used as control variables. Correlations between the key and control study variables are displayed in **Table 3**.

To test our hypotheses, we used the *a priori* model presented in **Figure 1**. In view of our non-clinical sample, as suggested from literature (e.g., Bifulco et al., 2005) we considered antipathy and neglect as observed indicators of the latent variable lack of care. This variable as well as psychological abuse and physical abuse represented the antecedent variables influencing the outcome variable propensity for suicide, both directly and indirectly by the mediating role of dependence, relatedness and self-criticism. Gender was controlled for by allowing it to predict all the mediating and outcome variables as well as the latent variable lack of care (given the significant correlation with neglect, as shown in **Table 2**), while age was controlled by allowing it to predict only the mediating variables. The covariation within the antecedent variables, on one hand, and the mediating variables, on the other, was also allowed. This model had a good fit, χ^2_{SB} (13) = 21.96, $p = 0.06$, CFI = 0.99, TLI = 0.97, RMSEA = 0.05, RMSEA 90% CI = 0.00–0.08, SRMR = 0.02.

Standardized coefficients are shown in **Figure 2**. Gender was significantly associated with lack of care as well as

TABLE 1 | Prevalence of the key study variables, calculated as the percentage of participants exceeding the cut-off scores for moderate or marked levels.

Observed variable	Cut-off scores for moderate or marked level	% (*N* = 301)
(1) Antipathy (scored 8–40)	≥25[a]	2.66
(2) Neglect (scored 8–40)	≥22[a]	6.64
(3) Psychological abuse (scored 0–102)	There is no established cut-off	–
(4) Physical abuse (scored 0 or 1)	≥1[a]	17.61
(5) Sexual abuse (scored 0 or 1)	≥1[a]	9.97
(6) Dependence (scored 10–70)	There is no established cut-off	–
(7) Relatedness (scored 8–56)	There is no established cut-off	–
(8) Self-criticism (factor derived scale score)	There is no established cut-off	–
(9) Propensity for suicide (scored 0–16)	≥8[b]	2.33
Suicidal ideation in the last year (scored 0 or 1)	≥1[b]	10.96
Suicidal planning in the last year (scored 0 or 1)	≥1[b]	5.65
Suicidal attempt in the last year (scored 0 or 1)	≥1[b]	0.66
More than one suicide attempt in the last year (scored 0 or 1)	≥1[b]	0.33
Suicidal ideation in the lifetime excluding the last year (scored 0 or 1)	≥1[b]	12.29
Suicidal planning in the lifetime excluding the last year (scored 0 or 1)	≥1[b]	6.98
Suicidal attempt in the lifetime excluding the last year (scored 0 or 1)	≥1[b]	2.33
More than one suicide attempt in the lifetime excluding the last year (scored 0 or 1)	≥1[b]	0.66

[a]*See Bifulco et al., 2005;* [b]*See Innamorati et al., 2011.*

TABLE 2 | Means, standard deviations, skewness, and kurtosis for the key study variables both in their original version and in their transformed version as well as including and excluding extreme outliers.

Observed variable	Transformation	*M*	*SD*	Skewness	Kurtosis	Min. stand.	Max. stand.
			Initial sample, *N* = 301				
(1) Antipathy (scored 8–40)	No	14.48	5.17	1.17	1.51	−1.45	3.87
(2) Neglect (scored 8–40)	No	13.57	4.74	1.26	2.01	−1.18	4.20
(3) Psychological abuse (scored 0–102)	No	4.38	7.46	2.85	10.41	−0.59	6.12
(4) Physical abuse (scored 0 or 1)	No	0.18	0.38	1.71	0.93	−0.46	2.16
(5) Sexual abuse (scored 0 or 1)	No	0.10	0.30	2.75	5.60	−0.33	3.06
(6) Dependence (scored 10–70)	No	42.19	8.62	0.12	−0.01	−2.69	2.76
(7) Relatedness (scored 8–56)	No	37.47	7.27	−0.31	−0.25	−2.95	2.55
(8) Self-criticism (factor-derived scale score)	No	−0.15	1.43	−0.03	0.54	−2.80	3.70
(9) Propensity for suicide (scored 0–16)	No	1.21	2.22	2.25	5.50	−0.55	5.76
			Final sample excluding extreme outliers, *N* = 293				
(1) Antipathy (scored 2.83–6.32)	Yes (square root)	3.71	0.60	0.59	−0.03	−1.77	3.53
(2) Neglect (scored 2.83–6.32)	Yes (square root)	3.61	0.58	0.72	0.43	−1.35	3.56
(3) Psychological abuse (scored 0–10.10)	Yes (square root)	1.30	1.49	0.89	−0.11	−0.87	3.29
(4) Physical abuse (scored 0 or 1)	No	0.16	0.37	1.83	1.34	−0.44	2.26
(5) Sexual abuse (scored 0 or 1)	No	0.10	0.29	2.77	5.69	−0.32	3.07
(6) Dependence (scored 10–70)	No	42.01	8.38	0.09	−0.07	−2.75	2.86
(7) Relatedness (scored 8–56)	No	37.40	7.08	−0.32	−0.29	−3.02	2.63
(8) Self-criticism (factor-derived scale score)	No	−0.18	1.37	−0.21	0.15	−2.90	2.94
(9) Propensity for suicide (scored 0–4)	Yes (square root)	0.60	0.89	1.19	0.18	−0.67	3.53

Min. stand., minimum value of standardized score; Max. stand., maximum value of standardized score.

TABLE 3 | Correlations for key and control study variables.

		1	2	3	4	5	6	7	8	9	10
(1)	Antipathy	–									
(2)	Neglect	0.73***	–								
(3)	Psychological abuse	0.61***	0.56***	–							
(4)	Physical abuse	0.38***	0.32***	0.36***	–						
(5)	Dependence	0.22***	0.14*	0.24***	0.16***	–					
(6)	Relatedness	0.15*	0.05	0.15**	0.04	0.69***	–				
(7)	Self-criticism	0.48***	0.32***	0.42***	0.23***	0.30***	0.20***	–			
(8)	Propensity for suicide	0.53***	0.40***	0.54***	0.25***	0.24***	0.16**	0.48***	–		
(9)	Gender	−0.09	−0.15*	0.01	−0.02	0.18**	0.21***	−0.04	−0.10	–	
(10)	Age	0.07	0.05	−0.01	0.06	−0.14*	−0.16**	−0.07	−0.05	−0.09	–

$*p < 0.05$, $**p < 0.01$, $***p < 0.001$.

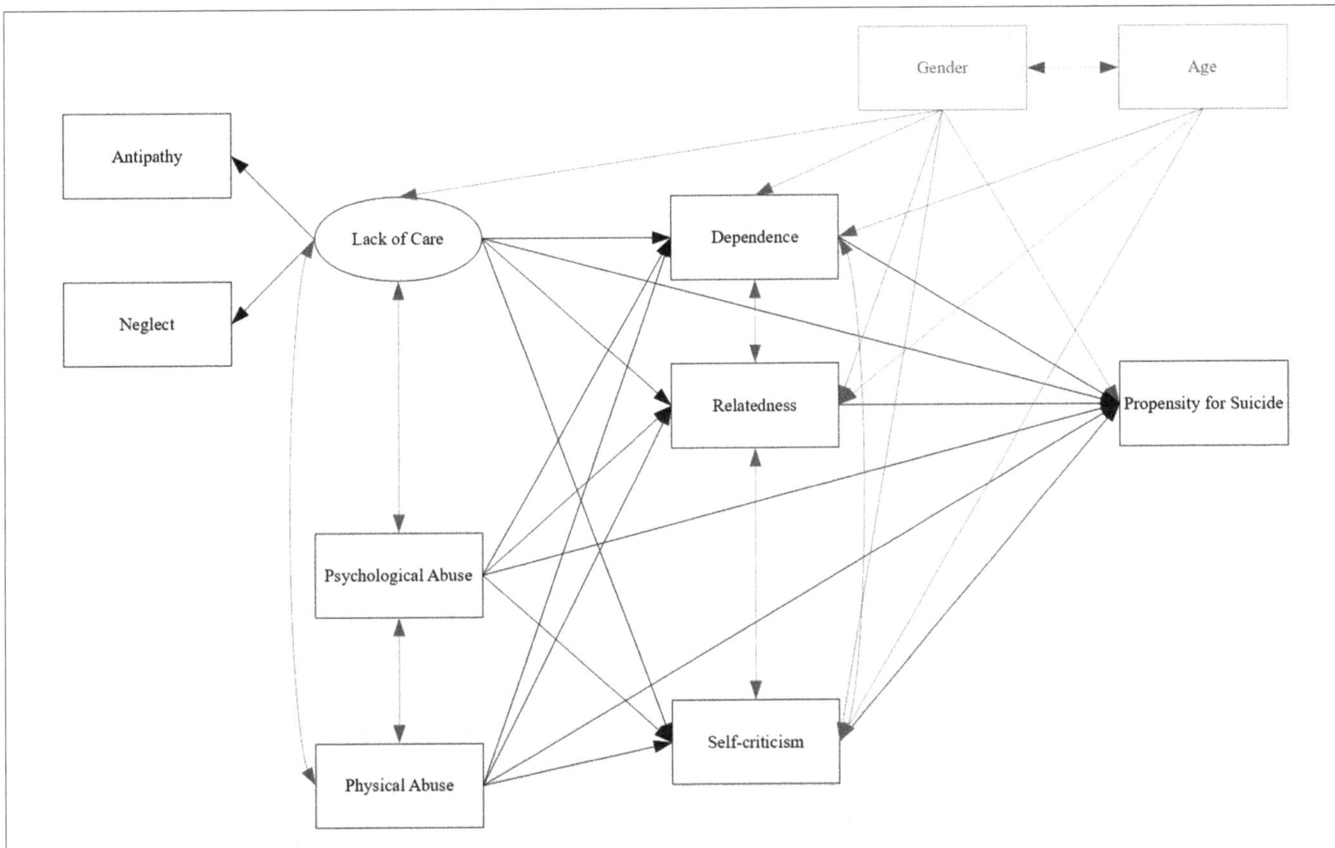

FIGURE 1 | The theoretical model of the study. Covariances, control variables, and their related paths are presented in light gray.

dependence and relatedness, such that experienced lower levels of lack of care and higher levels of dependence and relatedness than males. Age was significantly and negatively related to the mediating variables such that older participants showed lower levels of dependence, relatedness, and self-criticism. Over and above these effects, direct effects showed that lack of care (factor loadings linked to antipathy and neglect were adequate) and psychological abuse were significantly associated with propensity for suicide and higher levels of self-criticism, but not with dependence and relatedness. Self-criticism, but not dependence and relatedness, was significantly related to propensity for suicide. Physical abuse was not significantly linked to mediating or outcome variables. In summary, these results revealed that there was evidence of significant mediating effects of self-criticism in the relationships between lack of care, psychological abuse and suicidality. Specifically, while controlling for gender and age, lack of care, and psychological abuse were not only directly but also indirectly and positively related to propensity for suicide via self-criticism (respectively, $\beta = 0.08$, $p = 0.002$, 95% CI = 0.030–0.140, and $\beta = 0.04$, $p = 0.047$, 95% CI = 0.001–0.071).

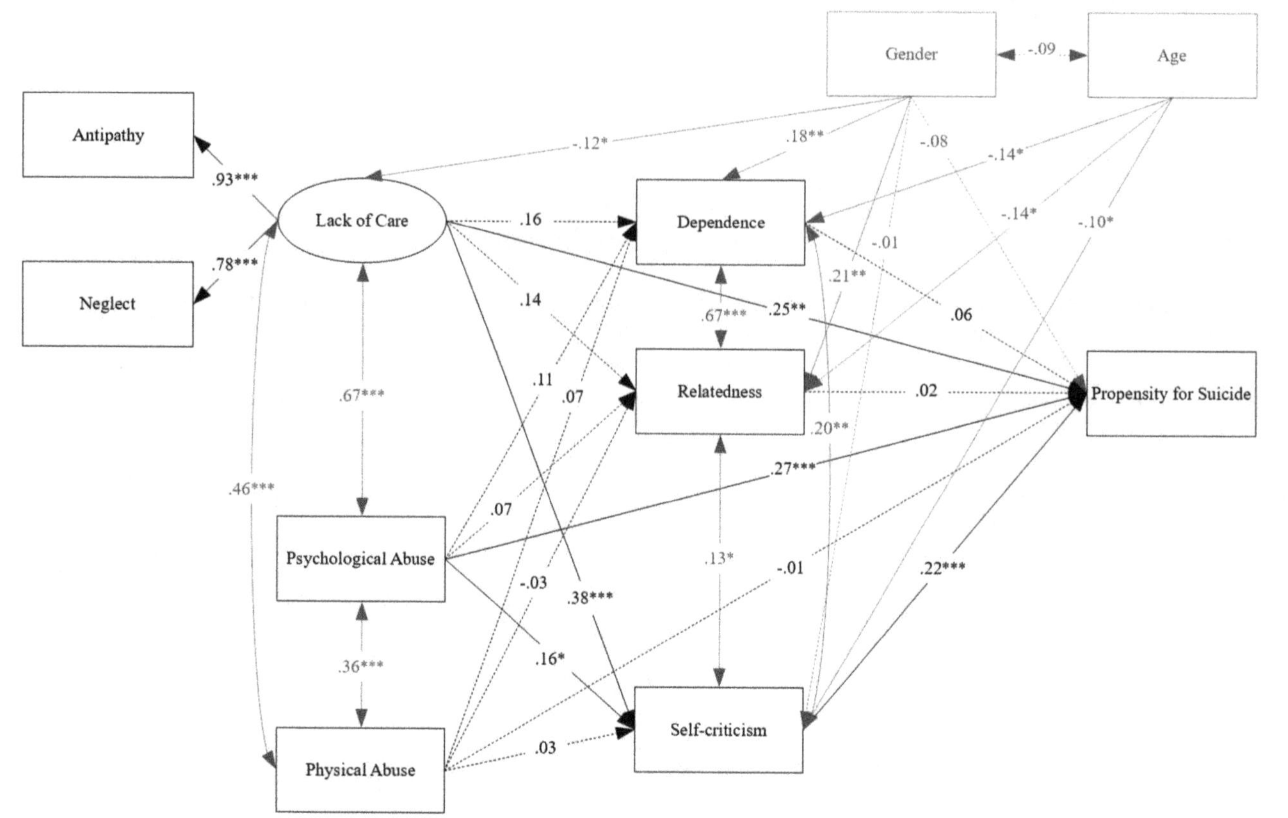

FIGURE 2 | Estimated structural equation model. Maximum likelihood standardized coefficients are shown. Solid lines represent significant pathways, dashed lines are non-significant. Covariances, control variables and their related paths are presented in light gray. $*p < 0.05$, $**p < 0.01$, $***p < 0.001$.

DISCUSSION

The current study examined whether self-criticism and dependence/relatedness mediated the relationship between different forms of childhood maltreatment and suicide risk in young adults. We found an association between lack of care (i.e., antipathy and neglect), psychological abuse, and suicide risk. Furthermore, self-criticism partially mediated this effect. No association was found between physical abuse and suicide risk. Finally, neither dependence nor relatedness mediated the relationship between different types of maltreatment and suicide risk.

Our results are consistent with prior studies reporting high correlations among experiences of hostility, rejection, humiliation and parental criticism and the development of a representation of the self that is characterized by feelings of low self-worth, shame, guilt, and propensity to adopt a punitive self-stance, as a consequence of an internalization of a highly critical family environment (Soffer et al., 2008; Kopala-Sibley and Zuroff, 2014; Baetens et al., 2015; Verrocchio et al., 2015). In a recent meta-analysis, Liu et al. (2017) found that emotional abuse had the strongest effect on suicidal behavior compared to other types of maltreatment. Glassman et al. (2007) found that people who experienced maltreatment during childhood including repeated insults, excessive criticism, or some form of physical abuse, may develop a self-critical cognitive style over time through internalizing the behavior of those who criticized and abused them, which may ultimately result in NSSI behaviors.

Finally, other studies found a relationship between emotional maltreatment and neglect and suicide attempts after controlling for other forms of abuse (physical and sexual abuse) among adults (de Araujo and Lara, 2016; Springe et al., 2016).

In sum, these findings suggest that the combined effect of specific forms of dysfunctional parental behavior (e.g., parental criticism and a lack of emotional and material support) and the development of rigid and dysfunctional negative self-schemas (e.g., self-criticism), may increase suicide risk (Wedig and Nock, 2007; Yates et al., 2008; Claes et al., 2012).

Despite Blatt et al.'s (1995) suggestion that there are two facets of the DEQ dependency factor, namely dependence and relatedness results show that these facets of dependency did not mediate the relationship between different types of adversities and suicide risk. According to published data (Soffer et al., 2008; Lassri and Shahar, 2012) this result indicates that dependency may be a relatively less maladaptive factor than self-criticism in that it may not be linked to childhood maltreatment or suicide risk. However, we should note that this is somewhat in contrast to other studies which have found dependency to be influenced by early childhood and adolescent parenting and peer relationships (e.g., Kopala-Sibley et al., 2012; Kopala-Sibley et al., 2015).

Regarding gender differences, it is important to note that the prevalence of females in our sample may limit the generalizability of findings to males. Nevertheless, results are consistent with previous studies (Blatt and Blass, 1996; Kuperminc et al., 1997; Henrich et al., 2000), showing that females scored higher on dependency and self-criticism than males. Furthermore, consistent with other studies (Dube et al., 2003; Puzia et al., 2014; Sachs-Ericsson et al., 2016), results indicate that males scored higher than females on neglect and antipathy. Finally, we found that older males and females showed lower levels of self-criticism and dependency. Indeed, several studies suggest a normative improvement in one's sense of relatedness and self-definition across the life span, as evidenced by age-related decreases in both self-criticism and dependency (Kopala-Sibley et al., 2013).

This study has several limitations. First, suicidality is linked to depression, although we did not measure depression in the current study. Thus, it is possible that symptoms of depression may account for some of the relationships found here, such as the association between self-criticism and suicidality. Second, like most research in this area, the present study is a cross-sectional investigation. This makes it impossible to document any causal relationship of child maltreatment and pathological personality traits with suicide risk. Third, all measures were self-reported, which might have inflated associations due to shared method variance. Moreover, childhood maltreatment was investigated retrospectively. Therefore, data did not necessarily reflect the full complement of omissive and commissive behaviors experienced by participants. Finally, a limitation involves the homogeneity of our sample of participants (all undergraduate-level students and enrolled in courses of Psychology, where there is a high female prevalence). A community sample would have increased the variability and strengthened the applicability of the results to the general population. This also raises the issue of whether college students might be an inappropriate comparison group against a clinical population, given age and other differences between these groups.

AUTHOR CONTRIBUTIONS

PM designed the computational framework for testing the model, analyzed the data, and contributed to the interpretation of the results. All authors participated in the concept and writing of this manuscript and approved the final version of the manuscript.

REFERENCES

1. Afifi, T. O., Taillieu, T., Zamorski, M. A., Turner, S., Cheung, K., and Sareen, J. (2016). Association of Child abuse exposure with suicidal ideation, suicide plans, and suicide attempts in military Personnel and the general population in Canada. *JAMA Psychiatry.* 73, 229–238. doi: 10.1001/jamapsychiatry.2015.2732 Agid, O., Shapira, B., Zislin, J., Ritsner, M., Hanin, B., Murad, H., et al. (1999). Environment and vulnerability to major psychiatric illness: a case control study of early parental loss in major depression, bipolar disorder and schizophrenia. *Mol. Psychiatry* 4, 163–172. doi: 10.1038/sj.mp.4000473
2. AlmaLaurea. (2017). *Caratteristiche dei Laureati al Momento dell'ingresso all'università.* Available at: http://www.almalaurea.it/sites/almalaurea.it/ files/docs/universita/profilo/Profilo2016/profilo2016_04_caratteristiche_dei_ laureati_al_momento_ingresso_universita.pdf
3. American Psychological Association [APA] (2010). *Ethical Principles of Psychologists and Code of Conduct.* Available at: http://www.apa.org/ethics/ code/principles.pdf
4. Anderson, P. L., Tiro, J. A., Price, A. W., Bender, M. A., and Kaslow, N. J. (2002). Additive impact of childhood emotional, physical, and sexual abuse on suicide attempts among low-income African American Women. *Suicide Life Threat. Behav.* 32, 131–138. doi: 10.1521/suli.32.2.131.24405
5. Baetens, I., Claes, L., Hasking, P., Smits, D., Grietens, H., Onghena, P., et al. (2015). The relationship between parental expressed emotions and non-suicidal self- injury: the mediating roles of self-criticism and depression. *J. Child Fam. Stud.* 24, 491–498. doi: 10.1007/s10826-013-9861-8
6. Barbosa, L. P., Quevedo, L., da Silva Gdel, G., Jansen, K., Pinheiro, R. T., Branco, J., et al. (2014). Childhood trauma and suicide risk in a sample of young individuals aged 14-35 years in southern Brazil. *Child Abuse Negl.* 38, 1191–1196. doi: 10.1016/j.chiabu.2014.02.008
7. Bentler, P. M. (1990). Comparative fit indexes in structural models. *Psychol. Bull.* 107, 238–246. doi: 10.1037/0033-2909.107.2.238
8. Bentler, P. M. (2006). *EQS 6 Structural Equations Program Manual.* Encino, CA: Multivariate Software, Inc.
9. Bentler, P. M., and Bonett, D. G. (1980). Significance tests and goodness of fit in the analysis of covariance structures. *Psychol. Bull.* 88, 588–606. doi: 10.1037/0033- 2909.88.3.588
10. Bifulco, A., Bernazzani, O., Moran, P. M., and Jacobs, C. (2005). The childhood experience of care and abuse questionnaire (CECA.Q): validation in a community series. *Br. J. Clin. Psychol.* 44, 563–581. doi: 10.1348/ 014466505X35344
11. Bifulco, A., Brown, G. W., and Harris, T. O. (1994). Childhood experience of care and abuse (CECA): a retrospective interview measure. *J. Child Psychol. Psychiatry* 35, 1419–1435. doi: 10.1111/j.1469-7610.1994.tb01284.x
12. Blatt, S. J. (1974). Levels of object representation in anaclitic and introjective depression. *Psychoanal. Study Child* 29, 107–157. doi: 10.1080/00797308.1974. 11822616
13. Blatt, S. J. (2004). *Experiences of Depression: Theoretical, Clinical, and Research Perspectives.* Washington, DC: American Psychological Association. doi: 10.1037/10749-000
14. Blatt, S. J. (2008). *Polarities of Experience: Relatedness and Self Definition in Personality Development, Psychopathology, and the Therapeutic Process.* Washington, DC: American Psychological Association.
15. Blatt, S. J., and Blass, R. B. (1996). "Relatedness and self-definition: a dialectic model of personality development," in *Development and Vulnerabilities in Close Relationships*, ed. G. G. Noam (Hillsdale, NJ: Erlbaum), 309–338.
16. Blatt, S. J., D'Afflitti, J. P., and Quinlan, D. M. (1976). Experiences of depression in normal young adults. *J. Abnorm. Psychol.* 85, 383–389. doi: 10.1037//0021- 843X.85.4.383
17. Blatt, S. J., Zohar, A. H., Quinlan, D. M., Zuroff, D. C., and Mongrain, M. (1995). Subscales within the dependency factor of the Depressive Experiences Questionnaire. *J. Pers. Assess.* 64, 319–339. doi: 10.1207/s15327752jpa6402
18. Blatt, S. J., and Zuroff, D. C. (1992). Interpersonal relatedness and self-definition: two prototypes for depression. *Clin. Psychol. Rev.* 12, 527–562. doi: 10.1016/ 0272-7358(92)90070-O
19. Bornstein, R., and O'Neill, R. M. (2000). Dependency and suicidality in psychiatric inpatients. *J. Clin. Psychol.* 56, 463–473. doi: 10.1002/(SICI)1097-4679(200004) 56:4<463::AID-JCLP2>3.0.CO;2-5
20. Brent, D. A. (2011). Preventing youth suicide: time to ask how. *J. Am. Acad. Child. Adolesc. Psychiatry* 50, 738–740. doi: 10.1016/j.jaac.2010.09.017
21. Brodsky, B. S., and Biggs, E. (2012). Adverse childhood experiences and suicidal behavior. *Suicidologi* 17, 16–21.
22. Brodsky, B. S., and Stanley, B. (2008). Adverse childhood experiences and suicidal behavior. *Psychiatr. Clin. North Am.* 31, 223–235. doi: 10.1016/j.psc.2008. 02.002
23. Browne, M. W., and Cudeck, R. (1993). "Alternative ways of assessing model fit," in *Testing Structural Equation Models*, eds K. A. Bollen and J. S. Long (Newbury Park, CA: Sage), 136–162.
24. Bruffaerts, R., Demyttenaere, K., Borges, G., Haro, J. M., Chiu, W. T., Hwang, I., et al. (2010). Childhood adversities as risk factors for onset and persistence of suicidal behaviour. *Br. J. Psychiatry* 197, 20–27. doi: 10.1192/bjp.bp.109.074716 Campos, R., Besser, A., Abreu, H., Parreira, T., and Blatt, S. (2014). Personality vulnerabilities in adolescent suicidality: the mediating role of psychological distress. *Bull. Menninger Clin.* 78, 115–139. doi: 10.1521/bumc.2014.78.2.115 Campos, R. C., Besser, A., and Blatt, S. J. (2010). The mediating role of self-criticism

25. and dependency in the association between perceptions of maternal caring and depressive. *Depress. Anxiety.* 27, 1149–1157. doi: 10.1002/da.20763
26. Campos, R. C., Besser, A., and Blatt, S. J. (2013). Recollections of parental rejection, self-criticism and depression in suicidality. *Arch. Suicide Res.* 17, 58–74. doi: 10.1080/13811118.2013.748416
27. Campos, R. C., and Holden, R. R. (2014). Suicide risk in a Portuguese non- clinical sample of adults. *Eur. J. Psychiatry* 28, 230–241. doi: 10.4321/S0213- 61632014000400004
28. Campos, R. C., and Mesquita, C. (2014). Testing a model of suicidality in community adolescents: a brief report. *J. Child Adolesc. Behav.* 147, 34–56. doi: 10.4172/2375-4494.1000147
29. Claes, L., Soenens, B., Vansteenkiste, M., and Vandereycken, W. (2012). The scars of the inner critic: Perfectionism and nonsuicidal self-injury in eating disorders. *Eur. Eat. Disord. Rev.* 20, 196–202. doi: 10.1002/erv.1158
30. Curran, P. J., West, S. G., and Finch, J. F. (1996). The robustness of test statistics to nonnormality and specification error in confirmatory factor analysis. *Psychol. Methods* 1, 16–29. doi: 10.1037/1082-989X.1.1.16
31. de Araujo, R. M., and Lara, D. R. (2016). More than words: the association of childhood emotional abuse and suicidal behavior. *Eur. Psychiatry* 37, 14–21. doi: 10.1016/j.eurpsy.2016.04.002
32. Dube, S. R., Felitti, V. J., Dong, M., Chapman, D. P., Giles, W. H., and Anda, R. F. (2003). Childhood abuse, neglect, and household dysfunction and the risk of illicit drug use: the adverse childhood experiences study. *Pediatrics* 111, 564–572. doi: 10.1542/peds.111.3.564
33. Dunn, E. C., McLaughlin, K. A., Slopen, N., Rosand, J., and Smoller, J. W. (2013). Developmental timing of child maltreatment and symptoms of depression and suicidal ideation in young adulthood: results from the National Longitudinal Study on Adolescent Health. *Depress Anxiety* 30, 1–15. doi: 10.1002/da.22102
34. Enns, M. W., Cox, B. J., Afifi, T. O., De Graaf, R., Ten Have, M., and Sareen, J. (2006). Childhood adversities and risk for suicidal ideation and attempts: a longitudinal population-based study. *Psychol. Med.* 36, 1–10. doi: 10.1017/ S0033291706008646
35. Falgares, G., Marchetti, D., De Santis, S., Carrozzino, D., Kopala-Sibley, D. C., Fulcheri, M., et al. (2017a). Attachment styles and suicide-related behaviors in adolescence: the mediating role of self-criticism and dependency. *Front. Psychiatry* 8:36. doi: 10.3389/fpsyt.2017.00036
36. Falgares, G., De Santis, S., Gullo, S., Carrozzino, D., Marchetti, D., Verrocchio, M. C., et al. (2017b). The Italian version of the depressive experiences questionnaire: psychometric properties and validation in students, community, and clinical groups. *Res. Psychother. Psychopathol. Process Outcome* 20, 81–90. doi: 10.4081/ripppo.2017.227
37. Faraci, P., and Musso, P. (2013). "La valutazione dei modelli di equazioni strutturali [The evaluation of structural equation models]," in *I Modelli di Equazioni Strutturali: Temi e Prospettive*, eds C. Barbaranelli and S. Ingoglia (Milano, IT: LED), 111–150. doi: 10.7359/649-2013-fara
38. Fazaa, N., and Page, S. (2003). Dependency and self-criticism as predictors of suicidal behavior. *Suicide Life Threat. Behav.* 33, 172–185. doi: 10.1521/suli.33. 2.172.22777
39. Fazaa, N., and Page, S. (2009). Personality style and impulsivity as determinants of suicidal subgroups. *Arch. Suicide Res.* 13, 31–45. doi: 10.1080/13811110802572122
40. Fehon, D. C., Grilo, C. M., and Martino, S. (2000). A comparison of dependent and self-critically depressed hospitalized adolescents. *J. Youth Adolesc.* 29, 93–106. doi: 10.1023/A:1005125322629
41. Gershon, A., Sudheimer, K., Tirouvanziam, R., Williams, L. M., and O'Hara, R. (2013). The long-term impact of early adversity on late-life psychiatric disorders. *Curr. Psychiatry Rep.* 15:352. doi: 10.1007/s11920-013-0352-9
42. Giannone, F., Schimmenti, A., Caretti, V., Chiarenza, A., Ferraro, A., Guarino, S., et al. (2011). Validità, attendibilità e proprietà psicometriche della versione Italiana dell'intervista CECA (Childhood Experience of Care and Abuse).[Validity, reliability and psychometric properties of the Italian translation of the CECA interview (Childhood experience of care and abuse)]. *Psichiatria Psicoter.* 30, 3–21.
43. Gilbert, R., Widom, C. S., Browne, K., Fergusson, D., Webb, E., and Janson, J. (2009). Burden and consequences of child maltreatment in high-income countries. *Lancet* 373, 68–81. doi: 10.1016/S0140-6736(08)61706-7
44. Glassman, L. H., Weierich, M. R., Hooley, J. M., Deliberto, T. L., and Nock, M. K. (2007). Child maltreatment, non-suicidal self-injury, and the mediating role of self-criticism. *Behav. Res. Ther.* 45, 2483–2490. doi: 10.1016/j.brat.2007.04.002
45. Grilo, C. M., Sanislow, C., Fehon, D. C., Martino, S., and McGlashan, T. H. (1999). Psychological and behavioral functioning in adolescent psychiatric inpatients who report histories of childhood abuse. *Am. J. Psychiatry* 156, 538–543. doi: 10.1176/ajp.156.4.538
46. Hahm, H. C., Lee, Y., Ozonoff, A., and Van Wert, M. J. (2010). The impact of multiple types of child maltreatment on subsequent risk behaviors among women during the transition from adolescence to young adulthood. *J. Youth Adolesc.* 39, 528–540. doi: 10.1007/s10964-009-9490-0
47. Hahs-Vaughn, D. L. (2016). *Applied Multivariate Statistical Concepts*. New York, NY: Taylor & Francis.
48. Henrich, C. C., Kuperminc, G. P., Sack, A., Blatt, S. J., and Leadbeater, B. J. (2000). Characteristics and homogeneity of early adolescent friendship groups: A comparison of male and female cliques and nonclique members. *Appl. Dev. Sci.* 4, 15–26. doi: 10.1207/S1532480XADS0401_2
49. Hu, L., and Bentler, P. M. (1999). Cutoff criteria for fit indexes in covariance structure analysis: Conventional criteria versus new alternatives. *Struct. Equa. Model.* 6, 1–55. doi: 10.1080/10705519909540118
50. Infurna, M. R., Brunner, R., Holz, B., Parzer, P., Giannone, F., Reichl, C., et al. (2016a). The specific role of childhood abuse, parental bonding, and family functioning in female adolescents with borderline personality disorder. *J. Pers. Disord.* 30, 177–192. doi: 10.1521/pedi_2015_29_186
51. Infurna, M. R., Reichl, C., Parzer, P., Schimmenti, A., Bifulco, A., and Kaess, M. (2016b). Associations between depression and specific childhood experiences of abuse and neglect: a meta-analysis. *J. Affect. Disord.* 190, 47–55. doi: 10.1016/ j.jad.2015.09.006
52. Innamorati, M., Pompili, M., Serafini, G., Lester, D., Erbuto, D., Amore, M., et al. (2011). Psychometric properties of the suicidal history self-rating screening scale. *Arch. Suicide Res.* 15, 87–92. doi: 10.1080/13811118.2011.540471
53. International Test Commission (2005). *International Guidelines on Test Adaptation*. Available at: https://www.intestcom.org/files/guideline_test_adaptation.pdf Italian Association of Psychology. (2015). *Codice Etico per la Ricerca in Psicologia [Ethical Code for Psychological Research]*. Available at: http://www.aipass.org/ node/11560
54. Kline, R. B. (2010). *Principles and Practice of Structural Equation Modeling*, 3rd Edn. New York, NY: Guilford Press.
55. Klomek, A., Orbach, I., Sher, L., Sommerfeld, E., Diller, R., Apter, A., et al. (2008). Quality of depression among suicidal inpatient youth. *Arch. Suicide Res.* 12, 133–140. doi: 10.1080/13811110701857160
56. Kopala-Sibley, D. C., Mongrain, M., and Zuroff, D. C. (2013). A lifespan perspective on dependency and self-criticism: age-related differences from 18 to 59. *J. Adult. Dev.* 20, 126–141. doi: 10.1007/s10804-013-9163-9
57. Kopala-Sibley, D. C., and Zuroff, D. C. (2014). The developmental origins of personality factors from the self-definitional and relatedness domains: a review of theory and research. *Rev. Gen. Psychol.* 18, 137–155. doi: 10.1037/gpr000 0013
58. Kopala-Sibley, D. C., Zuroff, D. C., Hankin, B. L., and Abela, J. R. (2015). The development of self-criticism and dependency in early adolescence and their role in the development of depressive and anxiety symptoms. *Pers. Soc. Psychol. Bull.* 41, 1094–1109. doi: 10.1177/0146167215590985
59. Kopala-Sibley, D. C., Zuroff, D. C., Leybman, M. J., and Hope, N. (2012). The developmental origins of dependency-related vulnerabilities to depression: recalled peer attachments and current levels of neediness and connectedness. *Can. J. Behav. Sci.* 44, 264–271. doi: 10.1037/a0028952
60. Kuperminc, G. P., Blatt, S. J., and Leadbeater, B. J. (1997). Relatedness, self-definition, and early adolescent adjustment. *Cognit. Ther. Res.* 21, 301–320. doi: 10.1023/A:1021826500037
61. Lassri, D., and Shahar, G. (2012). Self-criticism mediates the link between childhood emotional maltreatment and young adults' romantic relationships. *J. Soc. Clin. Psychol.* 31, 289–311. doi: 10.1521/jscp.2012.31.3.289
62. Liu, J., Fang, Y., Gong, J., Cui, X., Meng, T., Xiao, B., et al. (2017). Associations between suicidal behavior and childhood abuse and neglect: a meta-analysis. *J. Affect. Disord.* 220, 147–155. doi: 10.1016/j.jad.2017.03.060
63. Luyten, P., and Blatt, S. J. (2013). Interpersonal relatedness and self-definition in normal and disrupted personality development: retrospect and prospect. *Am. Psychol.* 68, 172–183. doi: 10.1037/a0032243
64. MacCallum, R. C., Browne, M. W., and Sugawara, H. M. (1996). Power analysis and determination of sample size in covariance structure modeling. *Psychol. Methods* 1, 130–149. doi: 10.1037/1082-989X.1.2.130
65. MacCallum, R. C., Zhang, S., Preacher, K. J., and Rucker, D. D. (2002). On the practice of dichotomization of quantitative variables. *Psychol. Methods* 7, 19–40. doi: 10.1037//1082-989X.7.1.19
66. Mendelson, T., Robins, C. L., and Johnson, C. S. (2002). Relations of sociotropy and autonomy to developmental experiences among psychiatric patients. *Cogn. Ther. Res.* 26, 189–198. doi: 10.1023/A:1014569703020
67. Mongrain, M., and Zuroff, D. C. (1994). Ambivalence over emotional expression and negative life events: Mediators of depressive symptoms in

dependent and self-critical individuals. *Pers. Individ. Dif.* 16, 447–458. doi: 10.1016/0191- 8869(94)90071-X

68. Muthén, B. O., and Muthén, L. K. (2014). *Mplus (Version 7.2) [Computer Software]*. Los Angeles, CA: Muthén & Muthén.
69. Nock, M. K. (2012). Future directions for the study of suicide and self-injury. *J. Clin. Child Adolesc. Psychol.* 41, 255–259. doi: 10.1080/15374416.2012.65 2001
70. O'Connor, R. C. (2007). The relations between perfectionism and suicidality: a systematic review. *Suic. Life Threat. Behav.* 37, 698–714. doi: 10.1521/suli.2007. 37.6.698
71. Pagura, J., Cox, B. J., Sareen, J., and Enns, M. W. (2006). Childhood adversities associated with self-criticism in a nationally representative sample. *Pers. Individ. Dif.* 41, 1287–1298. doi: 10.1016/j.paid.2006.05.003
72. Pompili, M., Innamorati, M., Lamis, D. A., Lester, D., Di Fiore, E., Giordano, G., et al. (2016). The interplay between suicide risk, cognitive vulnerability, subjective happiness and depression among students. *Curr. Psychol.* 35, 450– 458. doi: 10.1007/s12144-015-9313-2
73. Puzia, M. E., Kraines, M. A., Liu, R. T., and Kleiman, E. M. (2014). Early life stressors and suicidal ideation: mediation by interpersonal risk factors. *Pers. Individ. Dif.* 56, 68–72. doi: 10.1016/j.paid.2013.08.027
74. Rude, S. S., and Burnham, B. L. (1995). Connectedness and neediness: factors of the DEQ and SAS dependency scales. *Cogn. Ther. Res.* 19, 323–340. doi: 10.1007/BF02230403
75. Sachs-Ericsson, N. J., Rushing, N. C., Stanley, I. H., and Sheffler, J. (2016). In my end in my beginning: developmental trajectories of adverse childhood experiences to late-life suicide. *Aging Ment. Health.* 20, 139–165. doi: 10.1080/13607863. 2015.1063107
76. Schimmenti, A., and Bifulco, A. (2015). Linking lack of care in childhood to anxiety disorders in emerging adulthood: the role of attachment styles. *Child Adolesc. Ment. Health* 20, 41–48. doi: 10.1111/camh.12051
77. Shahar, G., and Priel, B. (2003). Active vulnerability, adolescent distress, and the mediating/suppressing role of life events. *Pers. Individ. Dif.* 35, 199–218. doi: 10.1016/S0191-8869(02)00185-X
78. Smith, N., Lam, D., Bifulco, A., and Checkley, S. (2002). Childhood experience of care and abuse questionnaire (CECA.Q). *Soc. Psychiatry Psychiatr. Epidemiol.* 37, 572–579. doi: 10.1007/s00127-002-0589-9
79. Soffer, N., Gilboa-Schechtman, E., and Shahar, G. (2008). The relationship of childhood emotional abuse and neglect to depressive vulnerability and low self-efficacy. *Int. J. Cogn. Ther.* 1, 151–162. doi: 10.1521/ijct.2008.1. 2.151
80. Speranza, M., Corso, M., Loas, G., Stéphan, P., Guilbaud, O., Perez-Diaz, F., et al. (2005). Depressive personality dimensions and alexithymia in eating disorders. *Psychiatry Res.* 135, 153–163. doi: 10.1016/j.psychres.2005.04.001
81. Springe, L., Pulmanis, T., Velika, B., Pudule, I., Grinberga, D., and Villerusa, A. (2016). Self-reported suicide attempts and exposure to different types of violence and neglect during childhood: Findings from a young adult population survey in Latvia. *Scand. J. Public Health* 44, 411–417. doi: 10.1177/ 1403494816631394
82. Steiger, J. S. (1990). Structural model evaluation and modification: an interval estimation approach. *Multivariate Behav. Res.* 25, 173–180. doi: 10.1207/ s15327906mbr2502_4
83. Tabachnick, B. G., and Fidell, L. S. (2013). *Using Multivariate Statistics*, 6th Edn. Boston, MA: Allyn and Bacon.
84. Verrocchio, M. C., Marchetti, D., and Baker, A. J. (2014). Assessment of psychological maltreatment: psychometric properties of the psychological maltreatment measure – Italian version. *Maltrattamento Abuso all'infanzia* 16, 57–75. doi: 10.3280/MAL2014-001004
85. Verrocchio, M. C., Marchetti, D., and Fulcheri, M. (2015). Perceived parental functioning, self-esteem, and psychological distress in adults whose parents are separated/divorced. *Front. Psychol.* 6:1760. doi: 10.3389/ fpsyg.2015.01760
86. Warner, R. M. (2012). *Applied Statistics: From Bivariate Through Multivariate Techniques: From Bivariate Through Multivariate Techniques.* Thousand Oaks, CA: Sage.
87. Wedig, M. M., and Nock, M. K. (2007). Parental expressed emotion and adolescent self-injury. *J. Am. Acad. Child Adolesc.* 46, 1171–1178. doi: 10.1097/chi. 0b013e3180ca9aaf
88. Witt, A., Münzer, A., Ganser, H. G., Fegert, J. M., Goldbeck, L., and Plener, P. L. (2016). Experience by children and adolescents of more than one type of maltreatment: association of different classes of maltreatment profiles with clinical outcome variables. *Child Abuse Negl.* 57, 1–11. doi: 10.1016/j.chiabu. 2016.05.001
89. World Medical Association (2001). Declaration of Helsinki. Ethical principles for medical research involving human subjects. *Bull. World Health Organ.* 79, 373–374.
90. Yates, T. M., Tracy, A. J., and Luthar, S. S. (2008). Nonsuicidal self-injury among "privileged" youths: longitudinal and cross-sectional approaches to developmental process. *J. Consult. Clin. Psychol.* 76, 52–62. doi: 10.1037/0022- 006X.76.1.52
91. Zuroff, D. C., Mongrain, M., and Santor, D. A. (2004). Conceptualizing and measuring personality vulnerability to depression: comment on Coyne and Whiffen (1995). *Psychol. Bull.* 130, 489–511. doi: 10.1037/0033-2909.130.3.489

10

Emotional Responses to Suicidal Patients: Factor Stucture, Construst and Predictive Validity of the Therapist Response Questionnaire-Suicide Form

Shira Barzilay[1†], Zimri S. Yaseen[1,2†], Mariah Hawes[2], Bernard Gorman[3], Rachel Altman[2], Adriana Foster[4], Alan Apter[5], Paul Rosenfield[6] and Igor Galynker[1,2]*

[1] *Department of Psychiatry, Icahn School of Medicine at Mount Sinai, New York City, NY, United States,* [2] *Department of Psychiatry and Behavioral Health, Mount Sinai Beth Israel Medical Center, New York City, NY, United States,* [3] *Gordon F. Derner School of Psychology, Adelphi University, Garden City, NY, United States,* [4] *Herbert Wertheim College of Medicine, Florida International University, Miami, FL, United States,* [5] *Feinberg Child Study Center, Schneider Children's Medical Center, Petach Tikva and Sackler Faculty of Medicine, Tel Aviv University, Tel Aviv, Israel,* [6] *Department of Psychiatry, Mount Sinai St. Luke's, New York City, NY, United States*

Correspondence:
Zimri S. Yaseen
zsyaseen@gmail.com

[†] *These authors have contributed equally to this work.*

Background: Mental health professionals have a pivotal role in suicide prevention. However, they also often have intense emotional responses, or countertransference, during encounters with suicidal patients. Previous studies of the Therapist Response Questionnaire-Suicide Form (TRQ-SF), a brief novel measure aimed at probing a distinct set of suicide-related emotional responses to patients found it to be predictive of near-term suicidal behavior among high suicide-risk inpatients. The purpose of this study was to validate the TRQ-SF in a general outpatient clinic setting.

Methods: Adult psychiatric outpatients (N = 346) and their treating mental health professionals (N = 48) completed self-report assessments following their first clinic meeting. Clinician measures included the TRQ-SF, general emotional states and traits, therapeutic alliance, and assessment of patient suicide risk. Patient suicidal outcomes and symptom severity were assessed at intake and one-month follow-up. Following confirmatory factor analysis of the TRQ-SF, factor scores were examined for relationships with clinician and patient measures and suicidal outcomes.

Results: Factor analysis of the TRQ-SF confirmed three dimensions: (1) affiliation, (2) distress, and (3) hope. The three factors also loaded onto a single general factor of negative emotional response toward the patient that demonstrated good internal reliability. The TRQ-SF scores were associated with measures of clinician state anger and anxiety and therapeutic alliance, independently of clinician personality traits after controlling for the state- and patient-specific measures. The total score and three subscales were associated in both concurrent and predictive ways with patient suicidal outcomes, depression severity, and clinicians' judgment of patient suicide risk, but not with global symptom severity, thus indicating specifically suicide-related responses.

Conclusion: The TRQ-SF is a brief and reliable measure with a 3-factor structure. It demonstrates construct validity for assessing distinct suicide-related countertransference to psychiatric outpatients. Mental health professionals' emotional responses to their patients are concurrently indicative and prospectively predictive of suicidal thoughts and behaviors. Thus, the TRQ-SF is a useful tool for the study of countertransference in the treatment of suicidal patients and may help clinicians make diagnostic and therapeutic use of their own responses to improve assessment and intervention for individual suicidal patients.

Keywords: suicide, countertransference, emotional response, risk assessment, suicidal ideation, suicide attempt, suicide prevention, TRQ

INTRODUCTION

Clinicians' emotional responses to their patients, broadly referred to as *countertransference*, have important implications for treatment outcomes (1, 2). Countertransference, which emerges in the context of a therapeutic relationship with the patient, has been extensively addressed in the theoretical and qualitative clinical literature (2–4). The concept of countertransference has developed over the years since Freud (1910) classical definition of countertransference as the therapist's own unresolved conflict-based reactions to the patient's transference, which are unbeneficial to treatment (5) to a "total" view of countertransference as comprising all of a clinician's emotional responses to a patient (6), an important source of information for understanding the patient's dynamics. Following the growing body of quantitative empirical research on countertransference over the past three decades, several recent studies have provided quantitative empirical evidence supporting the relation of countertransference to treatment outcomes (2, 7–9). Clinicians' feelings toward their patients may relate to treatment outcomes both as a causal force, influencing clinician behavior (3) and the therapeutic bond (4), and as a diagnostic signal, detecting patient patterns indicative of difficulties that will persist into the future (3, 10).

Assessing and treating patients at risk for suicide are clinical domains for which the study of countertransference is particularly pertinent, given the highly stressful nature of the interactions (11–14) and the concomitantly powerful feelings suicidal patients elicit, such as fear, anxiety, frustration, incompetence, helplessness, discouragement, sadness, and anger (15–18). The experience of bearing a patient's intense despair and hopelessness is extraordinarily difficult, and can erode clinicians' own sense of hope. For example, Pompili et al. (19) found that affective temperaments were significantly associated with hopelessness among patients with bipolar disorders, and hopelessness was associated with at least threefold odds for suicidal risk.

Suicide is one of the leading causes of death in the US and around the world (20), and much opportunity for prevention may be missed, as an estimated one-third of individuals (21) who die by suicide encounter a mental health-care provider within 1 month of their death (21–24). Thus, there is both a need for better understanding of the interactions between clinicians and suicidal patients, and for scalable and psychometrically sound ways of examining such interactions in large studies as well as clinical settings. Further, if areas of improvement in clinicians' management of emotional responses to patients can be identified and tracked, this will facilitate training and improve suicide outcomes.

To this end, we developed a brief questionnaire to specifically target countertransference that is potentially indicative of a patient's short-term suicide risk—the Therapist Response Questionnaire-Suicide Form (TRQ-SF). The questionnaire, described in detail in our previous study (25) comprises five items derived from the 79-item Therapist Response Questionnaire (TRQ; originally called the Countertransference Questionnaire (3, 26);) two items from the therapist form of the Working Alliance Inventory [WAI (27, 28)], and three rational items developed *de novo* by our group to capture distinctive emotional responses to high-risk suicidal patients (25). In our pilot study of this measure, the TRQ-SF was administered to first-year psychiatry residents treating patients psychiatrically hospitalized in the context of acute suicidal thoughts and behaviors [STB (25)]. In that study, although a two-factor model comprising dimensions of (a) Affiliation (vs. Rejection)—characterized by five items, and (b) Distress (vs. Comfort)—characterized by three items, fit the data, we also included a third countertransference dimension that was clinically and conceptually coherent: Hopefulness (vs. Hopelessness)—comprising two significantly correlated items with strong face validity that did not load robustly on either of the preceding factors. We found that level of patient STB in the 1–2 months following hospital discharge was significantly correlated with clinician Distress ($r = 0.27, p = 0.02$) and Hopefulness ($r = -0.25, p = 0.03$), and more robustly correlated with the interaction of Distress and Hopefulness ($r = 0.42$, $p < 0.001$). In addition, a composite total score for the TRQ-SF was found to predict post-discharge suicidal behavior among high-risk psychiatric inpatients (29), and clinicians' judgment of suicide risk in psychiatric outpatients (9).

While the initial results were promising, further research is needed to generalize these findings to other mental health professionals, patient populations, and treatment settings. Moreover, the previous study was limited by small sample size, and fully anonymous collection of clinician data that made accounting for individual clinician differences impossible. Therefore, in the present study, we seek to validate the TRQ-SF as a measure of suicide-risk associated countertransference in a general outpatient sample treated by a larger sample of clinicians varying in professional degree, experience and orientation. Specifically we aim to (a) confirm the previously proposed three-factor structure (b) provide further support for the reliability and validity of the scale and (c) evaluate the performance of the TRQ-SF in a different treatment setting with a larger, more diverse clinician and patient sample. We explore the following hypotheses:

1. factor Structure and Reliability:
   (a) the three-factor structure of the TRQ-SF proposed by Yaseen et al. (25) will be replicated in the current sample.
   (b) The TRQ-SF and its subscales will demonstrate good reliability evidenced by high Cronbach's alphas.
2. convergent and discriminant validity:
   The TRQ-SF will be associated with measures of clinician general emotional state and therapeutic alliance, while being unrelated to clinician personality traits.
3. concurrent and prospective criterion validity:
   The TRQ will demonstrate both cross-sectional and predictive relationships with patient suicide outcome measures, as well as robust associations with clinicians' concurrent judgment of patient suicide risk.

MATERIALS AND METHODS

Participants and Procedures

We recruited 346 patient and 48 clinician participants from adult psychiatric outpatient centers serving urban populations in New York City between January 2016 and June 2017. Patients presenting for intake or first visit with a new provider for any pharmacological or psychosocial treatment at one of three outpatient centers were referred by the evaluating clinician to an ongoing suicide risk study (MARIS) (29). Any mental health professional conducting patient intakes at one of the participating outpatient clinics was eligible to participate in the study. Eligible clinicians were approached at the onset of the study or of their employment at the clinic. Clinicians provided informed consent and completed a baseline packet of questionnaires assessing demographic and trait characteristics. Clinicians were instructed to identify patients who were potentially eligible to participate in the study at their first meeting with the patient. Clinicians then completed a packet including questionnaires about their clinical assessments, emotional responses, and emotional state when meeting with that particular patient. Of 81 potential clinicians, 64 (79%) consented to participate and 48 (59%) had at least one patient participant enrolled in the study.

Eligible patients who indicated to their clinician that they were interested in participating were contacted by an affiliate of the study and completed a baseline assessment following informed consent. Patients were eligible to participate in the study if they were over 18 years old and were meeting the referring clinician for the first time. Patients were excluded from the study if follow-up would be impaired—they were homeless or lacked collateral means of contact, were unable to understand the consent or did not speak English, or suffered a physical or mental impairment that might interfere with participation. Four hundred and ninety two patients were determined eligible for the study by their treating clinicians based on clinical evaluation and judgment of inclusion and exclusion criteria. Of potentially eligible patients, 346 patients (70%) consented and participated in initial assessment. Reasons for non-participation were primarily patients unwilling or unable to be reached. A few patients were excluded from the study prior to completing initial assessment due to inadequate English or language difficulties impeding their understanding the consent and/or study questions. At initial assessment, patients were administered questionnaires assessing demographics and trait characteristics, psychiatric symptomology, and STB. Patient participants were contacted one month after initial assessment for follow-up assessment of STB. Of the patient participants who completed the initial assessment, 276 (78.6%) completed follow-up assessment. The Icahn School of Medicine at Mount Sinai, Mount Sinai Beth Israel, and Mount Sinai St. Luke's—Roosevelt Institutional Review Boards approved this study.

Measures

Clinician Emotional Response

The Therapist Response Questionnaire-Suicide Form [TRQ-SF (25)] is a 10-item, Likert-type scale designed to capture clinicians' emotional responses to acutely suicidal patients. TRQ-SF individual item scores range from 0 (not at all) to 4 (extremely). Two factors were identified in previous study: affiliation (items 1, 2, 4, 8, and 10) and distress (items 3, 5, and 7) and a third *a priori* factor of hopefulness (items 6 and 9) (25). A total score of all TRQ items, with positively worded items reverse scored reflected negative emotional responses. Possible ranges for TRQ affiliation, distress, hope and total scores were 0–20, 0–12, 0–8, and 0–40, respectively.

STB Criteria

The Columbia Suicide Severity Rating Scale [CSSRS (30)] is a semi-structured interview of current and past STBs. The CSSRS outlines five progressively more severe levels of ideation, and three types of suicidal behaviors (SB) are defined: actual, interrupted and aborted suicide attempts. A composite variable of STBs on a 0–9 point scale was used: a score of 0–5 based on their peak level of suicidal ideation (SI) in the past month. Preparations for suicide without attempt received a score of 6. An aborted, interrupted, or actual suicide attempt in the past month received a score of 7–9, respectively (25, 31).

The Beck Scale for Suicide Ideation [BSS (32, 33)], a 21-item self-report measure of active and passive suicidal desires, was used. Because items 6–21 are completed only if items 4 and 5 are rated >0, we used BSS part 1 scores (items 1–5) in lieu of the total scale score. The possible range is 0–10. The BSS part 1 demonstrated good internal consistency in our sample ($\alpha = 0.83$).

The Clinician Prediction Scale [CPS (34, 35)] was used to measure clinician judgment of patient suicide risk. This single-item scale asks clinicians to rate the likelihood of their patients making a suicide attempt in the next 6 months if untreated, on a scale ranging from 0 (no likelihood) to 10 (very high likelihood).

Secondary Criteria

The Beck Depression Inventory [BDI (36, 37)] is a widely used 21-item self-report measure of severity of depressive symptoms. Total score ranges for severity have been recommended: 14–19 (mild), 20–28 (moderate), and 29–63 (severe). The BDI demonstrated excellent internal consistency in our sample ($\alpha = 0.91$).

The Brief Symptom Inventory [BSI (38)] is a 53-item self-report measure of psychiatric symptoms which provides a reliable measure of global severity of psychopathology. Patient participants completed the BSI at initial assessment only. The BSI demonstrated excellent internal consistency in our sample ($\alpha = 0.97$).

Convergent and Discriminant Validity Measures (Clinician Report)

The State-Trait Anxiety Inventory (39, 40) is a 40-item self-report assessment of state and trait levels of anxiety. Both subscales demonstrated good internal consistency (trait $\alpha = 0.84$, state $\alpha = 0.95$).

The Spielberger State-Trait Anger Expression Inventory [STAXI (41)] is a 44-item self-report assessment of state and trait anger and anger expression. Internal reliability of both the trait ($\alpha = 0.73$) and state ($\alpha = 0.85$) subscales was acceptable in our sample.

The Big Five Inventory (42) is a 44-item self-report assessment of the "Big Five" personality dimensions: Extraversion, Agreeableness, Conscientiousness, Neuroticism, and Openness. The five subscales demonstrated acceptable internal reliability in our study (α ranged from 0.77 to 0.84).

The WAI (28, 43) is a measure of patient-therapist alliance comprising three components: bond, and agreement on goals and tasks. For the current analyses we excluded the two items that were included in the TRQ-SF. Internal reliability ($\alpha = 0.93$) was excellent in our sample.

Statistical Analyses

Test of Assumptions

We conducted preliminary exploration of our data to identify any constraints in our sample that would impact our choice of statistical test. TRQ-SF responses were both univariate and multivariate non-normal, contraindicating the use of parametric techniques, thus all analyses were conducted with a parallel non-parametric test. Substantial TRQ-SF intraclass correlations (ICCs) suggested that there was appreciable variation in responses attributable to individual clinician differences (see "Results" for detail). While this would indicate the use of multilevel modeling given the clustering of patient TRQ-SF ratings within clinicians, this approach would not be appropriate due to Type I error inflation given the relatively small sample of clinicians and large proportion of clinicians referring only a few patients (44, 45). We, therefore, report only single-level model results. It is of note that the multilevel results did not substantively differ from the single-level results presented (available from the authors by request).

Analysis of Factor Structure

A Confirmatory Factor Analysis (CFA) was conducted to test our hypothesized factor structure. We used diagonally weighted least squares estimation, which is most appropriate for Likert scale and multivariate non-normal responses (46, 47). Absolute model fit was evaluated with the chi-squared statistic, which indicates the degree of agreement between the observed and expected covariance matrices and thus a non-significant test supports good model fit. Because of the sensitivity of the chi-squared test to sample and model size, additional indices of relative fit were evaluated, including the Comparative Fit Index (CFI) the Tucker-Lewis Index [TLI (48)], and the Root Mean Square Error of Approximation [RMSEA (49)]. Based on conventional standards, good fit is indicated by CFI and TLI values greater than 0.95 and an RMSEA value below 0.07 with a 90% confidence interval lower bound less than 0.05 and upper bound less than 0.10 (48, 50, 51). The CFA was conducted in the *lavaan* package of *R* statistical software (52).

Convergent, Discriminant, and Criterion Validity

Spearman's *rho* was used to investigate the 0-order rank correlations between the TRQ-SF subscales and total score and the convergent- and discriminant-related variables. A hierarchical linear regression analysis, with trait scales entered into the first step and state scales entered into the second step, was employed to evaluate whether clinicians' trait-variables predicted TRQ-SF scores controlling for clinician state-variables. Because TRQ-SF scores substantially deviated from the normal distribution, we used a computed *log* function of TRQ-SF as the dependent variable. To examine TRQ-SF scores, cross-sectional, and prospective associations with patient suicide outcome measures, and concurrent clinician assessments of patient suicide risk and psychopathological symptom severity, we performed another series of 0-order correlations by Spearman's *rho*. Convergent, discriminant, and criterion validity analyses were performed with SPSS version 24.0.

RESULTS

Participant Characteristics

Patient and clinician characteristics are described in **Table 1**.

Patients

The baseline sample included 346 subjects. Of those, 267 (77.2%) completed follow-up assessment 1 month following the initial assessment. Participants reached for follow-up were more likely to be older (mean difference 6.7 years, $p < 0.001$) and have, on average, 1 more year of education ($p = 0.04$) than those lost to follow-up. There were no other differences in sociodemographic characteristics. Descriptive statistics for all included scales are reported in **Table 1**. More than 40% of participants had made a suicide attempt in their lifetime. The average level of peak lifetime STB was active SI with plan and intent, while the average past-month level at intake was between passive wishes to be dead and active SI without methods, plan, or intent. On average, our participants fell into the moderate depressive severity range at both intake and follow-up. Participants lost to follow-up had been judged by clinicians to be at slightly higher risk for suicide ($p = 0.004$). There were no other differences in clinical characteristics between the groups, including measures

TABLE 1 | Patient demographics and descriptive measures.

Demographicsn(%) or mean (SD), as appropriate	Whole sample (N = 346)	Lost to follow-up (n = 79)	Followed-up (n = 267)	p-Value
Gender (female)	225 (65.0)	54(68.4)	171 (64.0)	0.74
Race				0.26
Asian	24 (6.9)	4 (5.1)	20 (7.5)	
Black	97 (28.0)	28 (35.4)	69 (25.8)	
White	124 (35.8)	21 (26.6)	103 (38.6)	
Other	93 (26.9)	24 (30.4)	69 (25.8)	
Age	39.29 (14.1)	34.09 (12.7)	40.78 (14.1)	<0.01
Annual household income				0.72
<$20,000	195 (56.4)	45 (57.0)	150 (56.2)	
$20–39,000	69 (19.9)	14 (17.7)	55 (20.6)	
$40–59,000	30 (8.7)	7 (8.9)	23 (8.6)	
$60–79,000	17 (4.9)	3 (3.8)	14 (5.2)	
$80–99,000	12 (3.5)	1 (1.3)	11 (4.1)	
>$100,000	15 (4.3)	5 (6.3)	10 (3.7)	
Years of education	14.3 (3.3)	13.6 (3.2)	14.5 (3.3)	0.04
Patient baseline clinical characteristics				
Primary diagnosis				0.08
Depressive disorder	156 (45.1)	29 (36.7)	127 (47.6)	
Anxiety disorder	34 (9.8)	5 (6.3)	29 (10.9)	
Bipolar disorder	44 (12.7)	8 (10.1)	36 (13.5)	
Psychotic disorder	26 (7.5)	5 (6.3)	21 (7.9)	
Trauma disorder	52 (15.0)	18 (22.8)	34 (12.7)	
Other	15 (4.3)	4 (5.5)	11 (4.1)	
Descriptivesn(%) or mean (SD), as appropriate. Observed response ranges reported				
Patient Baseline				
Lifetime SA[a]	144 (41.6)	27 (34.2)	117 (43.8)	0.13
SI[b] (range 0–9)	1.73 (2.3)	1.88 (2.5)	1.69 (2.2)	0.53
Depression (range 0–54)	22.44 (12.2)	23.25 (12.2)	22.21 (12.2)	0.52
Global Severity (range 53–424)	135.68 (47.7)	142.04 (42.4)	134.09 (47.7)	0.24
Lifetime STB[c] (range 0–9)	5.09 (3.5)	4.58 (3.5)	5.25 (3.5)	0.12
Past month STB[c] (range 0–9)	1.61 (2.2)	1.76 (2.6)	1.57 (2.1)	0.50
Patient follow-up				
SI[b] (range 0–8)			1.29 (1.9)	
Depression (range 0–50)			19.09 (11.6)	
STB[c] since baseline (range 0–9)			2.00 (1.7)	
Clinician patient-level ratings				
TRQ-SF[d] Total (range 0–33)	9.12 (5.2)	9.36 (6.0)	9.05 (5.0)	0.65
Affiliation (range 2–20)	13.84 (3.2)	13.65 (5.5)	13.90 (3.1)	0.55
Distress (range 0–9)	1.08 (1.7)	0.95 (1.8)	1.11 (1.6)	0.45
Hope (range 2–8)	6.14 (1.1)	6.05 (1.2)	6.17 (1.0)	0.40
Working alliance (range 13–84)	58.32 (14.2)	58.94 (15.3)	58.04 (13.9)	0.62
State Anxiety (range 20–64)	30.86 (9.5)	29.46 (10.9)	31.40 (9.0)	0.22
State Anger (range 15–35)	16.00 (2.4)	15.78 (2.2)	16.04 (2.4)	0.42
Assessment of Risk (range 0–8)	1.79 (1.7)	2.37 (2.2)	1.54 (1.4)	<0.01
Clinician traits				
Trait anxiety (range 27–55)	39.0 (7.0)			
Trait anger (range 10–26)	16.73 (3.6)			
Extraversion (range 14–38)	25.59 (6.3)			
Agreeableness (range 24–45)	35.51 (5.9)			
Conscientiousness (range 20–44)	34.85 (5.4)			
Neuroticism (range 9–31)	21.76 (5.7)			
Openness (range 25–57)	38.80 (6.7)			

(Continued)

TABLE 1 | Continued

[a]*Suicide Attempt assessed with the Columbia Suicide Severity Rating Scale (CSSRS).*
[b]*Suicidal Ideation (SI) assessed with the Beck Scale for Suicide Ideation.*
[c]*Suicidal Thoughts and Behaviors assessed with the CSSRS.*
[d]*Therapist Response Questionnaire-Suicide form.*

of global severity, depression, and SI, or in TRQ-SF responses, however.

Clinicians

The clinician sample consisted of 48 mental health trainees and professionals of whom 22 (45.8%) were women (4 participants were missing gender information), 20 (41.7%) were white, and 28 (58.3%) were born in the US. The participating clinicians were 83.3% psychiatrists (including 38 third-year psychiatry residents and two attending psychiatrists), 4.2% attending psychologists, and 4.2% social workers. The primary theoretical orientations reported by clinicians were 22.7% psychodynamic, 20.5% cognitive/behavioral, 13.6% integrative, 6.8% humanistic/supportive, and 4.5% interpersonal. The average reported length of clinical experience as a clinician was 4.05 years (SD = 4.79, range = 0–22).

Scores on the TRQ-SF were, in part, accounted for by clinician-level differences, as indicated by the ICCs. ICCs ranged from 0.16 (item 5: "I felt guilty about my feelings toward him/her") to 0.40 (item 6: "I thought life really might not be worth living for him/her"), indicating that between 16 and 40% of the total variance in ratings of each TRQ-SF item can be attributed to individual clinician differences (vs. individual patient differences).

Confirmatory Factor Analysis

A CFA was conducted to evaluate the proposed three-factor model (see **Table 2**) with a sample of 346 complete TRQ-SF ratings and the first indicator loading (i.e., item 1 in the affiliation factor, item 3 in the distress factor and item 9 in the hope factor) fixed to 1. All three of the approximate fit indexes (CFI, TLI, and RMSEA) exceeded the recommend threshold values for good fit, suggesting that the three-factor model fit the data well. The test of exact fit was significant, therefore not supporting exact model fit, $\chi^2(32) = 54.06$ ($p = 0.009$), which is unsurprising as the chi-square test is very sensitive to sample size.

As the three subscales were substantially correlated ($|r| = 0.55$ –0.68; $p < 0.001$), suggestive of a single general factor with three correlated subfactors, we conducted an additional CFA to test the model fit of the TRQ-SF as one-factor. The one-factor model also exceeded the recommend threshold values for good fit by approximate fit indexes (CFI, TLI, and RMSEA) but the test of exact fit was significant. A chi-square difference test revealed that the three-factor model provided slightly yet significantly better fit than the one-factor model, [$\chi^2(3) = 9.59$, $p = 0.022$], supporting the common factor with three subfactor interpretation. Factor loadings are reported in **Figure 1**.

We computed Cronbach's alpha for the three subscales in SPSS version 24. Alpha was adequate for the affiliation (0.83) and distress (0.71) subscales. However, alpha was low for the hope subscale (0.37), likely as a result of only two items being included in this subscale (53). For the total score, we computed both Cronbach's alpha and Revelle's beta (54) in the *psych* package for R (55) to evaluate internal consistency of the full scale. Beta is a lower bound estimate of reliability, whereas Cronbach's alpha is a measure of the average split-half reliability; therefore, minimal discrepancy between alpha and beta, specifically a discrepancy less than 15–20 points (56), suggests factorial homogeneity. This analysis produced an alpha value of 0.88 and a beta value of 0.75, indicating good internal consistency and scale unidimensionality. Taken together, these results suggest that there are three distinct, but highly correlated factors that combine into a meaningful general factor. We, therefore, found it appropriate to explore validity of both the TRQ-SF total score and all three subscales.

TABLE 2 | Goodness-of-fit indices for the TRQ-SF ($N = 346$).

Model	$\chi 2$	df	*p*-Value	CFI[a]	TLI[b]	RMSEA[c] (95% CI[d])
1 Factor[e]	63.65	35	0.002	0.979	0.973	0.049 (0.029, 0.067)
3 Factor[f]	54.06	32	0.009	0.984	0.977	0.045 (0.023, 0.065)
1 vs. 3[g]	9.59	3	0.022			

[a]*Comparative Fit Index [good fit indicated by Comparative Fit Index (CFI) > 0.95].*
[b]*Tucker-Lewis Index (good fit indicated by TLI > 0.95).*
[c]*Root Mean Square Error of Approximation (good fit indicated by RMSEA < 0.05).*
[d]*Confidence interval of RMSEA (good fit indicated by lower bound CI < 0.05, upper bound CI < 0.10).*
[e]*One-factor model of clinicians' emotional responses with all 10 items of the Therapist Response Questionnaire-Suicide form (TRQ-SF) serving as indicators.*
[f]*Three-factor model with correlated factors: affiliation (Items 1, 2, 4, 8, and 10), distress (Items 3, 5, and 7), and hope (Items 6 and 9).*
[g]*Comparison of the one- and three-factor models using the chi-square difference test.*

Examination of the descriptive statistics indicated there was somewhat of a floor-effect in terms of total scale and distress subscale ratings, with average responses falling in the "not at all" to "a little" range of the Likert scale. Average responses to the affiliation and hope subscale were more moderate, falling in the "somewhat" to "quite a bit" range.

Convergent and Discriminant Validity

To further examine the convergent and discriminant validity of the TRQ-SF general scale and subscales, we conducted 0-order correlation analyses. As shown in **Table 3**, the TRQ-SF total scores were positively related with clinicians' *state* anxiety and anger,

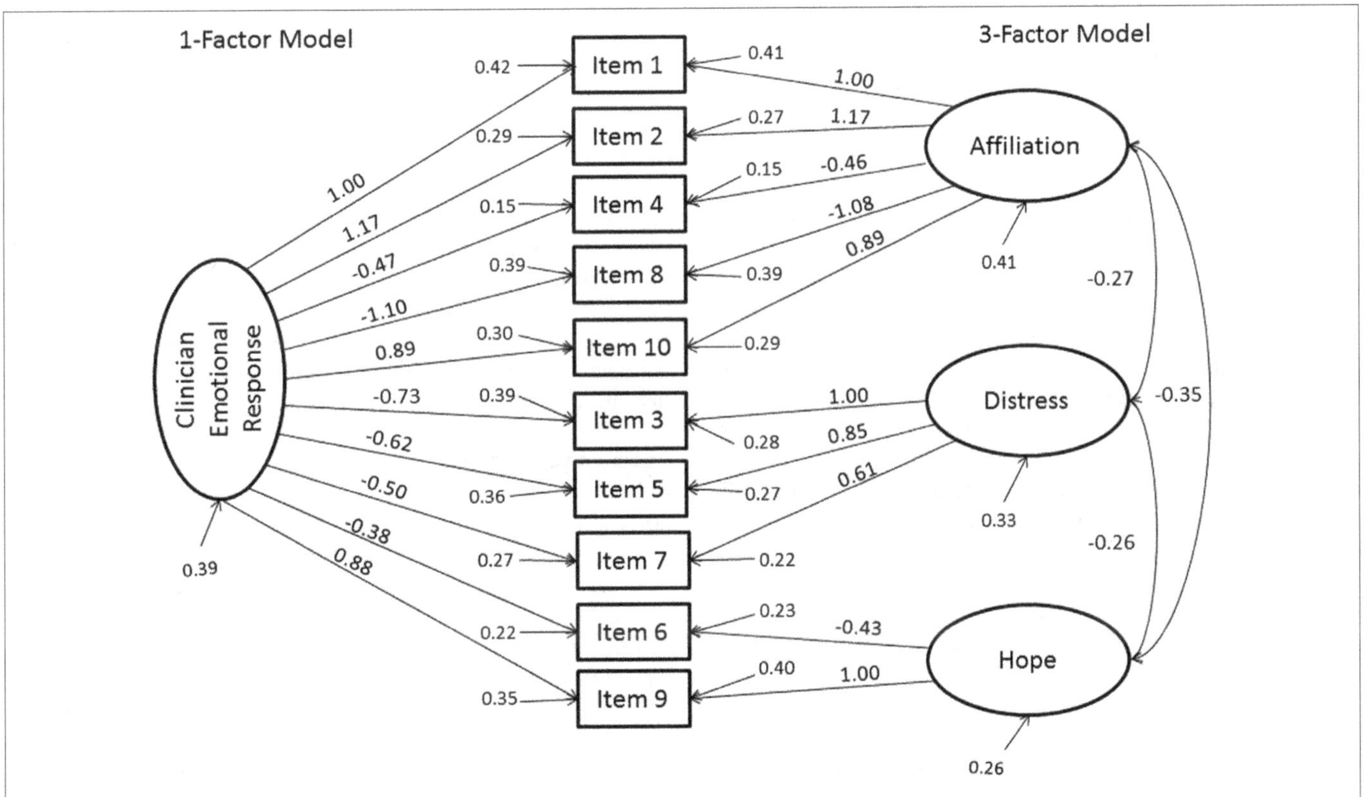

FIGURE 1 | Results of the confirmatory factor analyses of the one and three-factor models of Clinicians' Emotional Responses to their patients using items from the Therapist Response Questionnaire-Suicide Form (TRQ-SF). Factor loadings, variances, and covariances and indicator variances are reported. All factor loadings were significant in both models, as were the factor covariances in the three-factor model ($p < 0.001$).

TABLE 3 | Convergent/discriminant validity: 0-order correlations between clinicians' variables and TRQ-SF.

	Total score	Affiliation	Distress	Hope
State anxiety	0.51**	−0.42**	0.55**	−35**
Trait anxiety	0.17**	−0.10	0.23**	−0.18**
State anger	0.60**	−0.53**	0.55**	−0.35**
Trait anger	0.25**	−0.29**	0.14*	−0.10
Working alliance	−0.77**	0.74**	−0.50**	0.67**
Extroversion	−0.05	−0.04	−0.23**	0.04
Agreeableness	−0.24**	0.27**	−0.13*	0.13*
Conscientiousness	0.01	−0.04	−0.09	−0.01
Neuroticism	0.25**	−0.22**	0.20**	−0.24**
Openness	0.22**	−0.25**	0.05	−0.26**

*$p < 0.05$.
**$p < 0.01$.

TABLE 4 | TRQ-SF total convergent/discriminant associations with clinician traits and patient-specific states.

Predictor variable	*B*	SE *B*	β	*t*	Sig.
Model 1: clinician trait measures[a]					
Trait anxiety	−0.001	0.009	−0.014	−0.144	0.885
Trait anger	0.004	0.015	0.025	0.264	0.792
Extroversion	−0.022	0.007	−0.274	−3.316	0.001
Agreeableness	−0.023	0.009	−0.232	−2.477	0.014
Conscientiousness	−0.013	0.008	−0.123	−1.723	0.086
Neuroticism	0.016	0.011	0.141	1.387	0.167
Openness	0.019	0.006	0.262	3.300	0.001
Model 2: clinician state and trait measures[b]					
Trait anxiety	0.002	0.006	0.021	0.350	0.727
Trait anger	0.007	0.010	0.043	0.708	0.479
Extroversion	−0.001	0.004	−0.009	−0.166	0.868
Agreeableness	−0.004	0.006	−0.041	−0.684	0.495
Conscientiousness	0.002	0.005	0.016	0.347	0.729
Neuroticism	−0.012	0.007	−0.108	−1.668	0.097
Openness	0.006	0.004	0.087	1.711	0.088
State anxiety	0.013	0.004	0.214	3.403	0.001
State anger	0.017	0.010	0.086	1.640	0.102
Working alliance	−0.399	0.032	−0.621	−12.483	0.000

[a] $R^2 = 0.379$, $p < 0.001$.
[b] $R^2 = 0.820$, $p < 0.001$, $\Delta R^2 = 0.441$, $p < 0.001$.

and negatively correlated with clinician report of the therapeutic alliance. The magnitude of these associations was moderate to strong with high levels of significance (i.e., $p \leq 0.001$). TRQ-SF subscales demonstrated the same magnitude and significance of associations in the expected directions: affiliation and hope were negatively associated with clinician *state* anxiety and anger, and positively associated with therapeutic alliance scores. The results for the clinician trait variables showed that (a) the *trait* anxiety and anger were significantly negatively associated with TRQ-SF total scores and (b) TRQ-SF total scores were significantly negatively associated with clinician agreeableness and positively associated with clinician neuroticism and openness. The distress subscale showed comparable results as the total score, except for significant negative association with clinician extraversion, and non-significant association with openness. The affiliation and hope subscales demonstrated similar significance in the opposite direction of associations compared with the TRQ-total, except for a non-significant association between affiliation and clinician trait anxiety, and between hope and clinician trait anger. Overall, the associations between clinicians' traits and TRQ-SF were modest. Consistent with the pattern of these results, we sought to examine the contribution of clinician personality traits to TRQ-SF scores controlling for state-specific effects. We, therefore, conducted a hierarchical linear regression analysis predicting TRQ-SF total score. The results, presented in **Table 4**, show that among clinician traits included in the first step, clinician extroversion, and agreeableness were negatively associated with negative emotional responses to patients, while clinician openness was positively associated. On the second step, including state-specific measures, only state anxiety (*beta* = 0.214, $p = 0.001$) and clinician report of therapeutic alliance (*beta* = −0.621, $p < 0.001$) were independently associated with clinicians' overall negative emotional responses as measured by the TRQ-SF total score.

Criterion Validity

Concurrent and Prospective Criterion Validity

The TRQ-SF demonstrated statistically significant 0-order correlations with each of the criterion-related variables, except for the global psychopathological symptom severity. The associations ranged in value from.12 ($p < 0.05$) to 0.33 ($p < 0.01$) (see **Table 5**). Results, therefore, supported the concurrent and prospective criterion validity for the primary outcomes and demonstrate the relative specificity of the TRQ-SF response to clinician-perceived and patient-reported suicide risk.

Finally, we conducted exploratory analyses for the concurrent and predictive validity of each individual TRQ-SF item (see **Table 5**). Overall, results indicate significant cross-sectional associations between all the scale items and clinician judgment of patient suicide risk. None of the items associated with patient global symptom severity. Eight out of ten single items (except for items 3 and 4) were significantly associated with at least one of the concurrent suicidal severity measures. Items 3, 7, 8, and 9 were associated with SI at 1-month follow-up. Item 6 ("I thought life really might not be worth living for him/her") was exclusively associated with STB both at intake and at 1-month follow-up, while not associated with depression and global symptom severity, showing suicide-specific reaction.

DISCUSSION

This study replicated, validated and generalized the performance of the novel TRQ-SF for assessing a distinct suicide-related countertransference in a general outpatient clinic setting—a clinical sample with low and moderate short-term suicide risk. Adding to our previous reports on an acute inpatient sample (25, 29), these emotional responses are found to be related to patient risk for suicide as judged during the clinical assessment as well as predictive of short-term risk for SI and behavior. The current study results support the psychometric performance, construct and predictive validity of the TRQ-SF. Further, as they are generally consistent with our previous results in a high acuity patient population, our findings broadly support generalizability of the TRQ-SF across different clinical settings.

TABLE 5 | Criterion validity of the TRQ-SF total, three factors and individual items: 0-order correlations between patient variables and TRQ-SF.

	Concurrent (N = 346)						Prospective (N = 267)		
	Assessment of risk	**STB lifetime**	**STB recent**	**SI**	**Depression**	**Global severity**	**STB**	**SI**	**Depression**
TRQ-SF total	0.33**	0.21**	0.16**	0.21**	0.20**	0.10	0.12*	0.22**	0.25**
Affiliation	−0.29**	−0.20**	−0.16**	−0.20**	−0.20**	−0.10	−0.07	−0.16**	−0.20**
Distress	0.33**	0.12*	0.10	0.10	0.13*	0.07	0.06	0.18**	0.22**
Hope	−0.22**	−0.12*	−0.08	−0.09	−0.13*	−0.07	−0.13*	−0.16*	−0.19**
Individual items									
1-Feel good	−0.20**	−0.14**	−0.18**	−0.13*	−0.13*	−0.05	−0.10	−0.09	−0.12*
2-Liking	−0.24**	−0.14*	−0.11*	−0.14**	−0.20**	−0.09	−0.04	−0.10	−0.20**
3-In a bind	0.22**	0.08	0.09	0.07	0.08	0.01	0.05	0.13*	0.19**
4-Devalued	0.30**	−0.01	0.05	0.03	0.10	0.02	0.01	0.07	0.09
5-Guilty	0.29**	0.15**	0.06	0.10	0.12*	0.09	0.07	0.11	0.13
6-Not worth living	0.22**	0.12*	0.12*	0.07	0.05	−0.00	0.13*	0.10	0.04
7-Chills	0.25**	0.04	0.10	0.13*	0.15**	0.08	0.08	0.22**	0.18**
8-Forced self	0.23**	0.16**	0.04	0.10	0.17**	0.09	0.00	0.18**	0.18**
9-Confident	−0.20**	−0.08	−0.04	−0.07	−0.14*	−0.08	−0.09	−0.15*	−0.20**
10-Trust	−0.22**	−0.21**	−0.17**	−0.19**	−0.12*	−0.09	−0.08	−0.11	−0.11

*$p < 0.05$.
**$p < 0.01$.
STB, suicidal thoughts and behaviors; SI, suicidal ideation.

Thus, our findings suggest that the TRQ-SF may be of diagnostic and therapeutic use.

Factor Structure and Reliability

First, we found good fit for the hypothesized 3-factor model including affiliation, distress, and hope, thus supporting our predictions based on our previous study in a high suicide-risk inpatient sample (25). The results also supported the performance of the TRQ-SF as a general one-factor scale in assessing overall negative emotional responses toward the patient. While the three-factor model has slightly better fit compared to the one-factor model, the high inter-correlations between the three subscales and the high internal consistency indices that were found for the full scale support the meaningfulness and reliability of a scale total score. These results are in line with our previous studies using the TRQ-SF total score (9, 29). Findings, therefore, suggest that the TRQ-SF may be used as an overall scale to assess clinicians' emotional responses toward suicidal patients, as well as to assess specific dimensions of these emotional responses as indicated by the affiliation, distress, and hope subscales. While the brevity of the scale is one of its advantages for research and clinical use, given the small number of items, a larger item pool may be needed to reliably probe correlated subfactors.

Convergent and Discriminant Validity

Convergent and discriminant validity analyses primarily supported our predictions. Specifically, we found that the TRQ-SF associated significantly with related measures of general negative emotional states, i.e., anger and anxiety, and negative assessment of the therapeutic alliance. Patterns of correlation did not differ substantially between hypothesized subfactors, again supporting a generally unidimensional suicide-related countertransference, although some variation was observed, particularly in relation to clinician personality traits.

The considerable magnitude of the ICCs indicates that there was significant variation in responses attributable to individual clinician differences. Indeed, clinicians' emotional responses to patients as measured by the TRQ-SF were related to clinicians' individual tendencies to experience such emotions, as evidenced by the significant 0-order associations with clinician trait anxiety, anger, agreeableness, neuroticism, and openness. However, when accounting for state anger, anxiety, and therapeutic alliance as reported immediately following the clinical interaction with the patient, the contribution of any of the clinician's traits was no longer significant. This suggests that the effects of personality on clinician TRQ-SF responses are mediated by the specific emotional states to which they are prone. For example, we suggest that the association between trait anxiety and the TRQ-SF may be explained by the correlation between state anxiety and the TRQ-SF. The findings are consistent with a relational understanding of countertransference as clinicians' emotional responses cocreated in interaction with the patient; "The patient draws the therapist into playing a role that reflects the patient's internal world, but the specific dimensions of that role are colored by the therapist's own personality." [(6) p. 981]. It is of note that TRQ-SF scores were most strongly associated with clinician-reported state anxiety and lower therapeutic alliance. Both are robustly documented as prevalent in clinical interactions with suicidal individuals (14) as well as with poor treatment outcomes (2, 4, 7, 57).

Criterion Validity: Diagnostic and Prognostic Usefulness of the TRQ-SF

We found modestly sized but highly significant correlations of TRQ-SF total and its subscale scores with patient suicide outcomes. These correlations were stronger than associations with global severity of patient psychopathology, supporting a specifically suicide-related countertransference. Although similar associations with severity of depression were found, depression severity independent of clinical diagnosis is itself a robust predictor of SI and suicide (58). TRQ-SF scores were associated with suicide risk indices both as reported by the patient (i.e., STBs) and as assessed by the clinician (i.e., CPS). These findings support the potential utility of this scale for diagnosis and therapeutic interventions. This is in line with the body of psychological literature suggesting that evaluating therapists' countertransference is beneficial to understanding patients' intra-psychic and interpersonal dynamics (59–62). These results are also consistent with studies of countertransference measures, for example the Therapist Response Questionnaire, showing that countertransference reactions measured by clinician's self-report questionnaire were able to systematically capture patient personality and severe psychopathology regardless of therapeutic orientation (3, 63). Moreover, the prospective associations of the TRQ-SF with patient STB at 1-month following the initial intake demonstrate its potential clinical value in predicting short-term STB. These results support and extend our previous studies showing post-discharge SB among high-risk inpatients were predicted by clinicians' emotional responses as measured by the TRQ-SF (25, 29). This study, therefore, validates and generalizes our previous findings to a general psychiatric outpatient population with lower suicide-related acuity level. Hence, even in a sample with low base rate of SI and behaviors, clinicians' emotional responses measured by the TRQ-SF predict near-term STBs.

Exploratory examination of the criterion validity of individual TRQ-SF items suggests that items consistent with a projective identification process had very modest but significant prospective criterion validity, including feelings of entrapment ("My hands were tied or I was put in an impossible bind"), hopelessness ("I thought life really might not be worth living for him/her"), and helplessness ("I felt confident in my ability to help him/her", reversed) as well as unique affective-arousal ("patient gave me chills"). Items indicative of interpersonal rejection/difficulties (e.g., "I had to force myself to connect") also demonstrated modest concurrent criterion validity. Moreover, the item "I thought life really might not be worth living for him/her" showed unique suicide-specific associations and, therefore, future development may aim to better probe this emotional domain. Overall, the pattern of emotional reactions indicated by the individual items may relate to specific affective characteristics of the suicidal crisis as described in previous research (25, 64, 65). Joiner and Stanley (66) proposed that these suicidal affective states may activate an emotional contagion through non-verbal and perhaps unconscious mechanisms (66). Therefore, these intense reactions may alert a clinician to patient suicide risk independent of overtly evident risk factors such as declared suicidal intent, reported access to means, and so on. At the same time, negative emotional responses may result in less empathic communication, avoidance, and unwitting rejection of the patient (67–69) which are liable to damage the therapeutic alliance (70). Thus, further research is needed to elucidate the mechanisms by which clinicians' negative emotional responses are associated with patients' subsequent suicidal outcomes.

Implications

Our results are broadly consistent with the literature that suggests clinicians have negative emotional responses to patients presenting as at risk for suicide (14–18, 25, 67), and deepen this literature by characterizing specific responses that associate prospectively both individually and in aggregate with suicide-related outcomes and clinician judgment of suicide risk. Further, our results extend the growing body of literature that supports the potential diagnostic specificity of emotional responses (5, 6, 34, 44–48, 50, 53–56).

Mental health professional who routinely encounters patients at risk for suicide may benefit from recognizing and evaluating their emotional responses to their patients. Moreover, making meaning of emotional responses to patients is critical to managing them in a way that benefits the therapeutic relationship (59–62). Integrating explicit knowledge with the information coded in emotional cues to enhance understanding and care for suicidal individuals in training curricula and continuing education programs may facilitate assessment, intervention and ultimately reduce the risk of suicide. Training interventions for clinicians may focus on emotional self-awareness, such as mindfulness training for mental health professionals and trainees (71); relational therapy interventions that focus on the therapeutic alliance and managing counter-transference responses (72, 73) as well as novel training methods designed for improving empathic communication with psychiatric patients (74). In addition, existing training programs for suicide prevention (75) would benefit from including a component targeting emotional responses to suicidal individuals. Intervention emphasizing emotional self-awareness and the effect of clinicians' emotions on the clinical interaction may help clinicians to better recognize and assess the emotional response to their patients as well as to make use of this emotional awareness in a way that would benefit both evaluation and treatment.

Strengths and Limitations

This study has a number of strengths and limitations. Among the strengths of the study are the use of multiple validated measures of patient SI, assessment of both patient and clinician characteristics, moderately large sample size, and high rates of follow-up. Several limitations should also be noted. First, our analyses suggested that individual clinician differences are a considerable element of the TRQ-SF reports; however, multilevel modeling accounting for clinician individual differences was limited by the fact that many clinicians reported on only few patients, while a few clinicians reported on many patients. Further study is needed to evaluate the nature and extent of individual clinicians' effects. A second limitation of the study is the low rate of suicidal behavior at follow-up such that prediction of suicide attempts was not powered sufficiently to be tested. Third, while clinician responses were collected anonymously, social desirability bias cannot be ruled out. Finally, while we examined patient psychopathology symptoms, patient personality psychopathology was not broadly examined and accounted for in interpreting the results.

Conclusion

The primary implication of this study is that mental health professionals' emotional responses to their patients are indicative of severity of patients' STBs as well as predictive of the short-term development of these thoughts and behaviors. Our results support the potential utility of the TRQ-SF as a reliable, easily used and scored measure of clinicians' suicide-related countertransference. The brevity of this self-assessment may make it particularly useful in the clinical setting and for longitudinal clinical research as it may be comfortably administered on a repeated basis. Indeed, further study is warranted to understand how changes in countertransference over time such as might be assessed with the TRQ-SF in a series of patient encounters relate to changes in patient motivation for or liability to suicide.

AUTHOR CONTRIBUTIONS

SB and ZY conducted and contributed to the design of the experiment, designed the data analyses, analyzed the data, and wrote the paper. MH conducted the experiment and designed the data analyses, analyzed the data, and wrote the paper. BG designed the data analyses, analyzed the data, and contributed to writing the paper. RA, AF, and AA contributed to writing the paper. PR conducted the experiment. IG conducted and designed the experiment and contributed to writing the paper.

ACKNOWLEDGMENTS

This work was supported by the focus grant #RFA-1-015-14 from the American Foundation for Suicide Prevention. The content is solely the responsibility of the authors and does not necessarily represent the official views of the American Foundation for Suicide Prevention. The funders had no role in study design, data collection and analysis, decision to publish, or preparation of the manuscript. The authors would like to acknowledge Irina Kopeykina, Tal Ginsburg, Hae Joon Kim, and Firouz Ardalan, who contributed to the conduct of the study, MegAnn McGiness, Jenna Cohen, Kayla DeFazio, Sherilyn Wilman-Depena, Shoshana Linzer, Yael Shwartz, Nicolette Molina, Olivia Varas, Adina Chesir, Rachel Lerner, Rachel Altman, Joshua Starr, Olivia Tabaczyk, Radwa Mokhtar, Michelle Jeon, Dorin Levy, Vidal Yook, Cindy Forestal, Allison Shuck, Yuna Chang, Sarah Sperber, Tiffany Elchoueiri, and Michelle Hernanadez, who contributed to data collection and entry, as well as the participating patients and clinicians.

REFERENCES

1. Fauth J. Toward more (and better) countertransference research. *Psychotherapy* (2006) 43:16–31. doi:10.1037/0033-3204.43.1.16
2. Rossberg JI, Karterud S, Pedersen G, Friis S. Specific personality traits evoke different countertransference reactions: an empirical study. *J Nerv Ment Dis* (2008) 196:702–8. doi:10.1097/NMD.0b013e318186de80
3. Betan E, Heim AK, Conklin CZ, Westen D. Countertransference phenomena and personality pathology in clinical practice: an empirical investigation. *Am J Psychiatry* (2005) 162:890–8. doi:10.1176/appi.ajp.162.5.890
4. Hayes JA, Gelso CJ, Hummel AM. Managing countertransference. *Psychotherapy* (2011) 48:88–97. doi:10.1037/a0022182
5. Tishby O, Wiseman H. Types of countertransference dynamics: an exploration of their impact on the client-therapist relationship. *Psychother Res* (2014) 24:360–75. doi:10.1080/10503307.2014.893068
6. Gabbard GO. A contemporary psychoanalytic model of countertransference. *J Clin Psychol* (2001) 57:983–91. doi:10.1002/jclp.1065
7. Rossberg JI, Karterud S, Pedersen G, Friis S. An empirical study of countertransference reactions toward patients with personality disorders. *Compr Psychiatry* (2007) 48:225–30. doi:10.1016/j.comppsych.2007.02.002
8. Dahl HSJ, Høglend P, Ulberg R, Amlo S, Gabbard GO, Perry JC, et al. Does therapists' disengaged feelings influence the effect of transference work? A study on countertransference. *Clin Psychol Psychother* (2017) 24:462–74. doi:10.1002/cpp.2015
9. Barzilay S, Yaseen Z, Hawes M, Kopeykina I, Ardalan F, Rosenfield P, et al. Determinants and predictive validity of clinician assessment of short-term suicide risk. *Suicide Life Threat Behav* (2018). doi:10.1111/sltb.12462
10. Colli A, Tanzilli A, Dimaggio G, Lingiardi V. Patient personality and therapist response: an empirical investigation. *Am J Psychiatry* (2014) 171:102–8. doi:10.1176/appi.ajp.2013.13020224
11. Farber BA. Psychotherapists' perceptions of stressful patient behavior. *Prof Psychol Res Pract* (1983) 14:697. doi:10.1037/0735-7028.14.5.697
12. Deutsch CJ. Self-reported sources of stress among psychotherapists. *Prof Psychol Res Pract* (1984) 15:833. doi:10.1037/0735-7028.15.6.833
13. Rodolfa ER, Kraft WA, Reilley RR. Stressors of professionals and trainees at APA-approved counseling and VA medical center internship sites. *Prof Psychol Res Pract* (1988) 19:43. doi:10.1037/0735-7028.19.1.43
14. Pope KS, Tabachnick BG. Therapists' anger, hate, fear, and sexual feelings: national survey of therapist responses, client characteristics, critical events, formal complaints, and training. *Prof Psychol Res Pract* (1993) 24:142. doi:10.1037/0735-7028.24.2.142
15. Kleespies PM, Penk WE, Forsyth JP. The stress of patient suicidal behavior during clinical training: incidence, impact, and recovery. *Prof Psychol Res Pract* (1993) 24:293–303. doi:10.1037/0735-7028.24.3.293
16. Hendin H, Haas AP, Maltsberger JT, Koestner B, Szanto K. Problems in psychotherapy with suicidal patients. *Am J Psychiatry* (2006) 163:67–72. doi:10.1176/appi.ajp.163.1.67
17. Scocco P, Toffol E, Pilotto E, Pertile R. Psychiatrists' emotional reactions to patient suicidal behavior. *J Psychiatr Pract* (2012) 18:94–108. doi:10.1097/01.pra.0000413275.09305.d5
18. Yaseen ZS, Briggs J, Kopeykina I, Orchard KM, Silberlicht J, Bhingradia H, et al. Distinctive emotional responses of clinicians to suicide-attempting patients – a comparative study. *BMC Psychiatry* (2013) 13:230. doi:10.1186/1471-244X-13-230
19. Pompili M, Rihmer Z, Akiskal H, Amore M, Gonda X, Innamorati M, et al. Temperaments mediate suicide risk and psychopathology among patients with bipolar disorders. *Compr Psychiatry* (2012) 53:280–5. doi:10.1016/j.comppsych.2011.04.004
20. Kochanek KD. Deaths: final data for 2014. *Natl Vital Stat Rep* (2016) 65:1–122.
21. Schaffer A, Sinyor M, Kurdyak P, Vigod S, Sareen J, Reis C, et al. Population-based analysis of health care contacts among suicide decedents: identifying opportunities for more targeted suicide prevention strategies. *World Psychiatry* (2016) 15:135–45. doi:10.1002/wps.20321
22. Luoma JB, Martin CE, Pearson JL. Contact with mental health and primary care providers before suicide: a review of the evidence. *Am J Psychiatry* (2002) 159:909–16. doi:10.1176/appi.ajp.159.6.909
23. Ilgen MA, Conner KR, Roeder KM, Blow FC, Austin K, Valenstein M. Patterns of treatment utilization before suicide among male veterans with

substance use disorders. *Am J Public Health* (2012) 102:S88–92. doi:10.2105/AJPH.2011.300392

24. Ribeiro JD, Gutierrez PM, Joiner TE, Kessler RC, Petukhova MV, Sampson NA, et al. Health care contact and suicide risk documentation prior to suicide death: results from the Army Study to Assess Risk and Resilience in Servicemembers (Army STARRS). *J Consult Clin Psychol* (2017) 85:403. doi:10.1037/ccp0000178
25. Yaseen Z, Galynker II, Cohen LJ, Briggs J. Clinicians' conflicting emotional responses to high suicide-risk patients – association with short-term suicide behaviors: a prospective pilot study. *Compr Psychiatry* (2017) 76:69–78. doi:10.1016/j.comppsych.2017.03.013
26. Zittel Conklin C, Westen D. *The Therapist Response Questionnaire.* Atlanta, Georgia: Departments of Psychology and Psychiatry and Behavioral Sciences, Emory University (2003).
27. Tracey TJ, Kokotovic AM. Factor structure of the working alliance inventory. *Psychol Assess* (1989) 1:207. doi:10.1037/1040-3590.1.3.207
28. Busseri MA, Tyler JD. Interchangeability of the working alliance inventory and working alliance inventory, short form. *Psychol Assess* (2003) 15:193. doi:10.1037/1040-3590.15.2.193
29. Hawes M, Yaseen Z, Briggs J, Galynker I. The Modular Assessment of Risk for Imminent Suicide (MARIS): a proof of concept for a multi-informant tool for evaluation of short-term suicide risk. *Compr Psychiatry* (2017) 72:88–96. doi:10.1016/j.comppsych.2016.10.002
30. Posner K, Brown GK, Stanley B, Brent DA, Yershova KV, Oquendo MA, et al. The Columbia-Suicide Severity Rating Scale: initial validity and internal consistency findings from three multisite studies with adolescents and adults. *Am J Psychiatry* (2011) 168:1266–77. doi:10.1176/appi.ajp.2011.10111704
31. Cohen LJ, Ardalan F, Yaseen Z, Galynker I. Suicide crisis syndrome mediates the relationship between long-term risk factors and lifetime suicidal phenomena. *Suicide Life Threat Behav* (2017). doi:10.1111/sltb.12387
32. Beck AT, Kovacs M, Weissman A. Assessment of suicidal intention: the scale for suicide ideation. *J Consult Clin Psychol* (1979) 47:343. doi:10.1037/0022-006X.47.2.343
33. Beck AT, Steer RA. *BSI, Beck Scale for Suicide Ideation: Manual.* San Antonio, TX: Psychological Corporation (1991).
34. Nock MK, Park JM, Finn CT, Deliberto TL, Dour HJ, Banaji MR. Measuring the suicidal mind: implicit cognition predicts suicidal behavior. *Psychol Sci* (2010) 21:511–7. doi:10.1177/0956797610364762
35. Wang Y, Bhaskaran J, Sareen J, Bolton S-L, Chateau D, Bolton JM. Clinician prediction of future suicide attempts: a longitudinal study. *Can J Psychiatry* (2016) 61:428–32. doi:10.1177/0706743716645287
36. Beck AT, Ward CH, Mendelson M, Mock J, Erbaugh J. An inventory for measuring depression. *Arch Gen Psychiatry* (1961) 4:561–71. doi:10.1001/archpsyc.1961.01710120031004
37. Beck AT, Steer RA, Brown GK. Beck depression inventory-II. *San Antonio* (1996) 78:490–8.
38. Derogatis LR, Melisaratos N. The brief symptom inventory: an introductory report. *Psychol Med* (1983) 13:595–605. doi:10.1017/S0033291700048017
39. Rule WR, Traver MD. Test-retest reliabilities of State-Trait Anxiety Inventory in a stressful social analogue situation. *J Pers Assess* (1983) 47:276–7. doi:10.1207/s15327752jpa4703_8
40. Spielberger CD. *State-Trait Anxiety Inventory: A Comprehensive Bibliography.* Palo Alto, CA: Consulting Psychologists Press (1989).
41. Spielberger CD. *Staxi-2: State-Trait Anger Expression Inventory-2; Professional Manual.* Psychological Assessment Resources (1999).
42. John OP, Srivastava S. The big five trait taxonomy: history, measurement, and theoretical perspectives. *Handb Pers Theory Res* (1999) 2:102–38.
43. Horvath AO, Greenberg LS. Development and validation of the working alliance inventory. *J Couns Psychol* (1989) 36:223–33. doi:10.1037/0022-0167.36.2.223
44. Hox JJ, Maas CJ. The accuracy of multilevel structural equation modeling with pseudobalanced groups and small samples. *Struct Equ Model* (2001) 8:157–74. doi:10.1207/S15328007SEM0802_1
45. Maas CJ, Hox JJ. Sufficient sample sizes for multilevel modeling. *Methodology* (2005) 1:86–92. doi:10.1027/1614-2241.1.3.86
46. Mooney CZ, Duval RD. *Bootstrapping: A Nonparametric Approach to Statistical Inference.* London: SAGE (1993).
47. Mîndrila D. Maximum likelihood (ML) and diagonally weighted least squares (DWLS) estimation procedures: a comparison of estimation bias with ordinal and multivariate non-normal data. *Int J Digit Soc* (2010) 1:60–6. doi:10.20533/ijds.2040.2570.2010.0010
48. Bentler PM. Comparative fit indexes in structural models. *Psychol Bull* (1990) 107:238. doi:10.1037/0033-2909.107.2.238
49. Steiger J, Lind J. Statistically-based tests for the number of common factors. *Paper Presented at the Annual Spring Meeting of the Psychometric Society*, Iowa City (1980).
50. MacCallum RC, Browne MW, Sugawara HM. Power analysis and determination of sample size for covariance structure modeling. *Psychol Methods* (1996) 1:130. doi:10.1037/1082-989X.1.2.130
51. Hu L, Bentler P. Cut-off criteria for fit indexes in covariance structure analysis: conventional criteria versus new alternatives. Struct Equ Modeling. 6: 1–55. *Educ Psychol* (1999) 27:65–90.
52. Rosseel Y. *lavaan: An R Package for Structural Equation Modeling and More Version 0.4–9 (BETA).* Belgium: Ghent University (2011).
53. Streiner DL. Starting at the beginning: an introduction to coefficient alpha and internal consistency. *J Pers Assess* (2003) 80:99–103. doi:10.1207/S15327752JPA8001_18
54. Revelle W. Hierarchical cluster analysis and the internal structure of tests. *Multivariate Behav Res* (1979) 14:57–74. doi:10.1207/s15327906mbr1401_4
55. Revelle WR. *psych: Procedures for Personality and Psychological Research.* Software (2017).
56. Cooksey RW, Soutar GN. Coefficient beta and hierarchical item clustering: an analytical procedure for establishing and displaying the dimensionality and homogeneity of summated scales. *Organ Res Methods* (2006) 9:78–98. doi:10.1177/1094428105283939
57. Rossberg JI, Karterud S, Pedersen G, Friis S. Psychiatric symptoms and countertransference feelings: an empirical investigation. *Psychiatry Res* (2010) 178:191–5. doi:10.1016/j.psychres.2009.09.019
58. Barzilay S, Apter A. Predictors of suicide in adolescents and adults with mood and common comorbid disorders. *Neuropsychiatry* (2014) 4:81. doi:10.2217/npy.13.86
59. Tauber ES. Exploring the therapeutic use of countertransference data. *Psychiatry* (1954) 17:331–6. doi:10.1080/00332747.1954.11022978
60. Stern DB. Courting surprise: unbidden perceptions in clinical practice. *Contemp Psychoanal* (1990) 26:452–78. doi:10.1080/00107530.1990.10746672
61. Fauth J, Williams EN. The in-session self-awareness of therapist-trainees: hindering or helpful? *J Couns Psychol* (2005) 52:443. doi:10.1037/0022-0167.52.3.443
62. Fatter DM, Hayes JA. What facilitates countertransference management? The roles of therapist meditation, mindfulness, and self-differentiation. *Psychother Res* (2013) 23:502–13. doi:10.1080/10503307.2013.797124
63. Tanzilli A, Colli A, Del Corno F, Lingiardi V. Factor structure, reliability, and validity of the therapist response questionnaire. *Personal Disord* (2016) 7:147–58. doi:10.1037/per0000146
64. Hendin H, Maltsberger JT, Szanto K. The role of intense affective states in signaling a suicide crisis. *J Nerv Ment Dis* (2007) 195:363–8. doi:10.1097/NMD.0b013e318052264d
65. Galynker I, Yaseen ZS, Cohen A, Benhamou O, Hawes M, Briggs J. Prediction of suicidal behavior in high risk psychiatric patients using an assessment of acute suicidal state: the suicide crisis inventory. *Depress Anxiety* (2017) 34:147–58. doi:10.1002/da.22559
66. Joiner TE, Stanley IH. Can the phenomenology of a suicidal crisis be usefully understood as a suite of antipredator defensive reactions? *Psychiatry* (2016) 79:107–19. doi:10.1080/00332747.2016.1142800
67. Maltsberger JT, Buie DH. Countertransference hate in the treatment of suicidal patients. *Arch Gen Psychiatry* (1974) 30:625–33. doi:10.1001/archpsyc.1974.01760110049005
68. Hutchinson M, Jackson D. Hostile clinician behaviours in the nursing work environment and implications for patient care: a mixed-methods systematic review. *BMC Nurs* (2013) 12:25. doi:10.1186/1472-6955-12-25
69. Nilsen S, Malterud K. What happens when the doctor denies a patient's request? A qualitative interview study among general practitioners in Norway. *Scand J Prim Health Care* (2017) 35(2):201–7. doi:10.1080/02813432.2017.1333309
70. Ulberg R, Amlo S, Hersoug AG, Dahl HSJ, Høglend P. The effects of the therapist's disengaged feelings on the in-session process in psychodynamic psychotherapy. *J Clin Psychol* (2014) 70:440–51. doi:10.1002/jclp.22088

71. Davis DM, Hayes JA. What are the benefits of mindfulness? A practice review of psychotherapy-related research. *Psychotherapy* (2011) 48:198. doi:10.1037/a0022062
72. Safran JD, Muran JC, Eubanks-Carter C. Repairing alliance ruptures. *Psychotherapy* (2011) 48:80. doi:10.1037/a0022140
73. Wolf AW, Goldfried MR, Muran J. *Transforming Negative Reactions to Clients: From Frustration to Compassion*. Washington, DC: American Psychological Association (2013).
74. Foster A, Chaudhary N, Kim T, Waller JL, Wong J, Borish M, et al. Using virtual patients to teach empathy: a randomized controlled study to enhance medical students' empathic communication. *Simul Healthc* (2016) 11:181–9. doi:10.1097/SIH.0000000000000142
75. Schmitz WM, Allen MH, Feldman BN, Gutin NJ, Jahn DR, Kleespies PM, et al. Preventing suicide through improved training in suicide risk assessment and care: an American Association of Suicidology Task Force report addressing serious gaps in US mental health training. *Suicide Life Threat Behav* (2012) 42:292–304. doi:10.1111/j.1943-278X.2012.00090.x

11

Decision-Making in Suicidal Behavior: The Protective Role of Loss Aversion

Gergö Hadlaczky[1], Sebastian Hökby[1], Anahit Mkrtchian[1], Danuta Wasserman[1], Judit Balazs[2,3], Núria Machín[4], Marco Sarchiapone[5,6,7], Merike Sisask[8,9] and Vladimir Carli[1]*

[1] National Centre for Suicide Research and Prevention of Mental Ill-Health, Department of Learning, Informatics, Management and Ethics, Karolinska Institutet, Stockholm, Sweden, [2] Vadaskert Child Psychiatry Hospital and Outpatient Clinic, Budapest, Hungary, [3] Institute of Psychology, Eötövös Loránd University, Budapest, Hungary, [4] Skylark Health Research Ltd., London, United Kingdom, [5] Department of Medicine and Health Science, University of Molise, Campobasso, Italy, [6] National Institute for Health, Migration and Poverty, Rome, Italy, [7] Kazakh National Medical University, Almaty, Kazakhstan, [8] Estonian-Swedish Mental Health and Suicidology Institute, Tallinn, Estonia, [9] School of Governance, Law and Society, Tallinn University, Tallinn, Estonia

***Correspondence:**
Gergö Hadlaczky
gergo.hadlaczki@ki.se

Background: Loss aversion is a central and well operationalized trait behavior that describes the tendency for humans to strongly prefer avoiding losses to making equivalent gains. Human decision-making is thus biased toward safer choices.

Aim: The aim of this study was to explore the relationship between loss aversion and suicidal behavior in a large cohort of adolescents recruited in 30 schools of seven European countries for a longitudinal study (Current Controlled Trials ISRCTN65120704). We hypothesized that individuals with higher loss aversion would be less likely to attempt suicide.

Methods: A mixed monetary gamble task was used to generate loss aversion scores for each participant. Logistic regression was used to estimate the cross-sectional association between loss aversion and life-time suicide attempts in the baseline sample (N = 2,158; 156 attempters), and incident attempts were predicted in a 4-month prospective model (N = 1,763; 75 attempters). Multiple regression was used to estimate the association between loss aversion and suicidal ideation.

Results: Loss aversion was a significant predictor of attempted suicide in both the cross-sectional (OR = 0.79; P = 0.005) and prospective analysis (OR = 0.81; P = 0.040), adjusting for depression, anxiety, stress, and sex. The correlation between pre and post measures of loss aversion was r = 0.52 (P < 0.001). Interestingly, although depression, anxiety, and stress were associated with suicidal ideation, loss aversion was not (cross-sectional model: P = 0.092; Prospective model: P = 0.390). This suggests that the concept of loss aversion may be useful in understanding the transition from suicidal thoughts to attempts.

Conclusion: This and previous studies suggest that altered decision-making is involved in suicide attempts. In our study, we show the involvement of loss aversion in particular, and propose that individuals high in loss aversion are discouraged from carrying out the suicide attempt because of a greater focus on the negative consequences of the decision.

Keywords: loss aversion, decision-making, suicide, attempted, mental health, suicidal ideation

INTRODUCTION

Suicide and suicidal behavior is one of the leading causes of mortality and morbidity worldwide, making it a serious and significant public health problem (1). Perhaps, the most salient stressors implicated in suicidal behaviors are mental illnesses. Around 40–90% of suicide attempters suffer from depression, anxiety disorders, schizophrenia, and other mental health problems, such as alexithymia (2–5). Numerous other risk factors have been identified through association studies, such as a wide range of somatic illnesses [e.g., diabetes (6, 7), malignant neoplasms (8–10), and chronic pain (11)]; social difficulties, such as family conflicts (12, 13) and bullying (14, 15); and different socioeconomic factors, such as unemployment (16) and economic recession (17); not to mention a wide range of specific stressful life-events (18). A common denominator among these risk factors is that they often lead to suffering. However, despite their clear association to suicidality, the majority of individuals displaying these, or even a combination of these risk factors, never actually attempt suicide [see, for instance, Ref. (19–21)]. An important question is thus, what separates suffering individuals who attempt suicide from those who do not?

A number of putative mechanisms have been proposed to answer this question, from various scientific domains. A subset of behavioral studies has investigated the possible effects of decision-making on suicidal behavior. Jollant and colleagues (22), for instance, used the Iowa Gambling Task (IGT), to compare the performance of attempters, depressed non-attempters, and healthy controls. This task attempts to mimic real-life decision-making (23), and involves making a number of choices between four different decks of cards. Two of the decks are disadvantageous, as they entail large wins, but even larger losses, leading to a net loss. The losses and gains in the other two decks are smaller, but lead to a larger net profit in the long run. After sampling a few cards, healthy participants usually end up favoring the advantageous decks, while participants with for instance frontal cortex lesions underperform by selecting more cards from the high-risk decks (23–25). In the study of Jollant and colleagues (22), mood disorder patients with a history of suicide attempt performed significantly worse, both when compared to healthy controls and compared to mood disorder patients without a history of suicide attempts. In subsequent IGT studies, decreased performance was also found in bipolar patients with a history of suicidal behavior compared to other patient groups (26), or in adolescents with a previous history of suicide attempts (27). Although some studies have failed to replicate the IGT findings (28–31), a meta-analysis pooling all studies showed that suicide attempters exhibited substantially reduced performance (Hedge's $g = -0.47$) compared with control groups of varying composition (32). Altered decision-making in suicidal individuals has also been substantiated in studies using a conceptually similar task, the Cambridge Gamble Task, among older suicide attempters (33) and young adults with a history of suicide attempts (34) and those suffering from alexithymia (35). Examination of other components of decision-making, such as sunk cost bias (i.e., the continued investment in an action with a negative outcome) and delay-discounting (i.e., the preference for smaller, but immediate rewards compared to greater, but delayed rewards) and framing has also demonstrated impaired decision-making in suicidal individuals (36, 37).

However, as much as this literature supports the association between altered decision-making in suicidal behavior, the majority of these studies are cross-sectional, which makes it difficult to draw conclusions regarding the causal mechanism of altered decision-making and suicidal behavior. It is difficult to disentangle whether the impact of a suicide attempt alters decision-making, or whether the divergent decision-making leads to suicide attempts. Another problem is that, due to the complexity of the specific IGT task-paradigm, it is difficult to identify specific cognitive components that predict performance (38), which in turn could be used to characterize suicide attempters. Studies aimed at dissecting the IGT-paradigm identified several cognitive processes that are likely to drive performance. These include higher order processes involved in understanding and learning the structure of decks, including memory functioning, but also more basic features, such as impulsivity (39–42). Last, studies have found that IGT performance is influenced by participants' sensitivity to loss frequencies and loss magnitude (43, 44) by implicating loss aversion.

Loss aversion (45, 46) is one of the most robust and ubiquitous empirical findings in the behavioral sciences (47), which entails a strong human preference for avoiding losses, rather than making equivalent gains. In other words, the threat of a potential loss is more likely to influence human decisions compared to an opportunity for an equal gain. In tasks measuring loss aversion, participants may be offered various gambles with a 50% chance to either win or lose a certain amount of money [e.g., Ref. (48, 49)]. The magnitude of potential gains and losses are then varied for each gamble, and participants are asked to indicate whether they accept or reject them. Gambles will generally be rejected unless the potential gain is around twice the potential loss. For example, gambles offering a 50% chance to win \$30, but a 50% chance to lose \$20, will most often be rejected, despite the expected value being a gain of \$5. From an evolutionary perspective, loss aversion can be conceptualized as an automatic protective mechanism, which through biasing the decision-maker, guides him or her away from potential danger unless reward is valuable enough to warrant it.

It could be hypothesized that an individual with greater aversion to potential losses (e.g., the physical harm if the attempt fails, the sorrow afflicted on family members, etc.) would find the option of attempting suicide less advantageous. If the potential gains (i.e., the discontinuation of suffering) have a greater influence on the decision, the option of making an attempt may be perceived as something more advantageous. In this light, aversion to potential losses can be seen as a protective factor against suicide. Subsequently, individual differences in loss aversion could distinguish between suffering attempters and non-attempters.

In this study, we aimed at investigating the association between loss aversion and suicidal behavior. We used both cross-sectional and prospective analyses, to address issues of causal directionality that previous studies have not been able to. Our study is focused on a cohort of adolescents, since the suicide attempt rate in this age group is high (50). A mixed monetary gamble task (48) was used to investigate the association between individual differences in loss aversion and suicide attempts, and whether these differences may predict future suicide attempts.

MATERIALS AND METHODS

Study Design and Sampling Procedure

The current study utilized data from a randomized controlled trial (Current Controlled Trials ISRCTN65120704) conducted in 2012–2013 as a part of the Suicide Prevention through Internet and Media-Based Mental Health Promotion (SUPREME) project. The cluster-randomized trial used questionnaires to evaluate a mental health-promoting website among adolescents recruited from 30 randomly selected state schools in seven European countries. The intervention-effect was controlled in all prospective analyses in this study.

Adolescents were recruited from predefined catchment areas in each of the seven countries: West Viru County (Estonia; 3 schools, 416 participants), Budapest District II and District XII (Hungary; 6 schools, 413 participants), Molise (Italy; 3 schools, 311 participants), Vilnius City (Lithuania; 3 schools, 240 participants), Barcelona City (Spain; 3 schools, 182 participants), Stockholm County (Sweden; 9 schools, 337 participants), and Eastern England (United Kingdom; 3 schools, 387 participants). Eligible state schools in these areas were randomly arranged into a contact order, the order in which schools were contacted and asked to participate. If a school declined, the next school on the list was contacted. If a school accepted participation, a team of researchers went to the school and presented the background, aims, goals, and procedures of the study to the pupils verbally and through consent forms. Thus, the total baseline sample consisted of 2,286 school pupils, with 56% females and a mean age of 15.8 years (SD = 0.91 years).

Evaluation questionnaires were administered in three waves; at baseline (T1), at 2 months (T2), and at 4 months (T3). The questionnaires were administered in classrooms or computer labs during normal school hours, and after completion they also received information about the intervention. The questionnaires were administered on paper, or online if the schools could provide the pupils with laptops. The attrition rate between T1 and T2 was 20% (467 pupils), and between T2 and T3 it was 13% (244 pupils). Subjects were included in the longitudinal analyses if they had data from baseline and from either follow-up wave (T2 and/or T3). Written consent was obtained from all pupils who agreed to participate (as well as their parents', when applicable), and the study was approved by an ethics committee in all participating countries. The procedures involved in the SUPREME trial have been described in more detail elsewhere (51).

Measurements

Participants' levels of depression, anxiety, and stress were measured with the 42-item version of the Depression, Anxiety, and Stress Scale [DASS-42; (52)]. Scores on each subscale range between 0 and 42. Previous studies have confirmed the validity and reliability of this scale (52–55), but suggest that adolescents might differentiate less between the three factors compared to adults (56). High internal consistency was also achieved in the current sample (depression alpha = 0.93; anxiety alpha = 0.89; stress alpha = 0.91).

Suicidal ideation and attempts were measured with Paykel's suicide scale (57). Suicide attempts was measured with the question "Have you ever tried to take your own life?" to which participants could respond "No, never," "Yes, during the past 2 weeks," "Yes, between 2 weeks and 1 year ago," or "Yes, 1 year ago or earlier." A dichotomous "lifetime suicide attempt" variable was created for T1, T2, and T3, where all affirmative answers were coded as a "suicide attempt." Attempts at either of the follow-ups were pooled to create a variable indicating attempt at *either* T2 *or* T3 (positives at both T2 and T3 were coded as one attempt). This was done to increase the number of suicide attempts and thus power. Suicidal ideation was measured using the mean score of the four items that regard ideation on the Paykel's suicide scale (57). The item-response was a seven-point scale from "never" to "always" ("Have you felt, during the past two weeks, that life was not worth living?," "Have you wished, during the past two weeks, that you were dead – for instance, that you could go to sleep and not wake up?," "During the past two weeks, have you thought of taking your life, even if you would not really do it?," "During the past two weeks, have you reached the point where you seriously considered taking your life or perhaps made plans how you would go about doing it?"). For the prospective analyses, participants' pooled average at T2 and T3 was used. Individuals with missing values on either attempts or suicidal ideation at T1 or both follow-ups were excluded from the analyses. If they were missing on one follow-up only, data from the other follow-up was used.

Loss aversion at an individual level was measured using a mixed monetary gamble task (48), shown in **Figure 1** (when translating the questionnaire, the currency was adapted to each country so that the absolute amount of money would be approximately the same across settings). The potential gain always remained €6, but the potential losses were increased from €2 to €7, yielding a successively decreasing expected value for each gamble. A participant's loss aversion score was then defined as 0 minus the highest accepted gamble, thus producing a continuous variable with a score rage of −6 to 0, where a lower score indicates lower loss aversion.

Data Analysis

Independent samples *t*-tests and Chi-square tests were used to investigate sex differences in mental health, suicidality and loss aversion, and *t*-tests were used to examine differences in loss aversion between suicide attempters and non-attempters. A standard multiple regression was also calculated to examine how depression, anxiety, and stress (controlling for sex and intervention) was associated with loss aversion scores.

The main analyses consisted of one cross-sectional and one prospective (longitudinal) hierarchical binary logistic regression, where a life-time report of suicide attempt was used as the outcome variable (yes/no). The first model included only control variables: sex, depression, anxiety, and stress scores at T1, after which loss aversion scores from T1 was added in a second step to test if the model improved. In the prospective model, those who had reported a life-time attempt at T1 were excluded, and the outcome was thus incident suicide attempt at *either* T2 *or* T3

Alternatives	Accept	Reject
#1. If the coin turns up **heads**, you **lose €2**; if the coin turns up **tails**, you **win €6**.	□	□
#2. If the coin turns up **heads**, you **lose €3**; if the coin turns up **tails**, you **win €6**.	□	□
#3. If the coin turns up **heads**, you **lose €4**; if the coin turns up **tails**, you **win €6**.	□	□
#4. If the coin turns up **heads**, you **lose €5**; if the coin turns up **tails**, you **win €6**.	□	□
#5. If the coin turns up **heads**, you **lose €6**; if the coin turns up **tails**, you **win €6**.	□	□
#6. If the coin turns up **heads**, you **lose €7**; if the coin turns up **tails**, you **win €6**.	□	□

FIGURE 1 | Questionnaire item used to measure individual-level loss aversion. Imagine that a person wants to make a bet with you. He flips a coin, and if it turns up heads, you lose a certain amount of money, if it turns up tails, you win a certain amount. Which of the following offers do you accept?

(possible intervention effects were controlled for in this model). All non-binary variables (depression, anxiety, stress, and loss aversion scores) were standardized (Z-transformed) before analyses to simplify the interpretation and comparison of odds ratios.

Two further main analyses were performed with the same control variables, but using suicidal ideation as the outcome. Because this variable is continuous, standard multiple regression was used in both the cross-sectional and prospective analysis. In the prospective analysis, suicidal ideation at baseline was included as a control variable.

All analyses were performed in SPSS version 23, with $\alpha = 0.05$ (one-tailed on the main analyses). Missing data was treated using list-wise exclusion.

RESULTS

Prevalence of Depression, Anxiety, and Stress in the Sample

Baseline depression scores could be computed for 2,245 participants and the mean score was 7.47 (SD = 8.38). The average baseline anxiety score was 6.75 (SD = 6.96; N = 2,248) and the average stress score was 10.11 (SD = 8.38; N = 2,246). *T*-tests showed that females had higher scores than males on all three sub-scales (Depression: M difference = 3.25; $d = 0.40$; anxiety: M difference = 2.13; $d = 0.31$; stress: M difference = 3.72; $d = 0.46$; all *P*-values <0.001).

Prevalence of Suicidal Ideation and Behaviors in the Sample

Regarding suicide attempts, 156 (6.6%) participants reported a life-time attempt at baseline. When these subjects were excluded, there were 75 (3.4%) incident cases during the follow-up period. At baseline, females were more likely than males to have attempted suicide (females = 9.8%; males = 3.3%; $\chi^2_1 = 35.99$; $P < 0.001$; Phi = 0.13). There was no significant sex difference in prospective suicide attempts (females = 4.2%; males = 3.6%; $P = 0.546$). Regarding study drop-outs, participants who reported a lifetime suicide attempt at baseline were not less likely to participate at T2 (75.0 vs. 77.5%; $P = 0.488$), although they were less likely to participate at T3 (59.0 vs. 68.3%; $\chi^2_1 = 5.80$; $P = 0.021$; Phi = 0.05). However, this effect size was small.

Most participants did not report suicidal ideation. The average score at baseline was 1.47 (SD = 1.05; N = 2,223), and the average score at follow-up was 1.37 (SD = 0.87; N = 2,025). *T*-tests showed that females had more suicidal ideation than males at both baseline (M difference = 0.32; $t_{2,219} = 7.29$; $P < 0.001$; $d = 0.32$) and follow-up (M difference = 0.22; $t_{1,956} = 5.61$; $P < 0.001$; $d = 0.42$). *T*-tests showed that participants with higher levels of suicidal ideation were less likely to participate at T2 (M difference = 0.16; $t_{2,221} = 3.04$; $P = 0.006$; $d = 0.15$) and T3 (M difference = 0.16; $t_{2,221} = 3.22$; $P = 0.003$; $d = 0.14$), but this effect size was small.

A cross-sectional standard multiple regression showed that higher depression and lower stress was associated with more suicidal ideation, but not anxiety or sex (Model: $F_{4,\,2,187} = 570.88$; $P < 0.001$; $R^2_{adj} = 0.51$; sex: $P = 0.154$; depression: $\beta = 0.75$; $P < 0.001$; anxiety: $P = 0.068$; stress: $\beta = -0.09$; $P = 0.001$). A cross-sectional logistic regression further showed that higher suicidal ideation and female sex was associated with a higher likelihood of suicide attempt (Model Omnibus test: $\chi^2_2 = 310.11$; $P < 0.001$; Nagelkerke $R^2 = 0.33$; suicidal ideation: Wald = 236.94; OR = 2.52; $P < 0.001$; sex: Wald = 11.70; OR = 0.456; $P = 0.001$).

Loss Aversion

Baseline loss aversion scores could be calculated for a total of 2,203 participants. The median loss aversion score was −2 (mean = −2.22; SD = 1.79), corresponding to an implied acceptable loss of €3 for a prospective gain of €6. A small minority (less than 4.2%) of the subjects accepted the gamble with the negative expected value (an implied loss of €7 for a gain of €6). Overall, the distribution of loss aversion scores in this dataset (**Figure 2**) compare quite well to normative data in that approximately 75% of the sample rejected gambles in which the potential gains were lower than double that of the potential loss [e.g., Ref. (48, 58)]. Compared to Gächter and colleague's (48) sample, however, the proportion of individuals who rejected all bets was larger [16.6% in this sample compared to 1.8% in Ref. (48)]. *T*-tests showed that there was no difference in average loss aversion scores between participants who dropped out at T2 ($P = 0.695$) or T3 ($P = 0.859$), compared to participants who retained in the study. The test–retest reliability (Pearson correlation) of loss aversion was 0.54 between T1 and T2, and 0.52 between T1 and T3, and 0.63 between T2 and T3 (all *P*-values <0.001), indicating that loss aversion was relatively stable among participants over the course of 4 months.

An independent samples *t*-test showed that males had lower loss aversion scores compared to females (mean difference = 0.44; $t_{2,199} = 5.72$; $P < 0.001$; $d = 0.24$). No association was found between depression, anxiety, or stress and loss aversion

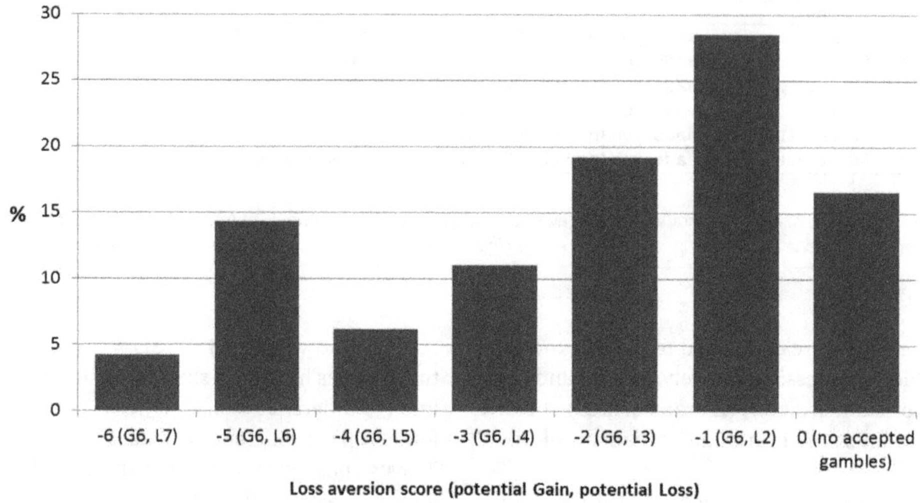

FIGURE 2 | Distribution of loss aversion scores in the baseline sample (N = 2,203). A participant's score is calculated as: 0 minus the highest (least profitable) accepted gamble. Thus, a score of −6 indicates very low loss aversion and a score of 0 indicates very high loss aversion. In parentheses, the potential gains (G) and losses (L) for the accepted gambles are shown. The probability of winning or losing the gamble is always 50%. Thus "G6, L7" means a 50–50% gamble with the possibility of a €6 gain and €7 loss.

scores after controlling for sex (Model: $F_{4,2,172} = 12.50$; $P < 0.001$; $R^2_{adj} = 0.02$; sex: $\beta = 0.14$, $P < 0.001$; depression: $P = 0.784$; anxiety: $P = 0.237$; stress: $P = 0.319$).

Importantly, independent samples t-test showed that baseline suicide attempters had lower loss aversion scores compared to non-attempters (mean difference = 0.43; $t_{2,180} = 2.59$; $P = 0.009$; d = 0.23). Moreover, in the prospective sample with baseline suicide attempters excluded, baseline loss aversion scores were significantly lower in participants who made an attempt at follow-up, compared to those who did not (mean difference = 0.44; $t_{1,780} = 2.02$; $P = 0.044$; $d = 0.25$). There was a small cross-sectional correlation between loss aversion scores and suicidal ideation scores ($r = -0.05$; $P = 0.016$), but there was no correlation between loss aversion scores and prospective suicidal ideation ($r = -0.03$; $P = 0.191$).

TABLE 1 | Results from logistic regressions predicting suicide attempts at baseline, and prospectively during the 4-month follow-up.

Model	Predictor	Wald	OR	95% CI	P-value
Cross-sectional	Sex[b]	12.64	0.44	0.30–0.64	<0.001*
	Depression	42.71	2.21	1.81–2.70	<0.001*
	Anxiety	2.27	1.21	0.98–1.48	0.066
	Stress	0.51	1.11	0.87–1.43	0.238
	Loss aversion score[c]	6.63	0.79	0.67–0.92	0.005*
Prospective[a]	Sex	0.00	1.02	0.66–1.56	0.475
	Depression	8.44	1.72	1.26–2.33	0.002*
	Anxiety	1.86	1.29	0.95–1.76	0.087
	Stress	1.51	0.76	0.53–1.10	0.110
	Loss aversion score[c]	3.09	0.81	0.66–0.99	0.040*

[a]*The prospective model controlled for the effect of experimental condition.*
[b]*In sex, female sex constitutes the reference category.*
[c]*Higher loss aversion scores indicates a greater aversion to losses.*
**Sig. at P < 0.05, one-sided.*

Main Analyses

The first hierarchical logistic regression was calculated to predict lifetime suicide attempts at baseline (N = 2,158). The first model which included sex, depression, anxiety, and stress was significant (Omnibus test: $\chi^2_4 = 257.35$; $P < 0.001$; Nagelkerke $R^2 = 0.29$). Adding loss aversion scores in the next step significantly improved the model (Omnibus test: $\chi^2_1 = 6.53$; $P = 0.011$; Nagelkerke $R^2 = 0.29$), with loss aversion as a significant predictor (OR = 0.79; $P = 0.005$; see **Table 1**). In the second hierarchical logistic regression analysis, the outcome variable was incident attempt at T2 or T3 (N = 1,763), and a sample where baseline suicide attempters were excluded (and intervention effects were controlled for). Similarly to the previous analysis, the first model which included only sex, baseline depression, anxiety, and stress, was significant (Omnibus test: $\chi^2_5 = 25.32$; $P < 0.001$; Nagelkerke $R^2 = 0.05$). Baseline loss aversion was also a significant predictor of future suicide attempts in this model (OR = 0.81; $P = 0.040$; see **Table 1**), but it did not significantly improve the model as a whole (Omnibus test: $\chi^2_1 = 3.02$; $P = 0.082$; Nagelkerke $R^2 = 0.06$).

The standardized OR = 0.79 (cross-sectional) or 0.81 (prospective) for loss aversion can be interpreted as follows: an increase of one SD (i.e., 1.79 points on the six-point scale) reduces the risk of suicide attempt with approximately 20%. Expressed in absolute values (not shown in table), this corresponds to a 12% reduction in suicide risk, when loss aversion is increased with 1 point (OR = 0.87 in the cross-sectional model, and OR = 0.89 in the prospective model).

Last, standard multiple regression was carried out to test if loss aversion is associated with suicidal ideation. In the cross-sectional model, sex and the DASS-42 subscales were found to be significant predictors, but loss aversion was not (Model: $F_{5,2,125} = 428.75$; $P < 0.001$; $R^2_{adj} = 0.50$; sex: $\beta = 0.03$; $P = 0.029$;

depression: $\beta = 0.74$; $P < 0.001$; anxiety: $\beta = 0.05$; $P = 0.042$; stress: $\beta = -0.09$; $P < 0.001$; loss aversion: $\beta = -0.02$; $P = 0.092$). In the prospective model, only the DASS-42 subscales and baseline suicidal ideation were significant predictors, but sex and loss aversion was not (Model: $F_{7, 1,828} = 145.14$; $P < 0.001$; $R^2_{adj} = 0.36$; sex: $\beta = 0.01$; $P = 0.240$; depression: $\beta = 0.18$; $P < 0.001$; anxiety: $\beta = 0.07$; $P = 0.011$; stress: $\beta = -0.07$; $P = 0.029$; baseline suicidal ideation score: $\beta = 0.44$; $P < 0.001$; loss aversion: $\beta = 0.01$; $P = 0.390$).

DISCUSSION

This study utilized a specific behavioral component of decision-making—loss aversion—to investigate its effect on suicidal behavior in a longitudinal sample of non-clinical adolescents; an age group in which the risk for attempted suicide is high. Loss aversion was hypothesized to be a protective factor against suicidal behavior. We found support for this hypothesis in that loss aversion was significantly lower among attempters compared to non-attempters, and this association remained significant even when controlling for mental health (depression anxiety and stress) and sex. Similar results were found in prospective analyses. Here, participants with no history of suicide attempts at baseline were selected, and an association was found between loss aversion scores at baseline, and attempts carried out in the subsequent 4 months (also controlling for sex and mental health). The prospective analyses strengthen the idea that altered decision-making, in particular loss aversion, is a precedent to attempt suicide, rather than being the result physical or psychological trauma followed by the attempt.

The results of our study are consistent with previous studies that implicate altered decision-making among suicide attempters [e.g., Ref. (59)]. A large body of literature reports that suicide attempters have decreased performance in IGT (32). A number of studies have argued that a key indicator in IGT performance is sensitivity to losses, that is, a preference for decks with low frequency of losses, rather than the intention of maximizing long-term gains [e.g., Ref. (60, 61)]. The lowered levels of loss aversion associated with suicide attempts are in line with these results and may thus explain this group's poor performance on the IGT. Interestingly, however, our results are inconsistent with a recent study investigating loss aversion in a clinical population (62). Here, depressed patients with a history of suicide attempts had significantly *increased* loss aversion compared to patients with depression, but without a history of attempts, as well as compared to healthy participants. This is difficult to reconcile with our findings, and also with the previous IGT studies, considering that an increased loss aversion would predict better IGT performance. However, it must be pointed out that the complexity of the IGT gives way for a number of mechanisms that may influence performance, and it is difficult to estimate how much influence each of the components exert.

Another component of decision-making which is often considered to be closely related to loss aversion is sunk cost fallacy. This refers to an individual's investment in a low probability pay-off because of a previously made irrecoverable investment. Szanto and colleagues (37) found that low-lethality attempters were more susceptible to sunk costs compared to non-psychiatric controls and suicidal ideators. No difference was found between high-lethality attempters and controls. The "bad investments" can be seen as the result of an aversion to the loss represented by the sunk cost. This interpretation would entail that the attempters in Szanto et al. (37) have *high* loss aversion (opposing our findings). However, the interpretation of Szanto and colleagues (37) is that low-lethality attempters are more affected by sunk costs, as a function of their proneness to emotional reactivity and impulsivity. We believe it is possible that these affect-driven components overshadow the effect of loss aversion when investigating sunk costs. For instance, older suicide attempters have shown to exhibit impaired reward/punishment-based learning compared to non-attempters and the low-lethality group with impulsive suicide attempts has been associated with enhanced discounting of delayed rewards, as well as impulsivity (63, 64). Another explanation to the discrepant findings in our study and that of Szanto and colleagues (37) may simply be that the connection between loss aversion and sunk cost bias is overestimated in general (65).

This study utilized a behavioral measure of loss aversion, but its neural underpinnings have been investigated in previous research. Loss aversion appears to be encoded in the ventromedial prefrontal cortex, orbitofrontal cortex, the ventral striatum, insula, thalamus, and the amygdala (49, 66–68), which are areas that overlap with regions found to be impaired in attempters (69–75). Neural measures of loss aversion appear to be highly consistent with behavioral measures, as shown by Tom et al. (49) (correlation of $r = 0.85$ between neural and behavioral measures). Thus, loss aversion may be an interesting endophenotype, and putative marker for future studies on suicide attempts. Also, loss aversion is often assumed to be a relatively stable and trait-like construct (76) with some empirical evidence supporting this assumption. For instance, Glöckner and Pachur (77) found a high consistency in the magnitude of loss aversion among participants' responses in a 1-week follow-up study. Zeisberger and colleagues (78) found high stability on an aggregate level, but instability in subset of their sample, during a 1-month follow-up. Finally, in our sample the three measures, 2 months apart during the 4-month period, correlated significantly, with repeated measures explaining about 27–40% of the variance. If loss aversion is a stable trait, not only could it be directly implicated in the decision to make a suicide attempt, it could also be hypothesized that individuals with lower levels of aversion are more often exposed to losses in life in general, which in turn may entail an indirect, long-term risk for suicidal behavior.

Previous studies suggest that suicide attempters may be oversensitive to the effect of incurred losses [e.g., Ref. (79)], and also to other types of negative feedback (80). In this light, it is important to underline that loss aversion relates to the anticipation of *potential* losses, rather than a reaction to *incurred* losses. In fact, a number of studies suggest that the effects of incurred losses, on for instance cognition or arousal, are independent of the aversion to potential losses (81, 82). It is, therefore, possible for an individual to have both a low aversion to potential losses, and at the same time a high sensitivity to incurred losses. This combination could constitute an even greater increase in suicide risk in the long term, where reduced aversion to potential losses increase an individuals' propensity for incurring losses, which is then exacerbated by an increased negative emotional reaction.

A mechanism by which loss aversion may affect the decision to make a suicide attempt is also proposed: For a suffering individual contemplating a suicide attempt, perhaps the most obvious desire, and most important "gain," is the discontinuation of suffering. The potential "loss" may be an injury if the attempt fails, sorrow to family members and friends if it is completed, death, and so on. In this situation, individuals with higher levels of loss aversion are protected from making an attempt, because their decisions are to a greater extent influenced by the potential losses. The aversion to these make the "proposition" less attractive and it is ultimately rejected. On the other hand, individuals with lower loss aversion are more likely to focus on immediate gains, such as the discontinuation of suffering, and may consequently carry out the act.

Interestingly, we found no association between loss aversion and suicidal thoughts, despite the high association between ideation and attempts. This finding suggests that loss aversion is to a greater extent involved in the actual decision to attempt (i.e., a direct effect), rather than the events proceeding up to the genesis of the ideation. It could be interesting to further explore the relationship between loss aversion, suicidal ideation and attempts, in order to explore if loss aversion could be used to distinguish between ideators that become attempters and those that do not.

Limitations

Given that our sample constitutes adolescents, it may be difficult to generalize the results to other age groups. Although there is some evidence to that loss aversion is similar between adolescents and adults (83), we know that suicidal behaviors are not. Attempts are usually overrepresented in the younger populations, while completed suicide is more common in older populations (1). Finally, although a prospective design was employed in this study, the validity of causal inferences may nevertheless be threatened by unmeasured confounders.

Conclusion

The results of this study support the involvement of loss aversion in attempted suicide, through both cross-sectional and longitudinal associations. We propose that individuals high in loss aversion are discouraged from carrying out the suicide attempt because of a greater focus on the negative consequences of the decision. There is some empirical evidence, including data presented here, for the over-time stability of loss aversion. If our findings are successfully replicated, loss aversion may be considered as a candidate for a highly measurable and specific endophenotype related to suicidal behavior.

AUTHOR CONTRIBUTIONS

GH conceived of the study. GH, SH, and AM carried out the analyses and wrote the manuscript, to which the other authors made important intellectual contributions. The other authors were responsible for the data collection in their respective countries. All authors approved of the submitted manuscript. We would like to thank Joakim Westerlund for his valuable consultation on the different aspects of this paper.

REFERENCES

1. World Health Organization. *Preventing Suicide: A Global Imperative*. Geneva, Switzerland: World Health Organization (2014).
2. Nock MK, Hwang I, Sampson N, Kessler RC, Angermeyer M, Beautrais A, et al. Cross-national analysis of the associations among mental disorders and suicidal behavior: findings from the WHO World Mental Health surveys. *PLoS Med* (2009) 6(8):e1000123. doi:10.1371/journal.pmed.1000123
3. Nock MK, Hwang I, Sampson NA, Kessler RC. Mental disorders, comorbidity and suicidal behavior: results from the National Comorbidity Survey Replication. *Mol Psychiatry* (2010) 15(8):868–76. doi:10.1038/mp.2009.29
4. Arsenault-Lapierre G, Kim C, Turecki G. Psychiatric diagnoses in 3275 suicides: a meta-analysis. *BMC Psychiatry* (2004) 4:37. doi:10.1186/1471-244X-4-37
5. De Berardis D, Fornaro M, Orsolini L, Valchera A, Carano A, Vellante F, et al. Alexithymia and suicide risk in psychiatric disorders: a mini-review. *Front Psychiatry* (2017) 8:148. doi:10.3389/fpsyt.2017.00148
6. Butwicka A, Frisén L, Almqvist C, Zethelius B, Lichtenstein P. Risks of psychiatric disorders and suicide attempts in children and adolescents with type 1 diabetes: a population-based cohort study. *Diabetes Care* (2015) 38(3):453–9. doi:10.2337/dc14-0262
7. Pompili M, Forte A, Lester D, Erbuto D, Rovedi F, Innamorati M, et al. Suicide risk in type 1 diabetes mellitus: a systematic review. *J Psychosom Res* (2014) 76(5):352–60. doi:10.1016/j.jpsychores.2014.02.009
8. Hem E, Loge JH, Haldorsen T, Ekeberg Ø. Suicide risk in cancer patients from 1960 to 1999. *J Clin Oncol* (2004) 22(20):4209–16. doi:10.1200/JCO.2004.02.052
9. Yousaf U, Christensen ML, Engholm G, Storm HH. Suicides among Danish cancer patients 1971–1999. *Br J Cancer* (2005) 92(6):995–1000. doi:10.1038/sj.bjc.6602424
10. Vyssoki B, Gleiss A, Rockett IR, Hackl M, Leitner B, Sonneck G, et al. Suicide among 915,303 Austrian cancer patients: who is at risk? *J Affect Disord* (2015) 175:287–91. doi:10.1016/j.jad.2015.01.028
11. Tang NK, Crane C. Suicidality in chronic pain: a review of the prevalence, risk factors and psychological links. *Psychol Med* (2006) 36(5):575–86. doi:10.1017/S0033291705006859
12. Kazan D, Calear AL, Batterham PJ. The impact of intimate partner relationships on suicidal thoughts and behaviours: a systematic review. *J Affect Disord* (2016) 190:585–98. doi:10.1016/j.jad.2015.11.003
13. Yip PS, Yousuf S, Chan CH, Yung T, Wu KC. The roles of culture and gender in the relationship between divorce and suicide risk: a meta-analysis. *Soc Sci Med* (2015) 128:87–94. doi:10.1016/j.socscimed.2014.12.034
14. van Geel M, Vedder P, Tanilon J. Relationship between peer victimization, cyberbullying, and suicide in children and adolescents: a meta-analysis. *JAMA Pediatr* (2014) 168(5):435–42. doi:10.1001/jamapediatrics.2013.4143
15. Holt MK, Vivolo-Kantor AM, Polanin JR, Holland KM, DeGue S, Matjasko JL, et al. Bullying and suicidal ideation and behaviors: a meta-analysis. *Pediatrics* (2015) 135(2):e496–509. doi:10.1542/peds.2014-1864

16. Milner A, Page A, LaMontagne AD. Long-term unemployment and suicide: a systematic review and meta-analysis. *PLoS One* (2013) 8(1):e51333. doi:10.1371/journal.pone.0051333
17. Frasquilho D, Matos MG, Salonna F, Guerreiro D, Storti CC, Gaspar T, et al. Mental health outcomes in times of economic recession: a systematic literature review. *BMC Public Health* (2016) 16:115. doi:10.1186/s12889-016-2720-y
18. Liu RT, Miller I. Life events and suicidal ideation and behavior: a systematic review. *Clin Psychol Rev* (2014) 34(3):181–92. doi:10.1016/j.cpr.2014.01.006
19. Isometsä E. Suicidal behaviour in mood disorders – who, when, and why? *Can J Psychiatry* (2014) 59(3):120–30. doi:10.1177/070674371405900303
20. Harris EC, Barraclough B. Suicide as an outcome for mental disorders. A meta-analysis. *Br J Psychiatry* (1997) 170:205–28. doi:10.1192/bjp.170.3.205
21. Latalova K, Kamaradova D, Prasko J. Suicide in bipolar disorder: a review. *Psychiatr Danub* (2014) 26(2):108–14.
22. Jollant F, Bellivier F, Leboyer M, Astruc B, Torres S, Verdier R, et al. Impaired decision making in suicide attempters. *Am J Psychiatry* (2005) 162(2):304–10. doi:10.1176/appi.ajp.162.2.304
23. Bechara A, Damasio AR, Damasio H, Anderson SW. Insensitivity to future consequences following damage to human prefrontal cortex. *Cognition* (1994) 50(1–3):7–15. doi:10.1016/0010-0277(94)90018-3
24. Bechara A, Damasio H, Tranel D, Damasio AR. Deciding advantageously before knowing the advantageous strategy. *Science* (1997) 275(5304):1293–5. doi:10.1126/science.275.5304.1293
25. Bechara A, Damasio H, Damasio AR, Lee GP. Different contributions of the human amygdala and ventromedial prefrontal cortex to decision-making. *J Neurosci* (1999) 19(13):5473–81.
26. Jollant F, Guillaume S, Jaussent I, Bellivier F, Leboyer M, Castelnau D, et al. Psychiatric diagnoses and personality traits associated with disadvantageous decision-making. *Eur Psychiatry* (2007) 22(7):455–61. doi:10.1016/j.eurpsy.2007.06.001
27. Bridge JA, McBee-Strayer SM, Cannon EA, Sheftall AH, Reynolds B, Campo JV, et al. Impaired decision making in adolescent suicide attempters. *J Am Acad Child Adolesc Psychiatry* (2012) 51(4):394–403. doi:10.1016/j.jaac.2012.01.002
28. LeGris J, Links PS, van Reekum R, Tannock R, Toplak M. Executive function and suicidal risk in women with borderline personality disorder. *Psychiatry Res* (2012) 196(1):101–8. doi:10.1016/j.psychres.2011.10.008
29. Gorlyn M, Keilp JG, Oquendo MA, Burke AK, John Mann J. Iowa gambling task performance in currently depressed suicide attempters. *Psychiatry Res* (2013) 207(3):150–7. doi:10.1016/j.psychres.2013.01.030
30. Loyo LS, Martinez-Velzquez ES, Ramos-Loyo J. Influence of emotions on executive functions in suicide attempters. *Suicidol Online* (2013) 4:42–55.
31. Pan L, Segreti A, Almeida J, Jollant F, Lawrence N, Brent D, et al. Preserved hippocampal function during learning in the context of risk in adolescent suicide attempt. *Psychiatry Res* (2013) 211(2):112–8. doi:10.1016/j.pscychresns.2012.07.008
32. Richard-Devantoy S, Berlim MT, Jollant F. A meta-analysis of neuropsychological markers of vulnerability to suicidal behavior in mood disorders. *Psychol Med* (2014) 44(8):1663–73. doi:10.1017/S0033291713002304
33. Clark L, Dombrovski AY, Siegle GJ, Butters MA, Shollenberger CL, Sahakian BJ, et al. Impairment in risk-sensitive decision-making in older suicide attempters with depression. *Psychol Aging* (2011) 26(2):321–30. doi:10.1037/a0021646
34. Chamberlain SR, Odlaug BL, Schreiber LR, Grant JE. Clinical and neurocognitive markers of suicidality in young adults. *J Psychiatr Res* (2013) 47(5):586–91. doi:10.1016/j.jpsychires.2012.12.016
35. Bibby PA. Loss-chasing, alexithymia, and impulsivity in a gambling task: alexithymia as a precursor to loss-chasing behavior when gambling. *Front Psychol* (2016) 7:3. doi:10.3389/fpsyg.2016.00003
36. Dombrovski AY, Hallquist MN. The decision neuroscience perspective on suicidal behavior: evidence and hypotheses. *Curr Opin Psychiatry* (2017) 30(1):7–14. doi:10.1097/YCO.0000000000000297
37. Szanto K, Bruine de Bruin W, Parker AM, Hallquist MN, Vanyukov PM, Dombrovski AY. Decision-making competence and attempted suicide. *J Clin Psychiatry* (2015) 76(12):e1590–7. doi:10.4088/JCP.15m09778
38. Buelow MT, Suhr JA. Construct validity of the Iowa gambling task. *Neuropsychol Rev* (2009) 19(1):102–14. doi:10.1007/s11065-009-9083-4
39. Bishara AJ, Pleskac TJ, Fridberg DJ, Yechiam E, Lucas J, Busemeyer JR, et al. Similar processes despite divergent behavior in two commonly used measures of risky decision making. *J Behav Decis Mak* (2009) 22(4):435–54. doi:10.1002/bdm.641
40. Pecchinenda A, Dretsch M, Chapman P. Working memory involvement in emotion-based processes underlying choosing advantageously. *Exp Psychol* (2006) 53:191–7. doi:10.1027/1618-3169.53.3.191
41. Lin CH, Chiu YC, Lee PL, Hsieh JC. Is deck B a disadvantageous deck in the Iowa gambling task? *Behav Brain Funct* (2007) 3:16. doi:10.1186/1744-9081-3-16
42. Fernie G, Tunney RJ. Some decks are better than others: the effect of reinforcer type and task instructions on learning in the Iowa gambling task. *Brain Cogn* (2006) 60:94–102. doi:10.1016/j.bandc.2005.09.011
43. Stocco A, Fum D, Napoli A. Dissociable processes underlying decisions in the Iowa gambling task: a new integrative framework. *Behav Brain Funct* (2009) 5:1. doi:10.1186/1744-9081-5-1
44. Weller JA, Levin IP, Bechara A. Do individual differences in Iowa gambling task performance predict adaptive decision making for risky gains and losses? *J Clin Exp Neuropsychol* (2010) 32(2):141–50. doi:10.1080/13803390902881926
45. Kahneman D, Tversky A. Prospect theory: an analysis of decision under risk. *Econometrica* (1979) 47:263–92. doi:10.2307/1914185
46. Tversky A, Kahneman D. Loss aversion in riskless choice: a reference-dependent model. *Q J Econ* (1991) 106:1039–61. doi:10.2307/2937956
47. Walasek L, Stewart N. How to make loss aversion disappear and reverse: tests of the decision by sampling origin of loss aversion. *J Exp Psychol Gen* (2015) 144(1):7–11. doi:10.1037/xge0000039
48. Gächter S, Johnson E, Herrmann A. Individual-level loss aversion in riskless and risky choices. *CeDEx Discussion Paper Series 2010–20* (2010). p. 1–26.
49. Tom SM, Fox CR, Trepel C, Poldrack RA. The neural basis of loss aversion in decision-making under risk. *Science* (2007) 315(5811):515–8. doi:10.1126/science.1134239
50. Nock MK, Borges G, Bromet EJ, Cha CB, Kessler RC, Lee S. Suicide and suicidal behavior. *Epidemiol Rev* (2008) 30:133–54. doi:10.1093/epirev/mxn002
51. Hökby S, Hadlaczky G, Westerlund J, Wasserman D, Balazs J, Germanavicius A, et al. Are mental health effects of internet use attributable to the web-based content or perceived consequences of usage? A longitudinal study of European adolescents. *JMIR Ment Health* (2016) 3(3):e31. doi:10.2196/mental.5925
52. Lovibond PF, Lovibond SH. The structure of negative emotional states: comparison of the Depression Anxiety Stress Scales (DASS) with the beck depression and anxiety inventories. *Behav Res Ther* (1995) 33(3):335–43. doi:10.1016/0005-7967(94)00075-U
53. Antony MM, Bieling PJ, Cox BJ, Enns MW, Swinson RP. Psychometric properties of the 42-item and 21-item versions of the Depression Anxiety Stress Scales in clinical groups and a community sample. *Psychol Assess* (1998) 10(2):176–81. doi:10.1037/1040-3590.10.2.176
54. Crawford JR, Henry JD. The Depression Anxiety Stress Scales (DASS): normative data and latent structure in a large non-clinical sample. *Br J Clin Psychol* (2003) 42(Pt 2):111–31. doi:10.1348/014466503321903544
55. Page AC, Hooke GR, Morrison DL. Psychometric properties of the Depression Anxiety Stress Scales (DASS) in depressed clinical samples. *Br J Clin Psychol* (2007) 46(Pt 3):283–97. doi:10.1348/014466506X158996
56. Szabó M. The short version of the Depression Anxiety Stress Scales (DASS-21): factor structure in a young adolescent sample. *J Adolesc* (2010) 33(1):1–8. doi:10.1016/j.adolescence.2009.05.014
57. Paykel ES, Myers JK, Lindenthal JJ, Tanner J. Suicidal feelings in the general population: a prevalence study. *Br J Psychiatry* (1974) 124:460–9. doi:10.1192/bjp.124.5.460
58. Novemsky BM, Kahneman D. The boundaries of loss aversion. *J Mark Res* (2005) 42:119–28. doi:10.1509/jmkr.42.2.119.62292
59. Gvion Y, Levi-Belz Y, Hadlaczky G, Apter A. On the role of impulsivity and decision-making in suicidal behavior. *World J Psychiatry* (2015) 5(3):255–9. doi:10.5498/wjp.v5.i3.255
60. Lin C-H, Song T-J, Chen Y-Y, Lee W-K, Chiu Y-C. Reexamining the validity and reliability of the clinical version of the Iowa gambling task: evidence from a normal subject group. *Front Psychol* (2013) 4:220. doi:10.3389/fpsyg.2013.00220
61. Steingroever H, Wetzels R, Horstmann A, Neumann J, Wagenmakers EJ. Performance of healthy participants on the Iowa gambling task. *Psychol Assess* (2013) 25(1):180–93. doi:10.1037/a0029929
62. Baek K, Kwon J, Chae JH, Chung YA, Kralik JD, Min JA, et al. Heightened aversion to risk and loss in depressed patients with a suicide attempt history. *Sci Rep* (2017) 7(1):11228. doi:10.1038/s41598-017-10541-5

63. Dombrovski AY, Szanto K, Siegle GJ, Wallace ML, Forman SD, Sahakian B, et al. Lethal forethought: delayed reward discounting differentiates high- and low-lethality suicide attempts in old age. *Biol Psychiatry* (2011) 70(2):138–44. doi:10.1016/j.biopsych.2010.12.025
64. Dombrovski AY, Szanto K, Clark L, Reynolds CF, Siegle GJ. Reward signals, attempted suicide, and impulsivity in late-life depression. *JAMA Psychiatry* (2013) 70(10):1. doi:10.1001/jamapsychiatry.2013.75
65. Tait VR. *Loss Aversion and Perspective Taking in the Sunk-Cost Fallacy [Doctoral Dissertation]*. Utah: Brigham Young University (2015).
66. De Martino B, Camerer CF, Adolphs R. Amygdala damage eliminates monetary loss aversion. *Proc Natl Acad Sci U S A* (2010) 107(8):3788–92. doi:10.1073/pnas.0910230107
67. Canessa N, Crespi C, Motterlini M, Baud-Bovy G, Chierchia G, Pantaleo G, et al. The functional and structural neural basis of individual differences in loss aversion. *J Neurosci* (2013) 33(36):14307–17. doi:10.1523/JNEUROSCI.0497-13.2013
68. Sokol-Hessner P, Camerer CF, Phelps EA. Emotion regulation reduces loss aversion and decreases amygdala responses to losses. *Soc Cogn Affect Neurosci* (2013) 8(3):341–50. doi:10.1093/scan/nss002
69. Mann JJ. Neurobiology of suicidal behaviour. *Nat Rev Neurosci* (2003) 4(10):819–28. doi:10.1038/nrn1220
70. Mann JJ, Huang YY, Underwood MD, Kassir SA, Oppenheim S, Kelly TM, et al. A serotonin transporter gene promoter polymorphism (5-HTTLPR) and prefrontal cortical binding in major depression and suicide. *Arch Gen Psychiatry* (2000) 57(8):729–38. doi:10.1001/archpsyc.57.8.729
71. Oquendo MA, Placidi GP, Malone KM, Campbell C, Keilp J, Brodsky B, et al. Positron emission tomography of regional brain metabolic responses to a serotonergic challenge and lethality of suicide attempts in major depression. *Arch Gen Psychiatry* (2003) 60(1):14–22. doi:10.1001/archpsyc.60.1.14
72. Desmyter S, van Heeringen C, Audenaert K. Structural and functional neuroimaging studies of the suicidal brain. *Prog Neuropsychopharmacol Biol Psychiatry* (2011) 35(4):796–808. doi:10.1016/j.pnpbp.2010.12.026
73. Jollant F, Lawrence NL, Olié E, Guillaume S, Courtet P. The suicidal mind and brain: a review of neuropsychological and neuroimaging studies. *World J Biol Psychiatry* (2011) 12(5):319–39. doi:10.3109/15622975.2011.556200
74. van Heeringen C, Bijttebier S, Godfrin K. Suicidal brains: a review of functional and structural brain studies in association with suicidal behaviour. *Neurosci Biobehav Rev* (2011) 35(3):688–98. doi:10.1016/j.neubiorev.2010.08.007
75. Zhang H, Chen Z, Jia Z, Gong Q. Dysfunction of neural circuitry in depressive patients with suicidal behaviors: a review of structural and functional neuroimaging studies. *Prog Neuropsychopharmacol Biol Psychiatry* (2014) 53:61–6. doi:10.1016/j.pnpbp.2014.03.002
76. Yechiam E, Ert E. Risk attitude in decision making: in search of trait-like constructs. *Top Cogn Sci* (2011) 3(1):166–86. doi:10.1111/j.1756-8765.2010.01126.x
77. Glöckner A, Pachur T. Cognitive models of risky choice: parameter stability and predictive accuracy of prospect theory. *Cognition* (2012) 123(1):21–32. doi:10.1016/j.cognition.2011.12
78. Zeisberger S, Vrecko D, Langer T. Measuring the time stability of prospect theory preferences. *Theory Decis* (2012) 72(3):359–86. doi:10.1007/s11238-010-9234-3
79. Olié E, Ding Y, Le Bars E, de Champfleur NM, Mura T, Bonafé A, et al. Processing of decision-making and social threat in patients with history of suicidal attempt: a neuroimaging replication study. *Psychiatry Res* (2015) 234(3):369–77. doi:10.1016/j.pscychresns.2015.09.020
80. Jollant F, Lawrence NS, Giampietro V, Brammer MJ, Fullana MA, Drapier D, et al. Orbitofrontal cortex response to angry faces in men with histories of suicide attempts. *Am J Psychiatry* (2008) 165(6):740–8. doi:10.1176/appi.ajp.2008.07081239
81. Hochman G, Yechiam E. Loss aversion in the eye and in the heart: the autonomic nervous system's responses to losses. *J Behav Decis Mak* (2011) 24:140–56. doi:10.1002/bdm.692
82. Yechiam E, Hochman G. Loss attention in a dual-task setting. *Psychol Sci* (2014) 25(2):494–502. doi:10.1177/0956797613510725
83. Barkley-Levenson EE, Van Leijenhorst L, Galván A. Behavioral and neural correlates of loss aversion and risk avoidance in adolescents and adults. *Dev Cogn Neurosci* (2013) 3:72–83. doi:10.1016/j.dcn.2012.09.007

12

Cognition as a Therapeutic Target in the Suicidal Patient Approach

Antônio Geraldo da Silva[1], Leandro Fernandes Malloy-Diniz[2,3]*, Marina Saraiva Garcia[4], Carlos Guilherme Silva Figueiredo[5], Renata Nayara Figueiredo[5], Alexandre Paim Diaz[6] and António Pacheco Palha[1]*

[1] Faculty of Medicine, University of Porto, Porto, Portugal, [2] Brazilian Society of Dual Pathology, Brasília, Brazil, [3] Universidade Federal de Minas Gerais, Belo Horizonte, Brazil, [4] Molecular Medicine Department, Universidade Federal de Minas Gerais, Belo Horizonte, Brazil, [5] Associação Brasileira de Psiquiatria, Rio de Janeiro, Brazil, [6] Universidade do Sul de Santa Catarina, Palhoça, Brazil

***Correspondence:**
Leandro Fernandes Malloy-Diniz
malloy.diniz@gmail.com

The current considerations about completed suicides and suicide attempts in different cultures call the attention of professionals to this serious public health problem. Integrative approaches have shown that the confluence of multiple biological and social factors modulate various psychopathologies and dysfunctional behaviors, such as suicidal behavior. Considering the level of intermediate analysis, personality traits and cognitive functioning are also of great importance for understanding the suicide phenomenon. About cognitive factors, we can group them into cognitive schemas of reality interpretation and underlying cognitive processes. On the other hand, different types of primary cognitive alterations are related to suicidal behavior, especially those resulting from changes in frontostriatal circuits. Among such cognitive mechanisms can be highlighted the attentional bias for environmental cues related to suicide, impulsive behavior, verbal fluency deficits, non-adaptive decision-making, and reduced planning skills. Attentional bias consists in the effect of thoughts and emotions, frequently not conscious, about the perception of environmental stimuli. Suicidal ideation and hopelessness can make the patient unable to find alternative solutions to their problems other than suicide, biasing their attention to environmental cues related to such behavior. Recent research efforts are directed to assess the possible use of attention bias as a therapeutic target in patients presenting suicide behavior. The relationship between impulsivity and suicide has been largely investigated over the last decades, and there is still controversy about the theme. Although there is strong evidence linking impulsivity to suicide attempts. Effective interventions address to reduce impulsivity in clinical populations at higher risk for suicide could help in the prevention. Deficits in problem-solving ability also seem to be distorted in patients who attempt suicide. Understanding cognitive changes in patients who attempt suicide open an important perspective in the approach of patients with mental disorders. Identifying cognitive deficits in these patients, along with personality traits, depressive symptoms, and suicidal cognitive schemas may indicate to the psychiatrist the need for emergency care. Behavioral and cognitive interventions have been associated with reductions in suicide ideation, as well as suicide attempts in different populations.

Keywords: suicide, cognition, impulsivity, attention bias, therapeutic target cognition, cognitive deficits, behavioral interventions, cognitive interventions

The current considerations about complete suicides and suicide attempts in different cultures call the attention of professionals from different areas to this serious public health problem. It is estimated that almost 1 million people commit suicide per year worldwide. In Brazil, there are 32 complete suicides every day from which about 96.8% had some identifiable mental disorder.

Suicidology is the field of interdisciplinary knowledge that brings together professionals from different specialties to enable them to construct proposals of prevention and acute intervention from the integration of different levels of analysis. Considering the levels of analysis derived from the basic sciences, the search for biomarkers related to suicidal behavior points, for example, to the participation of neural systems associated to the modulation of responses to stressors (e.g., hypothalamic–pituitary–adrenal axis and the noradrenergic system of the locus coeruleus), neuroinflammatory mechanisms system (e.g., increased levels of interleukins 1 and 6 in the frontopolar cortex), and also the serotonergic hypofunction (1). On the other hand, considering the levels of macroscopic analysis studied by Sociology, the relationship between the individual and society has been considered since the first trials to understand the phenomenon. Durkheim's classic works (2), for example, already predicted different types of suicide sociologically determined such as the anomic (suicidal behavior that happens because of the acute social chaos), fatalistic (suicide due to the lack of hope of overcoming oppression and of repression of individual freedom), altruistic (suicide motivated by an ideal that the subject considers him/herself as more important than his/her own life), and selfish (characterized by the chronicity of a weak bond between the person and the society).

More recently, integrative approaches have shown that the confluence of multiple biological and social factors modulate diverse psychopathologies and dysfunctional behaviors, such as suicidal behavior (3). Some of the results of the Dunedin longitudinal study clearly show that throughout life, biological vulnerability factors added to adverse social conditions increase the chance of ideation and suicide attempts (4). In this study, individuals who presented two copies of the short allele of this gene (related to a lower serotonergic function) and experienced more stressful situations presented a higher risk of showing ideation and suicide attempts. In this perspective, Brodsky (5), using the stress-diathesis model, suggests that adverse childhood experiences (e.g., family stress, abuse, and other types of violence) associated with biological characteristics (e.g., serotonergic hypofunction and HPA axis dysfunction) can create a vulnerability factor that, in adult life, in the face of stressful situations increases the risk of suicidal behavior. This, in its turn, involves self-aggression, suicidal preparation, the attempt and the act itself.

Considering the level of intermediate analysis, the one of individual differences, personality traits, and cognitive functioning, are also of great importance for understanding the suicidal phenomenon. For example, DeShong et al. (6) have demonstrated that personality traits can be considered important predictors of suicidal ideation. The results of this study indicate that high levels of neuroticism and low levels of extroversion are related to the current presence of suicidal ideation in a sample of university students. The authors also verified that high levels of neuroticism are positively and significantly correlated with two other personality traits that indicate the high risk for a suicide attempt: the perception of oneself as burdensomeness for the others (Perceived Burdensomeness) and the perception to be disconnected from society (Thwarted Belongingness). Moreover, the relationship between personality traits and the success of interventions has also been verified. For example, the extroversion trait seems to make the individual more sensitive to social support. In situations of low social support, extroversion tends to be significantly related to suicidal ideation (7).

COGNITION AND SUICIDE BEHAVIOR

In relation to cognitive factors, we can group them into cognitive schemas of reality interpretation and basic cognitive processes. Cognitive schemata of hopelessness (belief that the situation will not be resolved in the future) and intolerance to suffering are examples of interpretation patterns of reality in patients with suicidal ideation (8). On the other hand, different types of primary cognitive alterations are related to suicidal behavior, especially those resulting from changes in frontostriatal circuits (9). Among such cognitive mechanisms can be highlighted the attentional bias for environmental cues related to suicide, impulsive behavior, verbal fluency deficits, non-adaptive decision-making, and reduced planning skills.

Attentional bias consists in the effect of thoughts and emotions, frequently not conscious, about the perception of environmental stimuli. Attentional bias makes the individual to pay too much attention to specific environmental cues that are related to the psychiatric disorder he/she presents (10). According to Wenzel et al. (8), suicidal ideation and hopelessness can make the patient unable to find alternative solutions to their problems other than suicide, biasing their attention to environmental cues related to such behavior.

One of the most used tasks to evaluate attentional bias is the modified Stroop paradigm, involving processing of stimuli related to emotion. Stroop paradigms of an emotional nature usually require the patient to say, as quickly as possible, the name of the color with which certain words were written. These words may be neutral or have negative or positive emotional valence. In studies of attentional bias for suicide, neutral words, positive valence words, words with general negative valence, and words with negative valence related to suicide are generally used. As the patient processes more automatically read the word and give the desirable answer, that is, to name the color. Richard-Devantoy et al. (11) verified that patients with a history of suicide attempt perform poorly on emotional Stroop tasks when they have to process suicide-related words. Cha et al. (12), in a longitudinal study, found that the attentional bias for suicide-related stimuli is an important predictor of future attempts. In this study, the authors evaluated patients treated in the psychiatric emergency with a modified version of the Stroop test containing words with positive (e.g., happiness), negative (e.g., solitude), neutral valence (e.g., museum), and suicide related (e.g., death). Besides presenting a greater attention bias for words related to suicide, attentional bias was an important predictor of further attempts during the 6 months after the evaluation.

Bias in the processing of emotional information may also influence the way facial expressions are identified, even in individuals with subclinical depressive symptoms who have suicidal ideation. Maniglio et al. (13) verified, in a sample of subjects of the general population, that the presence of suicidal thoughts was related to the tendency to interpret neutral faces as they were expressing sadness.

Recent research efforts are directed to assess the possible use of attention bias as a therapeutic target in patients presenting suicide behavior. In a randomized control trial (RCT), a community sample of individuals who reported past month suicide ideation and inpatients admitted for suicide ideation or attempt were submitted to four training sessions of attentional bias modification (ABM) and their cognitive performance compared to a control group (14). The authors did not find significant differences between the groups even stratifying the analysis for severe suicide ideators. Possible reasons for the negative findings included number and duration of training sessions, lack of AMB efficacy for suicide-specific attentional bias, and type II error due to sample size (14). Other studies addressed the potential of AMB in alleviating clinical conditions that are known risk factors for suicide attempts. In a trial for testing the potential of ABM in reducing depressive symptoms in adolescents with depressive disorders, a major risk for suicidal behaviors (15), Yang et al. have compared active AMB intervention versus placebo ABM training (16). The former was associated with reduction on clinical-rated and self-reported depressive symptoms compared with the control group at 12-month follow-up assessment, as well as with higher remission rates (16). On the other hand, de Voogd et al., throughout a multi-center RCT with a non-clinical sample of adolescents, did not find significant differences regarding anxiety and depressive symptoms between intervention and control group (17). Insomnia, another clinical characteristic associated with suicidal behaviors (18, 19), was a target for ABM in a RCT by Lancee et al. (20). The results showed no evidence of efficacy for AMB in decreasing sleep symptoms problems, which may be related to the low level of attention bias at baseline (20). The discrepancy in the literature for the AMB as a potential therapeutic tool for treating suicidal thoughts as well as its risk factors, suggests that further studies exploring different protocols interventions and clinical sample characteristics should be performed.

The relationship between impulsivity and suicide has been largely investigated over the last decades and there is still controversy about the theme. Although there is strong evidence linking impulsivity to suicide attempts, and particularly to violent attempts [see, for example, Ref. (21)], Smith et al. (22) suggest that, if suicide is planned, the suicide behavior could not, in these cases, be explained by the impulsive tendency. Reyes-Tovilla et al. (23) verified important differences between people who attempt suicide in an inapposite way and those who premeditate the attempt. The second group tends to try in a more lethal way, has higher rates of comorbidity with alcoholism, and use cannabis besides having lower level of education. On the other hand, given the multidimensional nature of impulsivity, it is plausible to think that some specific types of impulsive manifestation would be more related to suicidal behavior. Thus, Malloy-Diniz et al. (24) and Neves et al. (25) verified that the impulsive and immediate decision-making is more related to the suicide attempts in bipolar patients. It is plausible to think here that even planned suicides could be understood by these results, yet planning would focus on the end of immediate suffering. These findings have been consistently replicated by other studies (11) showing that the decisional focus on psychiatric patients may be one of the risk factors for the suicide act.

Impulsivity can serve both as a moderator and mediator variable in the association between several diagnostic and clinical conditions with suicide ideation or attempts. Wang et al. (26) evaluated 162 patients with major depressive disorder and found that those with higher impulsivity, regardless depression severity, were more likely to present suicide ideation (26). In addition, specific neural circuits associated with impulsivity and aggression may mediate the lethality of suicidal behavior in patients with borderline personality disorder (27).

Thus, effective interventions address to reduce impulsivity in clinical populations at higher risk for suicide could help in the prevention. An internet-based psychoeducation approach was compared to a control group with no psychoeducation for the treatment of women with DSM-IV (28) criteria for borderline personality disorder. Among several others outcomes, the experimental group with psychoeducation showed significantly decrease in impulsivity scores (29). Thylstrup et al. (30) applied a different type of psychoeducational program for patients with substance use and antisocial personality disorder in a randomized trial. The Impulsive Lifestyle Counselling, with sessions that included linking "patients' impulsive behaviors to the immediate consequences," was associated with positive effects in reducing substance use behaviors, a major suicide risk factor (30, 31). Impulsivity was also decreased in a sample of high school students, an age group which suicide is the second main cause of dead (32), after a mindfulness training program (MTP). Ten weekly sessions of the MTP was associated with significantly reduction in cognitive, motor, and non-planning dimensions of impulsivity as compared to the control group (33).

As mentioned above, impulsive decision-making related to imediatistic focus regardless long-term consequences is frequently associated with suicide behavior. Oldershaw et al. (34) evaluated whether there was an association between improvements in decision-making and reduction on suicide ideation in adolescents with a history of self-harm, after a CBT treatment (34). According to the authors, the therapy has included elements with the aim of strength decision-making skills, measured in this study by the Iowa Gambling Task (IGT) (35). Despite improvements of IGT scores within the CBT group, changes in IGT scores did not correlate with suicide ideation (34).

Deficits in problem-solving ability also seem to be distorted in patients who attempt suicide. In particular, in situations of stress, problem-solving skills are important factors in minimizing the effect on mental health. In this perspective, Grover et al. (36) verified that deficits in problem-solving abilities in patients submitted to moderate and high situations of stress are related to suicidal behavior in adolescents. Khan et al. (37) found that university students who present productive strategies to manage stressful situations (work with the focus on the problem, maintaining optimism, seeking help and support from other people) and social support had lower chances to attempt suicide. In a study that evaluated the relationship between problem-solving skills and suicidal ideation in people who experienced childhood abuse, Kwok et al. (38) found that the rational style of problem-solving acts as a moderator in the relationship between abuse in childhood and suicide attempt in adulthood. Such association was described only in the women who participated in the study. The style of problem solving also seems to be related to suicidal behavior. Quinones et al. (39) found that patients who attempt suicide tend to present more passive strategies of solution of problems, that is, they are dependent on the action of other people, related to luck and chance or over time.

Cognitive-behavioral problem solving was compared to "treatment as usual" for several outcomes, including suicide ideation and attempts, in a sample of high-risk individuals, with positive findings, especially in short term (40). Cognitive therapy was also associated with a faster improvement in negative problem orientation among individuals with history of recent suicide attempt in another randomized controlled trial (41). Problem-solving therapy may be especially effective in older patients with depression and executive dysfunction. Gustavson et al. (42) reported lower frequency of reported suicide ideation in the experimental group in comparison to supportive therapy up to 36 weeks after treatment (42). At least part of the effectiveness of mindfulness-based interventions for suicide prevention has also been related by means of improvement in problem solving, as well as attentional dyscontrol and abnormal stress response (43). Thus, therapies with the aim of improve problem-solving abilities, especially active problem solving (39), should be considered in individuals at higher risk for suicide.

CONCLUSION

Evidences linking cognitive deficits and suicide behavior are consistent. Jollant et al. (9) group the main cognitive difficulties in people who attempt suicide in three categories that synthesize the above-mentioned findings and aggregate other described changes. The categories include

(1) Changes in the modulation and attribution of values to the experiences, which would involve an attentional and emotional biased response to environmental stimuli and less adaptive decisions in relation to the perception of environmental risks.

(2) Deficits in emotional and cognitive regulation including cognitive inflexibility, poor repertoire related to planning and problem solving, lowered verbal fluency affecting communicational ability.

(3) Behavioral facilitation in emotional contexts, characterized by impulsive response in situations of major stress and affective overload.

Moreover, cognitive deficits in psychiatric patients are important therapeutic targets, despite the paucity of intervention studies considering cognition as a therapeutic target in suicide patients, training self-regulatory processes, including decision-making skills, efficient problem solving, and impulse control present potential for clinical use in suicide prevention.

Behavioral and cognitive interventions has been associated with reductions on suicide ideation, as well as suicide attempts in different populations (1–4), probably by targeting different cognitive dysfunctions associated to suicide behaviors, in addition to anxiety and depressive symptoms. Thus, specific interventions toward these cognitive domains, such as attentional bias, impulsivity, problem solving, and decision-making, could help to maximize the efficacy of the available therapeutic options. Future studies are needed to evaluate the effectiveness of cognitive training for this purpose.

AUTHOR CONTRIBUTIONS

All authors listed have made substantial, direct, and intellectual contribution to the work and approved it for publication.

REFERENCES

1. Oquendo MA, Sullivan GM, Sudol K, Baca-Garcia E, Stanley BH, Sublette ME, et al. Toward a biosignature for suicide. *Am J Psychiatry* (2014) 171(12): 1259–77. doi:10.1176/appi.ajp.2014.14020194
2. Durkheim E. *Le suicide: Étude de sociologie*. Paris: Felix Alcan (1897).
3. Turecki G, Ota VK, Belangero SI, Jackowski A, Kaufman J. Early life adversity, genomic plasticity, and psychopathology. *Lancet Psychiatry* (2014) 2:461–6. doi:10.1016/S2215-0366(14)00022-4
4. Caspi A, Sugden K, Moffitt TE, Taylor A, Craig IW, Harrington HL, et al. Influence of life stress on depression: moderation by a polymorphism in the 5-HTT gene. *Science* (2003) 301(5631):386–9. doi:10.1126/science.1083968
5. Brodsky BS. Early childhood environment and genetic interactions: the diathesis for suicidal behavior. *Curr Psychiatry Rep* (2016) 18:86. doi:10.1007/s11920-016-0716-z
6. DeShong HL, Tucker RP, O'Keefe VM, Mullins-Sweatt SN, Wingate LR. Five factor model traits as a predictor of suicide ideation and interpersonal suicide risk in a college sample. *Psychiatry Res* (2015) 226(1):217–23. doi:10.1016/j.psychres.2015.01.002
7. Ayub N. Predicting suicide ideation through intrapersonal and interpersonal factors: the interplay of big-five personality traits and social support. *Personal Ment Health* (2015) 9(4):308–18. doi:10.1002/pmh.1301
8. Wenzel A, Brown GK, Beck AT. *Cognitive Therapy for Suicidal Patients: Scientific and Clinical Applications*. Washington: American Psychological Association (2015).
9. Jollant F, Lawrence NL, Olié E, Guillaume S, Courtet P. The suicidal mind and brain: a review of neuropsychological and neuroimaging studies. *World J Biol Psychiatry* (2011) 12(5):319–39. doi:10.3109/15622975.2011.556200
10. Aspen V, Darcy A, Lock J. A review of attention biases in women with eating disorders. *Cogn Emot* (2013) 27(5):820–38. doi:10.1080/02699931.2012.749777
11. Richard-Devantoy S, Turecki G, Jollant F. Neurobiology of elderly suicide. *Arch Suicide Res* (2016) 20(3):291–313. doi:10.1080/13811118.2015.1048397
12. Cha CB, Najmi S, Park JM, Finn CT, Nock MK. Attentional bias toward suicide-related stimuli predicts suicidal behavior. *J Abnorm Psychol* (2010) 119(3):616–22. doi:10.1037/a0019710
13. Maniglio R, Gusciglio F, Lofrese V, Belvederi MM, Tamburello A, Innamorati M. Biased processing of neutral facial expressions is associated with depressive

symptoms and suicide ideation in individuals at risk for major depression due to affective temperaments. *Compr Psychiatry* (2014) 55(3):518–25. doi:10.1016/j.comppsych.2013.10.008
14. Cha CB, Najmi S, Amir N, Matthews JD, Deming CA, Glenn JJ, et al. Testing the efficacy of attention bias modification for suicidal thoughts: findings from two experiments. *Arch Suicide Res* (2017) 21(1):33–51. doi:10.1080/13811118.2016
15. Bertolote JM, Fleischmann A. Suicide and psychiatric diagnosis: a worldwide perspective. *World Psychiatry* (2002) 1(3):181–5.
16. Yang W, Zhang JX, Ding Z, Xiao L. Attention bias modification treatment for adolescents with major depression: a randomized controlled trial. *J Am Acad Child Adolesc Psychiatry* (2016) 55(3):208–18e2. doi:10.1016/j.jaac.2015.12.005
17. de Voogd EL, Wiers RW, Prins PJ, de Jong PJ, Boendermaker WJ, Zwitser RJ, et al. Online attentional bias modification training targeting anxiety and depression in unselected adolescents: short- and long-term effects of a randomized controlled trial. *Behav Res Ther* (2016) 87:11–22. doi:10.1016/j.brat.2016.08.018
18. Pigeon WR, Pinquart M, Conner K. Meta-analysis of sleep disturbance and suicidal thoughts and behaviors. *J Clin Psychiatry* (2012) 73(9):e1160–7. doi:10.4088/JCP.11r07586
19. Bernert RA, Kim JS, Iwata NG, Perlis ML. Sleep disturbances as an evidence-based suicide risk factor. *Curr Psychiatry Rep* (2015) 17(3):554. doi:10.1007/s11920-015-0554-4
20. Lancee J, Yasiney SL, Brendel RS, Boffo M, Clarke PJF, Salemink E. Attentional bias modification training for insomnia: a double-blind placebo controlled randomized trial. *PLoS One* (2017) 12(4):e0174531. doi:10.1371/journal.pone.0174531
21. Swann AC, Dougherty DM, Pazzaglia PJ, Pham M, Steinberg JL, Moeller FG. Increased impulsivity associated with severity of suicide attempt history in patients with bipolar disorder. *Am J Psychiatry* (2005) 2(9):1680–7. doi:10.1176/appi.ajp.162.9.1680
22. Smith AR, Witte TK, Teale NE, King SL, Bender TW, Joiner TE. Revisiting impulsivity in suicide. *Behav Sci Law* (2008) 26(6):779–97. doi:10.1002/bsl.848
23. Reyes-Tovilla JE, Hernández Yánez HD, Peralta-Jiménez Y, Rámon-Frías T, Juárez-Rojop I, Pool-García S, et al. Differences between patients that made an impulsive or premeditated suicide attempt in a Mexican population. *Int J Psychiatry Med* (2015) 49(1):63–74. doi:10.2190/PM.49.1.e
24. Malloy-Diniz LF, Neve FS, Abrantes SS, Fuentes D, Corrêa H. Suicide behavior and neuropsychological assessment of type I bipolar patients. *J Affect Disord* (2009) 112(1–3):231–6. doi:10.1016/j.jad.2008.03.019
25. Neves FS, Malloy-Diniz LF, Romano-Silva MA, Aguiar GC, Matos LO, Correa H. Is the serotonin transporter polymorphism (5-HTTPLR) a potential marker for suicidal behavior in bipolar disorder patients? *J Affect Disord* (2010) 125(1–3):98–102. doi:10.1016/j.jad.2009.12.026
26. Wang YY, Jiang NZ, Cheung EFC, Sun HW, Chan RCK. Role of depression severity and impulsivity in the relationship between hopelessness and suicidal ideation in patients with major depressive disorder. *J Affect Disord* (2015) 183:83–9. doi:10.1016/j.jad.2015.05.001
27. Soloff P, White R, Diwadkar VA. Impulsivity, aggression and brain structure in high and low lethality suicide attempters with borderline personality disorder. *Psychiatry Res* (2014) 222(3):131–9. doi:10.1016/j.pscychresns.2014.02.006
28. American Psychiatric Association. *Diagnostic and statistical manual of mental disorders*. 4th ed. Washington, DC: American Psychiatric Association (2000).
29. Zanarini MC, Conkey LC, Temes CM, Fitzmaurice GM. Randomized controlled trial of web-based psychoeducation for women with borderline personality disorder. *J Clin Psychiatry* (in press). doi:10.4088/JCP.16m11153
30. Thylstrup B, Schroder S, Hesse M. Psycho-education for substance use and antisocial personality disorder: a randomized trial. *BMC Psychiatry* (2015) 15:283. doi:10.1186/s12888-015-0661-0
31. Suominen K, Isometsa E, Haukka J, Lonnqvist J. Substance use and male gender as risk factors for deaths and suicide – a 5-year follow-up study after deliberate self-harm. *Soc Psychiatry Psychiatr Epidemiol* (2004) 39(9):720–4. doi:10.1007/s00127-004-0796-7
32. Lozano R, Naghavi M, Foreman K, Lim S, Shibuya K, Aboyans V, et al. Global and regional mortality from 235 causes of death for 20 age groups in 1990 and 2010: a systematic analysis for the global burden of disease study 2010. *Lancet* (2012) 380(9859):2095–128. doi:10.1016/S0140-6736(12)61728-0
33. Franco C, Amutio A, Lopez-Gonzalez L, Oriol X, Martinez-Taboada C. Effect of a mindfulness training program on the impulsivity and aggression levels of adolescents with behavioral problems in the classroom. *Front Psychol* (2016) 7:1385. doi:10.3389/fpsyg.2016.01385
34. Oldershaw A, Simic M, Grima E, Jollant F, Richards C, Taylor L, et al. The effect of cognitive behavior therapy on decision making in adolescents who self-harm: a pilot study. *Suicide Life Threat Behav* (2012) 42(3):255–65. doi:10.1111/j.1943-278X.2012.0087.x
35. Bechara A, Damasio AR, Damasio H, Anderson SW. Insensitivity to future consequences following damage to human prefrontal cortex. *Cognition* (1994) 50(1–3):7–15. doi:10.1016/0010-0277(94)90018-3
36. Grover K, Green K, Pettit J, Monteith L, Garza M, Venta A. Problem Solving moderates the effects of life event stress and chronic stress on suicidal behaviors in adolescence. *J Clin Psychol* (2009) 65(12):1281–90. doi:10.1002/jclp.20632
37. Khan A, Hamdan AR, Ahmad R, Mustaffa MS, Mahalle S. Problem-solving coping and social support as mediators of academic stress and suicidal ideation among Malaysian and Indian adolescents. *Community Ment Health J* (2016) 52(2):245–50. doi:10.1007/s10597-015-9937-6
38. Kwok SYL, Yeung JWK, Low AYT, Lo HHM, Tam CHL. The roles of emotional competence and social problem-solving in the relationship between physical abuse and adolescent suicidal ideation in China. *Child Abuse Negl* (2015) 44(6):117–29. doi:10.1016/j.chiabu.2015.03.020
39. Quinones V, Jurska J, Fener E, Miranda R. Active and passive problem solving: moderating role in the relation between depressive symptoms and future suicidal ideation varies by suicide attempt history. *J Clin Psychol* (2015) 71(4):402–12. doi:10.1002/jclp.22155
40. Salkovskis PM, Atha C, Storer D. Cognitive-behavioural problem solving in the treatment of patients who repeatedly attempt suicide. A controlled trial. *Br J Psychiatry* (1990) 157:871–6. doi:10.1192/bjp.157.6.871
41. Ghahramanlou-Holloway M, Bhar SS, Brown GK, Olsen C, Beck AT. Changes in problem-solving appraisal after cognitive therapy for the prevention of suicide. *Psychol Med* (2012) 42(6):1185–93. doi:10.1017/S0033291711002169
42. Gustavson KA, Alexopoulos GS, Niu GC, McCulloch C, Meade T, Arean PA. Problem-solving therapy reduces suicidal ideation in depressed older adults with executive dysfunction. *Am J Geriatr Psychiatry* (2016) 24(1):11–7. doi:10.1016/j.jagp.2015.07.010
43. Chesin M, Interian A, Kline A, Benjamin-Phillips C, Latorre M, Stanley B. Reviewing mindfulness-based interventions for suicidal behavior. *Arch Suicide Res* (2016) 20(4):507–27. doi:10.1080/13811118.2016.1162244

13

Mediators Linking Childhood Adversities and Trauma to Suicidality in Individuals at Risk for Psychosis

Stefanie J. Schmidt[1,2*†], *Frauke Schultze-Lutter*[1,3†], *Sarah Bendall*[4,5], *Nicola Groth*[1], *Chantal Michel*[1,6], *Nadja Inderbitzin*[1], *Benno G. Schimmelmann*[1,7], *Daniela Hubl*[8] *and Barnaby Nelson*[4,5]

[1] *University Hospital of Child and Adolescent Psychiatry and Psychotherapy, University of Bern, Bern, Switzerland,* [2] *Department of Psychiatry and Psychotherapy, University of Cologne, Cologne, Germany,* [3] *Department of Psychiatry and Psychotherapy, Medical Faculty, Heinrich-Heine University, Düsseldorf, Germany,* [4] *Orygen, The National Centre of Excellence in Youth Mental Health, University of Melbourne, Melbourne, VIC, Australia,* [5] *Centre for Youth Mental Health, University of Melbourne, Melbourne, VIC, Australia,* [6] *Developmental Clinical Psychology Research Unit, Faculty of Psychology and Educational Sciences, University of Geneva, Geneva, Switzerland,* [7] *University Hospital of Child and Adolescent Psychiatry, University Hospital Hamburg Eppendorf, Hamburg, Germany,* [8] *University Hospital of Psychiatry and Psychotherapy, University of Bern, Bern, Switzerland*

***Correspondence:**
Stefanie J. Schmidt
stefanie.schmidt@upd.unibe.ch

†*Joint first authorship.*

Suicidality is highly prevalent in patients at clinical high risk (CHR) for psychosis. Childhood adversities and trauma are generally predictive of suicidality. However, the differential effects of adversity/trauma-domains and CHR-criteria, i.e., ultra-high risk and basic symptom criteria, on suicidality remain unclear. Furthermore, the underlying mechanisms and, thus, worthwhile targets for suicide-prevention are still poorly understood. Therefore, structural equation modeling was used to test theory-driven models in 73 CHR-patients. Mediators were psychological variables, i.e., beliefs about one's own competencies as well as the controllability of events and coping styles. In addition, symptomatic variables (depressiveness, basic symptoms, attenuated psychotic symptoms) were hypothesized to mediate the effect of psychological mediators on suicidality as the final outcome variable. Results showed two independent pathways. In the first pathway, emotional and sexual but not physical adversity/trauma was associated with suicidality, which was mediated by dysfunctional competence/control beliefs, a lack of positive coping-strategies and depressiveness. In the second pathway, cognitive basic symptoms but not attenuated psychotic symptoms mediated the relationship between trauma/adversity and suicidality. CHR-patients are, thus, particularly prone to suicidality if adversity/trauma is followed by the development of depressiveness. Regarding the second pathway, this is the first study showing that adversity/trauma led to suicidality through an increased risk for psychosis as indicated by cognitive basic symptoms. As insight is generally associated with suicidality, this may explain why self-experienced basic symptoms increase the risk for it. Consequently, these mediators should be monitored regularly and targeted by integrated interventions as early as possible to enhance resilience against suicidality.

Keywords: psychosis, mediation, depression, suicidality, basic symptoms, attenuated psychotic symptoms

INTRODUCTION

Suicide is defined as the deliberate act to take one's own life. With over 800,000 persons having completed suicide worldwide in 2012 (1), suicide is among the top 20 causes for mortality in the world. Notably, suicide rates in adolescents have increased in recent years, making suicide the second leading cause of death globally in individuals aged between 15 and 29 years (1). Non-lethal suicidality, including suicidal ideation (i.e., thinking about killing oneself) and suicide plans as well as attempts, is even more prevalent and substantially increases the risk of death by suicide (2). Among psychiatric patients, risk of suicidality is generally increased, in particular in patients with psychotic disorders (3). In psychosis, it is highest in the early stages of the disorder (4). Accordingly, the first meta-analysis of clinical high risk (CHR)-patients including 21 studies with 2,808 participants revealed high prevalence rates of 66.1% for current suicidal ideation and 17.7% for lifetime suicide attempts (5).

In both general population and psychiatric samples, childhood adversities and trauma are one of the main psychological predictors of suicidality (6–8). While suicidality seems to be related to childhood adversities and trauma in patients with first-episode psychosis (9, 10), this link has not yet been studied sufficiently in CHR-patients. Furthermore, most previous studies in general population, patient and in particular in CHR-samples have investigated potential predictors of suicidality in isolation without analyzing their interplay and their relative contributions to suicidality simultaneously. Consequently, we still have a limited understanding of the mechanisms linking adversities and trauma to suicidality (7). Therefore, based on the current literature, this study aimed to test theory-based models about potential mechanisms contributing to the relationship between childhood adversities/trauma and suicidality in a sample of CHR-patients. A CHR-state of psychoses was alternatively defined by the ultra-high risk (11) and the basic symptom criteria, including cognitive disturbances (COGDIS) and cognitive-perceptive basic symptoms (COPER) (12).

Experiences of adversities and trauma are highly prevalent in CHR-patients (13, 14). They are related to the development of psychopathology, including depressive and psychotic symptoms, which function as precipitants of suicidality (14–17). Models to explain this relationship in CHR-patients include stress-vulnerability and stress-sensitization models (14). They postulate that exposure to trauma as a major stressor interacts with an individual's vulnerability. This interaction leads to a dysregulation of the stress-response system and an increase in the susceptibility to develop psychopathology, such as psychotic symptoms. After an experience of first psychotic symptoms, the stress-threshold is lowered for the development of even more severe psychopathology (13, 18). Furthermore, the hopelessness theory of suicidality (19, 20) posits that early adversity can facilitate the development of a negative cognitive style as an enduring vulnerability factor characterized by external control beliefs (i.e., events are mainly controlled by others and outside of personal control) as well as negative self-evaluations (e.g., being worthless, lack of self-efficacy). Such a cognitive style has shown to trigger threat anticipation, paranoid ideas, depressive symptoms, and finally suicidal ideation (21, 22). The interpersonal theory of suicidality (20, 23, 24) suggests that the experience of adversities/trauma increases the risk for suicidality through thwarted belongingness and perceived burdensomeness, which are especially pronounced in patients with psychosis due to diminished social connectedness as well as stigma (20, 25) and experiences of being a burden on caregivers (26). In line with these current models of suicidality, childhood adversities and trauma were associated with poor emotion-focused coping, more distress, negative self-beliefs, and depressiveness in CHR-patients (27, 28). Suicidality was significantly related to poor self-esteem (29) and high levels of distress as well as depressiveness (30). However, all of these studies in CHR-patients have not yet integrated these potential mediator variables within one model. Furthermore, while studies demonstrated that a CHR-status, in particular defined by attenuated psychotic symptoms, was linked to childhood adversities as well as trauma and suicidality (30–32), basic symptom criteria have not yet been investigated for their potential association with suicidality.

Against this background, we hypothesized the following mechanisms: (1) childhood adversities and trauma are significantly associated with suicidality and (2) this relationship is mediated by psychological variables: dysfunctional coping and competence/control belief pattern. With regard to the second mechanism, it is noteworthy that social-learning theory and empirical results posit that having positive beliefs about one's own competencies (i.e., high self-efficacy) and about internal, personal controllability over events are associated with the use of more positive and less negative coping-strategies (33–35). However, some studies have also found the reverse sequence, i.e., positive coping-strategies being associated with high levels of positive competence-beliefs and perceived internal control (36, 37). Therefore, we examined both directions of the second assumed psychological mediators in alternative models. Furthermore, we hypothesized (3) that the mediation effect of psychological variables on suicidality is mediated through increased symptom levels [brief limited intermittent psychotic symptoms (BLIPSs), attenuated psychotic symptoms, COPER/COGDIS, and depressiveness]. Furthermore, potentially confounding variables (age, gender, educational level, current comorbid axis-I disorders) (5, 38) were included as covariates directly influencing suicidality.

MATERIALS AND METHODS

Sample

Clinical high risk-patients were aged between 8 and 40 years as this age-range is associated with the highest probability of psychotic development across gender (39). They were recruited from consecutive referrals to the Early Recognition and Intervention Center for mental crisis (FETZ) Bern between December 2010 and May 2016. Participants had to meet any ultra-high risk or basic symptom criterion. They were excluded if they had a medical, neurological, or substance use disorder accounting for their mental problems. To ensure excellent data quality, diagnostic assessments were performed by trained psychologists, who received weekly supervision. All participants provided written informed consent and parental consent, if they were under the age of 18. The ethics committee of the University of Bern approved the study.

Instruments

To avoid an age-bias, we administered the same tool when the respective instrument was validated for its application in adults as well as children/adolescents. When results of validation-studies suggested age-differences, we used well-validated children/adolescent- and adult-versions of the same instrument {i.e., Schizophrenia Proneness Instrument [SPI-A/SPI-CY (40, 41)]; German Stress-Coping-Questionnaires [SVF-120/SVF-KJ (42, 43)]; Mini International Neuropsychiatric Interview [MINI/MINI-KID (44, 45)]} or applied the age-adapted test norms available for the same instrument, i.e., German Competence and Control Beliefs Questionnaire [FKK (46)].

CHR for Psychosis

The Structured Interview for Psychosis-Risk Syndromes [SIPS (47)] was used to evaluate the presence of the ultra-high-risk criteria, including the attenuated psychotic symptom criterion, the BLIPS criterion, and the genetic risk and functional decline criterion. COPER and COGDIS were assessed by the Schizophrenia Proneness Instrument, adult [SPI-A (40)] and children/adolescent version [SPI-CY (41)]. A detailed description of the ultra-high-risk and basic symptom criteria can be found in Table S1 in Supplementary Material. Good interrater-reliability and construct-validity (48, 49) were reported for the assessments of CHR-criteria that also possess good test–retest reliability across short periods of time and assessment modes (48–51).

Childhood Adversities and Trauma

The Trauma And Distress Scale [TADS (52)] is a self-report questionnaire to assess retrospectively the frequency of five types of self-reported childhood adversities and trauma: emotional neglect, physical neglect, sexual abuse, emotional abuse, and physical abuse. Each of the 43 items is rated on a 5-point Likert-scale from "never" to "almost always." Higher values indicate more severe adversities and trauma. The TADS has been used in adolescent as well as adult samples (53, 54) and has been validated in a large general population study showing good internal consistency, inter-method reliability, and concurrent validity (52).

Coping

Coping-strategies were evaluated by the German Stress-Coping-Questionnaires using the version for adults [SVF-120 (42)] and children/adolescents [SVF-KJ (43)], which define coping-strategies as a person's habitual reactions to stressful events. The frequency of each coping-strategy is rated on a 5-point Likert-scale ranging from "not at all" to "in any case." Both versions allow the calculation of summary scores for positive and negative coping-strategies from 16 (SVF-120) and 9 (SVF-KJ) primary scales, respectively. Gender-adapted and age-adapted normative data are provided as T-values. Both age-adapted versions of the SVF have shown good internal consistency, retest reliability and construct, as well as criterion validity (42, 43, 55).

Competence and Control Beliefs

The German Competence and Control Beliefs Questionnaire [FKK (46)] is a 32-item questionnaire to assess a person's generalized expectations about own competencies and courses of action ("self-concept") as well as causal attributions of events to oneself ("internality"), to other persons ("social externality"), or to chance/situational factors ("fatalistic externality"). Each item is rated on a 6-point Likert-scale ranging from "totally false" to "totally true." Higher values indicate a stronger tendency for the respective competence/control belief. Age-adapted normative data are provided as T-values. Studies support the internal consistency, test–retest reliability and content, construct, concurrent, as well as predictive validity of the FKK in adolescents and adults (46).

Depressiveness

The Beck Depression Inventory [BDI-II (56)] is a 21-item self-assessment of depressiveness in the past 2 weeks. Each item is rated on a 4-point Likert-scale as described below. The summary score excluding suicidal ideation (item 9) was used with higher scores indicating more severe depressiveness. The BDI-II has been widely used among adolescents and adults (57, 58) to assess the severity of depressive symptoms with good psychometric properties in terms of internal consistency, retest reliability as well as content, construct, concurrent, and predictive validity (56, 59–61).

Suicidality

Suicidality was assessed by two measures to determine suicidality-domains: suicidal ideation and suicidal risk. The "suicidal ideation" item 9 of the BDI-II (56) was used to determine suicidal ideation in the past two weeks rated on a 4-point Likert-scale ranging from "absent" ("I don't have thoughts of killing myself") to "severe" ("I would kill myself if I had the chance"). The "suicidality scale" of the Mini International Neuropsychiatric Interview in its version for adults [MINI (44)] and children/adolescents [MINI-KID (45)] was used to determine suicidal risk with regard to suicidal ideation, plans, and attempts. In the MINI/MINI-KID, the interviewer asks yes–no questions about the presence of suicidal ideation, plans, and attempts within the past month. Points are granted for each question answered with "yes," while the number of points depends on the severity of the respective indicator for suicidality. The summary score was used to rate the current suicide risk as "not present" (0 points), "low" (1–8 points), "moderate" (9–16 points), or "high" (>17 points). Both instruments have shown to be reliable measures with good concurrent and predictive validity for assessing suicidality in children/adolescents and adults (44, 45, 62–65).

Statistical Analyses

All analyses were performed using Mplus version 7.4 with the weighted least squares mean and variance adjusted estimator (WLSMV) for categorical variables (66). Data (8.5%) were missing completely at random (MCAR) as indicated by Little's MCAR test [$\chi^2(88) = 97.25$, $p = 0.235$]. They were replaced through multiple imputations by creating 50 complete datasets that were used for all subsequent analyses (67).

Structural equation models were calculated to investigate the hypothesized mediation effects. Model fit was assessed by five commonly used indices: Chi-square test (χ^2), Comparative Fit Index (CFI), Tucker–Lewis Index (TLI), root-mean-square error of approximation (RMSEA), and the Weighted Root Mean Square Residual (WRMR). To generate measurement models, latent variables were formed for adversities and trauma (emotional abuse/neglect, physical abuse/neglect, sexual abuse), coping (positive/negative coping styles), competence/control beliefs (self-concept, internality, social externality, fatalistic externality), and suicidality-domains (MINI/MINI-KID suicidality subscale; BDI-II, item 9). The summary score of the BDI-II was used as a manifest indicator for current depressiveness; presence of any CHR-criterion was treated as binary manifest variable.

Following recommendations for assessing mediation effects (68, 69), we initially tested a basic model, which postulates a significant association between the independent variable "childhood adversities and trauma" and the dependent variable "suicidality" (hypothesis 1). To examine hypotheses 2 and 3, potential mediators needed to be associated with both the independent and dependent variable as a precondition to establish a mediation effect (Figures S1–S3A,B in Supplementary Material). Significance of indirect effects was tested by calculating bootstrapped, bias-corrected confidence intervals (CIs) of the indirect effect (70). Finally, potential socio-demographic and clinical confounding variables (age, gender, educational level, current comorbid axis-I disorders) were included as covariates. Additional models were calculated to test if the relationship between adversities/trauma and suicidality was also mediated by each mediator separately (Table S2 in Supplementary Material).

RESULTS

Sample Characteristics

The sample consisted of 73 CHR-patients aged between 9.5 and 35.3 years with the majority (84.9%, n = 62) falling within an age-range between 12 and 25 years (**Table 1**). 44 CHR-patients (60.3%) were younger than 18 years. Therefore, they completed the child/adolescent versions of the respective instruments, i.e., SPI-CY (41), SVF-KJ (43), and MINI-KID (45), while all other instruments were completed by the whole sample.

Table 1 shows sample characteristics and summary statistics for each model variable. With regard to childhood adversities and trauma, 35.8% (n = 24) CHR-patients reported clinically relevant levels of emotional abuse and emotional neglect, i.e., they scored more than 1 SD above the respective mean of the normative data provided (52); 31.3% (n = 21) reported physical neglect, 23.9% (n = 16) physical abuse and 21.5% (n = 14) sexual abuse. Furthermore, CHR-patients frequently demonstrated a lack of positive coping-strategies (48.4%, n = 30) and an excessive use of negative strategies (30.8%, n = 20) according to the test norms (42, 43). Moreover, they also showed deficits in competence and control beliefs in terms of a negative self-concept (28.8%, n = 19), low levels of internal attributions (33.3%, n = 22) as well as an excessive use of social external attributions (10.6%; n = 7) and fatalistic external attributions (15.2%, n = 10) according to the test norms (46). In addition, CHR-patients reported on average moderate levels of depressiveness with 66.2% (n = 45) having at least mild levels of suicidal ideation in the past 2 weeks as assessed by the BDI-II-item (56). Ten CHR-patients (13.6%) had at least a low risk for suicidality in the past month as assessed by the MINI/MINI-KID (44, 45). All of them also reported at least a minimal level of suicidal ideation.

Childhood Adversities/Trauma and Suicidality (Model 1)

Bivariate correlations among the measures are shown in **Table 2**. As expected, we found significant associations of several domains of childhood adversities and trauma, namely emotional abuse as well as neglect and sexual abuse, with both suicidality-domains. Consistent with our first hypothesis, childhood adversities and trauma were significantly associated with suicidality ($\beta = 0.50$, $p = 0.003$) with adequate model fit [$\chi^2(13) = 17.15$, $p = 0.192$; CFI = 0.95; TLI = 0.91; RMSEA = 0.07, p = 0.349; WRMR = 0.51]. Dropping the two domains of childhood adversities and trauma that were uncorrelated with either suicidality-domain (**Table 2**), i.e., physical abuse and neglect, from the model resulted in an excellent model fit (**Figure 1**), and the association between childhood adversities and trauma and suicidality was significant again ($\beta = 0.50, p = 0.002$). Consequently, we reduced the latent variable childhood adversities and trauma to three indicators (emotional abuse and neglect, sexual abuse) in subsequent models.

Psychological Mediators between Childhood Adversities/Trauma and Suicidality (Model 2)

A lack of positive coping-strategies was significantly associated with both emotional abuse and neglect, and suicidality-domains, while negative coping-strategies were unrelated to either suicidality-domain and to positive coping-strategies (**Table 2**). Consequently, no latent coping-variable could be formed, and negative coping-strategies were dropped from the model. With regard to competence/control beliefs, a negative self-concept was significantly associated with emotional abuse as well as neglect and suicidality-domains. An excessive use of social and fatalistic external beliefs was significantly correlated with both emotional abuse and neglect; a lack of internal beliefs with suicide risk. In line with our second hypothesis, both positive coping-strategies and dysfunctional competence/control beliefs functioned as mediators between childhood adversities as well as trauma and suicidality as indicated by significant indirect effects and adequate model fit (**Figure 2**, Figure S4).

Final Model with Symptomatic and Psychological Mediators (Model 3)

Testing our third hypothesis, including symptom levels as additional mediators of the identified indirect effects, higher levels of depressiveness were significantly correlated with various domains of childhood adversities and trauma, both suicidality-domains, and psychological mediators (**Table 2**). While presence of COGDIS was related to emotional abuse, COPER was related

TABLE 1 | Socio-demographic and clinical sample characteristics ($n = 73$).

Socio-demographic and clinical data		
Age in years, *mean (SD), median (quartiles), age categories in years, n (%)*	18.4 (4.6), 17.5 (15.7; 20.9), <12 years: 5 (6.8%); <18 years: 43 (58.9%), ≥18 years: 29 (39.7%); >25 years: 6 (8.2%)	
Gender, male, *n (%)*	38 (52.1%)	
Nationality, Swiss, *n (%)*	63 (86.3%)	
Highest ISCED score school (3ab), *n (%)*	15 (20.6%)	
Functional outcome, SOFAS, mean (SD)	61.0 (11.3)	
Axis-I diagnoses[a], *n (%)*		
Current major depressive episode	12 (17.4%)	
Past major depressive episode	28 (40.6%)	
Recurrent episodes of major depression	15 (22.1%)	
Current substance use disorders	14 (20.3%)	
Current anxiety disorders	18 (24.7%)	
Past anxiety disorders	13 (19.1%)	
Model variables	**With missing values**	**With imputed values**[b]
Childhood adversities and trauma		
TADS, mean (SD)		
Emotional neglect	7.7 (4.9)	7.8 (4.8)
Physical neglect	5.4 (3.3)	5.4 (3.3)
Sexual abuse	1.7 (3.7)	1.7 (3.6)
Emotional abuse	6.6 (4.9)	6.7 (4.8)
Physical abuse	3.0 (3.1)	3.0 (3.1)
Competence and control beliefs		
FKK, summary T-scores, mean (SD)		
Self-concept	45.8 (9.7)	45.9 (9.7)
Internality	44.9 (10.1)	44.9 (10.0)
Social externality	49.6 (9.6)	49.5 (9.5)
Fatalistic externality	50.6 (8.7)	50.5 (8.6)
Coping-strategies		
SVF, summary T-scores, mean (SD)		
Positive coping-strategies	41.3 (11.4)	40.5 (11.8)
Negative coping-strategies	54.7 (12.9)	54.6 (12.8)
Depressiveness		
BDI-II, summary score, mean (SD)	23.3 (11.6)	23.4 (11.5)
Suicidality		
BDI-II, item 9, n (%)		
No suicidal ideation (0)	23 (31.5%)	26 (35.6%)
Mild ideation (1)	34 (46.6%)	35 (47.9%)
Severe ideation (2)	9 (12.3%)	10 (13.7%)
Very severe ideation (3)	2 (2.7%)	2 (2.7%)
MINI/-KID, suicidality risk, n (%)		
Absent	58 (79.5%)	62 (84.9%)
Low	5 (6.8%)	5 (6.8%)
Moderate	–	1 (1.4%)
High	5 (6.8%)	5 (6.8%)

APS, attenuated psychotic symptom criterion; BDI-II, Beck Depression Inventory (56); BLIPS, brief limited intermittent psychotic symptom criterion; COGDIS, cognitive disturbances criterion; COPER, cognitive-perceptive basic symptoms criterion; FKK, Competence and Control Belief Questionnaire (46); GRFD, genetic risk and functional decline criterion; ISCED, International Standard Classification of Education; MINI/-KID, Mini-Neuropsychiatric Interview for adults and children (44, 45); SOFAS, Social and Occupational Functioning Assessment Scale (71); SVF, Stress-Coping-Questionnaires for adults and children (42, 43); TADS, Trauma And Distress Scale (52).

[a]*Multiple diagnoses were possible; ≥5% of individuals fulfilled the diagnostic criteria for the respective mental disorder.*

[b]*For categorical variables, the most frequent imputation pattern is reported. No data were missing for clinical high-risk criteria.*

to emotional/physical abuse and emotional/physical neglect. However, only COGDIS was significantly correlated with both suicidality-domains and, therefore, included in the model.

Presence of any attenuated psychotic symptom was significantly associated with physical abuse but unrelated to either suicidality-domain (**Table 2**). With regard to single attenuated psychotic symptoms, we found a significant relationship between the presence of any persecutory idea (P2-item of the SIPS) and emotional abuse ($r = 0.25$, $p = 0.042$) as well as between perceptual abnormalities as well as attenuated hallucinations (P4-item of the SIPS) and suicidal ideation ($r = 0.29$, $p = 0.017$). However, SIPS-P4 was unrelated to all other model variables, thus making a mediation effect impossible. When used as a predictor instead of a mediator variable, SIPS-P4 was not significantly associated with suicidality in the model ($r = 0.29$, $p = 0.071$), and, therefore, dropped from the final model. Associations between presence of

TABLE 2 | Bivariate correlations between model variables with imputed values.

Model variables	1	2	3	4	5	6	7	8	9	10	11	12	13	14	15	16	17
1. Emotional abuse	–																
2. Emotional neglect	0.79**	–															
3. Physical abuse	0.45**	0.57**	–														
4. Physical neglect	0.59**	0.69**	0.64***	–													
5. Sexual abuse	0.15	0.20	0.38**	0.11	–												
6. Positive coping	−0.25*	−0.35**	−0.06	−0.16	−0.14	–											
7. Negative coping	0.24	0.24	0.20	0.24	0.32*	0.15	–										
8. Self-concept	−0.31*	−0.25*	0.11	0.05	−0.19	0.52**	−0.24	–									
9. Internal beliefs	−0.14	−0.18	0.03	0.05	−0.05	0.46**	0.12	0.34**	–								
10. Social-external beliefs	0.33**	0.20	0.07	0.13	0.22	−0.17	0.27*	0.39**	−0.01	–							
11. Social-fatalistic beliefs	0.32**	0.24*	0.24	0.17	0.21	−0.38**	0.20	−0.50**	0.03	0.44**	–						
12. Depressiveness	0.47**	0.53**	0.25*	0.23	0.36**	−0.57**	0.17	−0.58**	−0.24*	0.30*	0.44**	–					
13. Cognitive disturbances	0.31*	0.27	0.09	0.09	−0.19	−0.27	0.03	−0.11	−0.17	0.10	0.33*	0.20	–				
14. Cognitive-perceptive basic symptoms	0.39*	0.42**	0.34*	0.43**	−0.23	−0.10	0.15	−0.15	0.05	0.22	0.38*	0.12	0.46**	–			
15. Attenuated psychotic symptoms	0.03	0.00	0.26*	−0.19	0.02	−0.12	−0.06	−0.17	−0.21	−0.16	−0.06	0.13	−0.14	−0.44**	–		
16. Suicidal ideation[a]	0.33**	0.32**	0.05	0.06	0.21	−0.27*	0.10	−0.25*	−0.18	0.20	0.21	0.68**	0.32*	0.02	0.04	–	
17. Suicide risk[b]	0.23	0.29*	0.19	0.11	0.31*	−0.28*	0.08	−0.27*	−0.25*	0.18	0.15	0.51**	0.35*	0.14	−0.03	0.45**	–

[a] *Assessed by the Beck Depression Inventory II, item 9 (BDI-II; 56).*

[b] *Assessed by the Mini-Neuropsychiatric Interview for adults and children (MINI/MINI-KID; 44, 45).*

$*p < 0.05$.

$**p < 0.01$.

$***p < 0.001$.

BLIPS and any other model variable could not be investigated because only three CHR-patients (4.1%) met this criterion.

Thus, two independent mediation pathways were detected in the final model. One pathway ran from experiences of childhood adversities and trauma through more dysfunctional competence/control beliefs and a lack of positive coping-strategies to more depressiveness and from there to an increased risk for suicidality (**Figure 3**). This indirect effect was significant. The second pathway was weaker and led from experiences of childhood adversities and trauma through an increased probability to meet COGDIS to an increased risk for suicidality. This indirect effect was also significant. The same pattern of results was observed when the sequence of the psychological mediators was changed (Figure S5). The final model had a good fit to the data. Additional structural equation models, which included each mediator (i.e., dysfunctional beliefs, lack of positive coping, depressiveness, and COGDIS) separately, could confirm the relevance of each variable to explain this relationship between adversities/trauma and suicidality as indicated by significant indirect effects (Table S2 in Supplementary Material).

No changes were suggested by the modification indices that would turn the single pathway from childhood adversities and trauma on suicidality through psychological mediators into a dual pathway (e.g., through a separate path for coping and competence/control beliefs). None of the included covariates had a significant effect on suicidality and all of the identified pathways remained stable when they were included in the final model.

DISCUSSION

The results of this study extend the current literature on psychological and symptomatic mediation effects between childhood adversities and trauma and suicidality to patients at CHR for psychosis as well as to the effects of attenuated psychotic symptoms and basic symptoms. We found in our first model that childhood adversities and trauma were significantly related to suicidality. This relationship was mainly conveyed by sexual and emotional abuse as well as emotional neglect, while inclusion of physical abuse and neglect led to worse model fit. Only one study so far (72) has investigated this relationship in CHR-patients; it revealed no effect of trauma on the number of suicide attempts. Yet, this study had assessed only trauma but not adversities and only suicide attempts but not suicidal ideation, which we found to be highly prevalent and interrelated in our study. Furthermore, trauma was treated as a single entity (72), which may have masked actual associations because our results suggest a differential relationship of different domains of childhood adversities and trauma with suicidality. With regard to our data, the lack of an association between physical adversities as well as trauma and suicidality was not explained by a lower prevalence of physical compared to emotional adversities/trauma because the most infrequent domain sexual abuse was nevertheless significantly associated with suicidality. This is well in line with the literature (8, 73). Furthermore, the strong effect of emotional adversity and trauma in our study corresponds to previous studies that investigated the differential effects of various domains of childhood adversities and trauma and reported

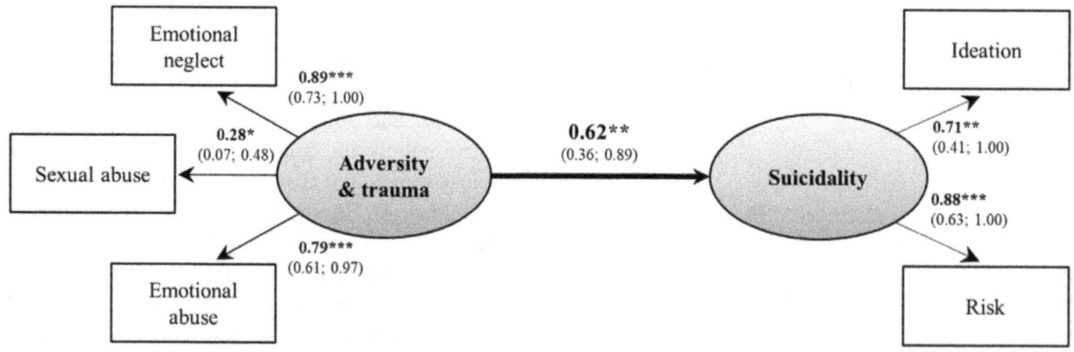

FIGURE 1 | Basic model between childhood adversities/trauma and suicidality. Model fit indices: $\chi^2(4) = 3.61$, $p = 0.461$; Comparative Fit Index = 1.00; Tucker–Lewis Index = 1.02; root-man-square error of approximation = 0.00, $p = 0.552$; Weighted Root Mean Square Residual = 0.34. Rectangles present observed manifest variables, ovals unobserved latent variables; values are standardized path coefficients and 95% confidence intervals of parameter estimates. $^*p < 0.05$, $^{**}p < 0.01$, $^{***}p < 0.001$.

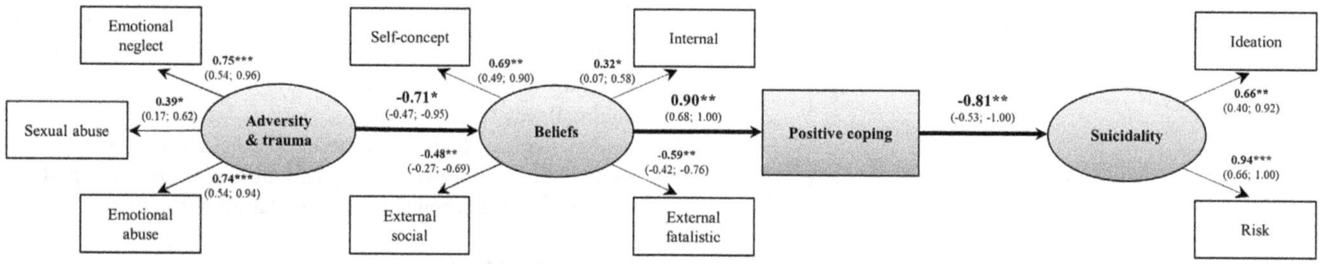

FIGURE 2 | Psychological mediators between childhood adversities/trauma and suicidality. Model fit indices: $\chi^2(33) = 43.41$, $p = 0.106$; Comparative Fit Index = 0.90; Tucker–Lewis Index = 0.87; root-mean-square error of approximation = 0.06, $p = 0.300$; Weighted Root Mean Square Residual = 0.61. Standardized indirect effect, IE = 0.54; 95% confidence intervals (Cis) = 0.27; 0.82; $p = 0.005$. Rectangles present observed manifest variables, ovals unobserved latent variables; values are standardized path coefficients and 95% CIs of parameter estimates. $^*p < 0.05$, $^{**}p < 0.01$, $^{***}p < 0.001$.

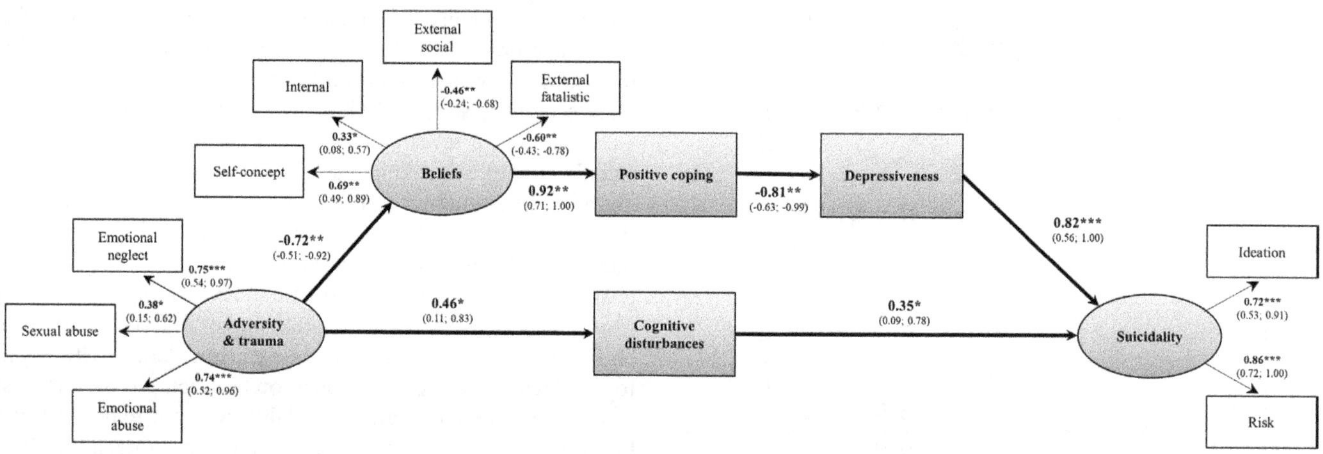

FIGURE 3 | Psychological and symptomatic mediators between childhood adversities/trauma and suicidality. Model fit indices: $\chi^2(51) = 59.68$, $p = 0.190$; Comparative Fit Index = 0.95; Tucker–Lewis Index = 0.94; root-mean-square error of approximation = 0.046, $p = 0.496$; Weighted Root Mean Square Residual (WRMR) = 0.59. Standardized indirect effect through beliefs–coping–depressiveness: IE = 0.44; 95% CIs = 0.10; 0.78; $p < 0.001$ and through cognitive disturbances: IE = 0.16, 95% confidence intervals (Cis) = 0.01; 0.34; $p = 0.045$. Rectangles present observed manifest variables, ovals unobserved latent variables; values are standardized path coefficients values are standardized path and 95% CIs of parameter estimates. $^*p < 0.05$, $^{**}p < 0.01$, $^{***}p < 0.001$.

emotional neglect to have the strongest association with suicidality (74, 75). This is consistent with the assumption of the interpersonal–psychological theory of suicide (24) that adversities and trauma increase the desire for suicide by augmenting feelings of perceived burdensomeness and decreased belongingness. Such feelings are assumed to result from all forms of adversities and trauma but seem to be especially amplified in the presence of high levels of negative emotions, which are an integral part of emotional neglect and abuse (23).

With regard to the second model, as expected the relationship between childhood adversities as well as trauma and suicidality was mediated by dysfunctional competence/control beliefs and coping. Yet, unexpectedly, the role of coping on suicidality was only conveyed by positive coping-strategies but not additionally by negative coping-strategies, which were not significantly correlated with each other. This is in contrast to previous results (76, 77) and might be caused by the fact that our CHR-patients rather reported a lack of positive coping-strategies than an excessive use of negative strategies. Furthermore, severe forms of trauma, such as sexual abuse that were predominately linked to an excessive use of negative coping-strategies were rare in our sample. In addition, our assessment was not limited to abuse but included neglect, which is thought to exert a less detrimental effect on coping and suicidality than abuse (78).

With regard to the sequence of competence/control beliefs and coping, both alternative models (competence/control beliefs first and coping second as well as *vice versa*) were supported by our data. Models placing competence/control beliefs first posit that individuals, who perceive themselves to be less competent and events to be predominantly controlled by external factors, are less likely to initiate and sustain positive coping behavior (34, 79). Models with the reverse sequence, however, state that exposure to childhood adversities and trauma has an adverse effect on cognitive development (80), which results in poor coping skills (81). Ineffective coping skills lead to long-standing difficulties when faced with future stressors, which increases the risk to develop dysfunctional competence/control beliefs as well as depressiveness and suicidality (77, 82–84). Our results argue for a more complex and synergistic view in that both constructs mutually influence each other, i.e., beliefs about low controllability and few competences reduce the probability to apply positive coping-strategies, which leads to even more dysfunctional beliefs and *vice versa*. The high path coefficients of the relationship between competence/control beliefs and coping in our models suggest that both constructs represent a higher-order phenomenon known as "coping-efficacy" (85), which refers to an individual's beliefs about the efficacy of coping in the future based on previous coping-experiences. In line with our results, coping-efficacy mediated the relationship between childhood adversities as well as trauma and depression (86) and was linked to suicidality (87).

With regard to the other mediators and covariates in model 3, none of the assumed covariates had a significant direct relationship to suicidality, while of the symptomatic mediators only depressiveness and COGDIS but not attenuated psychotic symptoms and COPER became significant. Thereby, depressiveness followed competence/control beliefs and coping and had a direct impact on suicidality. COGDIS was an independent mediator between childhood adversities as well as trauma and suicidality, introducing a second, yet weaker pathway.

The first pathway implies that childhood adversities and trauma act as a catalyst in the suicidal process by triggering the development of dysfunctional competence/control beliefs. This belief pattern is often referred to as "hopelessness" (46) and may set back the application of positive coping-strategies, which then leads to depressiveness and finally to suicidality. This model is consistent with integrated hopelessness and interpersonal-psychological theories of suicidality and related empirical findings. They suggest that childhood adversities and trauma confer risk for the development of a negative and hopeless cognitive style (defined as low control beliefs for negative events and negative self-evaluations) with the consequence that a person is hopeless about the future and develops depressiveness and suicidality (7, 88). In line with our results, in particular emotional abuse and neglect were reported to be associated with the development of such a negative cognitive style, possibly because the abuser directly supplies the abused individual with self-blaming statements (e.g., "I believe that I am a bad person"; TADS-item 14) often involved in suicidal ideation (7). Furthermore, the relationship between emotional adversities/trauma and poor coping reported in our and other studies may be explained by the fact that maltreating parents/care-givers are likely inappropriate role models due to their own coping deficits, who cannot provide a supportive environment to learn adequate coping-strategies (7, 76). This pathway has often been described in the development of depression (89, 90) and may reflect the high percentage of depressiveness in our sample and in CHR-patients in general (91).

With regard to attenuated psychotic symptoms, presence of any attenuated psychotic symptom was significantly associated with childhood adversities and trauma in terms of physical abuse but not with suicidality. With regard to single attenuated psychotic symptoms, persecutory ideas were significantly associated with emotional abuse. This is in line with results in patients with psychosis (92) that also found this specific relationship. However, only perceptual abnormalities and attenuated hallucinations were significantly associated with suicidality. This specific association is in accordance with studies on psychotic-like experiences (29, 77) and on patients with psychosis (93). However, no significant mediation effect of any attenuated psychotic symptom between childhood adversities as well as trauma and suicidality was found in this study. This suggests that childhood adversities and trauma may not be specific for the development of psychotic symptoms as other symptomatic mediators, in particular depressiveness, were more influential in conveying the link between adversities/trauma and suicidality. This is supported by the result that childhood adversities and trauma contribute to a shared vulnerability for both the development of psychosis and in particular of depression, with the latter being the strongest predictor of suicidality (94). Furthermore, other factors may have a stronger impact on suicidality than (attenuated) psychotic symptoms, which is supported by the result that suicidality in patients with first-episode psychosis is highest in the remission phase (95).

In light of the missing mediation effect through attenuated psychotic symptoms in our study and inconclusive results about the relationship between higher cognitive functions and suicidality in schizophrenia (10), the role of COGDIS is especially noteworthy. COGDIS includes subtle, subclinical disturbances in thinking that are self-experienced with immediate full insight into their abnormal nature (12). One possible explanation focuses on the full insight when experiencing basic symptoms. This was reported to lead to increased levels of affective tension that decrease when (attenuated) psychotic symptoms develop (96). Therefore, basic symptoms may be more closely linked to suicidality than attenuated psychotic symptoms. Furthermore, it has been suggested that insight may result in a negative change in self-image and/or an exaggerated awareness of consequences related to a possible mental disorder and feelings of stigma. Thereby high levels of insight, in particular prior to treatment, increase risk for suicidality (10, 97). This might link our results on COGDIS to findings of increased levels of social isolation and feelings of burdensomeness and belongingness as the main predictors of suicidality (24, 30). While there is a large overlap between COGDIS and COPER, the latter was only significantly associated with childhood adversities and trauma but not with suicidality. This may be due to the lower specificity of COPER in predicting conversion to psychosis (98, 99).

Apart from the strengths of our study (e.g., detailed examination of adversity-/trauma- and CHR-domains), some limitations have to be discussed. First, we used only a cross-sectional design, which does not allow firm conclusion about the causality between the investigated variables. In particular, it was not possible to disentangle cause and effect or continuous interaction between competence/control beliefs and coping, which highlights the need for more longitudinal studies. Furthermore, due to the large age-range, younger individuals might still be exposed to childhood adversities and trauma in contrast to older ones, which also challenges the assumption of a unidirectional sequence of the model variables. In addition, although age was not significantly associated with suicidality as the outcome of interest in our model and did not affect the relationships between the model variables when included as a covariate, future studies with a more homogeneous sample or with larger samples-sizes in each age-group should be conducted to test for potential age-effects using more sophisticated analyses (e.g., multiple-group comparisons). Yet, our age-range might also be an advantage as the effect of recent or even still on-going childhood adversities and trauma might be even stronger than the effect of past ones. Furthermore, we used a theory-driven approach, which clearly suggests that childhood adversities and trauma contributes to the formation of dysfunctional belief- and coping-pattern and the development of depressiveness and suicidality. Second, we were interested in answering the question how childhood adversities and trauma and suicidality are linked to each other. However, alternative models may fit the data equally well, e.g., that high levels of self-efficacy and positive coping moderate the relationship between childhood adversities and trauma and suicidality (100). Together with the fact that we made *post hoc* modifications on the model, this clearly warrants a cross-validation and comparison of alternative models in a larger sample. This seems also indicated as our sample size was rather small within the context of structural equation modeling, which is associated with a higher risk of detecting spurious effects as well as of not detecting true but small effects and with larger CIs for estimation of the indirect effect limiting the generalizability of our results (69). Thus, our results and conclusions are only preliminary and need to be interpreted cautiously. Third, the fact that we assessed depressiveness and suicidal ideation with the same measurement scale may have increased the correlation between them. However, we did not rely on a single item to assess suicidality as many previous studies but additionally applied the suicidality subscale of a structured clinical interview. Both instruments have demonstrated good predictive validity to assess suicidality in adolescents and adults (62–65).

Despite these limitations, our study has important clinical implications. It suggests that interventions to prevent suicidality in CHR-patients should focus on both reducing COGDIS and disrupting the detrimental cascading effect through poor coping skills, dysfunctional belief pattern, and depressiveness as early as possible. In order to identify CHR-patients at risk for suicidality, childhood adversities and trauma as well as competence/control beliefs and coping styles should be routinely assessed, monitored, and targeted if necessary. Trauma-focused interventions for CHR-patients should be supplemented by interventions to enhance positive beliefs about own competencies and controllability over events as well as to increase the repertoire of positive coping-strategies, such as re-attribution and coping-strategy enhancement techniques (101, 102) to increase resilience against depressiveness and suicidality (88, 100).

In summary, our results identified psychological and symptomatic mechanisms that contribute to the explanation why individuals exposed to childhood adversities and trauma develop suicidality. Therefore, these mediators should be monitored regularly and should be targeted therapeutically in addition to trauma-focused interventions as early as possible to enhance resilience against suicidality.

ETHICS STATEMENT

The authors assert that all procedures contributing to this work comply with the ethical standards of the relevant national and institutional committees on human experimentation and with the Helsinki Declaration of 1975, as revised in 2008, as well as with the Swiss Federal Act on Research involving Human Beings as of 2011. All participants and, in case of minors, their care-givers were evaluated for their capacity to provide informed consent before giving written informed consent to the further use of their clinical data for research. The ethics committee of the University of Bern approved the procedure.

AUTHOR CONTRIBUTIONS

SS, FS-L, BS, and DH designed the study. CM and NI managed the data and the recruitment. All authors managed the literature searches and analyses. SS, NI, and BN undertook the statistical analyses. SS and FS-L wrote the first draft of the manuscript. All authors contributed to and have approved the final manuscript.

ACKNOWLEDGMENTS

The FETZ Bern is a cooperation between the University Hospitals of Child and Adolescent Psychiatry and Psychotherapy, and of Psychiatry and Psychotherapy of the Unive rsity of Bern, and the Soteria Bern.

REFERENCES

1. World Health Organization. *Prevention of Mental Disorders: Effective Interventions and Policy Options*. Geneva: World Health Organization (2014). 376 p.
2. Chan MK, Bhatti H, Meader N, Stockton S, Evan J, O'Connor RC, et al. Predicting suicide following self-harm: systematic review of risk factors and risk scales. *Br J Psychiatry* (2016) 209(4):277–83. doi:10.1192/bjp.bp.115.170050
3. Kelleher I, Ramsay H, DeVylder J. Psychotic experiences and suicide attempt risk in common mental disorders and borderline personality disorder. *Acta Psychiatr Scand* (2017) 135(3):212–8. doi:10.1111/acps.12693
4. Palmer BA, Pankratz VS, Bostwick JM. The lifetime risk of suicide in schizophrenia: a reexamination. *Arch Gen Psychiatry* (2005) 62(3):247–53. doi:10.1001/archpsyc.62.3.247
5. Taylor PJ, Hutton P, Wood L. Are people at risk of psychosis also at risk of suicide and self-harm? A systematic review and meta-analysis. *Psychol Med* (2015) 45(05):911–26. doi:10.1017/S0033291714002074
6. Liu RT, Miller I. Life events and suicidal ideation and behavior: a systematic review. *Clin Psychol Rev* (2014) 34(3):181–92. doi:10.1016/j.cpr.2014.01.006
7. Sachs-Ericsson NJ, Rushing NC, Stanley IH, Sheffler J. In my end is my beginning: developmental trajectories of adverse childhood experiences to late-life suicide. *Aging Ment Health* (2016) 20(2):139–65. doi:10.1080/1360 7863.2015.1063107
8. Castellví P, Miranda-Mendizábal A, Parés-Badell O, Almenara J, Alonso I, Blasco MJ, et al. Exposure to violence, a risk for suicide in youths and young adults. A meta-analysis of longitudinal studies. *Acta Psychiatr Scand* (2017) 135(3):195–211. doi:10.1111/acps.12679
9. Hassan AN, Stuart EA, De Luca V. Childhood maltreatment increases the risk of suicide attempt in schizophrenia. *Schizophr Res* (2016) 176(2):572–7. doi:10.1016/j.schres.2016.05.012
10. Ventriglio A, Gentile A, Bonfitto I, Stella E, Mari M, Steardo L, et al. Suicide in the early stage of schizophrenia. *Front Psychiatry* (2016) 7:116. doi:10.3389/fpsyt.2016.00116
11. Yung AR, Phillips LJ, McGorry PD, McFarlane CA, Francey S, Harrigan S, et al. Prediction of psychosis: a step towards indicated prevention of schizophrenia. *Br J Psychiatry* (1998) 172:14–20.
12. Schultze-Lutter F. Subjective symptoms of schizophrenia in research and the clinic: the basic symptom concept. *Schizophr Bull* (2009) 35(1):5–8. doi:10.1093/schbul/sbn139
13. Gibson LE, Alloy LB, Ellman LM. Trauma and the psychosis spectrum: a review of symptom specificity and explanatory mechanisms. *Clin Psychol Rev* (2016) 49:92–105. doi:10.1016/j.cpr.2016.08.003
14. Mayo D, Corey S, Kelly LH, Yohannes S, Youngquist AL, Stuart BK, et al. The role of trauma and stressful life events among individuals at clinical high risk for psychosis: a review. *Front Psychiatry* (2017) 8:55. doi:10.3389/fpsyt.2017.00055
15. Johnson J, Gooding P, Tarrier N. Suicide risk in schizophrenia: explanatory models and clinical implications, The Schematic Appraisal Model of Suicide (SAMS). *Psychol Psychother* (2008) 81(1):55–77. doi:10.1348/1476083 07X244996
16. Sachs-Ericsson NJ, Stanley IH, Sheffler JL, Selby E, Joiner TE. Non-violent and violent forms of childhood abuse in the prediction of suicide attempts: direct or indirect effects through psychiatric disorders? *J Affect Disord* (2017) 215:15–22. doi:10.1016/j.jad.2017.03.030
17. Turecki G, Brent DA. Suicide and suicidal behavior. *Lancet* (2016) 387(10024):1227–39. doi:10.1016/S0140-6736(15)00234-2
18. Trotman HD, Holtzman CW, Walker EF, Addington JM, Bearden CE, Cadenhead KS, et al. Stress exposure and sensitivity in the clinical high-risk syndrome: initial findings from the North American Prodrome Longitudinal Study (NAPLS). *Schizophr Res* (2014) 160(1–3):104–9. doi:10.1016/j.schres.2014.09.017
19. Abramson LY, Metalsky GI, Alloy LB. Hopelessness depression: a theory-based subtype of depression. *Psychol Rev* (1989) 96(2):358–72. doi:10.1037/0033-295X.96.2.358
20. Huang X, Fox KR, Ribeiro JD, Franklin JC. Psychosis as a risk factor for suicidal thoughts and behaviors: a meta-analysis of longitudinal studies. *Psychol Med* (2017):1–2. doi:10.1017/S0033291717002136
21. Bentall RP, Fernyhough C. Social predictors of psychotic experiences: specificity and psychological mechanisms. *Schizophr Bull* (2008) 34(6):1012–20. doi:10.1093/schbul/sbn103
22. Hutcheson C, Fleming MP, Martin CR. An examination and appreciation of the dimensions of locus of control in psychosis: issues and relationships between constructs and measurement. *J Psychiatr Ment Health Nurs* (2014) 21(10):906–16. doi:10.1111/jpm.12160
23. Anestis MD, Joiner TE. Examining the role of emotion in suicidality: negative urgency as an amplifier of the relationship between components of the interpersonal–psychological theory of suicidal behavior and lifetime number of suicide attempts. *J Affect Disord* (2011) 129(1):261–9. doi:10.1016/j.jad.2010.08.006
24. Van Orden KA, Witte TK, Cukrowicz KC, Braithwaite SR, Selby EA, Joiner TE Jr. The interpersonal theory of suicide. *Psychol Rev* (2010) 117(2):575–600. doi:10.1037/a0018697
25. Lee S, Lee MT, Chiu MY, Kleinman A. Experience of social stigma by people with schizophrenia in Hong Kong. *Br J Psychiatry* (2005) 186(2):153–7. doi:10.1192/bjp.186.2.153
26. Papastavrou E, Charalambous A, Tsangari H, Karayiannis G. The burdensome and depressive experience of caring: what cancer, schizophrenia, and Alzheimer's disease caregivers have in common. *Cancer Nurs* (2012) 35(3):187–94. doi:10.1097/NCC.0b013e31822cb4a0
27. Addington J, Stowkowy J, Cadenhead KS, Cornblatt BA, McGlashan TH, Perkins DO, et al. Early traumatic experiences in those at clinical high risk for psychosis. *Early Interv Psychiatry* (2013) 7(3):300–5. doi:10.1111/eip.12020
28. Laloyaux J, Dessart G, Van der Linden M, Lemaire M, Larøi F. Maladaptive emotion regulation strategies and stress sensitivity mediate the relation between adverse life events and attenuated positive psychotic symptoms. *Cogn Neuropsychiatry* (2013) 21(2):116–29. doi:10.1080/13546805.2015.11 37213
29. DeVylder JE, Hilimire MR. Suicide risk, stress sensitivity, and self-esteem among young adults reporting auditory hallucinations. *Health Soc Work* (2015) 40(3):175–81. doi:10.1093/hsw/hlv037
30. Pyle M, Stewart SL, French P, Byrne R, Patterson P, Gumley A, et al. Internalized stigma, emotional dysfunction and unusual experiences in young people at risk of psychosis. *Early Interv Psychiatry* (2013) 9(2):133–40. doi:10.1111/eip.12098
31. Kraan T, van Dam DS, Velthorst E, de Ruigh EL, Nieman DH, Durston S, et al. Childhood trauma and clinical outcome in patients at ultra-high risk of transition to psychosis. *Schizophr Res* (2015) 169(1):193–8. doi:10.1016/j.schres.2015.10.030

32. Veling W, Counotte J, Pot-Kolder R, van Os J, van der Gaag M. Childhood trauma, psychosis liability and social stress reactivity: a virtual reality study. *Psychol Med* (2016) 46(16):3339–48. doi:10.1017/S0033291716002208
33. Aldwin CM. Does age affect the stress and coping process? Implications of age differences in perceived control. *J Gerontol* (1991) 46(4):174–80. doi:10.1093/geronj/46.4.P174
34. Bandura A. Perceived self-efficacy in cognitive development and functioning. *Educ Psychol* (1993) 28(2):117–48. doi:10.1207/s15326985ep2802_3
35. Lefcourt HM. Locus of control and the response to aversive events. *Can Psychol Rev* (1976) 17(3):202–9. doi:10.1037/h0081839
36. Haythornthwaite JA, Menefee LA, Heinberg LJ, Clark MR. Pain coping strategies predicting perceived control over pain. *Pain* (1998) 77(1):33–9. doi:10.1016/S0304-3959(98)00078-5
37. Keefe FJ, Kashikar-Zuck S, Robinson E, Salley A, Beaupre P, Caldwell D, et al. Pain coping strategies that predict patients' and spouses' ratings of patients' self-efficacy. *Pain* (1997) 73(2):191–9. doi:10.1016/S0304-3959(97)00109-7
38. Hor K, Taylor M. Suicide and schizophrenia: a systematic review of rates and risk factors. *J Psychopharmacol* (2010) 24(4):81–90. doi:10.1177/1359786810385490
39. Kirkbride JB, Fearon P, Morgan C, Dazzan P, Morgan K, Tarrant J, et al. Heterogeneity in incidence rates of schizophrenia and other psychotic syndromes: findings from the 3-center AeSOP study. *Arch Gen Psychiatry* (2006) 63(3):250–8. doi:10.1001/archpsyc.63.3.250
40. Schultze-Lutter F, Addington J, Ruhrmann S, Klosterkötter J. *Schizophrenia Proneness Instrument, Adult Version (SPI-A)*. Rome: Fioriti (2007).
41. Schultze-Lutter F, Koch E. *Schizophrenia Proneness Instrument, Child and Youth Version (SPI-CY)*. Rome: Fioriti (2010).
42. Janke W, Erdmann G, Kallus KW. *Stressverarbeitungsfragebogen SVF-120*. Göttingen: Hogrefe (1997).
43. Hampel P, Petermann F, Dickow B. *Stressverarbeitungsfragebogen von Janke und Erdmann angepasst für Kinder und Jugendliche*. Göttingen: Hogrefe (2001).
44. Sheehan DV, Lecrubier Y, Sheehan KH, Sheehan K, Amorim P, Janavs J, et al. The Mini-International Neuropsychiatric Interview (M.I.N.I.): the development and validation of a structured diagnostic psychiatric interview for DSM-IV and ICD-10. *J Clin Psychiatry* (1998) 59:22–33.
45. Sheehan DV, Sheehan KH, Shytle RD, Janavs J, Bannon Y, Rogers JE, et al. Reliability and validity of the Mini International Neuropsychiatric Interview for Children and Adolescents (MINI-KID). *J Clin Psychiatry* (2010) 71(3):313–26. doi:10.4088/JCP.09m05305whi
46. Krampen G. *Fragebogen zu Kompetenz-und Kontrollüberzeugungen (FKK)*. Göttingen: Hogrefe (1991).
47. McGlashan T, Walsh B, Woods S. *The Psychosis-Risk Syndrome. Handbook for Diagnosis and Follow-Up*. New York: Oxford University Press (2010). 256 p.
48. McGlashan TH, Miller TJ, Woods SW, Rosen JL, Hoffman RE, Davidson L. *Structured Interview for Prodromal Syndromes*. New Haven: PRIME Research Clinic, Yale School of Medicine (2001).
49. Schultze-Lutter F, Ruhrmann S, Fusar-Poli P, Bechdolf A, Schimmelmann B, Klosterkotter J. Basic symptoms and the prediction of first-episode psychosis. *Curr Pharm Des* (2012) 18(4):351–7. doi:10.2174/138161212799316064
50. Fux L, Walger P, Schimmelmann BG, Schultze-Lutter F. The schizophrenia proneness instrument, child and youth version (SPI-CY): practicability and discriminative validity. *Schizophr Res* (2013) 146(1–3):69–78. doi:10.1016/j.schres.2013.02.014
51. Michel C, Schimmelmann BG, Kupferschmid S, Siegwart M, Schultze-Lutter F. Reliability of telephone assessments of at-risk criteria of psychosis: a comparison to face-to-face interviews. *Schizophr Res* (2014) 153(1):251–3. doi:10.1016/j.schres.2014.01.025
52. Salokangas RK, Schultze-Lutter F, Patterson P, von Reventlow HG, Heinimaa M, From T, et al. Psychometric properties of the Trauma and Distress Scale, TADS, in an adult community sample in Finland. *Eur J Psychotraumatol* (2016) 7:30062. doi:10.3402/ejpt.v7.30062
53. Baryshnikov I, Joffe G, Koivisto M, Melartin T, Aaltonen K, Suominen K, et al. Relationships between self-reported childhood traumatic experiences, attachment style, neuroticism and features of borderline personality disorders in patients with mood disorders. *J Affect Disord* (2017) 210:82–9. doi:10.1016/j.jad.2016.12.004
54. Luutonen S, Tikka M, Karlsson H, Salokangas RK. Childhood trauma and distress experiences associate with psychotic symptoms in patients attending primary and psychiatric outpatient care. Results of the RADEP study. *Eur Psychiatry* (2013) 28(3):154–60. doi:10.1016/j.eurpsy.2011.11.005
55. Hampel P. Brief report: coping among Austrian children and adolescents. *J Adolesc* (2007) 30(5):885–90. doi:10.1016/j.adolescence.2007.04.005
56. Beck AT, Steer RA, Brown GK. *Manual for the Beck Depression Inventory-II*. San Antonio, TX: Psychological Corporation (1996).
57. Ford KA, Wammes M, Neufeld RW, Mitchell D, Théberge J, Williamson P, et al. Unique functional abnormalities in youth with combined marijuana use and depression: an FMRI study. *Front Psychiatry* (2014) 5:130. doi:10.3389/fpsyt.2014.00130
58. Stockings E, Degenhardt L, Lee YY, Mihalopoulos C, Liu A, Hobbs M, et al. Symptom screening scales for detecting major depressive disorder in children and adolescents: a systematic review and meta-analysis of reliability, validity and diagnostic utility. *J Affect Disord* (2015) 174:447–63. doi:10.1016/j.jad.2014.11.061
59. Lee EH, Lee SJ, Hwang ST, Hong SH, Kim JH. Reliability and validity of the Beck Depression Inventory-II among Korean adolescents. *Psychiatry Investig* (2017) 14(1):30–6. doi:10.4306/pi.2017.14.1.30
60. Osman A, Barrios FX, Gutierrez PM, Williams JE, Bailey J. Psychometric properties of the Beck Depression Inventory-II in nonclinical adolescent samples. *J Clin Psychol* (2008) 64(1):83–102. doi:10.1002/jclp.20433
61. Wang YP, Gorenstein C. Psychometric properties of the Beck Depression Inventory-II: a comprehensive review. *Rev Bras Psiquiatr* (2013) 35(4): 416–31. doi:10.1590/1516-4446-2012-1048
62. Brown GK. *A Review of Suicide Assessment Measures for Intervention Research with Adults and Older Adults*. Philadelphia: University of Pennsylvania (2000).
63. Green KL, Brown GK, Jager-Hyman S, Cha J, Steer RA, Beck AT. The predictive validity of the Beck Depression Inventory suicide item. *J Clin Psychiatry* (2015) 76(12):1683–6. doi:10.4088/JCP.14m09391
64. Roaldset JO, Linaker OM, Bjørkly S. Predictive validity of the MINI suicidal scale for self-harm in acute psychiatry: a prospective study of the first year after discharge. *Arch Suicide Res* (2012) 16(4):287–302. doi:10.1080/13811118.2013.722052
65. Straub J, Plener PL, Koelch M, Keller F. Konkordanz zwischen Selbst-und Klinikerurteil hinsichtlich depressiver Symptomatik bei Jugendlichen am Beispiel von BDI-II und CDRS-R. *Z Kinder Jugendpsychiatr Psychother* (2014) 42:243–52. doi:10.1024/1422-4917/a000297
66. Brown TA. *Confirmatory Factor Analysis for Applied Researchers*. New York, NY: Guilford Press (2006).
67. Asparouhov T, Muthén B. *Multiple Imputation with Mplus 2010*. (2016). 25 p. Available from: http://www.statmodel.com/download/Imputations7.pdf
68. Baron RM, Kenny DA. The moderator-mediator variable distinction in social psychological research: conceptual, strategic, and statistical considerations. *J Pers Soc Psychol* (1986) 51(6):1173–82. doi:10.1037/0022-3514.51.6.1173
69. Little TD. *Longitudinal Structural Equation Modelling*. New York: The Guilford Press (2013). 386 p.
70. Preacher KJ, Hayes AF. SPSS and SAS procedures for estimating indirect effects in simple mediation models. *Behav Res Methods Instrum Comput* (2004) 36(4):717–31. doi:10.3758/BF03206553
71. American Psychiatric Association, editor. Social and Occupational Functioning Assessment Scale (SOFAS). *Diagnostic and Statistical Manual of Mental Disorders*. Washington, DC: American Psychiatric Association (2000).
72. Preti A, Meneghelli A, Pisano A, Cocchi A. Risk of suicide and suicidal ideation in psychosis: results from an Italian multi-modal pilot program on early intervention in psychosis. *Schizophr Res* (2009) 113(2):145–50. doi:10.1016/j.schres.2009.06.007
73. Soloff PH, Lynch KG, Kelly TM. Childhood abuse as a risk factor for suicidal behavior in borderline personality disorder. *J Personal Disord* (2009) 16(3):201–14. doi:10.1521/pedi.16.3.201.22542
74. Barbosa LP, Quevedo L, da Silva GD, Jansen K, Pinheiro RT, Branco J, et al. Childhood trauma and suicide risk in a sample of young individuals aged 14-35 years in southern Brazil. *Child Abuse Negl* (2014) 38(7):1191–6. doi:10.1016/j.chiabu.2014.02.008
75. De Araújo RM, Lara DR. More than words: the association of childhood emotional abuse and suicidal behavior. *Eur Psychiatry* (2016) 37:14–21. doi:10.1016/j.eurpsy.2016.04.002

76. Futa KT, Nash CL, Hansen DJ, Garbin CP. Adult survivors of childhood abuse: an analysis of coping mechanisms used for stressful childhood memories and current stressors. *J Fam Violence* (2003) 18(4):227–39. doi:10.1023/A:1024068314963
77. Martin MS, Dykxhoorn J, Afifi TO, Colman I. Child abuse and the prevalence of suicide attempts among those reporting suicide ideation. *Soc Psychiatry Psychiatr Epidemiol* (2016) 51(11):1477–84. doi:10.1007/s00127-016-1250-3
78. Joiner TE, Sachs-Ericsson NJ, Wingate LR, Brown JS, Anestis MD, Selby EA. Childhood physical and sexual abuse and lifetime number of suicide attempts: a persistent and theoretically important relationship. *Behav Res Ther* (2007) 45(3):539–47. doi:10.1016/j.brat.2006.04.007
79. Shikai N, Uji M, Chen Z, Hiramura H, Tanaka N, Shono M, et al. The role of coping styles and self-efficacy in the development of dysphoric mood among nursing students. *J Psychopathol Behav Assess* (2007) 29(4):241–8. doi:10.1007/s10862-007-9043-3
80. Berthelot N, Paccalet T, Gilbert E, Moreau I, Mérette C, Gingras N, et al. Childhood abuse and neglect may induce deficits in cognitive precursors of psychosis in high-risk children. *J Psychiatry Neurosci* (2015) 40(5):336–43. doi:10.1503/jpn.140211
81. Wilder-Willis KE, Shear PK, Steffen JJ, Borkin J. The relationship between cognitive dysfunction and coping abilities in schizophrenia. *Schizophr Res* (2002) 55(3):259–67. doi:10.1016/S0920-9964(01)00211-0
82. Aldao A, Nolen-Hoeksema S, Schweizer S. Emotion-regulation strategies across psychopathology: a meta-analytic review. *Clin Psychol Rev* (2010) 30(2):217–37. doi:10.1016/j.cpr.2009.11.004
83. Canetti D, Kimhi S, Hanoun R, Rocha GA, Galea S, Morgan CA III. How personality affects vulnerability among Israelis and Palestinians following the 2009 Gaza conflict. *PLoS One* (2016) 11(7):e0156278. doi:10.1371/journal.pone.0156278
84. Law KC, Khazem LR, Anestis MD. The role of emotion dysregulation in suicide as considered through the ideation to action framework. *Curr Opin Psychol* (2015) 3:30–5. doi:10.1016/j.copsyc.2015.01.014
85. Sandler IN, Tein JY, Mehta P, Wolchik S, Ayers T. Coping efficacy and psychological problems of children of divorce. *Child Dev* (2000) 71(4):1099–118. doi:10.1111/1467-8624.00212
86. Asselmann E, Wittchen HU, Lieb R, Höfler M, Beesdo-Baum K. Does low coping efficacy mediate the association between negative life events and incident psychopathology? A prospective-longitudinal community study among adolescents and young adults. *Epidemiol Psychiatr Sci* (2016) 25(02):171–80. doi:10.1017/S204579601500013X
87. Li D, Zhang W, Li X, Li N, Ye B. Gratitude and suicidal ideation and suicide attempts among Chinese adolescents: direct, mediated, and moderated effects. *J Adolesc* (2012) 35(1):55–66. doi:10.1016/j.adolescence.2011.06.005
88. Kleiman EM, Riskind JH, Schaefer KE. Social support and positive events as suicide resiliency factors: examination of synergistic buffering effects. *Arch Suicide Res* (2014) 18(2):144–55. doi:10.1080/13811118.2013.826155
89. Dennison MJ, Sheridan MA, Busso DS, Jenness JL, Peverill M, Rosen ML, et al. Neurobehavioral markers of resilience to depression among adolescents exposed to child abuse. *J Abnorm Psychol* (2016) 125(8):1201–12. doi:10.1037/abn0000215
90. Morris MC, Kouros CD, Fox KR, Rao U, Garber J. Interactive models of depression vulnerability: the role of childhood trauma, dysfunctional attitudes, and coping. *Br J Clin Psychol* (2014) 53(2):245–63. doi:10.1111/bjc.12038
91. Fusar-Poli P, Nelson B, Valmaggia L, Yung AR, McGuire PK. Comorbid depressive and anxiety disorder in 509 individuals with an at-risk mental state: impact on psychopathology and transition to psychosis. *Schizophr Bull* (2014) 40(1):120–31. doi:10.1093/schbul/sbs136
92. Hardy A, Emsley R, Freeman D, Bebbington P, Garety PA, Kuipers EE, et al. Psychological mechanisms mediating effects between trauma and psychotic symptoms: the role of affect regulation, intrusive trauma memory, beliefs, and depression. *Schizophr Bull* (2016) 42(Suppl 1):S34–43. doi:10.1093/schbul/sbv175
93. Fujita J, Takahashi Y, Nishida A, Okumura Y, Ando S, Kawano M, et al. Auditory verbal hallucinations increase the risk for suicide attempts in adolescents with suicidal ideation. *Schizophr Res* (2015) 168(1):209–12. doi:10.1016/j.schres.2015.07.028
94. Van Dam DS, van Nierop M, Viechtbauer W, Velthorst E, van Winkel R, Bruggeman R, et al. Childhood abuse and neglect in relation to the presence and persistence of psychotic and depressive symptomatology. *Psychol Med* (2015) 45(7):1363–77. doi:10.1017/S0033291714001561
95. Barrett EA, Sundet K, Faerden A, Nesvåg R, Agartz I, Fosse R, et al. Suicidality before and in the early phases of first episode psychosis. *Schizophr Res* (2010) 119(1):11–7. doi:10.1016/j.schres.2010.03.022
96. Klosterkötter J. The meaning of basic symptoms for the genesis of the schizophrenic nuclear syndrome. *Jpn J Psychiatry Neurol* (1992) 46(3):609–30. doi:10.1111/j.1440-1819.1992.tb00535.x
97. Massons C, Lopez-Morinigo JD, Pousa E, Ruiz A, Ochoa S, Usall J. Insight and suicidality in psychosis: a cross-sectional study. *Psychiatry Res* (2017) 252:147–53. doi:10.1016/j.psychres.2017.02.059
98. Schultze-Lutter F, Debbané M, Theodoridou A, Wood SJ, Raballo A, Michel C, et al. Revisiting the basic symptoms concept: toward translating risk symptoms for psychosis into neurobiological targets. *Front Psychiatry* (2016) 7:9. doi:10.3389/fpsyt.2016.00009
99. Schultze-Lutter F, Michel C, Schmidt SJ, Schimmelmann BG, Maric NP, Salokangas RK, et al. EPA guidance on the early detection of clinical high risk states of psychoses. *Eur Psychiatry* (2015) 30(3):405–16. doi:10.1016/j.eurpsy.2015.01.010
100. Johnson J, Wood AM, Gooding P, Taylor PJ, Tarrier N. Resilience to suicidality: the buffering hypothesis. *Clin Psychol Rev* (2011) 31(4):563–91. doi:10.1016/j.cpr.2010.12.007
101. Waite P, McManus F, Shafran R. Cognitive behaviour therapy for low self-esteem: a preliminary randomized controlled trial in a primary care setting. *J Behav Ther Exp Psychiatry* (2012) 43(4):1049–57. doi:10.1016/j.jbtep.2012.04.006
102. Walsh K, Fortier MA, DiLillo D. Adult coping with childhood sexual abuse: a theoretical and empirical review. *Aggress Violent Behav* (2010) 15(1):1–13. doi:10.1016/j.avb.2009.06.009

14

Serious Suicide Attempts: Systematic Review of Psychological Risk Factors

Yari Gvion[1] and Yossi Levi-Belz[2]*

[1] Bar-Ilan University, Ramat Gan, Israel, [2] Ruppin Academic Center, Emek Hefer, Israel

***Correspondence:**
Yari Gvion
yari@kadi.co.il

Background: One of the main obstacles in studying suicide risk factors is the difference between cases in which the individual died by suicide and those in which the individual engaged in suicidal behavior. A promising strategy that overcomes this obstacle is the study of survivors of *serious suicide attempt* (SSA), i.e., an attempt that would have been lethal had it not been for the provision of rapid and effective emergency treatment. Serious suicide attempters are epidemiologically very much like those who died by suicide, and thus may serve as valid proxies for studying suicides. This paper aims to define the specific risk factors for SSAs by conducting a qualitative data synthesis of existing studies.

Methods: Following Preferred Reporting Items for Systematic Reviews and Meta-Analyses guidelines, we conducted a systematic search of the literature in PubMed, ProQuest, and Psychlit electronic research-literature databases. Search terms were "serious" "OR" "near lethal," combined with the Boolean "AND" operator with "suicide*." In addition, we performed a manual search on Google Scholar for further studies not yet identified.

Results: The preliminary search identified 683 citations. A total of 39 research reports that met the predefined criteria were analyzed. Mental pain, communication difficulties, decision-making impulsivity, and aggression, as well as several demographic variables, were found to be major risk factors for SSAs.

Limitations: We found a variability of definitions for SSA that hamper the ability to draw a model for the risk factors and processes that facilitate it. Moreover, the role of suicide intent and planning in SSA is still unclear. Further studies should aim to clarify and refine the concepts and measures of SSA, thereby enabling more specific and concrete modeling of the psychological element in its formation.

Conclusion: SSA is a distinguishable phenomenon that needs to be addressed specifically within the scope of suicidal behavior. Interpersonal problems, as well as impulsivity and aggression, seem to facilitate SSA when mental pain serves as a secondary factor. Healthcare professionals should be aware of SSA, and familiar with its specific risk factors. Moreover, psychological and suicidal risk assessment should include a designated evaluation of these risk factors as part of intervention and prevention models for SSA.

Keywords: suicide, medical lethality, suicide intent, mental pain, decision making, interpersonal, systematic review

INTRODUCTION

While the significance of identification, assessment, and intervention in the prevention of suicide attempts (SAs), and particularly, of suicide completion is undisputed, suicide completion is still recurrent at an annual yearly global age-standardized rate of 11.4 per one hundred thousand. Furthermore, approximately 10 times this rate attempt suicide annually (1). Thus, suicidologists are still faced with the challenge of identifying the factors leading to suicide (2, 3).

The first step toward identifying risk factors for suicide is to determine how to study this phenomenon. In general, suicidal behavior comprises a diverse set of behaviors, including suicidal thoughts, non-suicidal self-injuries, SAs, and actual death by suicide (4). Other related behaviors are deliberate self-harm, parasuicide, and non-suicidal self-injury (5). Given the significant differences between these behavioral categories, suicidologists are aware that the generalizability of research findings is dramatically affected by the population selected for study (4, 6). To date, one of the most prevalent methods for studying suicide is the psychological autopsy (7, 8). This strategy allows for very detailed information about the patient, including psychiatric records, police investigations, military records, etc. (9). However, while this approach can be informative as to certain suicide features, such as sociodemographic characteristics and psychiatric disorders, a serious limitation remains its lack of access to information pertaining to the subject's difficulties, problems, and processes, particularly those of a more personal nature (10).

Serious Suicide Attempt (SSA) Strategy

An alternative and promising strategy for investigating suicide focuses on the study of SSA survivors. As a concept, SSA is an SA which would have been fatal without the provision of speedy and effective first-aid care, other forms of emergency treatment or, in some cases, mere coincidence (11, 12).

Thus, SSA is an SA that requires hospitalization for more than 24 h and meets one of the following treatment criteria: (a) treatment in specialized units, including the intensive care unit; (b) surgery under general anesthesia; and (c) extensive medical treatment, including antidotes for drug overdose, telemetry, or repeated tests or investigations. In addition, attempted suicide by methods carrying a high-fatality risk (e.g., hanging or gunshot) is also defined as medically serious suicide attempt (MSSA) if the attempt led to hospitalization for over 24 h (13, 14). Individuals who have made SSAs may serve as valid proxies for studying suicides given that they are epidemiologically very much like those who complete suicide (13, 15), and twice as liable as other suicide attempters to subsequently complete suicide (16, 17).

Due to its emphasis on access to SSA survivors, this approach has several important advantages which have broadened the scope of potential research areas (14, 18, 19). Studying individuals who have survived a potentially lethal incident of self-harm enables a comprehensive inquiry into both the psychological processes leading up to the suicidal act, and the influence of early and current experiences that serve as catalysts for suicide (20, 21). Moreover, this approach may provide some insight into many first attempt suicide completers, who mental health professionals have so far neglected. Another advantage is the ability to follow patients who survived near-fatal attempts and explore their treatment outcomes (21, 22). To conclude, as Hawton postulated, "investigating survivors of SSAs can develop into a key research strategy in the study of suicidal behavior" [(20), p. 3].

Throughout the history of suicide research, authors have operationalized SSA's definition in various ways, using widely differing criteria (e.g., hospitalization, suicide intent more than zero, violent method, etc.). This diversity of definitions, as well as of measures used and populations studied, make arriving at aggregate conclusions rather difficult.

Thus, the crucial question is how to best identify serious suicide attempters for studies of this kind. Drawing on Levi-Belz and Beautrais' review (21) and several different studies in the field (13, 14, 18, 19), in this study we conceptualized SSA in terms of the attempt's *actual medical lethality*. Medical lethality can be inferred from two different, but overlapping, dimensions: the suicidal act's physiological consequences, and post-attempt medical procedures. Thus, we defined SSA as an SA that causes a significant physical injury requiring intensive, substantial medical treatment. Accordingly, we aimed to systematically review more recent studies whose definitions of SSA are based solely on these criteria. Our goal was to illuminate the psychological risk factors that relate to, or even facilitate, SSA, such as data regarding correlations, mediating roles, predictions, and comparisons between variables associated with SSA. As no such systematic review has been executed to date, we are hopeful that the results of this study will enhance knowledge of specific risk factors and psychological processes. This knowledge, in turn, may then facilitate SSA prediction, and enable researchers and clinicians to customize treatment programs for those at risk for SSA and suicide.

METHODS

Information Databases and Searches

A comprehensive digital search strategy was applied to identify peer-reviewed articles on the relation between SSA and a wide range of psychological factors. This strategy is in line with Preferred Reporting Items for Systematic Reviews and Meta-Analyses (23). We also searched PubMed and Psycnet databases. Search terms were "serious" "OR" "near lethal" in combination with the Boolean "AND" operator with "suicide." In addition, a manual search in Google Scholar was performed for hitherto unidentified studies.

Study Selection

Studies were eligible if they were original, written in English, and presented data regarding a wide range of psychological factors associated with SSA. To focus solely on recent studies, we included studies from 2000. This time frame is also consistent with the emergence of the SSA strategy first proposed by Beautrais in studies from 1996 and 1999. Thus, we searched papers dating from January 1, 2000 to October 31, 2017. Case studies, reviews, book chapters, conference papers, and incomplete studies were excluded.

Data Analysis

As studies on SSA risk factors are highly heterogeneous, with different study designs, measures, and sample types, they could not be combined into a singular meta-analysis study. Consequently, we conducted a systematic review of the results of each study. Studies were first categorized based on clusters of risk factors (e.g., mental pain, interpersonal factors, impulsivity, etc.), and then summarized while highlighting the information unique for each study, as well as features common to the studies in each cluster.

RESULTS

The database search yielded a total of 683 citations. Based on both inclusion and exclusion criteria, a total of 39 original research studies were identified and included in the systematic review (see flowchart in **Figure 1**). In what follows, we present the literature review results, which have been sub-grouped according to common risk factor themes. A detailed description of reviewed studies is presented in **Table 1**.

Psychopathology

Given its strong linkages with suicide (58–60), psychopathology was most likely to constitute a risk factor for SSAs. Several studies have examined the relationships between SSA and specific DSM mental disorders (depressive disorder, borderline personality disorder, etc.). Led by Beautrais, The Canterbury Suicide Project in New Zealand was one of the pioneer studies in the field of SSAs (13, 14). Beautrais (14) examined 125 young (under 25) individuals who made SSAs, and compared them to 151 healthy controls. Also in the framework of this project, Beautrais et al. (61) found that those who executed SSAs had high levels of mental disorders (according to the DSM-III-R diagnoses) and psychiatric comorbidity at the time of the SA. More specifically, they found that the probability that SSA attempters were diagnosed with major depressive disorder (MDD), anxiety disorders, and anti-social behaviors was higher when compared with non-suicidal subjects (14). In another study, Beautrais (26) found similar results: current mood disorders elevated the risk for SSAs mostly among older adults [odd ratio (OR) = 179]. Psychiatric hospital admission within the previous year was also found to elevate the risk for SSAs [OR = 24.4 (26)]. Interestingly, the strong relationship between depression and suicidal behavior, and SSAs was even found on the temperamental level, whereas Rihmer et al. (62) found that four of the five affective temperaments contained depressive components (i.e., depressive, cyclothymic, irritable, and anxious).

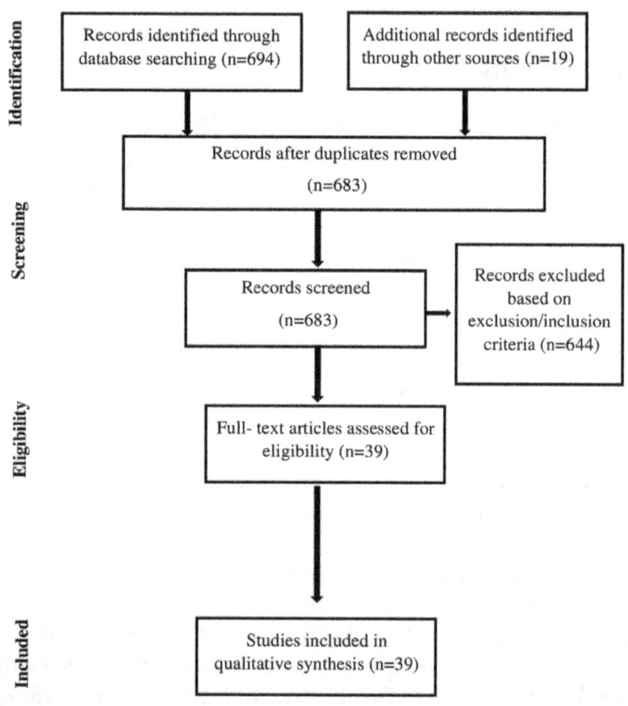

FIGURE 1 | Dataset selection process.

Rivlin et al. (48) focused on male prisoners who made SSAs, and compared them to 60 prisoners who had never performed near-lethal SAs in prison (control group). The results showed that psychiatric disorders and specific mood disorders are highly common among serious suicide attempters. Specifically, psychiatric disorders were present in all SSA cases, while present in only 62% of the controls. The current psychiatric disorders most associated with SSAs included major depression (OR = 42.0), psychosis (OR = 15.0), and anxiety disorders (OR = 6.0). Marzano et al. (43) employed the same design on 60 female prisoners and on controls. Here too, the strongest associations were between SSAs and current depression (OR = 23.7), and with the history of psychiatric in-patients' admissions (OR = 25.4). Other studies reached similar results (32, 35). Lopez-Castroman et al. (41) investigated 726 adult patients who had attempted suicide, of which 104 met SSA criteria. The authors found that individuals who made SSAs had a significantly higher probability of receiving a diagnosis of PTSD (OR = 1.86). Interestingly, when combined with a lifetime diagnosis of PTSD, individuals who experienced different types of childhood abuse (emotional, physical, and/or sexual) showed an increased risk for serious attempts (up to OR of 4.14).

Another factor for SSA is substance abuse disorders, including alcohol, cannabis, cocaine, and opiate abuse/dependence. The research clearly shows that substance abuse is strongly correlated with suicidal behavior. Thus, cannabis use/dependence is commonly attributed to suicide attempters or completers who reported some additional risk factors for suicide, such as mood disorders, stressful life events, interpersonal problems, poor social support, loneliness, and feelings of hopelessness (63).

Although there are numerous studies on the linkage between suicide behavior and substance use disorder (SUD), the literature regarding the association between SUD and SSA has been limited since Beautrais, Joyce, and Mulder's pioneering study in 1999 (11). In this study, 302 instances of SSA were compared with 1,028 healthy controls from the local community. 16.2% of those who performed SSAs met DSM criteria for cannabis abuse/dependence at the time of the SA, while among the control group, only 1.9% met DSM criteria for cannabis abuse/dependence.

TABLE 1 | Characteristics of studies used in the review.

Number	Study	Title	Aim	Sample information
1.	Apter et al. (24)	Relationship between self-disclosure and serious suicidal behavior	To study the influence of self-disclosure on suicide attempters and completers	Sample size: 80 divided into four groups; G1 patients with suicidal thoughts but no suicidal behavior (20); G2 patients who made a mild SA (20); G3 patients who made an SSA (20); G4 patients who had no suicidal behavior (20) Mean age: G1 = 38.3 (SD = 15.0) years; G2 = 36.7 (SD = 17.2) years; G3 = 39.7 (SD = 18.9) years; G4 = 40.5 (SD = 16.1) years Female: G1 = 55%; G2 = 55%; G3 = 55%; G4 = 50%
2.	Barnes et al. (25)	Help-seeking behavior prior to nearly lethal suicide attempts	To define various help-seeking behaviors prior to a nearly lethal suicide attempt in a population of adolescents and young adults and to examine the association between these behaviors and nearly lethal suicide attempts	Sample size: 666 divided into two groups; G1 hospitalized after an NLSA (153); G2 controls from population-based sample (513) Mean age: NA Female: G1 = 46%; G2 = 57%
3.	Beautrais (13)	Suicides and serious suicide attempts: two populations or one?	To compare suicides and serious suicide attempts in terms of known risk factors for suicidal behavior	Sample size: 1,461 divided into three groups; G1 individuals who died by suicide (202); G2 individuals who made an MSSA (275); G3 control subjects (984) Mean age: G1 = 36.8 (SD = 16.2) years; G2 = 30.0 (SD = 14.2) years; G3 = NA Female: G1 = 22.3%; G2 = 54.9%; G3 = NA
4.	Beautrais (26)	A case–control study of suicide and attempted suicide in older adults	To provide a descriptive profile of the sociodemographic, mental, and physical health characteristics and life circumstances of older people who make serious suicide attempts or die by suicide, and, using a case–control design, to compare these characteristics with those of a randomly selected community comparison series of adults of similar age	Sample size: 322 divided into three groups; G1 individuals who made an MSSA (22); G2 individuals who died by suicide (31); G3 comparison subjects (269) Mean age: G1 = 66.3 (SD = 9.2) years; G2 = 65.2 (SD = 8.2); G3 = 67.6 (SD = 8.5) years Female: G1 = 68.2%; G2 = 35.5%; G3 = NA
5.	Beautrais (14)	Suicide and serious suicide attempts in youth: a multiple-group comparison study	To compare risk factors for suicide and medically serious non-fatal suicide attempts among youth under 25 years of age	Sample size: 336 divided into three groups; G1 individuals who committed suicide (60); G2 individuals who made an MSSA (125); G3 non-suicidal individuals (151) Mean age: G1 = 19.98 (SD = 2.53) years; G2 = 19.31 (SD = 3.1); G3 = 21.43 (SD = 1.52) years Female: G1 = 18.3%; G2 = 54.4%; G3 = 48.3%
6.	Beautrais et al. (27)	Unemployment and serious suicide attempts	To examine the association between unemployment and risk of medically serious suicide attempt	Sample size: 1,330 divided into two groups; G1 individuals who made an MSSA (302); G2 non-suicidal individuals (1,028) Mean age: G1 = 30.4 (SD = 14.2) years; G2 NA Female: G1 = 53.6%; G2 = NA
7.	Beautrais et al. (11)	Cannabis abuse and serious suicide attempts	To compare the relationship between cannabis abuse/dependence and risk of medically serious suicide attempts in individuals making serious suicide attempts and randomly selected comparison subjects	Sample size: 1,330 divided into two groups; G1 individuals who made an MSSA (302); G2 non-suicidal individuals (1,028) Mean age: NA Female: NA
8.	Conner et al. (28)	Risk factors for suicide and medically serious suicide attempts among alcoholics: analyses of Canterbury Suicide Project data	To identify risk factors for serious suicidal behavior among individuals with alcohol dependence	Sample size: 146 participants with alcohol dependence divided into three groups; G1 completed suicide (38); G2 individuals who made an MSSA (62); G3 community controls (46) Mean age: NA Female: NA
9.	Conner et al. (29)	Moderators of the relationship between alcohol dependence and suicide and medically serious suicide attempts: analyses of Canterbury Suicide Project data	To evaluate potential moderators of the relationship between alcohol dependence and suicide and medically serious suicide attempts by using case–control data gathered in the Canterbury region of New Zealand for the Canterbury Suicide Project	Sample size: 1,417 divided into three groups; G1 suicide decedents (193); G2 individuals who made an MSSA (240); G3 community controls (984) Mean age: G1 = 37.7 (SD = 15.9) years; G2 = 32.1 (SD = 14.0); G3 = 43.5 (SD = 17.7) years Female: G1 = 22.8%; G2 = 52.5%; G3 = 51.6%

(Continued)

TABLE 1 | Continued

Number	Study	Title	Aim	Sample information
10.	Doihara et al. (30)	Trait aggression in suicide attempters: a pilot study	To investigate aggression in medically serious suicide attempters at an emergency department in Japan	Sample size: 126 divided into two groups; G1 hospitalized for an MSSA (55); G2 healthy control group (71) Mean age: G1 = 39.0 (SD = 16.6) years; G2 = 34.3 (SD = 11.3) years Female: G1 = 60%; G2 = 71.8%
	Dombrovski et al. (31)	Lethal forethought: delayed reward discounting differentiates high- and low-lethality suicide attempts in old age	To examine the hypothesis that individuals who make less serious suicide attempts would show a preference for immediate rewards, whereas those who plan and carry out the most serious attempts would be more patient	Sample size: 80 divided into five groups; G1 individuals who made high-lethality SA (15); G2 individuals who made low-lethality SA (14); G3 "ideators" (12); G4 non-suicidal depressed (42); G5 psychiatrically healthy (31) Mean age: G1 = 67.4 (SD = 7.1) years; G2 = 66.1 (SD = 8.1) years; G3 = 69.5 (SD = 8.7) years; G4 = 70.3 (SD = 8.6) years; G5 = 68.1 (SD = 5.8) Female: G1 = 46.7%; G2 = 64.3%; G3 = 33.3%; G4 = 64.3%; G5 = 45.2%
11.	Donald et al. (32)	Risk and protective factors for medically serious suicide attempts: a comparison of hospital-based with population-based samples of young adults	To investigate risk and protective factors for medically serious suicide attempts among young Australian adults	Sample size: 475 divided into two groups; G1 hospitalized after an SA (95); G2 matched controls from population-based sample (380) Mean age: NA Female: G1 = 48.4%; G2 = 48%
12.	Durant et al. (33)	Racial differences in hopelessness as a risk factor for a nearly lethal suicide attempt	To explore the relationship between hopelessness, race, and suicidal behavior	Sample size: 327 divided into two groups; G1 hospitalized after an NLSA (153); G2 controls from population-based sample (513) Mean age: NA Female: G1 = 45%; G2 = 64%
13.	Elliott et al. (34)	A profile of medically serious suicide attempts	To identify factors associated with medically serious suicide attempts (requiring medical hospitalization)	Sample size: 97 divided into two groups; G1 individuals who made an MSSA (65); G2 individuals who made an MNSSA (32) Mean age: NA Female: NA
14.	Fowler et al. (35)	Risk factors for medically serious suicide attempts: evidence for a psychodynamic formulation of suicidal crisis	To explore a psychodynamic model for suicide risk by examining risk factors for medically serious suicide attempts, including assessments of affect flooding, negative self-schema/fragmentation, and impaired reality testing, closely approximating Maltsberger's psychodynamic formulation of suicide crisis	Sample Size: 75 divided into three groups; G1 inpatients with an MSSA (25); G2 inpatients with no suicidal activity (25); G3 outpatients with no suicidal activity (25) Mean age: G1 = 32.2 (SD = 11.3) years; G2 = 31.3 (SD = 14.7) years; G3 = 30.9 (SD = 14.4) years Female: G1 = 76%; G2 = 68%; G3 = 68%
15.	Gvion et al. (19)	Aggression-impulsivity, mental pain, and communication difficulties in medically serious and medically non-serious suicide attempters	To evaluate the relative effects of aggression and impulsivity on the lethality of suicide attempts	Sample size: 196 divided into four groups; G1 hospitalized for MSSA (43); G2 MNSSA (49); G3 psychiatric control group (47); G4 healthy control group (57) Mean age: G1 = 37.37 (SD = 13.31) years; G2 = 40.31 (SD = 13.76) years; G3 = 40.96 (SD = 14.07) years; G4 = 37.28 (SD = 12.34) years Female: G1 = 39.5%; G2 = 30.6%; G3 = 29.8%; G4 = 45.6%
16.	Gvion (36)	Aggression, impulsivity and their predictive value on medical lethality of suicide attempts: a follow-up study on hospitalized patients	To study the role of aggressive impulsive variants and suicide history in predicting the medical severity of follow-up suicide attempts	Sample size: 97 divided into three groups; G1 history of MSSA (33); G2 history of MNSSA (29); no history of suicide (35) Mean age: NA Female: NA
17.	Horesh et al. (37)	Medically serious versus non-serious suicide attempts: relationships of lethality and intent to clinical and interpersonal characteristics	To investigate the relationship of intent and lethality in medically serious and medically non-serious suicide attempts and to examine relationship of specific psychological and clinical variables with the subjective and objective components of suicide intent	Sample size: 102 divided into two groups; G1 patients after an MSSA (35); G2 patients after an MNSSA (67) Mean age: G1 = 39.7 (SD = 15.3) years; G2 = 37.3 (SD = 14.0) years Female: G1 = 48.6%; G2 = 53.7%

(Continued)

TABLE 1 | Continued

Number	Study	Title	Aim	Sample information
18.	Levi et al. (38)	Mental pain and its communication in medically serious suicide attempts: an "impossible situation"	To test the hypothesis that mental pain is a general risk factor for suicidal behavior and communication difficulties are a particular risk factor for medically serious suicidal behavior	Sample size: 173 divided into three groups; G1 hospitalized for an MSSA (35); G2 MNSSA (67); G3 without psychiatric diagnosis or history of suicidal behavior (71) Mean age: G1 = 39.7 (SD = 15.3) years; G2 = 37.3 (SD = 14.0) years; G3 = 36.5 (SD = 14.0) years Female: G1 = 48.6%; G2 = 53.7%; G3 = 47.9%
19.	Levi-Belz et al. (39)	Attachment patterns in medically serious suicide attempts: the mediating role of self-disclosure and loneliness	To examine the associations between attachment patterns to severe suicidal behavior	Sample size: 102 divided into two groups; G1 patients after an MSSA (35); G2 patients after an MNSSA (67) Mean age: G1 = 39.7 (SD = 15.3) years; G2 = 37.3 (SD = 14.0) years Female: G1 = 48.6%; G2 = 53.7%
20.	Levi-Belz et al. (18)	Mental pain, communication difficulties, and medically serious suicide attempts: a case–control study	To assess the role of mental pain and communication difficulties in MSSA	Sample size: 336 divided into four groups; G1 hospitalized for MSSA (78); G2 MNSSA (116); G3 psychiatric control group (47); G4 healthy control group (95) Mean age: G1 = 38.5 (SD = 14.2) years; G2 = 38.5 (SD = 13.9) years; G3 = 40.9 (SD = 14.0) years; G4 = 38.5 (SD = 14.2) years Female: G1 = 43.6%; G2 = 56.0%; G3 = 70.2%; G4 = 45.3%
21.	Lohner and Konrad (40)	Deliberate self-harm and suicide attempt in custody: distinguishing features in male inmates' self-injurious behavior	To find differences between self-injurious behavior of "low seriousness" (i.e., low-lethality and low-suicidal intent) and of "high seriousness," by inmates while under custodial authority	Sample size: 49 male inmates exhibiting self-injurious behavior and high-lethal suicide attempts Mean age: 27.1 (SD = 9.152) years
22.	Lopez-Castroman et al. (41)	Post-traumatic stress disorder following childhood abuse increases the severity of suicide attempts	To investigate the association of PTSD and childhood abuse to suicide attempts	Sample size: 726 suicide attempters Mean age: NA (median) Female: 74.4%
23.	Lopez-Castroman et al. (42)	Heavy tobacco dependence in suicide attempters making recurrent and medically serious attempts	To investigate, specifically, the association between the level of tobacco dependence and the severity of suicidal outcomes among suicide attempters, as well as the relationship of impulsivity with both conditions	Sample size: 542 hospitalized patients in a unit for affective disorders and suicidal behavior Mean age: NA (median—41.1) Female: 73.6%
24.	Marzano et al. (43)	Psychiatric disorders in women prisoners who have engaged in near-lethal self-harm: case–control study	To investigate prevalence of psychiatric disorders in women prisoners who had recently engaged in near-lethal self-harm (cases) and others who had never carried out near-lethal attempts in prison (controls)	Sample size: 120 female prisoners divided into two groups; G1 made an NLSA (60); G2 matched controls (60) Mean age: NA (median: G1-25.5, G2-26)
25.	Marzano et al. (44)	Psychosocial influences on prisoner suicide: a case–control study of near-lethal self-harm in women prisoners	To examine the psychosocial influences on female prisoner suicide by carrying out a study of near-lethal self-harm	Sample size: 120 female prisoners divided into two groups; G1 made an NLSA (60); G2 matched controls (60) Mean age: NA (median)
26.	McGirr et al. (45)	Deterministic learning and attempted suicide among older depressed individuals: cognitive assessment using the Wisconsin Card Sorting Task	To characterize the relationship between suicidal behavior and cognitive control during learning in a complex environment among older individuals	Sample size: 93 divided into four groups; G1 individuals who made high-lethality SA (14); G2 individuals who made low-lethality SA (20); G3 non-suicidal depressed (29); G4 healthy controls (30) Mean age: G1 = 68.86 (SD = 7.53) years; G2 = 66.80 (SD = 8.15) years; G3 = 70.30 (SD = 9.03) years; G4 = 69.77 (SD = 6.76) years Female: G1 = 50%; G2 = 50%; G3 = 65.5%; G4 = 46.7%
27.	Potter et al. (46)	The influence of geographic mobility on nearly lethal suicide attempts	To understand the relationship between mobility and suicidal behavior by studying the association at the individual level of analysis, in a large sample, and using a rigorous measure of suicidal behavior	Sample size: 666 divided into two groups; G1 cases of NLSA (153); G2 control subjects (513) Mean age: NA (range 13–34) Female: G1 = 45.8%; G2 = 56.9%

(*Continued*)

TABLE 1 | Continued

Number	Study	Title	Aim	Sample information
28.	Powell et al. (47)	Alcohol consumption and nearly lethal suicide attempts	To examine various pathways that may link alcohol consumption and suicide, which might be used to identify persons at higher risk of suicide	Sample size: 666 divided into two groups; G1 hospitalized after an NLSA (153); G2 controls from population-based sample (513) Mean age: NA Female: G1 = 45.8%; G2 = 56.9%
29.	Rivlin et al. (48)	Psychiatric disorders in male prisoners who made near-lethal suicide attempts: case–control study	To investigate the association of psychiatric disorders with near-lethal suicide attempts in male prisoners	Sample size: 120 male prisoners divided into two groups; G1 made an NLSA (60); G2 matched controls (60) Mean age: NA
30.	Rivlin et al. (49)	The suicidal process in male prisoners making near-lethal suicide attempts	To identify the psychological problems and processes leading up to, and following, suicide attempts in order to identify key opportunities for prevention	Sample size: 60 male prisoners who had made NLSA Mean age: NA (median—29 years)
31.	Simon et al. (50)	Characteristics of impulsive suicide attempts and attempters. Suicide and life-threatening behavior	To test four hypotheses concerning the characteristics of individuals who make impulsive and non-impulsive suicide attempts	Sample size: 666 divided into two groups; G1 cases of NLSA (153); G2 control subjects (513) Mean age: NA (range 13–34) Female: NA
32.	Soloff et al. (51)	High-lethality status in patients with borderline personality disorder	To identify risk factors for suicide within a BPD sample by comparing patients with high-and low-lethality attempts	Sample size: 113 borderline personality disorder attempters divided into two groups; G1 high-lethality attempters (44); G2 low-lethality attempters (69) Mean age: G1 = 31.3 (SD = 8.8) years; G2 = 27.5 (SD = 7.6) years Female: G1 = 63.6%; G2 = 76.8%
33.	Swahn and Potter (52)	Factors associated with the medical severity of suicide attempts in youths and young adults	To determine how demographic factors, symptoms of mental health problems, help-seeking behaviors, and the characteristics of the suicide attempts are associated with the severity of outcomes from non-fatal suicide attempts	Sample size: 200 suicide attempters divided into two groups; G1 with NLSA (153); G2 with LLSA (47) Mean age: NA (range 13–34) Female: G1 = 45.8%; G2 = 61.7%
34.	Swann et al. (53)	Increased impulsivity associated with severity of suicide attempt history in patients with bipolar disorder	To investigate the relationship between impulsivity and severity of past suicidal behavior, a potential predictor of eventual suicide, in patients with bipolar disorder	Sample size: 48 subjects with bipolar personality disorder divided into three groups; G1 history of an MSSA (8); G2 history of an MNSSA (16); G3 without history of SA Mean age: G1 = 34.3 (SD = 5.5) years; G2 = 35.1 (SD = 8.3) years; G3 = 35.0 (SD = 12.1) years Female: G1 = 62.5%; G2 = 68.8%; G3 = 37.5%
35.	Szanto et al. (54)	The cost of social punishment and high-lethality suicide attempts in the second half of life	To understand the role of social decision making in suicide, our study focused on older adults because of the high proportion of medically serious suicide attempts in this age group	Sample size: 103 divided into four groups; G1 individuals who made high-lethality SA (26); G2 individuals who made low-lethality SA (20); G3 non-suicidal depressed (35); G4 non-psychiatric controls (22) Mean age: G1 = 62.8 (SD = 10.1) years; G2 = 62.5 (SD = 6.4) years; G3 = 66.9 (SD = 7.2) years; G4 = 64.6 (SD = 11.0) years Female: G1 = 35%; G2 = 40%; G3 = 60%; G4 = 53%
36.	Szanto et al. (55)	Decision-making competence and attempted suicide	To examine the susceptibility of low-lethality and high-lethality suicide attempters to common decision biases, which may ultimately obscure alternative solutions and deterrents to suicide in a crisis	Sample size: 171 divided into five groups; G1 individuals who made high- lethality SA (31); G2 individuals who made low-lethality SA (29); G3 "ideators" (30); G4 non-suicidal depressed (53); G5 psychiatrically healthy (28) Mean age: G1 = 64.0 (SD = 9.6) years; G2 = 62.0 (SD = 7.4) years; G3 = 65.1 (SD = 10.7) years; G4 = 69.4 (SD = 8.7) years; G5 = 68.4 (SD = 12.0) Female: G1 = 48%; G2 = 48%; G3 = 40%; G4 = 55%; G5 = 57%
37.	Trakhtenbrot et al. (22)	Predictive value of psychological characteristics and suicide history on medical lethality of suicide attempts: a follow-up study of hospitalized patients	To examine the role of mental pain, communication difficulties, and suicide history in predicting the medical severity of follow-up suicide attempts	Sample size: 153 divided into three groups; G1 hospitalized for an MSSA (53); G2 hospitalized for an MNSSA (64); G3 inpatients without a history of suicide (36) Mean age: G1 = 37.60 (SD = 12.25) years; G2 = 37.74 (SD = 13.05) years; G3 = 40.27 (SD = 13.26) years Female: G1 = 42%; G2 = 39%; G3 = 31%

(Continued)

TABLE 1 | Continued

Number	Study	Title	Aim	Sample information
38.	Vanyukov et al. (56)	Perceived burdensomeness is associated with low-lethality suicide attempts, dysfunctional interpersonal style, and younger rather than older age	To answer the questions: does a high level of perceived burdensomeness differentiate medically serious suicidal acts, most closely resembling death by suicide, from less serious ones? How is perceived burdensomeness related to dysfunctional personality dimensions implicated in suicide?	Sample size: 165 aged over 42 divided into five groups; G1 individuals who made high-lethality SA (32); G2 individuals who made low-lethality SA (32); G3 suicidal ideators (34); G4 non-suicidal depressed individuals (37); G5 non-psychiatric controls (30) Mean age: G1 = 65.50 (SD = 11.0) years; G2 = 61.25 (SD = 7.1) years; G3 = 64.47 (SD = 10.1) years; G4 = 66.68 (SD = 5.9) years; G5 = 67.57 (SD = 11.7) Female: G1 = 44%; G2 = 50%; G3 = 38%; G4 = 38%; G5 = 60%
39.	Wiktorsson et al. (57)	Medically serious and non-serious suicide attempts in persons aged 70 and above	To compare clinical and psychosocial characteristics in older adult attempters (70+) with and without medically serious suicide attempts	Sample size: 101 older adult suicide attempters divided into two groups; G1 with MSSA (28); G2 without MSSA (73) Mean age: G1 = 79.5 years; G2 = 79.8 years Female: G1 = 60.7%; G2 = 50.7%

In another study, conducted in the framework of the Canterbury Suicide Project, Conner et al. (29) used case–control data to assess potential moderators for the connection between alcohol dependence and suicide or MSSAs. The psychological autopsy methodology was used to collect data on 193 suicide decedents, 240 individuals who engaged in MSSAs, and 984 adult community controls. The correlation between alcohol dependence and suicide (excluding high-lethal attempts) was intensified with increased age. Neither mood disorder nor gender moderated the relationship between alcohol dependence and suicide. Increased age strengthened the association between mood disorder and suicide, while decreased age amplified the association between mood disorder and near-lethal attempts.

Another study in the same project (28) looked for risk factors for serious suicidal behavior among individuals with alcohol dependence. The cohort included 38 completed suicides, 62 individuals whose SSAs had medical repercussions, and 46 community controls who had experienced alcohol dependence in the past month. Mood disorders and financial problems were more frequent among MSSA attempters compared with the controls. Individuals who had completed suicides, mostly older males, were more prone to mood disorders, partner/relationship difficulties, and other interpersonal life events than the controls.

Powell et al. (47) assessed the linkage between SSAs, lethal SAs, and aspects of alcohol consumption (drinking frequency and quantity, binge drinking, alcoholism, drinking within 3 h prior to the SA, and the age one began drinking) among patients aged 13–34. All measures were found to be related to near-lethal SAs. Odds ratios ranged from 2.4 for alcoholism to 7.0 for drinking within 3 h prior to the attempt. All exposure variables, except the age one started drinking, exhibited a J-shaped relationship between alcohol exposure and near-lethal SAs. Once controlling for potential confounders and other measures of alcohol exposure, drinking within 3 h prior to the attempt remained most strongly associated (ORs > 6) with the seriousness of the attempt.

Lopez-Castroman et al. (42) aimed to investigate the specific association between the tobacco dependence level and the severity of suicidal outcomes. A cohort of 542 adult suicide attempters was assessed, of them 107 who made SSAs. SSA attempters were characterized as smokers, compared with non-smokers. The authors concluded that high or very high levels of tobacco dependence could point to a specific vulnerability leading to more severe SAs.

To conclude, the paucity of research regarding the relation between substance abuse/dependence and SSA calls attention to the need for further research to understand the impact of substance abuse/dependence on SSA.

Mental Pain Levels: Experiences of Depression, Anxiety, Hopelessness, and Distress

As Shneidman postulated in his seminal book, "*Suicide is caused by psychache*" (Shneidman, 1993, p. 51), mental pain is one of the main facilitators of SAs in general, and particularly in suicide. Hence, the proliferation of literature on the relationships between the subjective experience of mental pain, the phenomenological experience of depression, anxiety, and hopelessness, and SSAs.

Several studies have shown that SSAs are characterized by high levels of mental pain, specifically hopelessness, when compared with healthy controls. Examining several personality traits and psychological states, Beautrais et al. (11) demonstrated that hopelessness is a main risk factor for SSA, as well as neuroticism and low-self-esteem. Other studies arrived at similar results. Durant et al. (33), for example, conducted a case-control study of SSAs in the United States to reveal racial differences. They compared 105 SSA attempters with 395 controls selected through a random-digit-dial telephone survey. Compared with the controls, the SSA attempters, especially young African Americans, reported significantly higher levels of hopelessness.

While these studies demonstrated that hopelessness levels are significantly higher among SSA attempters than in the general population, results were different when SSA subjects were compared with a more suitable comparison group, such as hospitalized patients or individuals who made SAs that were not considered serious. When SSA patients were compared with patients with no history of suicidality, different result patterns pertaining to psychopathology levels emerged. In the

Center for Disease Control and Prevention Project in Houston, Swahn and Potter (52) compared 153 nearly lethal attempters with 47 less lethal attempters on several demographic and psychological variables. They found that the percentage of subjects who experienced severe depression (not a DSM definition) in both groups was significantly high—86% of SSA attempters and 98% of those who made less lethal attempts. Moreover, depression was statistically associated with a lower risk for SSAs.

Like the Houston project, the Israeli SSAs project investigated 78 SSA attempters and compared them with 116 suicide attempters whose attempts were less serious, 47 psychiatric controls with no past accounts of suicidal behavior, and 95 healthy controls (18). While depression experience levels measured by the Beck Depression Inventory were considerably higher in the SSA group than in the psychiatric or healthy control group, no differences related to depression were found when comparing individuals who executed SSAs with those whose attempts were less medically serious. A similar tendency was found when overlapping aspects of distress—mental pain, anxiety, and hopelessness—were examined [e.g., Ref. (19)]. For example, while hopelessness was identified as a predictor of SSAs when compared with controls, it was unable to predict medical lethality when SSA attempters were compared with non-SSA attempters [(38), see also (64)]. Mental pain experience, measured by the OMMP scale (65), yielded the same result pattern.

Wiktorsson et al. (57) comparison between older adult attempters with ($n = 28$) and without ($n = 73$) SSAs, produced comparable results. They found that while major depression was common in both groups, SSA attempters were higher on the anxiety scale. When asked about the reasons for attempting suicide, SAA attempters ascribed the attempt to interpersonal social problems and functioning difficulties more often than the non-suicidal group.

Vanyukov et al. (56) examined the perceived burdensomeness factor associated with the interpersonal theory of suicide (66) alongside other psychological factors (e.g., Big Five factors, impulsivity, and anger rumination). They compared levels of perceived burdensomeness among depressed suicidal subjects with a history of both high- and low-lethality attempts, depressed subjects with suicidal ideation, non-suicidal depressed subjects, and psychiatrically healthy controls. Surprisingly, perceived burdensomeness was higher among low-lethality suicide attempters compared with all the other groups, including SSA attempters. Older adults SSA attempters scored very low on perceived burdensomeness, implying that, contrary to thwarted belongingness, the perceived burdensomeness factor does not figure significantly in the SA's lethality.

Lohner and Konrad (40) examined several risk factors among inmates who were high- and low-lethality suicide attempters while under custodial authority. The seriousness of the attempt was positively correlated with measures of depression, and negatively correlated with the psychopathy factor, measured by the Psychopathy Checklist—revised (67). No other psychopathological or mental pain factors were found to be related to seriousness of the attempt (hopelessness, cluster B personality disorder, etc.).

Regarding suicide intent, Horesh et al. (37) showed that high levels of mental pain was a significant factor in the prediction of the subjective components of the suicide intent scale which measures the intent to die. However, mental pain did not predict the objective components of suicide intent, thereby bearing a significant association with lethality of the suicidal attempt.

Together, these results highlight that while distress and mental pain levels are high among suicide attempters, they do not characterize only SSA attempters, as non-SSA attempters also report high-distress levels (which may lead them to attempt suicide in the first place). In other words, while psychopathology, as well as mental pain variables (e.g., hopelessness), are important risk factors for SAs in comparison with the general population, they are not indicative of differences between SAs' low and high levels of seriousness. Although, as Shneidman (68) argued, psychological pain is the common stimulus for both suicide and suicidal attempts, it is only when high levels of mental pain are accompanied by other psychological dimensions, such as interpersonal difficulties, impulsivity, or decision-making deficits, that they can increase the risk for SSAs. Found in several studies, these interactions (19, 38) will be elaborated on later in this review.

Interpersonal Factors

Several studies examined the contribution of different factors to SSAs within the interpersonal context. First and foremost, interpersonal and communication difficulties were found to be strongly related to SSAs. Levi et al. (38) investigated 35 SSA attempters and compared them with two control groups: suicide attempters whose attempts were less serious, and healthy controls. They found that self-disclosure and perceived loneliness are unique predictors of SSAs, above and beyond mental pain levels (i.e., depression and hopelessness). Specifically, levels of self-disclosure, represented by difficulties in sharing intimate information with significant others, was considerably lower among SSA attempters in comparison with the other two control groups. Moreover, self-disclosure was the sole predictor that contributed both to the attempt's medical lethality, and to the type and extent of the medical treatment received after the attempt. Perceived loneliness was highly predictive of the attempt's severity. Thus, the authors proposed a model which they coined "an impossible situation" to describe instances that involve individuals who are unable to ask for help (hence "impossible"). In these cases, the matching of the predisposition for mental pain with other factors can provoke an SA with serious medical ramifications or an actual suicide (38). Apter et al. (24) arrived at similar results in their investigation of depressed patients. In particular, they found that self-disclosure was significantly lower among SSA attempters than among non-SAA attempters, suicide ideators, and patients without a history of suicide.

In a more recent study, Levi-Belz et al. (18) demonstrated that the communication difficulties dimension impacted both the distinction between MSSA attempters and non-MSSA attempters, and from psychiatric controls. Interestingly, the interaction between mental pain and communication difficulties accounted for 23% of the suicide lethality variance, above and beyond each component's individual contribution. These findings demonstrated that the severity of the attempt depends on the individual's ability to communicate their distress to others. Schizoid tendency and loneliness were the most valid sole predictors within the communication difficulties dimension. Gvion et al. (19) confirmed the results pertaining to the interaction between mental pain and schizoid tendency in a larger sample of MSSA and non-MSSA attempters.

In another study from the Israeli project, Horesh et al. (37) showed that difficulties in self-disclosure contributed significantly to the prediction of the objective components of the suicide intent scale, which in turn, determined the attempt's medical lethality. Thus, low-interpersonal communication abilities facilitated higher medical lethality and higher intent that were reflected in objective circumstances related to the attempt (including preparation and steps taken to avoid discovery). In line with these results, it was found that among suicide attempters over 70-years-old, SSA attempters were more likely to attribute their attempts to social problems than non-SSA attempters (57).

When examining the core personality factors that may facilitate communication difficulties, Levi-Belz et al. (39) showed that attachment style significantly predicted the severity of the suicidal attempt, above and beyond the contribution of mental pain. Specifically, the more avoidant the subject's attachment style was, the higher the level of their attempt's medical lethality was. The authors also confirmed a structured equation model in which avoidant attachment facilitated medical lethality through the mediation of social support and self-disclosure. Interestingly, Signoretta et al. (69). found that subjects with communication difficulties and low-social interaction were mostly characterized by depressive temperament traits. This may highlight the interchange relationship between mental pain features and interpersonal factors which are main factors in our model for SSAs.

Other studies explored more directly the ability of SSA attempters to ask for help. Beautrais (14) employed a series of personality and cognitive style measures to assess SSA attempters (n = 125) and non-suicidal community comparison subjects (n = 151). SSA attempters were characterized by significantly lower levels of actual social interaction. When dichotomized, those with low levels of social interaction had elevated odds (up to eight times more) for SSA than controls.

Barnes et al. (25) study focused solely on subjects seeking help from others. They found that 153 subjects aged 13–34 who made SSAs had been less likely than the random sample of 513 control subjects to seek help from any consultant, including psychologists and physicians, in the past month.

To conclude, difficulties in interpersonal communication—reflected by a low ability to disclose oneself, resulting in loneliness and low-social support—seem to play an important role in more lethal SAs associated with high-objective suicide intent. At the basis of these difficulties are characteristics of avoidant attachment style, as well as schizoid tendency. Most of the studies indicated that interpersonal difficulties become risk factors when there is a high level of distress, depression, and mental pain in the background, thereby pointing to the interaction between mental pain and interpersonal problems as an important risk factor for SSAs.

Decision-Making Factors

Over the last five decades, the fields of psychiatry and psychology have been influenced by economic theories that study patterns of decision making. Decision-making processes result in choosing a course of action or perception from several alternatives. To make optimal choices, our brain screens, gathers, and analyzes information prior to each decision. Recently, studies have begun to look at the impulsivity factor of suicidal behavior as a construct that involves a failure of higher-order control, that is, a deficit in decision making (19, 31). Thus, poor decision making can ultimately obscure alternative solutions and lead to suicidal behavior in times of crisis or depression.

The association between decision making and attempt lethality is mostly studied among middle-aged and elderly subjects who traditionally have high rates of both significantly lethal attempts and suicide (55). In Dombrovski et al. (31) seminal study, four groups of depressed participants aged 60 and older were assessed: 15 high-lethality suicide (SAA) attempters, 14 low-lethality suicide attempters, 12 who contemplated suicide, and 42 depressed subjects with no history of suicidal thoughts. The reference group comprised of 31 psychiatrically fit elders. To measure the preference for smaller immediate versus larger delayed rewards, participants were tested on Kirby's Monetary Choice Questionnaire. Interestingly, the SSA attempters were more disposed to delay future rewards than the low-lethality attempters. Moreover, low-lethality attempters exhibited an exaggerated preference for immediate rewards compared with the two control groups. These effects were stable also after accounting for several possible covariates, such as education, global cognitive function medications, and possible brain injury. In another study, McGirr et al. (45) assessed older suicide attempters of varying medical lethality. All participants completed the Wisconsin Card Sorting Test that examines cognitive control during rule learning. Cognitive control is a mental process that underlies rule learning by integrating feedback with past knowledge of contingency and environment structure. In contrast to low-lethality attempters and healthy controls, high-lethality attempters exhibited poorer conceptual reasoning and increased rates of perseverative errors and total errors. Moreover, high-lethality attempters made more conceptual errors than non-suicidal depressed participants. Thus, this study highlights that high-lethality SAs in older people are related to impaired cognitive control during rule learning. This liability may contribute to serious or even fatal suicidal acts in old age.

To better define and map the diversity in SA lethality in terms of specific decision-making deficits, Szanto et al. (55) evaluated 31 older and middle-aged SSA attempters, and compared them, on decision biases, with 29 low-lethality suicide attempters, 30 suicide ideators, 53 non-suicidal depressed subjects, and 28 psychiatrically well participants. Attempters, ideators, and non-suicidal depressed subjects had unipolar non-psychotic major depression. The authors found that all attempters (both SSAs and those with lower lethality) were more susceptible to *framing effects* (i.e., made decisions affected by irrelevant variations in how information is presented) in comparison with the control groups. Thus, it seems that SSA attempters and low-lethality attempters are similar in their tendency to make decisions influenced by irrelevant variations in the way information is presented to them. This may indicate that suicidal behavior, but not its severity, reflects a lack of ability to make a decision from an objective standpoint during a crisis.

In another study, Szanto et al. (54) used the *Ultimatum Game* in which players decide whether or not to accept dubious monetary offerings from another player. Participants were older adults suffering from depression with a past of high-lethality SAs, low-lethality SAs, and no suicidal attempts. The control group consisted of healthy controls. Participants in all groups penalized their counterparts in response to inequitable monetary offers. Yet, low-lethality attempters, non-suicidal depressed participants, and healthy controls decreased the extent of penalty they inflicted as the level of punishment inflicted upon them increased—they accepted more unfair offers as the risks grew higher. SSA attempters did not modify their choices in accordance with stake magnitude, and penalized unjust offers regardless of the cost. 66% of the difference between the low-lethality attempters and non-psychiatric controls was explained in terms of individual differences in fairness judgments: the comparison group judged offer fairness as a combined function of inequality and magnitude, whereas the SSA attempters judged offer fairness based on inequality.

To conclude, decision-making impairments are risk factors for suicide behaviors in general. Nevertheless, specific difficulties, i.e., the lack of ability to calculate the positive and negative consequences of one's actions, and the impaired ability to modify choices when making decisions regarding actions, are related to more serious suicide behaviors. As most research on decision making and SSAs focuses on the elderly population, generalization of conclusions is limited.

Impulsivity–Aggression Factors

Under the concept of aggression, the literature employs diverse terms, such as violence, aggression, irritability, and hostility. These constructs have common aspects and are highly correlated (5, 70). Thus, we will relate to these constructs interchangeably. Several studies have highlighted the importance of aggression and related concepts to SSAs. Doihara et al. (30) studied the aggression dimension in 55 MSSA attempters in a hospital's emergency room, and compared them with a control group of 71 healthy individuals. It was found that aggression and hostility scores were significantly higher in the SSA attempters when compared with controls.

The study of aggression is usually associated with the study of impulsivity as some researchers suggest that the overlap between these constructs is strong, and therefore they should be viewed as a single phenotype [for review see Ref. (5)]. Accordingly, Soloff et al. (51) evaluated 44 high-lethality attempters and 69 low-lethality attempters. Impulsivity, aggression, and state hostility failed to distinguish between high- and low-lethality attempters. Gvion et al. (19) studied 43 MSSA attempters, 49 medically non-SSA attempters, 47 psychiatric patients who had not attempted suicide, and 57 healthy control subjects. Among other variables, participants were assessed for aggression–impulsivity. The data revealed that although aggressive variables (e.g., anger-in, anger-out, and violence) and impulsivity differentiated between suicide attempters and non-attempters, they did not differentiate between high- and low-lethality attempters.

Interestingly, in a recent follow-up study (2017), Gvion examined the role of aggressive-impulsive variants and suicide history in foreseeing the medical severity of follow-up SAs. Anger-out, violence, and impulsivity were significantly and positively correlated with medical severity of follow-up SAs. Impulsive–aggressive variables accounted for 10.6% of the variance, over and above the contribution of personal factors, medical severity of index SA, and hopelessness. Moreover, interactions between medical acuteness levels of the index SA and impulsivity, self-disclosure, and anger-in, accounted for 16.4% of the variance, over and beyond each component alone. The findings further indicate that although impulsivity and aggression do not necessarily account for the seriousness of the original attempt (19), they do facilitate the ability to attempt a more lethal suicide in the future. This is especially true among those who originally made an SSA.

An interesting distinction in the literature relates to state or trait characteristic of impulsivity (71). A common way to operationalize state impulsivity is to examine the degree of objective signs of planning. Rivlin et al. (49) investigated 60 prisoners who performed near-lethal SAs. Although 73% indicated that they had intended to die, 40% of the acts were impulsive. The prisoners said they had thought about and planned the act for only a very short period of time (typically less than 3 h). Moreover, very few prisoners took any precautions against detection, left a suicide note, made plans or arrangements for suicide, or thought about the timing of the act.

Simon et al. (50) studied 153 subjects aged 13–34 who made nearly lethal suicide attempts. 24% of survivors contemplated their attempt for under 5 min. Those who executed their attempt within 5 min of the decision were less likely to have considered another method of suicide.

Swann et al. (53) compared bipolar SSA attempters, non-SSA attempters, and bipolar non-attempters. Subjects were assessed using the Barratt Impulsiveness Scale (BIS) and behavioral laboratory performance measures (immediate memory/delayed memory tasks). While no difference was found between the groups on BIS scores, impulsivity as manifested in behavioral laboratory performance measures was greatest in those with the most serious medical attempts. These results can also be explained in terms of the difference between trait and state aspects of impulsivity.

To summarize, aggressive–impulsive variables play a role in suicide behavior in general. Regarding SSA, data are sparse and limited. Looking at aggression and impulsivity in SSAs may differ significantly from studying aggression and impulsivity among SA repeaters and/or those who make low-lethality attempts. The extent of preparation and planning is a significant factor in determining the seriousness of the attempt, and is generally used as an indicator of state impulsivity. Nonetheless, many people die by suicide or make high-lethal acts performed on the spur of the moment with no or limited planning. The lethality of these attempts depends also on circumstantial factors (like availability of means). The findings further indicate that although impulsivity and aggression do not necessarily account for the lethality of the original attempt, they are factors in the ability to attempt a more lethal suicide in the future. This is especially true among those who originally made an SSA.

Other Risk Factors for SSA

In this section, our focus is on specific and more isolated factors, rather than on risk factor clusters. Considering these factors' scarcity, we have also included studies published 5 years prior to 2000. It goes without saying that more research is needed to fully appreciate the accuracy and specific impact of these variables as risk factors for SSA.

Negative life events were one of the factors suggested to be an isolated risk factor for SSAs. In the Canterbury Suicide Project, Beautrais (14) found a higher number of stressful life events among young people who made SSAs compared with controls with no history of suicidal behavior. Specifically, childhood and family adversities (e.g., sexual abuse or poor parenting) were significantly higher among the SSA group. Similar results were found in Elliott et al. (34) study that examined demographic and psychiatric factors associated with serious suicide attempters when compared with 32 non-medically serious attempters admitted to emergency rooms. Serious suicide attempters were found to have a higher rate of sexual and physical abuse, and in general, higher numbers of traumatic life events. They were also found to have higher rates of borderline personality disorder.

Other studies that investigated the relationship between medical lethality and life events among specific groups had similar results. Marzano et al. (44) studied 60 imprisoned male serious suicide attempters and compared them with inmates who had not attempted suicide. The Childhood Trauma Questionnaire was used to assess accounts of past emotional, physical, and sexual abuse, and emotional and physical neglect. Compared with controls, SSA attempters reported higher levels of adverse life events and criminal history factors. Being bullied in prison was significant even in multivariate analyses of several factors. While adverse life events were common among the prisoners, bullying, hopelessness, and a parent or sibling's death were significantly higher among SSA attempters. Bullying was found to be significant even after controlling for other factors in the multivariate analysis.

Another single study investigated the association between geographic mobility and SSAs. Potter et al. (46) found that geographic mobility (changing residence over the past 12 months) among young adults was highly associated with SSAs while only weakly associated with non-SSAs. However, the adjusted odds ratio of this result was relatively low (2.1, with 95% confidence interval of 1.4–3.3). When looking more specifically at the risk factor—recent (in the past 3 months) or three or more relocations over the past 12 months—the OR rises to 6.2 (3.0–13.3). Thus, it seems that recent and frequent geographic mobility are more refined risk factors for SSA.

Although unemployment is a common stressful event often leading to various experiences of psychopathologies, we found only one study (from 1998) that evaluated the link between unemployment and SSAs. Beautrais et al. (27) studied 302 SSA attempters and compared them to 1,028 randomly selected community control subjects. They found that SSA attempters reported higher rates of current unemployment (OR = 4.2) compared with controls. This correlation was similar for males and females. Following adjustment for preexisting childhood, familial, and educational factors, the association between unemployment and risk of SSA decreased, but remained significant (OR = 2.1). Nevertheless, when both preceding family and childhood factors, and psychiatric morbidity were considered, unemployment was not significantly related to risk of SSA. The authors concluded that the link between unemployment and suicidal behavior was to a large extent non-causal, and reflected mutual or correlated factors contributing to risks of both unemployment and suicidal behavior. Any remaining association between unemployment and SA risk appeared to result from the correlation between unemployment and psychiatric disorder.

DISCUSSION

Most studies regard SAs as a unified phenomenon, while neglecting to consider differences between levels of suicidal behaviors. Disregarding these distinctions impedes the detection of those at high risk for suicide. This is also partly because these studies tend to draw conclusions from findings regarding attempters to suicide completers.

To overcome this obstacle, researchers have developed the SSA strategy, which focuses on individuals who made definite, near-fatal attempts but who did not die from suicide due to intensive medical intervention. This group seems to resemble suicide victims quite closely (14, 20). Therefore, it may provide some insight into the large group of suicide completers whose first attempt is fatal, and who have hitherto been neglected by mental health professionals. More specifically, the SSA approach can provide insight into understanding the personal and interpersonal characteristics, circumstances, and psychological processes leading to SAs. However, to the best of our knowledge, no study has systematically reviewed the empirical data accumulated in this field to date.

In what follows, we would like first to summarize and integrate the main findings of our review. Next, we will highlight methodological limitations akin to the study of SSA.

Risk Factors for SSA: Toward an Integration of a Model

Drawing on the SSA approach, several projects and studies [e.g., (14, 18, 48, 72)] highlighted important psychological characteristics and variables that can serve as risk factors of SSA. In this paper, we aimed to systematically review the empirical data accumulated thus far regarding the psychological risk factors for severe SAs.

In general, several categories of psychological risk factors and warning signs for SSA were identified: psychopathology and mental pain, interpersonal relationships, impulsivity and aggressiveness, decision making, and several-specific isolated factors, such as negative life events. High levels of psychopathology [e.g., Ref. (14)] and unbearable mental pain were found to be conditions of susceptibility to SSAs, and to play a major role in creating the basis for suicide acts. Specifically, the review findings revealed the unique value of mental illness, particularly the diagnoses of MDD, anxiety disorder, PTSD, anti-social personality disorder, substance abuse/dependence disorders, and psychiatric comorbidity as predictors of SSAs (14, 41, 48). Along with psychopathology, psychological pain [including hopelessness and depression experience (64)] was a distinguishing factor between serious suicide attempters and healthy populations in various studies. In other words, levels of psychopathology and mental pain were associated with an increased risk for SSA compared with controls. These recurring results emphasize that psychopathology and mental pain may serve as vulnerability factors that need to be considered when attempting to predict SSAs in large community populations.

However, when comparing SSA attempters to those with lower severity, psychopathology, and mental pain dimensions alone cannot effectively predict SSAs (38, 52, 57). Nonetheless, several studies found that these dimensions play a critical role in cases where the individual is unable to regulate or adjust the experienced emotional pain (18, 19). In other words, if mental pain is high, its effect on suicide severity depends on other psychological factors that serve as facilitators, or protective factors against SSAs.

The most essential factor that was found to moderate the facilitation of mental pain and should serve as critical risk factor to SSAs was the interpersonal abilities dimension. Several studies emphasized that in instances in which mental pain is combined with an inability to communicate stress, painful feelings remain unaddressed, thereby resulting in more serious forms of suicidal behavior with higher severity levels of the suicide intent's objective components (18, 37, 38). Put differently, combined with mental pain, interpersonal, and communication difficulties expressed by loneliness, schizoid traits, alexithymia, lack of social support (18), insecure attachment style (39), low-actual social interaction (14), limited help-seeking behaviors (25), and inability to disclose emotions and thoughts (19) interact to facilitate SSAs (18).

Another important psychological risk factor for SSAs is the impaired cognitive control during rule learning, which may explain some of the reasons for choosing highly lethal suicide methods leading in turn, to medically severe SAs. In several studies, individuals who made SSAs were found to be more inclined to delay rewards (31), had poorer conceptual reasoning, and more conceptual errors. Interestingly, SSA attempters were found to decide and choose without considering the cost and implications of their decisions (55). It seems that while some decision-making impairments are associated with suicidal behavior in general, specific difficulties are related to more serious suicide behaviors. These difficulties can be categorized as the lack of ability to calculate costs and gains as a result of one's behavior, and the reluctance to modify choices when deciding on actions (e.g., willingness to delay rewards and high-punishment regardless of the costs). Thus, these impairments should be carefully considered when attempting to assess the probability for SSAs. It should be noted, however, that the research on decision making and SSAs focuses mainly on elderly populations. No data are available on this relationship among young and young adult participants. Obviously, more research is needed to generalize and refine these results in terms of other SSA attempter populations.

The impulsivity–aggressive dimension was also investigated as a possible risk factor for SSAs. In general, the impulsivity, aggression, and hostility factors were found to differentiate between suicide attempters from non-attempters, but in most studies, both impulsivity and the related constructs failed to account for differences between high- and low-lethality attempters. Thus, it seems that this dimension is a more general risk factor for suicidality than it is a specific factor related to severe SAs. It can be concluded that while characteristics of planning and preparation are important factors related to the seriousness of the attempt, highly lethal acts depend also on circumstantial factors (like availability of means) and are often performed on the spur of the moment with limited planning. Interestingly, in a follow-up study (36), impulsivity, anger-out, and violence were found to have significant positive correlations with medical severity of follow-up SAs among those who made SSAs in the index attempt. Thus, the impulsivity–aggressive dimension does play some role in the potential for higher lethal SAs among subjects with a history of SSAs. One can conclude, therefore, that when a person has made SSAs in the past, the potential for a repeated serious attempt is higher, especially when the decision is impulsive and made on the spur of the moment.

Some studies found that recurrent stressful life events can also serve as SSA risk factors. Among particularly traumatic events, the evidence points to childhood sexual abuse (14, 44), geographic mobility, and unemployment.

Taking together, and in line with Levi et al. (38) model, we propose an integrative model of psychological risk factors for SSAs. This model contains vulnerability factors, immanent factors, and facilitating factors in three stages of occurrence (see **Figure 2**). In the first stage of the proposed model, mental pain experience, psychopathology, and drug and substance abuse converge to create an atmosphere of unbearable mental pain, which is similarly manifested among all suicide attempters. Notably, the combination of this personal state with lack of interpersonal and communications abilities, as well as with impairments in decision making and specific negative life events, seems to generate an "impossible situation," which in turn may provoke an SSA. In other words, the combination of vulnerability factors with the critical risk factors for SSAs in stage 2 (and other demographic factors), render the probability for SSAs profoundly higher. In this devastating state of "impossible situation," higher levels of impulsivity and aggression may act as facilitators and aggravate suicidality levels to highly lethal SAs.

This systematic review highlights that while personal factors and psychopathology are the main risk factors for SAs in general, the critical elements that facilitate higher levels of dangerous suicidal acts are difficulties in communication and impaired decision making. The insights from these results are twofold: first, in order to accurately assess those at risk for SSA and even more dangerous suicidal acts, it is important to examine the patient's levels of communication and social connectedness, as well their decision-making processes with emphasis on their lack of cognitive control. Second, these dimensions should be at the crux of all therapy goals. Several therapeutic protocols

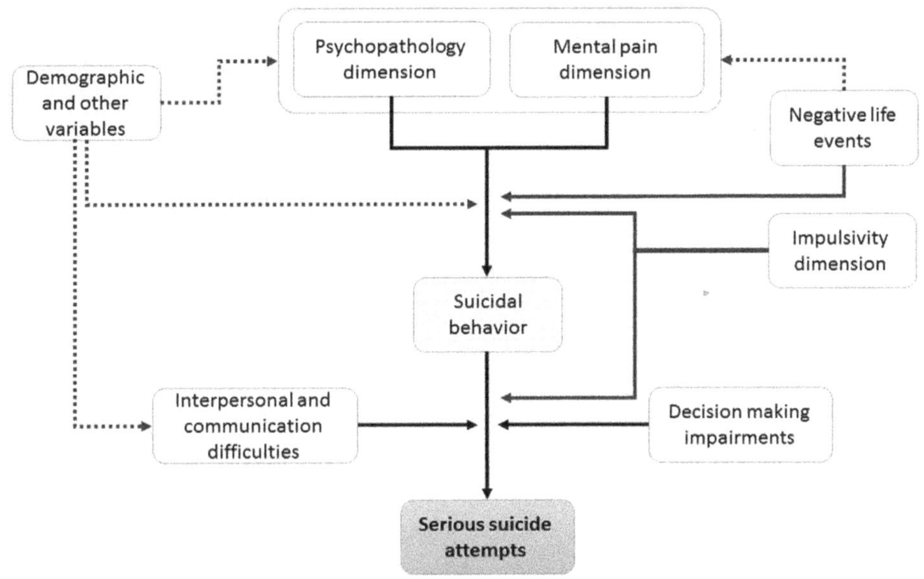

FIGURE 2 | Proposed psychological model of risk factors to serious suicide attempts.

(e.g., interpersonal psychotherapy), focused on these dimensions are already available.

Methodological Limitations to the Study of SSA

One of the main complications associated with the study of SSA is participant recruitment. The definition of SSA entails the understanding that the attempter was saved merely by chance and/or due to intensive medical intervention. This explains the scarce data and small SSA samples. Moreover, several studies reviewed here [e.g., Ref. (31, 55)] restricted assessment to specific groups (e.g., elderly people), thereby limiting the ability to generalize conclusions.

Another important drawback lies with the definition of, and criteria for, SSA. Most studies employ the terminology of severe suicidality; however, given that the criteria for SSA are highly variable, in practice researchers often apply non-stringent criteria (e.g., lethality rating scale >3). This decreases the ability to infer data regarding SSAs, whereas the reliance on a strict and consistent definition makes it possible, to a large extent (13, 14), to infer information from SSAs, thereby increasing the ability to identify the risk factors for suicide.

This study stems from the awareness that near lethal attempters are a unique group, distinct from non-SSA attempters. Nevertheless, the literature survey revealed that only a few studies compared SSAs to non-SSAs. A large portion of the studies reviewed here compared SSAs to non-suicidal psychiatric and/or general population controls rather than use non-serious suicide attempters as a comparison group. This weakens the ability to draw conclusions about the SSAs group.

An important limitation of the SSAs strategy is related to the use of medical lethality as a central criterion. While most studies adopted this criterion [e.g., Ref. (18, 19)], its main drawback is that it does not take into consideration that the outcome of any suicide method is heavily influenced by chance factors and circumstances. Put differently, while the post-SA physical condition is an objective criterion with several advantages, it may be greatly influenced by the method's availability or imprecise knowledge of the employed method's lethality (73). For example, the extent and nature of physical harm aligned with medication overdoses is significantly contingent on the type of medication: SSRI antidepressants cause limited physical damage, whereas use of tricyclic drugs will most probably warrant intensive hospital care. Considering, however, that the choice of medication is usually limited to the attempter's prescription drugs—of which they are ignorant as to potentially lethal effects—it is not closely related to the actual seriousness of the intent to die. Thus, in future studies it is important to assess actual suicidal intent and take it into account when defining SSAs that closely resemble actual suicides (20). Incorporating an intent factor can also help refine the definition for SSA as limited to particularly severe SAs (21).

Lastly, a broad limitation is the use of retrospective self-report measures for collecting data on the majority of psychological factors mentioned in this review. These measures may introduce a familiar range of biases triggered by factors such as mood dependent recall, forgetfulness, cathartic effect, and social desirability.

Implications for Research and Treatment

Serious suicide attempts are a valid proxy for completed suicides, and therefore, the variables that predict severe suicidal behavior should be at the forefront of the research and clinical efforts when assessing risk groups for suicide. Future studies need to consider the importance of strict and consistent definition criteria for SSAs to improve research strategies, assessment, and preventive efforts. This review also highlights the importance for mental health professionals and clinicians to further assess patients who present psychopathology and distress. Those patients should be asked about their support circles, and ability to recruit the environment for help. As decision-making processes have been found to increase the risk of serious medical suicidal behavior when distress is in the background, it is important to evaluate the patient's ability to make flexible decisions, to calculate the consequences of his behavior (e.g., suicide), and to modify his choices accordingly.

CONCLUSION

Overall, our findings provide a foundation for future research regarding the combined role of psychopathology, mental pain, communication difficulties, decision-making patterns, and facets of impulsivity and aggression, in the occurrence of near-lethal SAs. Moreover, our review suggests that the developmental paths culminating in suicidal behavior are heterogeneous, and that different mechanisms or processes are more likely in play for those who commit suicide as opposed to those who attempt non-lethal suicidal attempts. Regardless of the limited scope of research and available data, it is important that health care professionals consider these risk factors when assessing the risk of future severe SAs and suicide.

AUTHOR CONTRIBUTIONS

We were both involved in the initiation of the subject, searching the web, categorizing and integrating the data, and in writing the paper.

REFERENCES

1. World Health Organization. *Preventing Suicide: A Global Imperative*. (2014). Available from: http://www.who.int/mental_health/publications/prevention_suicide_2012/en
2. Hawton K, Saunders KE, O'Connor RC. Self-harm and suicide in adolescents. *Lancet* (2012) 379(9834):2373–82. doi:10.1016/S0140-6736(12)60322-5
3. Pickles A, Aglan A, Collishaw S, Messer J, Rutter M, Maughan B. Predictors of suicidality across the life span: the isle of Wight study. *Psychol Med* (2010) 40(9):1453–66. doi:10.1017/S0033291709991905
4. Silverman MM, Berman AL, Sanddal ND, O'Carroll PW, Joiner ET. Rebuilding the tower of Babel: a revised nomenclature for the study of suicidal behavior: part I: background, rationale and methodology. *Suicide Life-Threatening Behav* (2007) 37(3):264–77. doi:10.1521/suli.2007.37.3.248
5. Gvion Y, Apter A. Aggression, impulsivity and suicide behavior: a review of the literature. *Arch Suicide Res* (2011) 15:93–112. doi:10.1080/13811118.2011.565265
6. O'Carroll PW, Berman AL, Maris RW, Moscicki EK, Tanney BL, Silverman MM. Beyond the tower of babel: a nomenclature for suicidology. *Suicide Life-Threatening Behav* (1996) 26(3):237–52.
7. Conner KR, Beautrais AL, Brent DA, Conwell Y, Phillips MR, Schneider B. The next generation of psychological autopsy studies. *Suicide Life-Threatening Behav* (2011) 41(6):594–613. doi:10.1111/j.1943-278X.2011.00057.x
8. Cavanagh JT, Carson AJ, Sharpe M, Lawrie SM. Psychological autopsy studies of suicide: a systematic review. *Psychol Med* (2003) 33:395–405. doi:10.1017/S0033291702006943
9. Wong A, Escobar M, Lesage A, Loyer M, Vanier C, Sakinofsky I. Are UN peacekeepers at risk for suicide? *Suicide Life Threat Behav* (2001) 31(1):103–12. doi:10.1521/suli.31.1.103.21305
10. Hawton K, Appleby L, Platt S, Foster T, Cooper J, Malmberg A, et al. The psychological autopsy approach to studying suicide: a review of methodological issues. *J Affect Disord* (1998) 50(2–3):269–76.
11. Beautrais AL, Joyce PR, Mulder RT. Cannabis abuse and serious suicide attempts. *Addiction* (1999) 94(8):1155–64. doi:10.1046/j.1360-0443.1999.94811555.x
12. Potter LB, Kresnow MJ, Powell KE, O'Carroll PW, Lee RK, Briscoe MG. Identification of nearly fatal suicide attempts: self-inflicted injury severity form. *Suicide Life-Threatening Behav* (1998) 28(2):174–86.
13. Beautrais AL. Suicides and serious suicide attempts: two populations or one? *Psychol Med* (2001) 31(5):837–45. doi:10.1017/S0033291701003889
14. Beautrais AL. Suicide and serious suicide attempts in youth: a multiple-group comparison study. *Am J Psychiatry* (2003) 160(6):1093–9. doi:10.1176/appi.ajp.160.6.1093
15. Mościcki EK. Epidemiology of completed and attempted suicide: toward a framework for prevention. *Clin Neurosci Res* (2001) 1(5):310–23. doi:10.1016/S1566-2772(01)00032-9
16. Rosen DH. The serious suicide attempt. *JAMA* (1976) 235(19):2105–9. doi:10.1001/jama.235.19.2105
17. Beautrais AL. Further suicidal behavior among medically serious suicide attempters. *Suicide Life-Threatening Behav* (2004) 34(1):1–11. doi:10.1521/suli.34.1.1.27772
18. Levi-Belz Y, Gvion Y, Horesh N, Fischel T, Treves I, Or E, et al. Mental pain, communication difficulties and medically serious suicide attempts: a case-control study. *Arch Suicide Res* (2014) 18(1):74–87. doi:10.1080/13811118.2013.809041
19. Gvion Y, Horesh N, Levi-Belz Y, Fischel T, Treves I, Weiser M, et al. Aggression–impulsivity, mental pain, and communication difficulties in medically serious and medically non-serious suicide attempters. *Compr Psychiatry* (2014) 55(1):40–50. doi:10.1016/j.comppsych.2013.09.003
20. Hawton K. Studying survivors of nearly lethal suicide attempts: an important strategy in suicide research. *Suicide Life-Threatening Behav* (2002) 32(1):76–84. doi:10.1521/suli.32.1.5.76.24215
21. Levi-Belz Y, Beautrais A. Serious suicide attempts: towards an integration of terms and definitions. *J Crisis Intervention Suicide Prevention* (2016) 37(4):299–309. doi:10.1027/0227-5910/a000386
22. Trakhtenbrot R, Gvion Y, Levi-Belz Y, Horesh N, Fischel T, Weiser M, et al. Predictive value of psychological characteristics and suicide history on medical lethality of suicide attempts: a follow-up study of hospitalized patients. *J Affect Disord* (2016) 199:73–80. doi:10.1016/j.jad.2016.03.054
23. Moher D, Liberati A, Tetzlaff J, Altman DG, Prisma Group. Preferred reporting items for systematic reviews and meta-analyses: the PRISMA statement. *PLoS Med* (2009) 6(7):e1000097. doi:10.1371/journal.pmed.1000097
24. Apter A, Horesh N, Gothelf D, Graffi H, Lepkifker E. Relationship between self-disclosure and serious suicidal behavior. *Compr Psychiatry* (2001) 42(1):70–5. doi:10.1053/comp.2001.19748
25. Barnes LS, Ikeda RM, Kresnow MJ. Help-seeking behavior prior to nearly lethal suicide attempts. *Suicide Life-Threatening Behav* (2002) 32(s1):68–75. doi:10.1521/suli.32.1.5.68.24217
26. Beautrais AL. A case control study of suicide and attempted suicide in older adults. *Suicide Life-Threatening Behav* (2002) 32(1):1–9. doi:10.1521/suli.32.1.1.22184
27. Beautrais AL, Joyce PR, Mulder RT. Unemployment and serious suicide attempts. *Psychol Med* (1998) 28(1):209–18. doi:10.1017/S0033291797005990
28. Conner KR, Beautrais AL, Conwell Y. Risk factors for suicide and medically serious suicide attempts among alcoholics: analyses of Canterbury suicide project data. *J Stud Alcohol* (2003) 64(4):551–4. doi:10.15288/jsa.2003.64.551
29. Conner KR, Beautrais AL, Conwell Y. Moderators of the relationship between alcohol dependence and suicide and medically serious suicide attempts: analyses of Canterbury suicide project data. *Alcohol Clin Exp Res* (2003) 27(7):1156–61. doi:10.1097/01.ALC.0000075820.65197.FD

30. Doihara C, Kawanishi C, Yamada T, Sato R, Hasgawa H, Furuno T, et al. Trait aggression in suicide attempters: a pilot study. *Psychiatry Clin Neurosci* (2008) 62(3):352–4. doi:10.1111/j.1440-1819.2008.01804.x
31. Dombrovski AY, Szanto K, Siegle GJ, Wallace ML, Forman SD, Sahakian B, et al. Lethal forethought: delayed reward discounting differentiates high-and low-lethality suicide attempts in old age. *Biol Psychiatry* (2011) 70(2):138–44. doi:10.1016/j.biopsych.2010.12.025
32. Donald M, Dower J, Correa-Velez I, Jones M. Risk and protective factors for medically serious suicide attempts: a comparison of hospital-based with population-based samples of young adults. *Aust N Z J Psychiatry* (2006) 40(1):87–96. doi:10.1080/j.1440-1614.2006.01747.x
33. Durant T, Mercy J, Kresnow MJ, Simon T, Potter L, Hammond WR. Racial differences in hopelessness as a risk factor for a nearly lethal suicide attempt. *J Black Psychol* (2006) 32(3):285–302. doi:10.1177/0095798406290468
34. Elliott AJ, Pages KP, Russo J, Wilson LG. A profile of medically serious suicide attempts. *J Clin Psychiatry* (1996) 57(12):567–71. doi:10.4088/JCP.v57n1202
35. Fowler JC, Hilsenroth MJ, Groat M, Biel S, Biedermann C, Ackerman S. Risk factors for medically serious suicide attempts: Evidence for a psychodynamic formulation of suicidal crisis. *J Am Psychoanal Assoc* (2012) 60(3):555–76. doi:10.1177/0003065112442240
36. Gvion Y. Aggression, impulsivity, and their predictive value on medical lethality of suicide attempts: a follow-up study on hospitalized patients. *J Affect Disord* (2018) 227:840–6. doi:10.1016/j.jad.2017.11.033
37. Horesh N, Levi Y, Apter A. Intent, lethality and interpersonal characteristics of medically serious suicide attempters. *J Affect Disord* (2012) 136(3):286–93. doi:10.1016/j.jad.2011.11.035
38. Levi Y, Horesh N, Ficshel Z, Or E, Apter A. Mental pain and its communication in medically serious suicide attempts: an impossible situation. *J Affect Disord* (2008) 111(2):244–50. doi:10.1016/j.jad.2008.02.022
39. Levi-Belz Y, Gvion Y, Horesh N, Apter A. Attachment patterns in medical serious suicide attempts: the mediating role of self-disclosure and loneliness. *Suicide Life-Threatening Behav* (2013) 43(5):511–22. doi:10.1111/sltb.12035
40. Lohner J, Konrad N. Deliberate self-harm and suicide attempt in custody: distinguishing features in male inmates' self-injurious behavior. *Int J Law Psychiatry* (2006) 29(5):370–85. doi:10.1016/j.ijlp.2006.03.004
41. Lopez-Castroman J, Jaussent I, Beziat S, Guillaume S, Baca-Garcia E, Olié E, et al. Posttraumatic stress disorder following childhood abuse increases the severity of suicide attempts. *J Affect Disord* (2015) 170:7–14. doi:10.1016/j.jad.2014.08.010
42. Lopez-Castroman J, Cerrato L, Beziat S, Jaussent I, Guillaume S, Courtet P. Heavy tobacco dependence in suicide attempters making recurrent and medically serious attempts. *Drug Alcohol Depend* (2016) 160:177–82. doi:10.1016/j.drugalcdep.2016.01.004
43. Marzano L, Fazel S, Rivlin A, Hawton K. Psychiatric disorders in women prisoners who have engaged in near-lethal self-harm: case-control study. *Br J Psychiatry* (2010) 197(3):219–26. doi:10.1192/bjp.bp.109.075424
44. Marzano L, Hawton K, Rivlin A, Fazel S. Psychosocial influences on prisoner suicide: a case-control study of near-lethal self-harm in women prisoners. *Soc Sci Med* (2011) 72(6):874–83. doi:10.1016/j.socscimed.2010.12.028
45. McGirr A, Dombrovski AY, Butters MA, Clark L, Szanto K. Deterministic learning and attempted suicide among older depressed individuals: cognitive assessment using the Wisconsin card sorting task. *J Psychiatr Res* (2012) 46(2):226–32. doi:10.1016/j.jpsychires.2011.10.001
46. Potter LB, Kresnow MJ, Powell KE, Simon TR, Mercy JA, Lee RK, et al. The influence of geographic mobility on nearly lethal suicide attempts. *Suicide Life-Threatening Behav* (2002) 32(s1):42–8. doi:10.1521/suli.32.1.5.42.24216
47. Powell KE, Kresnow JM, Mercy JA, Potter LB, Swann AC, Frankowski RF, et al. Alcohol consumption and nearly lethal suicide attempts. *Suicide Life-Threatening Behav* (2002) 32(s1):30–41. doi:10.1521/suli.32.1.5.30.24208
48. Rivlin A, Hawton K, Marzano L, Fazel S. Psychiatric disorders in male prisoners who made near-lethal suicide attempts: case-control study. *Br J Psychiatry* (2010) 197(4):313–9. doi:10.1192/bjp.bp.110.077883
49. Rivlin A, Fazel S, Marzano L, Hawton K. The suicidal process in male prisoners making near-lethal suicide attempts. *Psychol Crime Law* (2013) 19(4):305–27. doi:10.1080/1068316X.2011.631540
50. Simon OR, Swann AC, Powell KE, Potter LB, Kresnow MJ, O'Carroll PW. Characteristics of impulsive suicide attempts and attempters. *Suicide Life-Threatening Behav* (2001) 32:49–59. doi:10.1521/suli.32.1.5.49.24212
51. Soloff PH, Fabio A, Kelly TM, Malone KM, Mann JJ. High-lethality status in patients with borderline personality disorder. *J Pers Disord* (2005) 19(4): 386–99. doi:10.1521/pedi.2005.19.4.386
52. Swahn MH, Potter LB. Factors associated with the medical severity of suicide attempts in youths and young adults. *Suicide Life-Threatening Behav* (2002) 32(s1):21–9. doi:10.1521/suli.32.1.5.21.24214
53. Swann AC, Dougherty DM, Pazzaglia PJ, Pham M, Steinberg JL, Moeller FG. Increased impulsivity associated with severity of suicide attempt history in patients with bipolar disorder. *Am J Psychiatry* (2005) 162(9):1680–7. doi:10.1176/appi.ajp.162.9.1680
54. Szanto K, Clark L, Hallquist M, Vanyukov P, Crockett M, Dombrovski AY. The cost of social punishment and high-lethality suicide attempts in the second half of life. *Psychol Aging* (2014) 29(1):84–94. doi:10.1037/a0035339
55. Szanto K, Bruine de Bruin W, Parker AM, Hallquist MN, Vanyukov PM, Dombrovski AY. Decision-making competence and attempted suicide. *J Clin Psychiatry* (2015) 76(12):e1590–7. doi:10.4088/JCP.15m09778
56. Vanyukov PM, Szanto K, Hallquist M, Moitra M, Dombrovski AY. Perceived burdensomeness is associated with low-lethality suicide attempts, dysfunctional interpersonal style, and younger rather than older age. *Int J Geriatr Psychiatry* (2017) 32(7):788–97. doi:10.1002/gps.4526
57. Wiktorsson S, Olsson P, Waern M. Medically serious and non-serious suicide attempts in persons aged 70 and above. *Geriatrics* (2016) 1(3):23. doi:10.3390/geriatrics1030023
58. Mann JJ. A current perspective of suicide and attempted suicide. *Ann Intern Med* (2002) 136(4):302–11. doi:10.7326/0003-4819-136-4-200202190-00010
59. Mann JJ, Apter A, Bertolote J, Beautrais A, Currier D, Mehlum L. Suicide prevention strategies: a systematic review. *JAMA* (2005) 294(16):2064–74. doi:10.1001/jama.294.16.2064
60. O'Connor RC, Nock MK. The psychology of suicidal behavior. *Lancet Psychiatry* (2014) 1(1):73–85. doi:10.1016/S2215-0366(14)70222-6
61. Beautrais AL, Joyce PR, Mulder RT. Psychiatric illness in a New Zealand sample of young people making serious suicide attempts. *N Z Med J* (1998) 11(1060):44–8.
62. Rihmer A, Rozsa S, Rihmer Z, Gonda X, Akiskal KK, Akiskal HS. Affective temperaments, as measured by TEMPS-A, among nonviolent suicide attempters. *J Affect Disord* (2009) 116(1):18–22. doi:10.1016/j.jad.2008.10.024
63. Serafini G, Pompili M, Innamorati M, Rihmer Z, Sher L, Girardi P. Can cannabis increase suicide risk in psychosis? a critical review. *Curr Pharm Des* (2012) 18(32):5165–87. doi:10.2174/138161212802884663
64. Levi-Belz Y, Gvion Y, Grisaru S, Apter A. When the pain becomes unbearable: case-control study of mental pain characteristics among medically serious suicide attempters. *Arch Suicide Res* (2017) 8:1–14. doi:10.1080/13811118.2017.1355288
65. Orbach I, Mikulincer M, Sirota P, Gilboa-Schechtman E. Mental pain: a multidimensional operationalization and definition. *Suicide Life-Threatening Behav* (2003) 33(3):219–30. doi:10.1521/suli.33.3.219.23219
66. Van Orden KA, Witte TK, Cukrowicz KC, Braithwaite SR, Selby EA, Joiner TE. The interpersonal theory of suicide. *Psychol Rev* (2010) 117(2):575–600. doi:10.1037/a0018697
67. Hare RD. *The Hare Psychopathy Checklist–Revised (PCL-R)*. Toronto, ON: MultiHealth Systems (1991).
68. Shneidman ES. *Definition of Suicide*. Northvale, New Jersey: Jason Aronson (1985).
69. Signoretta S, Maremmani I, Liguori A, Perugi G, Akiskal HS. Affective temperament traits measured by TEMPS-I and emotional-behavioral problems in clinically-well children, adolescents, and young adults. *J Affect Disord* (2005) 85(1):169–80. doi:10.1016/S0165-0327(03)00100-9
70. Buss AH, Perry M. The aggression questionnaire. *J Pers Soc Psychol* (1992) 63:452–9. doi:10.1037/0022-3514.63.3.452
71. Baca-Garcia E, Diaz-Sastre C, Resa EG, Blasco H, Conesa DB, Oquendo MA, et al. Suicide attempts and impulsivity. *Eur Arch Psychiatry Clin Neurosci* (2005) 255(2):152–6. doi:10.1007/s00406-004-0549-3
72. Kresnow MJ, Ikeda RM, Mercy JA, Powell KE, Potter LB, Simon TR, et al. An unmatched case-control study of nearly lethal suicide attempts in Houston, Texas: research methods and measurements. *Suicide Life-Threatening Behav* (2002) 32(S1):7–20. doi:10.1521/suli.32.1.5.7.24210

73. Brown GK, Henriques GR, Sosdjan D, Beck AT. Suicide intent and accurate expectations of lethality: predictors of medical lethality of suicide attempts. *J Consult Clin Psychol* (2004) 72(6):1170–74. doi:10.1037/0022-006X.72.6.1170

15

Epidemiology of Suicidal Behavior in Malaga (Spain): An Approach From the Prehospital Emergency Service

Berta Moreno-Küstner[1,2], José del Campo-Ávila[3], Ana Ruíz-Ibáñez[1,2], Ana I. Martínez-García[4], Serafina Castro-Zamudio[1,2], Gonzalo Ramos-Jiménez[3] and José Guzmán-Parra[2,5]*

[1] Departamento de Personalidad, Evaluación y Tratamiento Psicológico, Universidad de Málaga, Málaga, Spain, [2] Grupo Andaluz de Investigación Psicosocial (GAP) (CTS-945), Instituto de Biomedicina de Málaga (IBIMA), Málaga, Spain, [3] Departamento de Lenguajes y Ciencias de la Computación, Universidad de Málaga, Málaga, Spain, [4] Unidad de Gestión Clínica del Dispositivo de Cuidados Críticos y Urgencias del Distrito Sanitario Málaga-Coín-Guadalhorce, Málaga, Spain, [5] Unidad de Salud Mental del Hospital Regional Universitario de Málaga, Málaga, Spain

Correspondence:
Berta Moreno-Küstner
bertamk@uma.es

Objective: This study aims to analyse the number and characteristics of calls made to the Málaga Prehospital Emergency Service (PES) for suicidal behavior based on sociodemographic, temporal, and health care variables.

Method: This is a retrospective, descriptive study that records all calls made to the PES due to suicidal behavior (suicide attempts and completed suicides) in 2014. Sociodemographic variables (age, sex, and health district), variables related to the calls (time-slot, degree of sunlight, type of day, month, season of the year, prioritization, and number of resources mobilized) were extracted from these calls. The number of cases and percentages were presented for the qualitative variables. The rates per 100,000 were calculated by sex and health district and presented with the corresponding 95% confidence interval (CI).

Results: Of the total valid calls to PES (n = 181,824), 1,728 calls were made due to suicidal behavior (0.9%). The mean age was 43.21 (±18) years, 57.4% were women, and the rate was 112.1 per 100,000 inhabitants. The calls due to suicidal behavior were in the younger-middle age segment, in the time-slot between 16 and 23 h and during daylight hours, on bank holidays, in spring and summer in comparison with winter, and with a peak of calls in August. The majority of these calls were classified as undelayable emergencies and mobilized one health resource.

Conclusions: Prehospital emergency services are the first contact to the sanitary services of persons or families with suicide attempts. This information should be a priority to offer a complete overview of the suicide behavior.

Keywords: prehospital emergency services, suicide, suicide attempt, epidemiology, suicidal behavior, risk factors

INTRODUCTION

The World Health Organization (WHO) recognizes suicide as a public health priority (1). Approximately 800,000 people commit suicide worldwide each year, resulting in an overall mortality rate of 16 per 100,000 inhabitants and with the number of suicides in an ever-increasing rise (2). In 2014, the suicide rate was 11.25 per 100,000 inhabitants in Europe (3) and 9.5 per 100,000 inhabitants in Spain (4). Suicide is the leading external cause of death in men (5). The southern Spanish region of Andalusia also recorded a suicide rate of 9.34 per 100,000 inhabitants in 2014 (6).

However, these figures do not include suicide attempts that did not actually result in death. A previous suicide attempt is the most important and predictive risk factor for suicide as indicated by Bostwick et al. (7), who estimated that people with a history of self-injury were 25 times more likely to commit suicide than others. Moreover, it has been estimated that for every completed suicide, there are 20 previous attempts, so identifying and following up on these events should be critical for suicide prevention (2). In Andalusia (Spain), suicide attempts have increased following the economic recession that began in 2008 (8).

Considering the importance of identifying suicide attempts and related behavior, more studies should be conducted in the health services, specifically in emergency services, both in hospital and prehospital services, as these are the first places where the person arrives, and much information can be collected on suicide attempts and related behavior. Hence, there is increased importance acquired by pre-hospital emergencies. In an emergency service in the Spanish region of Galicia, Vázquez-Lima et al. (9) found that previous suicide attempts were present in almost half of the patients who completed suicide, a finding that coincides with subsequent studies (10, 11).

Given the results from previous studies in the same research area, we consider it of utmost interest to continue analyzing and updating information where differential characteristics were found in the calls made to the Malaga Prehospital Emergency Service (PES) due to suicidal behavior (12, 13).

The present research aims to study the number and characteristics of calls made to the Malaga PES due to suicidal behavior (including threats, attempts, and completed suicide) by reviewing records of the public emergency healthcare database.

METHODS

Study Design

The research consists of a descriptive, observational, and cross-sectional study of the calls made to the PES due to suicidal behavior in the province of Malaga during 2014. The population of the Malaga province at the time was roughly 1,541,831 inhabitants. The study met the ethical criteria for research and was approved by the Malaga Ethics and Research Committee.

Sources of Information and Selection of Records

The information recorded in the computerized database of the Malaga Urgencies and Emergency Coordination Centre (UECC), including the calls made to the PES (number 061 or 112) of this province was considered to carry out this study. The procedure followed by the Malaga UECC is that once the telephone call has been made, the operator and unit doctor record all information on the event to choose the best-suited resource (ambulance, helicopter, etc.) according to the reason and priority of the call. If deemed necessary, a medical team will travel to the scene to attend to the person calling for service.

In the process of selecting the cases to be included in this study, the following information collected at three different levels was considered: (1) the type of call according to the UECC classification given by the operator or coordinator doctor at the time of the call, (2) the "Clinical Judgement" offered by the health professionals attending the patient at the scene, and (3) the type of outcome when the PES team arrives at the scene. These three levels are:

1) The classification made by the UECC operator consists of 14 categories (**Table 1**). Within these, the category called *psychiatric calls* includes elements such as nervousness, incoherence/confusion, opposition, sadness, violence, and anxiety, among others. Calls recorded in this category related to suicidal behavior (such as self-injury and suicidal tendency, suicidal thoughts, suicide threat, and suicide) were included in the suicidal behavior category (**Table 1**).
2) Concerning information regarding "Clinical Judgement," the calls whose International Classification of Diseases (ICD-9) codes were related to suicidal behavior were selected. These codes were V62.84, including those referring to suicidal ideation, and codes from E950 to E959, referring to suicide and self-inflicted injuries. These codes are listed in **Table 1**.
3) Finally, cases where the PES team directly visit the site and the outcome was fatal (*exitus*) were selected.

Study Variables

The outcomes of suicidal behavior include self-injury and suicidal tendency, suicidal thoughts, suicide threat, and consummated suicide (or *exitus*).

The variables considered for users were sex (female/male) and age (categorized in intervals: 0–17, 18–29, 30–44, 45–59, 60–75, and 75+). The health district in which the person calling the service lives was also analyzed (Ronda, Antequera, Axarquía, Coín-Guadalhorce, Costa del Sol, or Malaga city).

The temporal variables of the calls were: time-slot (from 0:00 to 7:59, 8:00 to 15:59, or 16:00 to 23:59), degree of sunlight (sunrise or sunset), type of day (working days or bank holidays), month of the year, and seasonal distribution (winter, autumn, spring, or summer).

Finally, health care information was analyzed according to the prioritization of the call, from highest to lowest priority (4: emergency, 3: undelayable emergency, 2: delayable emergency, or 1: not urgent) and the number of resources mobilized (one or more), where the mobilized resource is understood to be the intervention of an ambulance.

Statistical Analysis

Rates were calculated based on the total population of the province of Málaga and by health district and presented by 100,000 inhabitants. The reference population was provided by the Andalusian Health Service relating to the health cards of 2014 distributed by health district in the province of Malaga. Rates were calculated using the direct method and the confidence interval:

$$t = \frac{n}{N}$$

where t = gross rate, n = number of cases, and N = person-years.

The following formula was used to calculate the confidence intervals:

$$t \pm 1.96\sqrt{\frac{t \times (1 - t)}{N}}$$

where t = gross rate and N = person-years.

The arithmetic mean and standard deviation (SD) were used to describe the quantitative variables. Qualitative variables were expressed with the number of cases and percentage. For percentages, the confident intervals were built using bootstrapping (1,000 samples). All confident intervals were at 95%. The SPSS statistical package (version 17) and Excel were used in a Windows operating system.

RESULTS

The analyzed database consisted of 299,405 calls. For this study, calls unrelated to health (those that did not involve assistance to people with health needs; n = 56,273) and those not classified in any specific category by the UECC (n = 30,198) were eliminated from the sample. The database was also subject to a quality control process in which duplicate records (records that matched the identification number, date, and time) and registry errors (n = 31,110) were eliminated from the sample.

Of the 181,824 valid calls to the PES in the Malaga province, 1,728 (0.9%) were due to suicidal behavior. Further information on the sample selection process is shown in **Figure 1**.

With respect to sociodemographic variables, the mean age of people with suicidal behavior was 43.21 (SD = 18.26). The 30–44 age group proved to make the most calls due to suicidal behavior, followed by the 45–59 group (**Table 2**). Women made 1.3 times more calls than men (56.5% [95% CI: 54.2 to 58.7] vs. 43.5% [95%CI: 41.3 to 45.8]).

The rate of suicidal behavior calls made to the Malaga PES in 2014 was 112.07 per 100,000 inhabitants. Regarding health districts of residence, Malaga city recorded the highest total suicide rate (121.70 per 100,000 inhabitants), and Ronda had the lowest rate (94.62 per 100,000 inhabitants; **Table 3**). There were no statistically significant differences between the different regions regarding suicide rate. When comparing rates by sex, there was a higher overall rate in women (118.88 per 100,000 inhabitants) compared to men (96.29 per 100,000 inhabitants; $p < 0.05$) with a ratio of 1.2.

Regarding the temporality variables of suicidal behavior calls (**Table 4**), more calls were made for suicidal behavior in the timeslot between 16:00 and 23:59 (48.1%). Considering the solar calendar, more calls were made at sunrise (57.3%) than at sunset. Regarding the months, there were more calls in the month of August compared to January and February and more in October compared to February ($p < 0.05$). There was a higher percentage of calls in the spring and summer compared to winter ($p < 0.05$).

The mean number of calls due to suicidal behavior on bank holidays and working days was calculated based on the number of calls in each case. There were 300 working days and 65 bank holidays in 2014, and the average number of calls on bank holidays was 8.69, but on working days it was 3.87.

Finally, regarding care information about the functioning of PES, it was noted that 89.1% of calls were classified as undelayable emergencies (priority level 3), while 0.3% were classified as not

TABLE 1 | Classification of the Urgencies and Emergencies Coordinating Center of Malaga and classification of suicidal behaviors according to the International Classification of Diseases (ICD-9).

Classification of the urgencies and emergency coordinating center of malaga	
Non-traumatic pain	
Neurological and/or level of consciousness	
Dyspnoea	
Trauma	
Alteration of vital signs	
Psychiatric illness*	
Traffic accidents	
Gastrointestinal	
Nursing calls	
Poisoning/allergies	
Hemorrhages	
Gynecological/obstetric/urinary	
Environmental Emergencies/external agents	
Others	
Code	**Definition**
INTERNATIONAL CLASSIFICATION OF DISEASES, 9TH REVISION	
V.62.84	Suicide ideation
E950	Suicide and self-inflicted poisoning by solid or liquid substances
E951	Suicide and self-inflicted poisoning by gases in domestic use
E952	Suicide and self-inflicted poisoning by other gases and vapors
E953	Suicide and self-inflicted injury by hanging, strangulation and suffocation
E954	Suicide and self-inflicted injury by submersion (drowning)
E955	Suicide and self-inflicted injury by firearms, air guns and explosives
E956	Suicide and self-inflicted injury by cutting and piercing instrument
E957	Suicide and self-inflicted injury by jumping from high places
E958	Suicide and self-inflicted injury by other and unspecified means
E959	Late effects of self-inflicted injury

In this category, calls related to "self-injury and suicidal tendency, suicidal thoughts, suicide threated and suicide were selected for this study.

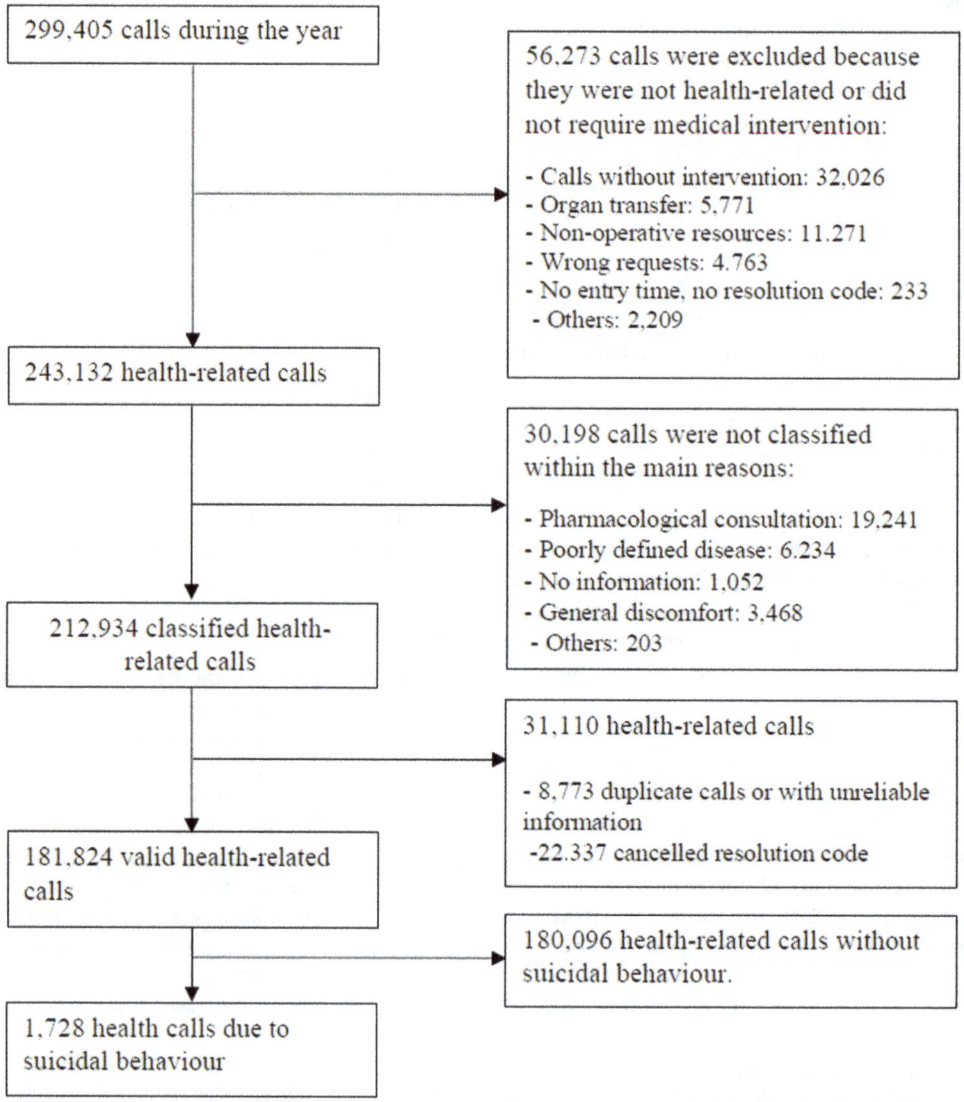

FIGURE 1 | Flow chart of the study sample selection process.

urgent (priority level 1). In terms of the number of resources mobilized (ambulances), 97% used one resource and 3% used more than one resource.

DISCUSSION

The main result of this study is that calls made to the PES due to suicidal behavior in the province of Malaga accounted for 0.9% of all calls ($n = 1,728$) and presented a suicide behavior rate of 112.07 per 100,000 inhabitants. Our figure is higher (0.8%) than that reported by Jiménez-Hernández et al. (13) in the same area in 2008. A possible explanation for the increase in this figure is that in the Jiménez-Hernández et al. study, they selected only calls classified by the operator as suicidal behavior, while in our study, we also selected the calls classified by the sanitary staff who attended the caller *in situ* and indicated a clinical judgement of ICD-9 code of suicidal behavior. Comparing our results with studies that used information from PES, the suicide behavior rate we obtained (112.07 per 100,000 inhabitants) in our region was higher than those found in other parts of Spain [76.1 per 100,000 inhabitants found by Vázquez-Lima et al. (9)]. A recent study developed by Mejías et al. (14) offered a figure of 34.7 per 100,000 inhabitants in the whole region of Andalusia, and it presented the highest rate in the province of Malaga (60.0 per 100,000 inhabitants). An explanation for our high results, which are nearly double those found by Mejías et al. (14), is that they have included only calls automatically labeled with the code X84 (intentional self-harm by unspecified means) of the ICD-10, while this code was not used automatically in Malaga in 2014, so we included all calls with terms related to suicidal behavior such as self-injury, suicidal tendency, suicidal thoughts, and suicide threat. This comparison must be made with caution

TABLE 2 | Distribution of the suicidal behavior calls made to the Prehospital Emergency Service according to age and sex.

Age groups	Total			Men			Women		
	n	%	CI 95%	*n*	%	CI 95%	*n*	%	CI 95%
<18 years	71	4.3	3.4–5.3	16	2.2	1.3–3.3	55	5.9	4.4–7.4
18–29 years	246	14.9	13.2–16.6	127	17.6	14.9–2.5	119	12.7	10.4–14.8
30–44 years	622	37.6	35.3–39.9	295	40.9	37.4–44.5	327	35.0	31.8–38.2
45–59 years	519	31.3	28.9–33.5	200	27.7	24.6–30.8	319	34.1	31.4–37.0
60–75 years	141	8.6	7.2–9.9	47	6.5	4.7–8.3	94	10.1	8.2–11.9
>75 years	57	3.4	2.6–4.4	37	5.1	3.7–6.8	20	2.1	1.3–3.1
Total	1656	100		722	100		934	100	

Missing data n = 72.

TABLE 3 | Distribution of the suicidal behavior calls made to the Prehospital Emergency Service by health district.

Health district	Population	Total calls	Suicidal calls	Rate x 100,000	CI 95%	% of total calls
Ronda	53,901	8,088	51	94.62	68.66–120.57	0.6
Antequera	109,678	15,001	109	99.38	80.73–118.03	0.7
Axarquía	150,033	22,070	161	107.31	90.74–123.88	0.7
Coín- Guadalhorce	134,944	14,701	144	106.71	89.29–124.13	1.0
Costa del Sol	475,354	46,304	511	107.50	98.18–116.81	1.1
Málaga Capital	617,921	75,520	752	121.70	113.01–130.39	1.0
Total	1,541,831	181,684	1728	112.07	106.79–117.36	0.9

CI: Confidence Interval.

and awareness that we were very inclusive in order to detect as many cases of suicide attempt as possible. However, in USA a study found a rate between 163.1 and 173.8 per 100,000 (15) which were higher in comparison with the results of this study.

Suicidal behavior in our study was higher in women (56.5%) than in men. The same trend was also found in other studies in the literature in which women used emergency services more frequently due to suicidal behavior or suicidal ideation (9, 14, 16, 17). The average age of our sample (43.2 years) is similar to previous studies (14–16) but higher than that of Vázquez-Lima et al. (9). In line with previous studies (12, 13), differences according to age were found with more suicide calls being made by people between the ages of 30 and 44 and between 45 and 59.

Regarding the time interval, our study shows an increase in suicide attempts in the time slot between 16:00 and 23:59, which is in accordance with other studies (14, 16). Doganay et al. (18) also found that suicide attempts were more frequent between 18:00 and 21:00 in men and between 15:00 and 18:00 in women, . Incidentally, we also found an increase in suicidal calls at sunrise (57.3%).

We further observed that there were proportionally more calls on bank holidays than on working days, as noted by Mejías et al. (14). However, there is an inconsistency of results in most of the publications in terms of distribution by months and of the year (9, 13, 16), and homogeneous behavior has not been found. Our results offer a higher frequency of suicide behavior calls during the summer, as observed in previous studies (14, 15, 19, 20). Our findings corroborate the temporal distribution of the current body of knowledge in the field.

As for the priority level, a high percentage of calls were classified as urgent and non-deferrable (89.1%), which is to say priority level 3 (the maximum being level 4), due to the severity of these calls and the danger of the emergency being fatal in accordance with figures reported by Mejías et al. (14) for all of Andalusia. Finally, a higher proportion of calls mobilizing one health resource was found with its implicit economic cost. This result was similar to that of Jiménez-Hernández et al. (13), who asserted that most suicidal behavior emergencies entailed a high economic cost because they mobilized one ambulance.

In conclusion, the results suggest that people who made suicidal behavior calls to the PES in Malaga were in the younger-middle age segment, more frequently women, both sexes called more frequently in the time-slot between 16:00 and 23:59 and during the daylight hours, there were more calls due to suicidal behavior on bank holidays than working days, and there were more calls in spring and summer than in winter with a peak of calls in August. In addition, the clear majority of these calls were classified as priority level 3 (non-deferrable emergencies) and frequently mobilized one health resource.

Limitations

Several limitations must be highlighted in this study. The most significant limitation relates to the problems arising from the cross-sectional study design. A second limitation is the scarcity of validated clinical information recorded by emergency health personnel, as there is a possibility that some suicide attempts might not have been included in the sample due to coding errors on the part of the operator. An example could be cataloging a

TABLE 4 | Distribution of suicidal behavior calls made to Prehospital Emergency Service by temporal and care variables.

Variables	Suicidal behavior calls		
	n	%	CI 95%
TIME SLOT			
0:00–7:59	307	18.8	16.0–19.6
8:00–15:59	589	34.1	31.9–36.5
16:00–23:59	832	48.1	45.7–50.5
DEGREE OF SUNLIGHT			
Sunrise	990	57.3	55.0–59.6
Sunset	738	42.7	40.4–45.0
MONTHS OF THE YEAR			
January	123	7.1	5.9–8.4
February	112	6.5	5.4–7.7
March	151	8.7	7.5–10.1
April	131	7.6	6.4–9.0
May	152	8.8	7.6–10.2
June	148	8.6	7.2–9.9
July	152	8.8	7.3–10.1
August	172	10.0	8.5–11.3
September	156	9.0	7.7–10.4
October	167	9.7	8.3–11.2
November	125	7.2	6.0–8.4
December	139	8.0	6.8–9.4
SEASONS			
Winter	375	21.7	19.7–23.6
Spring	445	25.8	23.7–27.7
Summer	474	27.4	25.3–29.5
Autumn	434	25.1	23.0–27.1
PRIORITY			
Emergencies	148	8.6	7.3–9.8
Non-deferrable emergencies	1539	89.1	87.6–90.5
Deferrable emergencies	35	2.0	1.3–2.7
Not urgent	6	0.3	0.1–0.6
NO OF RESOURCES MOBILIZED			
One	1682	97.3	96.6–98.1
More than one	46	2.7	1.9–3.4
TYPE OF DAY			
Working day	1163	67.3 (3.87*)	64.8–69.3
Bank holiday	565	32.7 (8.69*)	30.7–35.2

Mean calls per day based on 65 bank holidays and 300 working days during 2014.

call as drug intoxication even though the person might actually be attempting suicide. In this case, this call would not have been included in the analysis. However, although this is a considerable limitation, the study also has the advantage that the data analyzed were collected from daily clinical practice in the prehospital emergency service and correspond to all calls made in the province of Malaga. It can, therefore, be considered that these data accurately represent the calls made to the PES in this province.

Another significant limitation of our study has to do with the Malaga UECC's classification system, which does not follow an international classification method, and there are no homogeneous registration methods for suicide attempts. Therefore, the data obtained should be compared with caution with those of other communities or international studies. Regarding the comparison between different regions of Malaga, the small populations compared increase the probability of type II errors. Finally, inter-rater reliability between UECC operators is not reported and could be an important issue for estimating the rate of behavior suicide calls. However, one of our main strengths is that this study is closer to the real number of calls made to the PES due to suicidal behavior.

CONCLUSION

Research studies based on pre-hospital clinical databases are very scarce. As pre-hospital services are the first contact to the sanitary services of persons or families with suicidal behavior, this information should be a priority in order to offer a complete overview of the suicide behavior, as it is closely related to suicide completion. As Málaga presents a higher rate of suicide attempts compared with other parts of Spain, further investigations are needed in this province in order to find possible explanations for these findings.

AUTHOR CONTRIBUTIONS

BM-K and JG-P were involved in the conception, design, interpretation of data, and drafting the article. JdC-A and GR-J were involved in the design, analysis, interpretation of data, and drafting the article. AR-I, AM-G, and SC-Z were involved in the interpretation of data and drafting the article. All authors provided final approval of the version to be published.

ACKNOWLEDGMENTS

We thank Cristobalina Guillén Benítez from the pre-hospital emergency service of Málaga-Guadalhorce and Distrito Sanitario Málaga. We also thanks to I Plan Propio de la Universidad de Málaga.

REFERENCES

1. World Health Organization. *Suicide.* (2017). Available online at: http://www.who.int/mediacentre/factsheets/fs398/es/ (Accessed December 15, 2017).
2. World Health Organization. *Suicide Prevention: A Global Imperative* (2014).
3. *Eurostat.* (2014). Available online at: http://ec.europa.eu/eurostat/tgm/refreshTableAction.do?tab=table&plugin=1&pcode=tps00122&language=en (Accessed December 29, 2017).
4. Santurtún M, Santurtún A, Zarrabeitia MT. Does the environment affect suicide rates in Spain? A spatiotemporal analysis. *Rev Psiquiatr Salud Ment.* (2017). 11:192–98.doi: 10.1016/j.rpsm.2017.05.001
5. Instituto Nacional de Estadística. *Defunciones Según Causa de Muerte.* (2015) Available online at: http://www.ine.es/jaxiT3/Tabla.htm?t=7947 (Accessed December 15, 2017)

6. Junta de Andalucía Instituto de Estadística y Cartografía de Andalucía. *Conserjería de Economía y Conocimiento* (2016). Available online at: http://www.juntadeandalucia.es/institutodeestadisticaycartografia (Accessed December 29, 2017)
7. Bostwick JM, Pabbati C, Geske JR, McKean AJ. Suicide attempt as a risk factor for completed suicide: even more lethal than we knew. *Am J Psychiatry.* (2016) 173:1094–100. doi: 10.1176/appi.ajp.2016.15070854
8. Córdoba-Doña JA, San Sebastián M, Escolar-Pujolar A, Martínez-Faure JE, Gustafsson PE. Economic crisis and suicidal behaviour: the role of unemployment, sex and age in Andalusia, Southern Spain. *Int J Equity Health.* (2014) 13:13–55. doi: 10.1186/1475-9276-13-55
9. Vázquez Lima MJ, Alvarez Rodríguez C, López-Rivadulla Lamas M, Cruz Landeira A, Abellás Alvarez C. Epidemiology of suicide attempts in a public health care area: the perspective of an emergency medical service. *Emergencias.* (2012) 24:121–5.
10. Parra-Uribe I, Blasco-Fontecilla H, Garcia-Parés G, Martínez-Naval L, Valero-Coppin O, Cebrià-Meca A, et al. Risk of re-attempts and suicide death after a suicide attempt: a survival analysis. *BMC Psychiatry.* (2017) 17:163. doi: 10.1186/s12888-017-1317-z
11. Bilén K, Ponzer S, Ottosson C, Castrén M, Owe-Larsson B, Ekdahl K, Pettersson H. Can repetition of deliberate self-harm be predicted? A prospective multicenter study validating clinical decision rules. *J Affect Disord.* (2013) 149:1–3. doi: 10.1016/j.jad.2013.01.037
12. Guzmán-Parra J, Martínez-García AI, Guillén-Benítez C, Castro-Zamudio S, Jiménez-Hernández M, Moreno-Küstner B. Factores asociados con las demandas psiquiátricas a los servicios de emergencias extra-hospitalarios de Malaga (Spain) [Factors associated with psychiatric demands for prehospital emergency care services in Málaga (Spain)]. *Salud Ment.* (2016) 39:287–94. doi: 10.17711/SM.0185-3325.2016.033
13. Jiménez-Hernández M, Castro-Zamudio S, Guzmán-Parra J, Martínez-García AI, Guillén-Benítez C, Moreno-Küstner B. Las demandas por conducta suicida a los servicios de urgencias prehospitalarios de Málaga: características y factores asociados [Calls due to suicidal behaviour made to the prehospital, emergency department in Málaga: Characteristics and associated factor. *An Sist Sanit Navar.* (2017) 40:379–89. doi: 10.23938/ASSN.0047
14. Mejías-Martín Y, Martí-García C, Rodríguez-Mejías C, Valencia-Quintero JP, García-Caro MP, de Dios Luna J. Suicide attempts in Spain according to prehospital healthcare emergency records. *PLoS ONE.* (2018) 13:e0195370. doi: 10.1371/journal.pone.0195370
15. Canner JK, Giuliano K, Selvarajah S, Hammond ER, Schneider EB. Emergency department visits for attempted suicide and self harm in the USA: 2006-2013. *Epidemiol Psychiatr Sci.* (2018) 27:94–102. doi: 10.1017/S20457960 16000871
16. Mejías Y, Garcia Caro M, Schmidt J, Quero A, Gorlat B. Estudio preliminar de las características del intento de suicidio en la provincia de Granada [Preliminary study of the characteristics of attempted suicide in the province of Granada]. *An Sist Sanit Navar.* (2011) 34:431–41. doi: 10.4321/S1137-66272011 000300009
17. Wei S, Yan H, Chen W, Liu L, Bi B, Li H, Hou J, Tan S, Chen X, Dong G, et al. Gender-specific differences among patients treated for suicide attempts in the emergency departments of four general hospitals in Shenyang, China. *Gen Hosp Psychiatry.* (2013) 35:54–8. doi: 10.1016/j.genhosppsych.2012. 10.007
18. Doganay Z, Tevfik Sunter A, Guz H, Ozkan A, Altintop L, Kati C, et al. Climatic and diurnal variation in suicide attempts in the ED. *Am J Emerg Med.* (2003) 21:271–25. doi: 10.1016/S0735-6757(03) 00039-1
19. Dixon PG, Sinyor M, Schaffer A, Levitt A, Haney CR, Ellis KN, Sheridan SC. Association of weekly suicide rates with temperature anomalies in two different climate types. *Int J Environ Res Public Health.* (2014) 11:11627–44. doi: 10.3390/ijerph111111627
20. Hiltunen L, Suominen K, Lönnqvist J, Partonen T. Relationship between daylength and suicide in Finland. *J Circadian Rhythms.* (2011) 9:10. doi: 10.1186/1740-3391-9-10

16

Suicidal Risk, Psychopathology and Quality of Life in a Clinical Population of Adolescents

Judit Balazs[1,2]*, *Monika Miklosi*[1,3], *Jozsef Halasz*[2,4], *Lili Olga Horváth*[1,5], *Dóra Szentiványi*[1,5] *and Péter Vida*[1,6]

[1] *Institute of Psychology, Eötvös Loránd University, Budapest, Hungary,* [2] *Vadaskert Child Psychiatry Hospital, Budapest, Hungary,* [3] *Heim Pál Paediatric Hospital, Centre of Mental Health, Budapest, Hungary,* [4] *Alba Regia Technical Faculty, Obuda University, Szekesfehervar, Hungary,* [5] *Doctoral School of Psychology, Eötvös Loránd University, Budapest, Hungary,* [6] *School of Ph.D. Studies, Semmelweis University, Budapest, Hungary*

Correspondence:
Judit Balazs
judit.agnes.balazs@gmail.com

Background: According to literature data, psychopathology is associated with both quality of life (QoL) and suicidal risk in adolescents, but the literature does not fully support a direct association between psychopathology and suicidal thoughts and behaviors. The aim of this study was to investigate the possible mediational role of QoL in the relationship between psychopathology and level of suicidal risk in a clinical sample of adolescents.

Method: The authors examined a clinical population of 134 adolescents, aged 13–18 years. Suicidal risk—having any current suicidal ideations and/or previous suicide attempt—was assessed by the Mini International Neuropsychiatric Interview. QoL was evaluated by the adolescent self-rated versions of "Das Intervertar zur Erfassung der Lebensqualität Kindern und Jugendlichen" (ILK: Measure of Quality of Life for Children and Adolescents) and psychopathology was measured by adolescent self-rated versions of the Strengths and Difficulties Questionnaire (SDQ). A mediational model, in which QoL mediated the relationship between psychopathology and suicidal risk controlling for gender and age, was tested by means of regression analyses.

Results: Gender and age were both associated with suicidal risk. Self-reported QoL significantly mediated the relationships between emotional problems (=1.846; 95% BCa CI: 0.731–2.577), as well as peer problems (=0.883; 95% BCa CI: 0.055–1.561) and suicidal risk: more emotional and peer problems were associated with lower QoL, which in turn was related to higher level of suicidal risk.

Conclusion: Based on this study, which aims to make further steps in suicidal prevention, our findings suggest that clinicians should routinely screen the QoL of their patients, especially in adolescents with emotional and peer problems. Furthermore, it is important to focus intervention and treatment efforts on improving the QoL of adolescents with emotional and peer problems.

Keywords: suicidal risk, psychopathology, quality of life, adolescent

INTRODUCTION

It is well known that about 90% of suicidal adolescents, similar to adults, have at least one psychiatric disorder [e.g., Ref. (1–4)].

During the last decade, several studies showed that children with psychiatric disorders have poorer quality of life (QoL) than their healthy peers [e.g., Ref. (5–10)]. QoL is a multidimensional construct, which aims to describe an individual's well-being by summarizing his/her physical, mental, and social functioning (11). Though QoL includes mental state, it seeks information only about general well-being and does not screen psychopathology based on externalizing and internalizing symptoms.

On the basis of the aforementioned data, researchers aim to study the possible association between QoL and suicide, but there are conflicting available data.

There are both non-clinical and clinical studies, which support the association between QoL and suicide. A cross-sectional population study showed that adolescents above age 15 and adults with suicidal thoughts reported significantly poorer QoL than people without suicidal thoughts (12). A case–control study found that the QoL of adult suicide attempters was significantly lower than the QoL of matched controls (13). A study on a randomly selected community population found that poorer QoL was associated with higher odds of suicide ideation onset (14). A study on young adult college students also found that those with poorer QoL were more likely to endorse suicidal ideation (15). Performing a logistic regression to assess the impact of sociodemographic (e.g., age, gender, ethnicity, living satisfaction, living situation, and family SES) and clinical factors (e.g., depression) on the likelihood that young adult college students would endorse suicidality, Farabaugh et al. (15) found that poorer QoL was still a significant predictor of suicidal ideation. The results of a longitudinal epidemiological study showed that adults' baseline self-reported life dissatisfaction was associated with a higher risk of completed suicide throughout the 20-year follow-up (16). A psychological autopsy study found that low QoL within the month before death was a significant predictor of completed suicide (17). Musyimi et al. (18) reported that based on their cross-sectional epidemiological survey conducted over a period of 3 months among adult patients seeking care from traditional and faith healers in rural Kenya, regression analysis indicated that depression, suicidal ideation, and being married predicted lower overall QoL controlling for other variables.

Investigating a clinical population, Alves Vde et al. (19) found that patients who had a mental disorder and risk of suicide attempts had lower QoL than patients without the risk of suicide attempt. Further clinical studies found that patients diagnosed with depressive disorder (20), bipolar disorder (21), or epilepsy (22) and current suicidal ideation had worse QoL than patients with the same diagnoses and without suicidal ideation. Ponizovsky et al. (23) and Xiang et al. (24) reported that the differences in the QoL of schizophrenic patients with and without previous suicide attempt remained significant after adjusting for clinical factors, e.g., age of onset of the disorder, psychiatric history, and current comorbid psychopathology variables (i.e., depressive symptoms). Moreover, both child and adult bipolar patients and adult schizophrenic patients with a history of previous suicide attempt had poorer QoL than those schizophrenic and bipolar patients who had never attempted suicide (21, 23–27). Moreover, examining epileptic patients, Andrade-Machado et al. (22) reported that in a multivariate analysis lower QoL of epileptic patients significantly increased the probability of having higher suicidal risk, next to depression. Furthermore, examining a special patient-group, depressed, or anxious family caregivers of patients with cancer, Park et al. (28) found that low QoL of family caregivers was associated with their increased odds of suicidal ideation.

However, further investigating the associations between QoL and suicidal thoughts and behaviors, there are non-supportive evidence in the literature as well. Though Kao et al. (29) found that among schizophrenia patients there is a significant association between QoL and suicidal behavior—including both previous suicide attempt and current suicidal thought—this association became non-significant while controlling for depressive symptoms, with the exception of the social domain of QoL. Moreover, the study by Yan et al. (30) reported that adult schizophrenic patients with prior suicide attempt had higher social QoL than schizophrenic patients with no history of suicide attempt. Hecimovic et al. (31) reported that low QoL of epileptic patients was not related to suicide ideation in multivariate analysis, only depression.

Most of the above described studies on the role of QoL in suicidal thoughts and behaviors focused on adults; there are only very limited data on children under 18. Moreover, only a few studies investigated the role of QoL in psychopathology and suicide risk relationship and additionally these data are conflicting. Therefore, based on the knowledge gap, the aim of our study was to examine the possible mediational role of QoL—according to the above described WHOQOL Group's definition (1995) measuring adolescents well-being by summarizing their somatic and mental health and social functioning (i.e., school, family, peer relations, and being alone)—in the relationship between psychopathology and level of suicidal risk—having any current suicidal ideations and/or previous suicide attempt—in a clinical sample of adolescents.

MATERIALS AND METHODS

Sample

The study population was adolescents who had been referred for psychiatric assessment at the Vadaskert Child Psychiatric Hospital and Outpatient Clinic, Budapest, Hungary. Referral was done most often by parents (based on there own opinion or suggested by teachers) or pediatricians, but sometimes by patients themselves or child protection. Both symptoms of externalizing (e.g., attention deficit hyperactivity disorder, conduct disorder, oppositional disorder) and internalizing disorders (e.g., major depressive disorder, anxiety disorders) were among the reasons for referral. Subjects were recruited from inpatient side of this Institution. Adolescents over 13 and under 18 years old were included. An exclusion criterion was mental retardation in the medical history.

The study was approved by the Ethical Committee of the Medical Research Council, Hungary (ETT-TUKEB). The parents of each adolescent and adolescents older than 14 years included in this study provided written informed consent after being informed of the nature of the study.

Measures

Suicidal risk—having any current suicidal ideations and/or previous suicide attempt—was evaluated with the suicidal module of the *Mini International Neuropsychiatric Interview KID (MINI KID)* 2.0, Hungarian version (32–35). The MINI KID identifies current suicidal risk *via* the following questions: "In the past month did you: wish you were dead?" "Want to hurt yourself?" "Think about killing yourself?" "Think of a way to kill yourself?" "Attempt suicide?" All the questions had to be answered with "yes" or "no" by the adolescents, "yes" answers scored 1, while "no" was 0. A score of 0 was considered as no risk, scores between 1 and 5 were considered as low risk, scores between 6 and 9 were considered as medium risk, and scores ≥10 were considered as high risk. To ensure inter-rater reliability, all interviewers had participated in a training course before the study, and during the study, the interviewers were regularly supervised.

Quality of life was evaluated with the Hungarian, adolescent self-reported version of the Erfassung der Lebensqualität Kindern und Jugendlichen (ILK) (Measure of Quality of Life for Children and Adolescents) scale (36, 37). ILK assesses QoL in six different domains: school, family, peer relations, being alone, somatic health, and mental state. It uses a 5-point Likert scale, where a higher value indicates worse QoL.

Psychopathology was assessed by the Hungarian, self-reported version of the Strengths and Difficulties Questionnaire (SDQ) (38–41). SDQ is a brief screening questionnaire. SDQ consists of five scales, each with five items: (1) hyperactivity/inattention, (2) emotional symptoms, (3) conduct problems, (4) peer relationship problems scale, and (5) prosocial behavior. The first four scales constitute the Difficulties Scales. The total difficulties score is generated by summing the scores of the Difficulties scales. Each item can be answered as "not true," "somewhat true," and "certainly true." Higher scores indicate higher levels of psychopathology.

Statistical Analyses

Descriptive statistics and intercorrelations of study variables by means of Pearson's correlations are reported. Gender differences were explored using independent *t*-tests. According to the level of suicidal risk, we created two groups for further analyses and compared adolescents with no/low risk and medium/high risk. To test the mediational role of QoL reported on ILK in the relationships between psychopathology reported on SDQ and the level of suicidal risk measured by MINI KID, we conducted multiple logistic regression analyses using the PROCESS procedure (42). Gender and age were included as covariates throughout the analyses. Our hypothetical model is presented in **Figure 1**.

RESULTS

Participants

A clinical sample of 134 adolescents, 72 (53.7%) boys and 62 (46.3%) girls participated in the study. Mean age was 14.48 years (SD = 1.34, range 13–18 years).

According to the MINI KID, 54 (40.3%) adolescents showed no suicidal risk, 24 (17.9%) showed low risk, 14 (10.4%) showed medium risk, and 42 (31.3%) adolescents high suicidal risk.

Descriptive Statistics, Intercorrelations, and Reliabilities of Study Variables

Intercorrelations and reliabilities of study variables are shown in **Table 1**. Except for the SDQ Conduct problems scale, all measures showed acceptable to good internal consistencies.

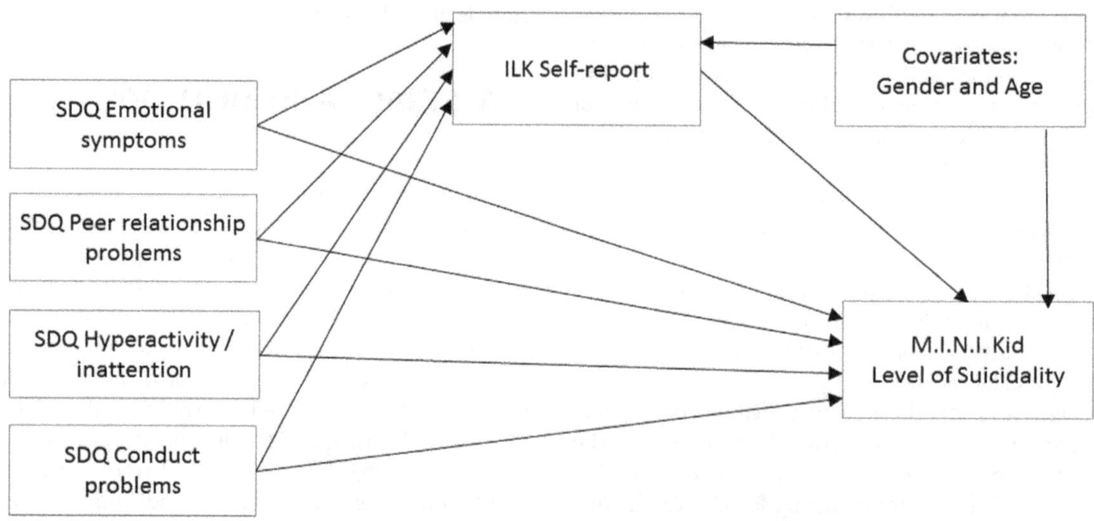

FIGURE 1 | Our hypothetical mediational model: the relationship between psychopathology and level of suicidal risk (suicidal risk) as mediated by self-reported quality of life. Abbreviations: ILK, Inventar zur Erfassung der Lebensqualität von Kindern und Jugendlichen; SDQ, Strengths and Difficulties Questionnaire; MINI KID, Mini International Neuropsychiatric Interview Kid.

TABLE 1 | Reliabilities and bivariate relationships of study variables.

	α	skew	2.	3.	4.	5.	6.	7.
1. Child's age	–	–	0.11	−0.02	−0.20	−22	0.10	0.19
2. SDQ emotional problems	0.78	0.07	–	0.33*	0.29*	0.24*	0.76*	0.65*
3. SDQ peer problems	0.67	0.55		–	0.02	0.20	0.61*	0.40*
4. SDQ attention deficit/hyperactivity problems	0.61	0.20			–	0.40*	0.63*	0.21
5. SDQ conduct problems	0.49	0.39				–	0.63*	0.29*
6. SDQ total difficulties	0.77	0.04					–	0.61*
7. ILK self-report	0.76	0.10						–

N = 134.

*ILK, Inventar zur Erfassung der Lebensqualität von Kindern und Jugendlichen; SDQ, Strengths and Difficulties Questionnaire. *p < 0.008 (= 0.05/6 using Bonferroni corrections).*

TABLE 2 | Descriptive statistics of study variables for the total sample and for no/low and medium/high suicidal risk and gender subgroups.

	Mean (SD)						
	Total sample (*N* = 134)	No/low suicidal risk (*N* = 78)	Medium/high suicidal risk (*N* = 56)	*t*(*p*) *df* = 132	Girls (*N* = 62)	Boys (*N* = 72)	*t*(*p*) *df* = 132
1. Child's age	14.48 (1.34)	14.01 (1.14)	15.13 (1.33)	5.190 (<0.001)	14.69 (1.32)	14.30 (1.34)	1.681 (0.095)
2. SDQ emotional problems	4.60 (2.79)	3.53 (2.59)	6.10 (2.59)	5.822 (<0.001)	5.71 (2.78)	3.65 (2.44)	4.554 (<0.001)
3. SDQ peer problems	3.55 (2.42)	3.00 (2.11)	4.32 (2.62)	3.225 (0.002)	3.68 (2.61)	3.44 (2.26)	1.093 (0.580)
4. SDQ attention deficit/hyperactivity problems	4.74 (2.28)	4.47 (2.07)	4.75 (2.55)	0.016 (0.987)	4.81 (2.53)	4.69 (2.05)	0.283 (0.778)
5. SDQ conduct problems	3.27 (1.82)	3.33 (1.82)	3.17 (1.84)	0.483 (0.630)	3.39 (1.98)	3.17 (1.69)	0.696 (0.487)
6. SDQ total difficulties	16.17 (6.18)	14.62 (5.71)	18.34 (6.20)	3.593 (<0.001)	17.58 (6.65)	14.96 (5.50)	2.499 (0.014)
7. ILK self-report	22.44 (5.95)	19.22 (4.63)	26.95 (4.49)	9.650 (<0.001)	24.34 (6.20)	20.82 (5.24)	3.561 (0.001)

ILK, Invertar zur Erfassung dcr Lchcnsqualitat von Kindcrn und Jugcnd lichen; SDQ, Strengths and Difficulties Questionnaire.

Inventar zur Erfassung der Lebensqualität von Kindern und Jugendlichen scores showed significant positive correlations of large effect size with SDQ Emotional problems and Total difficulties subscale scores and significant positive correlations of medium effect size with SDQ peer problems and Conduct problems scores (**Table 1**).

Descriptive statistics of the study variables for the total sample, and for the no/low and medium/high suicidal risk subgroups are presented in **Table 2**. Adolescents showing medium/high level of suicidal risk were older showed higher scores on the SDQ emotional problem scale, SDQ peer problems scale, SDQ total difficulties scale, and ILK self-report than adolescents with no/low level of suicidal risk, but no differences were found in SDQ conduct problems and SDQ ADHD subscales (**Table 2**).

Girls reported more emotional problems on SDQ and scored higher on ILK, indicating lower QoL (**Table 2**). Gender differences were found in suicidal risk as well, more girls (*N* = 46; 74.2%) than boys (*N* = 10; 13.9%) showed medium/high level of suicidal risk [$\chi^2(1) = 49.802$ $p < 0.001$].

TABLE 3 | Results of the multiple regression analyses with ILK Self-report scale as dependent.

	a	SE	t	p
Intercept	3.124	4.672	0.505	0.505
Gender (0 = girls, 1 = boys)	−0.843	0.810	−1.041	0.300
Age	0.771	0.296	2.609	0.010
SDQ emotional problems	1.040	0.163	6.401	<0.001
SDQ peer problems	0.498	0.167	2.982	0.003
SDQ attention deficit/hyperactivity problems	0.087	0.189	0.464	0.644
SDQ conduct problems	0.498	0.233	2.139	0.034
Model	$R^2 = 0.503$, $F(6,127) = 21.413$, $p < 0.001$			

N = 134.

a, unstandardized regression coefficient; ILK, Inyontar zur Erfassung dcr Lchcnsqualitat von Kindcrn und Jugcnd lichen; SDQ, Strengths and Difficulties Questionnaire.

Results of the Mediational Analyses

Results of the multivariate analyses are shown in **Tables 3** and **4**. ILK Self-report scores were related to age, as well as SDQ emotional problems, peer problems, and conduct problems subscale scores (**Table 3**). On the other hand, the level of suicidal risk was significantly associated with gender, age, SDQ emotional problems, and conduct problems subscale scores, as well as ILK self-report scores (**Table 4**).

Inventar zur Erfassung Lebensqualität von Kindern und Jugendlichen self-report scores significantly mediated the relationships between SDQ Emotional problems (=1.846; 95% BCa CI: 0.731–2.577), as well as SDQ peer problems (=0.883; 95% BCa CI: 0.055–1.561) and suicidal risk: more emotional and peer problems were associated with lower QoL, which in turn was related to higher level of suicidal risk. The relationship between SDQ ADHD subscale (=0.155; 95% BCa CI: −0.598 to 0.855), as well as SDQ Conduct problems (=0.884; 95% BCa CI: −0.425 to 1.987) and suicidal risk was not mediated by ILK self-report (**Figure 2**).

DISCUSSION

Due to the fact that the QoL measure gains more information about daily functioning and impairment than simple symptom

TABLE 4 | The logistic model with level of suicidal risk according to M.I.N.I. Kid (0 = no/low, 1 = medium/high) as dependent.

	b	SE	z	p
Step 1				
Intercept	−26.164	5.514	−4.745	<0.001
Gender (0 = girls, 1 = boys)	−4.153	0.828	5.014	<0.001
Age	1.180	0.293	4.022	<0.001
SDQ emotional symptoms	0.305	0.125	2.450	0.014
SDQ peer relationship problems	0.505	0.163	3.099	0.002
SDQ attention deficit/hyperactivity problems	−0.013	0.154	−0.082	0.935
SDQ conduct problems	−0.237	0.174	−1.363	0.173
Model	$\chi^2(6) = 103.786$ $p < 0.001$; Cox and Snell $R^2 = 0.539$; Nagelkerke $R^2 = 0.725$			
Step 2				
Intercept	−61.724	19.542	−3.159	0.002
Gender (0 = girls, 1 = boys)	−9.954	2.992	−3.329	0.001
Age	2.417	0.808	2.993	0.003
SDQ emotional problems	−0.847	0.372	−2.277	0.023
SDQ peer problems	0.130	0.299	0.432	0.666
SDQ attention deficit/hyperactivity problems	−0.477	0.288	−1.655	0.098
SDQ conduct problems	−1.431	0.545	−2.624	0.009
ILK self-report	1.773	0.571	3.103	0.002
Model	$\chi^2(7) = 160.361$ $p < 0.001$; Cox and Snell $R^2 = 0.693$; Nagelkerke $R^2 = 0.932$			

N = 134.
b, unstandardized regression coefficient; ILK, Inventar zur Erfassung Lebensqualität von Kindern und Jugendlichen; SDQ, Strengths and Difficulties Questionnaire; M.I.N.I. Kid, Mini International Neuropsychiatric Interview Kid.

scoring—while it also includes non-health-related domains of functioning—there has recently been growing interest in the QoL of children with psychiatric disorders [e.g., Ref. (6, 43–45)]. However, to the best of our knowledge, this study is the first to explore QoL as a possible mediator in the relationship between externalizing/internalizing psychopathology and level of suicidal risk in a clinical sample of adolescents.

Our results are consistent with those previous studies that stated that there are gender differences already at adolescent age in several aspects: girls have more internalizing (emotional problems) psychopathology (46, 47), lower QoL (48, 49), and higher level of suicidal risk (47, 50) than adolescents' boys.

The findings of this study are in line with previous studies as well, indicating that higher level of suicidal risk is significantly associated with both internalizing (emotional problems) and externalizing (conduct problems) psychopathology (1–4), with peer relation problems, with total difficulties (i.e., emotional + conduct + hyperactivity + peer problems) and with poorer QoL.

The very new result of this study is that QoL significantly mediates the relationships between internalizing psychopathology (i.e., emotional problems) as well as peer problems and suicidal risk: more internalizing and peer problems were associated with lower QoL, which in turn was related to higher suicidal risk.

Our data support that psychopathology and QoL are related but conceptually different constructs, showing Spearman's correlations of small to medium effect sizes between SDQ subscales and single domains of QoL, e.g., SDQ peer problems and QoL in the peer (rho = 0.48) and being alone domains (rho = 0.01);

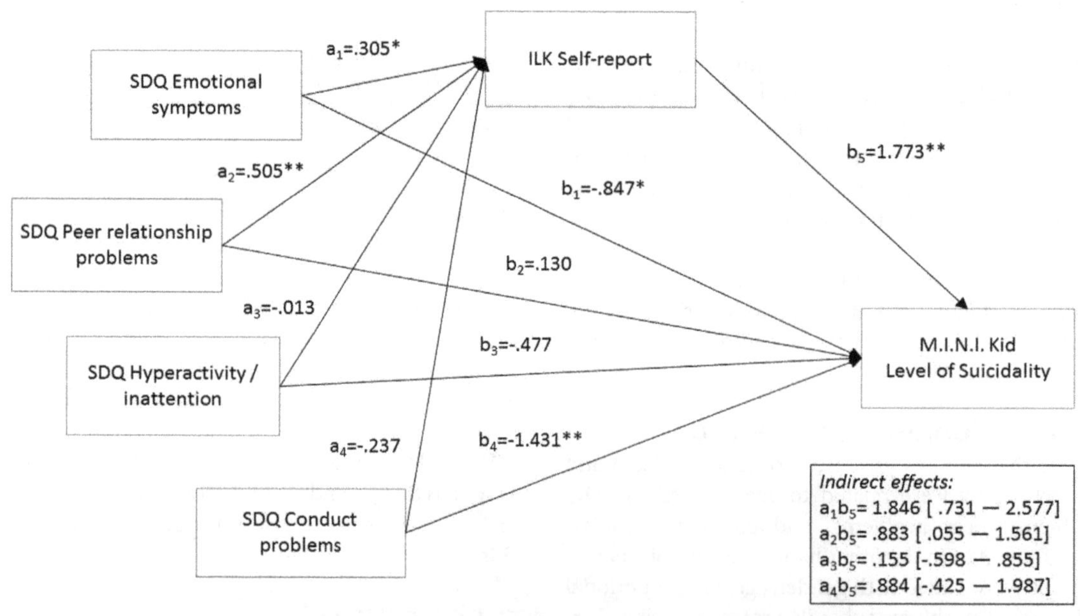

FIGURE 2 | Results of the mediational analysis. *$p < 0.05$, **$p < 0.01$. a_i, b_i: unstandardized regression coefficients. Abbreviations: ILK, Inventar zur Erfassung der Lebensqualität von Kindern und Jugendlichen; SDQ, Strengths and Difficulties Questionnaire; M.I.N.I. Kid, Mini International Neuropsychiatric Interview Kid. Gender and age were included as covariates, but are not presented in Figure because of reasons of clarity.

SDQ emotional problems and QoL somatic health (rho = 0.32) and mental state (rho = 0.47).

In this study, we measured psychopathology in a dimensional way, why we share the those researchers' opinion who have suggested during the last decade that next to categorical approaches of diagnoses, what the classification systems—i.e., Diagnostic and Statistical Manual of Mental Disorders 5th Edition (51) and International Classification of Diseases, Tenth Edition (52)—mostly follow, dimensional approaches are important for both clinical work and research (53–56). Moreover, this study supports the results of two of our previous studies, which found that subthreshold disorders—those who do not fulfill all the criteria—increase suicidal risk in children, both in the population and clinical groups of adolescents (47, 57).

These results have implications for suicide prevention. While the importance of the recognition and appropriate treatment of both internalizing and externalizing psychopathology and peer problems are well known in suicide prevention, the role of the direct measure of QoL as a possible screening method in suicide prevention is less highlighted for clinicians. Internalizing problems of a child is often less evident to others and these children often do not receive proper professional help [e.g., Ref. (58)]. The same is often true for children with peer problems, for example, victims of bullying are often ashamed and hide that they are being bullied (59, 60), additionally bullying is an important risk factor of suicide (61, 62). Based on the results of this study, screening QoL can be a marker of suicidal risk as well. Moreover, this study suggests that an improvement of the QoL, especially in the case of those who have internalizing and/or peer problems, can have a suicide prevention role. Further studies should investigate which aspects of QoL mediate the relationship between psychopathology and suicidal risk, and interventions could focus on them.

At first sight, it could be a surprising result that QoL did not mediate the relationships between hyperactivity/impulsivity/conduct symptoms and suicidal risk. However, when we made further analyses, we found that hyperactivity/impulsivity symptoms were related to more emotional symptoms and conduct problems, additionally more emotional symptoms and/or peer relationship problems were associated with higher level of suicidal risk.

We have found the same results in this study as we did in our previous study on a different clinical group of adolescents (57): the association between ADHD symptoms and suicidal risk was fully mediated by internalizing symptomatology, however it was not mediated by conduct problems. The new result is that the association between ADHD symptoms and suicidal risk was not mediated by peer problems either. All these results highlight the importance of careful assessment of comorbid internalizing symptomatology in adolescents with ADHD.

This study should be interpreted in the context of its limitations. First, the study was cross-sectional, which made us unable to consider any causal relationship among psychopathology, QoL, and suicidal risk. Second, the study population included a clinical sample. Third, although SDQ measures a wide range of adolescent psychopathology, it does not assess all of them. Third, we used self-rated scales for the assessment of QoL and psychopathology. Finally, low internal consistency of the Conduct problem subscale of the SDQ also limits the validity of the results.

In summary, according to our results, QoL significantly mediates the relationships between internalizing psychopathology, peer problems and suicidal risk. Our data indicate that suicide prevention strategies should involve assessing QoL in clinically referred adolescents, in particular in adolescents with emotional and peer problems.

AUTHOR CONTRIBUTIONS

JB: designed the study, trained the study staff, formulated the study questions, interpreted the results, and wrote the manuscript. MM: statistical analyses and wrote the manuscript. JH: participated in the study designed and approved the final manuscript. LH: supervised the data collection, participated in the data collection, and approved the final manuscript. DS: supervised the data collection, participated in the data collection, supervised the data collection, participated in the data entry, and approved the final manuscript. PV: participated in the data collection, supervised the data collection, participated in the data entry, and approved the final manuscript.

REFERENCES

1. Gould MS, Greenberg T, Velting DM, Shaffer D. Youth suicide risk and preventive interventions: a review of the past 10 years. *J Am Acad Child Adolesc Psychiatry* (2003) 42:386–405. doi:10.1097/01.CHI.0000046821.95464.CF
2. Henriksson MM, Aro HM, Marttunen MJ, Heikkinen ME, Isometsa ET, Kuoppasalmi KI, et al. Mental disorders and comorbidity in suicide. *Am J Psychiatry* (1993) 150:935–40. doi:10.1176/ajp.150.6.935
3. Marttunen MJ, Aro H, Henriksson M, Lönngvist JK. Mental disorders in adolescent suicide: DSM-III-R axes I and II diagnoses in suicides among 13- to 19- year-olds in Finland. *Arch Gen Psychiatry* (1991) 48:834–9. doi:10.1001/archpsyc.1991.01810330058009
4. Shaffer D, Gould MS, Fisher P, Trautman P, Moreau D, Kleinman M, et al. Psychiatric diagnosis in child and adolescent suicide. *Arch Gen Psychiatry* (1996) 53:339–48. doi:10.1001/archpsyc.1996.01830040075012
5. Bastiaansen D, Koot HM, Ferdinand RF. Determinants of quality of life in children with psychiatric disorders. *Qual Life Res* (2005) 14:1599–612. doi:10.1007/s11136-004-7711-2
6. Dallos Gy, Miklósi M, Keresztény A, Velő Sz, Szentiványi D, Gádoros J, et al. Self- and parent-rated quality of life of a treatment naïve sample of children

with ADHD: the impact of age, gender, type of ADHD, and comorbid psychiatric conditions according to both a categorical and a dimensional approach. *J Atten Disord* (2017) 21(9):721–30. doi:10.1177/1087054714542003
7. Freeman AJ, Youngstrom EA, Michalak E, Siegel R, Meyers OI, Findling RL. Quality of life in pediatric bipolar disorder. *Pediatrics* (2009) 123:e446–52. doi:10.1542/peds.2008-0841
8. Lack CW, Storch EA, Keeley ML, Geffken GR, Ricketts ED, Murphy TK, et al. Quality of life in children and adolescents with obsessive-compulsive disorder: base rates, parent-child agreement, and clinical correlates. *Soc Psychiatry Psychiatr Epidemiol* (2009) 44:935–42. doi:10.1007/s00127-009-0013-9
9. Moreira H, Carona C, Silva N, Frontini R, Bullinger M, Canavarro MC. Psychological and quality of life outcomes in pediatric populations: a parent-child perspective. *J Pediatr* (2013) 163:1471–8. doi:10.1016/j.jpeds.2013.06.028
10. Sawyer MG, Whaites L, Rey JM, Hazell PL, Graetz BW, Baghurst P. Health-related quality of life of children and adolescents with mental disorders. *J Am Acad Child Adolesc Psychiatry* (2002) 41:530–7. doi:10.1097/00004583-200205000-00010
11. The WHOQOL Group. The World Health Organization Quality of Life Assessment (WHOQOL): position paper from the World Health Organization. *Soc Sci Med* (1995) 10:1403–9.
12. Goldney RD, Fisher W, Wilson DH, Cheok F. Suicidal ideation and health-related quality of life in the community. *Med J Aust* (2001) 175:546–649.
13. Kumar PN, George B. Life events, social support, coping strategies, and quality of life in attempted suicide: a case-control study. *Indian J Psychiatry* (2013) 55:46–51. doi:10.4103/0019-5545.105504
14. Fairweather-Schmidt AK, Batterham PJ, Butterworth P, Nada-Raja S. The impact of suicidality on health-related quality of life: a latent growth curve analysis of community-based data. *J Affect Disord* (2016) 31:14–21. doi:10.1016/j.jad.2016.05.067
15. Farabaugh A, Bitran S, Nyer M, Holt DJ, Pedrelli P, Shyu I, et al. Depression and suicidal ideation in college students. *Psychopathology* (2012) 45:228–34. doi:10.1159/000331598
16. Koivumaa-Honkanen H, Honkanen R, Viinamäki H, Heikkilä K, Kaprio J, Koskenvuo M. Life satisfaction and suicide: a 20-year follow-up study. *Am J Psychiatry* (2001) 158:433–9. doi:10.1176/appi.ajp.158.3.433
17. Phillips MR, Yang G, Zhang Y, Wang L, Ji H, Zhou M. Risk factors for suicide in China: a national case-control psychological autopsy study. *Lancet* (2002) 360:1728–36. doi:10.1016/S0140-6736(02)11681-3
18. Musyimi C, Mutiso VN, Nayak SS, Ndetei DM, Henderson DC, Bunders J. Quality of life of depressed and suicidal patients seeking services from traditional and faith healers in rural Kenya. *Health Qual Life Outcomes* (2017) 5:95. doi:10.1186/s12955-017-0657-1
19. Alves Vde M, Francisco LC, Belo FM, de-Melo-Neto VL, Barros VG, Nardi AE. Evaluation of the quality of life and risk of suicide. *Clinics (Sao Paulo)* (2016) 71:135–9. doi:10.6061/clinics/2016(03)03
20. Berlim MT, Mattevi BS, Pavanello DP, Caldieraro MA, Fleck MP. Suicidal ideation and quality of life among adult Brazilian outpatients with depressive disorders. *J Nerv Ment Dis* (2003) 191:193–7. doi:10.1097/01.NMD.0000055081.29002.C0
21. Algorta GP, Youngstrom EA, Frazier TW, Freeman AJ, Youngstrom JK, Findling RL. Suicidality in pediatric bipolar disorder: predictor or outcome of family processes and mixed mood presentation? *Bipolar Disord* (2011) 13:76–86. doi:10.1111/j.1399-5618.2010.00886.x
22. Andrade-Machado R, Ochoa-Urrea M, Garcia-Espinosa A, Benjumea-Cuartas V, Santos-Santos A. Suicidal risk, affective dysphoric disorders, and quality-of-life perception in patients with focal refractory epilepsy. *Epilepsy Behav* (2015) 45:254–60. doi:10.1016/j.yebeh.2015.01.005
23. Ponizovsky AM, Grinshpoon A, Levav I, Ritsner MS. Life satisfaction and suicidal attempts among persons with schizophrenia. *Compr Psychiatry* (2003) 44:442–7. doi:10.1016/S0010-440X(03)00146-9
24. Xiang YT, Weng YZ, Leung CM, Tang WK, Ungvari GS. Socio-demographic and clinical correlates of lifetime suicide attempts and their impact on quality of life in Chinese schizophrenia patients. *J Psychiatr Res* (2008) 42: 495–502. doi:10.1016/j.jpsychires.2007.06.001
25. de Abreu LN, Nery FG, Harkavy-Friedman JM, de Almeida KM, Gomes BC, Oquendo MA, et al. Suicide attempts are associated with worse quality of life in patients with bipolar disorder type I. *Compr Psychiatry* (2012) 53:125–9. doi:10.1016/j.comppsych.2011.03.003
26. Huang RR, Chen YS, Chen CC, Chou FH, Su SF, Chen MC, et al. Quality of life and its associated factors among patients with two common types of chronic mental illness living in Kaohsiung City. *Psychiatry Clin Neurosci* (2012) 66:482–90. doi:10.1111/j.1440-1819.2012.02380.x
27. Studart P, Galvão-de Almeida A, Bezerra-Filho S, Caribé A, Reis Afonso N, Daltro C, et al. Is history of suicidal behavior related to social support and quality of life in outpatients with bipolar I disorder? *Psychiatry Res* (2016) 30:796–802. doi:10.1016/j.psychres.2016.10.045
28. Park B, Kim SY, Shin JY, Sanson-Fisher RW, Shin DW, Cho J, et al. Suicidal ideation and suicide attempts in anxious or depressed family caregivers of patients with cancer: a nationwide survey in Korea. *PLoS One* (2013) 8:e60230. doi:10.1371/journal.pone.0060230
29. Kao YC, Liu YP, Cheng TH, Chou MK. Subjective quality of life and suicidal behavior among Taiwanese schizophrenia patients. *Soc Psychiatry Psychiatr Epidemiol* (2012) 47:523–32. doi:10.1007/s00127-011-0361-0
30. Yan F, Xiang YT, Hou YZ, Ungvari GS, Dixon LB, Chan SS, et al. Suicide attempt and suicidal ideation and their associations with demographic and clinical correlates and quality of life in Chinese schizophrenia patients. *Soc Psychiatry Psychiatr Epidemiol* (2013) 48:447–54. doi:10.1007/s00127-012-0555-0
31. Hecimovic H, Santos JM, Carter J, Attarian HP, Fessler AJ, Vahle V, et al. Depression but not seizure factors or quality of life predicts suicidality in epilepsy. *Epilepsy Behav* (2012) 24:426–9. doi:10.1016/j.yebeh.2012.05.005
32. Balázs J, Bíró A, Dálnoki D, Lefkovics E, Tamás Z, Nagy P, et al. A Gyermek M.I.N.I. kérdőív magyar nyelvű változatának ismertetése. *Psychiatr Hung* (2004) 19:358–64.
33. Lecrubier Y, Sheehan DV, Weiller E, Amorim P, Bonora L, Sheehan HK, et al. The MINI International Neuropsychiatric Interview (M.I.N.I.). A short diagnostic structured interview: reliability and validity according the CIDI. *Eur Psychiatry* (1997) 12:224–31. doi:10.1016/S0924-9338(97)83296-8
34. Sheehan DV, Lecrubier Y, Sheehan KH, Amorim P, Janavs J, Weiller E, et al. The Mini-International Neuropsychiatric Interview (M.I.N.I.): the development and validation of a structured diagnostic psychiatric interview for DSM-IV and ICD-10. *J Clin Psychiatry* (1998) 59(Suppl 20):34–57.
35. Sheehan DV, Sheehan KH, Shytle RD, Janavs J, Bannon Y, Rogers JE, et al. Reliability and validity of the Mini International Neuropsychiatric Interview for Children and Adolescents (MINI-KID). *J Clin Psychiatry* (2010) 71:313–26. doi:10.4088/JCP.09m05305whi
36. Kiss E, Baji I, Mayer L, Skulteti D, Benak I, Vetro A. Validity and psychometric properties of a quality of life questionnaire in a Hungarian child and adolescent population. *Psychiatr Hung* (2007) 22:33–42.
37. Mattejat F, Remschmidt H. Zur Erfassung der Lebensqualität bei psychischgestörten Kindern und Jugendlichen – Eine Übersicht. *Z Kinder Jugendpsychiatr Psychother* (1998) 26:183–96.
38. Birkás E, Lakatos K, Tóth I, Gervai J. [Screening childhood behavior problems using short questionnaires I.: the Hungarian version of the strengths and difficulties questionnaire]. *Psychiatr Hung* (2007) 23:358–65.
39. Goodman R, Meltzer H, Bailey V. The strengths and difficulties questionnaire: a pilot study on the validity of the self-report version. *Eur Child Adolesc Psychiatry* (1998) 7:125–30. doi:10.1007/s007870050057
40. Turi E, Toth I, Gervai J. [Further examination of the strengths and difficulties questionnaire (SDQ-Magy) in a community sample of young adolescents]. *Psychiatr Hung* (2010) 26:415–26.
41. Turi E, Gervai J, Aspan N, Halasz J, Nagy P, Gadoros J. [Validation of the Hungarian version of the strengths and difficulties questionnaire in an adolescent clinical population]. *Psychiatr Hung* (2012) 28:165–79.
42. Hayes AF. *Introduction to Mediation, Moderation, and Conditional Process Analysis: A Regression-Based Approach*. New York, NY: Guilford Press (2013).
43. Bastiaansen D, Koot HM, Bongers IL, Varni JW, Verhulst FC. Measuring quality of life in children referred for psychiatric problems: psychometric properties of the PedsQLTM 4.0 generic core scales. *Qual Life Res* (2004) 13:489–95. doi:10.1023/B:QURE.0000018483.01526.ab
44. Klassen AF, Miller A, Fine S. Health-related quality of life in children and adolescents who have a diagnosis of attention-deficit/hyperactivity disorder. *Pediatrics* (2004) 114(5):E541–7. doi:10.1542/peds.2004-0844
45. Mattejat F, Simon B, König U, Quaschner K, Barchewitz C, Felbel D, et al. Lebensqualität bei psychisch kranken Kindern und Jugendlichen. (Quality of life of children and adolescents with mental health disorders).

Z Kinder Jugendpsychiatr Psychother (2003) 31(4):293–303. doi:10.1024/1422-4917.31.4.293

46. Angold A, Costello EJ, Worthman CM. Puberty and depression: the roles of age, pubertal status and pubertal timing. *Psychol Med* (1998) 28:51–61. doi:10.1017/S003329179700593X
47. Balazs J, Miklosi M, Kereszteny A, Hoven CW, Carli V, Wasserman C, et al. Adolescent subthreshold-depression and anxiety: psychopathology, functional impairment and increased suicide risk. *J Child Psychol Psychiatry* (2013) 54:670–7. doi:10.1111/jcpp.12016
48. Cavallo F, Zambon A, Borraccino A, Raven-Sieberer U, Torsheim T, Lemma P. Girls growing through adolescence have a higher risk of poor health. *Qual Life Res* (2006) 15:1577–85. doi:10.1007/s11136-006-0037-5
49. Michel G, Bisegger C, Fuhr DC, Abel T; KIDSCREEN Group. Age and gender differences in health-related quality of life of children and adolescents in Europe: a multilevel analysis. *Qual Life Res* (2009) 18:1147–57. doi:10.1007/s11136-009-9538-3
50. Wunderlich U, Bronisch T, Wittchen HU, Carter R. Gender differences in adolescents and young adults with suicidal behaviour. *Acta Psychiatr Scand* (2001) 104:332–9. doi:10.1111/j.1600-0447.2001.00432.x
51. American Psychiatric Association. *Diagnostic and Statistical Manual of Mental Disorders*. 5th ed. Washington, DC: American Psychiatric Association (2013).
52. World Health Organization. *ICD-10 Classifications of Mental and Behavioural Disorder: Clinical Descriptions and Diagnostic Guidelines*. Geneva: World Health Organization (1992).
53. Helmchen H, Linden M. Subthreshold disorders in psychiatry: clinical reality, methodological artifact and double-threshold problem. *Compr Psychiatry* (2000) 41(Suppl 1):1–7. doi:10.1016/S0010-440X(00)80001-2
54. Lecrubier Y. Refinement of diagnosis and disease classification in psychiatry. *Eur Arch Psychiatry Clin Neurosci* (2008) 258(Suppl 1):6–11. doi:10.1007/s00406-007-1003-0
55. Möller HJ. Systematic of psychiatric disorders between categorical and dimensional approaches: Kraepelin's dichotomy and beyond. *Eur Arch Psychiatry Clin Neurosci* (2008) 258(Suppl 2):48–73. doi:10.1007/s00406-008-2004-3
56. Okasha A. Would the use of dimensions instead of categories remove problems related to subthreshold disorders? *Eur Arch Psychiatry Clin Neurosci* (2009) 259(Suppl 2):129–33. doi:10.1007/s00406-009-0052-y
57. Balazs J, Miklosi M, Kereszteny A, Dallos G, Gadoros J. Attention-deficit hyperactivity disorder and suicidality in a treatment naive sample of children and adolescents. *J Affect Disord* (2014) 152-154:282–7. doi:10.1016/j.jad.2013.09.026
58. Wagner R, Silove D, Marnane C, Rouen D. Delays in referral of patients with social phobia, panic disorder and generalized anxiety disorder attending a specialist anxiety clinic. *J Anxiety Disord* (2006) 20:363–71. doi:10.1016/j.janxdis.2005.02.003
59. Duarte C, Pinto-Gouveia J, Rodrigues T. Being bullied and feeling ashamed: implications for eating psychopathology and depression in adolescent girls. *J Adolesc* (2015) 44:259–68. doi:10.1016/j.adolescence.2015.08.005
60. Vie TL, Glasø L, Einarsen S. How does it feel? Workplace bullying, emotions and musculoskeletal complaints. *Scand J Psychol* (2012) 53:165–73. doi:10.1111/j.1467-9450.2011.00932.x
61. Alavi N, Reshetukha T, Prost E, Antoniak K, Patel C, Sajid S, et al. Relationship between bullying and suicidal behaviour in youth presenting to the emergency department. *J Can Acad Child Adolesc Psychiatry* (2017) 26:70–7.
62. Barzilay S, Brunstein Klomek A, Apter A, Carli V, Wasserman C, Hadlaczky G, et al. Bullying victimization and suicide ideation and behavior among adolescents in Europe: a 10-country study. *J Adolesc Health* (2017) 61:179–86. doi:10.1016/j.jadohealth.2017.02.002

17

Attachment to Parents as a Moderator in the Association Between Sibling Bullying and Depression or Suicidal Ideation among Children and Adolescents

*Jasmin Bar-Zomer and Anat Brunstein Klomek**

Baruch Ivcher School of Psychology, Interdisciplinary Center (IDC), Herzliya, Israel

Correspondence:
Anat Brunstein Klomek
bkanat@idc.ac.il

Bullying is one of the most widespread phenomenon in childhood and adolescence. Interestingly, most research on bullying focuses on bullying at school and not on bullying among siblings at home. Sibling bullying is the most frequent form of repeated aggression that children experience in their lifetime. Furthermore, previous studies indicate that sibling bullying is associated with depression and self-harm behavior. However, the association between sibling bullying and suicidal ideation was never previously examined. Attachment to parents is one variable that can moderate the association between sibling bullying and depression/suicide ideation. To our knowledge, there is no existing study that examines the association between sibling bullying and attachment patterns. In addition, no previous study has examined the moderating role of attachment on the association between sibling bullying and depression or suicidal ideation among adolescents. The current study includes 279 Israeli students aged 10–17 (M = 13.5; SD = 1.98; 164, 58.8% females) who completed self-report questionnaires regarding school and sibling bullying, attachment to mother and father, depression, and suicidal ideation. The results indicated an association between bullying among siblings and school bullying. In addition, children and adolescents who were consistently involved in sibling bullying were at greater risk for depression and suicide ideation when compared to children and adolescents who were not involved in sibling bullying. A secure attachment to one's father (but not to one's mother) moderated the association between sibling bullying and depression/suicide ideation. It should be noted that when suicide ideation was examined above and beyond depression, attachment to one's father did not moderate the association between sibling bullying involvement and suicide ideation. This finding indicates that depression plays a central role in the association between sibling bullying and suicide ideation. These results suggest that sibling bullying is a risk factor for depressive symptoms and suicide ideation and that secure attachment to one's father may serve as a protective role. Future bullying prevention programs should include sibling bullying and encourage the increased availability of paternal emotional support. Other theoretical and applied implications for prevention of both sibling bullying and suicide are discussed.

Keywords: bullying, sibling, attachment, depression, suicidal ideation, adolescence

INTRODUCTION

Bullying is a subtype of aggression (1). Research on sibling relationships rarely defines sibling violence as a form of bullying (2). However, violence between siblings often meets the three criteria for bullying: a situation in which a child is exposed to unwanted aggression that is intended to induce fear, distress or harm; frequently repeats itself; and an unbalanced distribution of power between the aggressor and the aggressed (1, 3). Furthermore, an important literature review, conducted by Wolke et al. (4), suggests that we should relate to sibling bullying as we do to peer bullying. Therefore, it seems appropriate to categorize those involved in sibling bullying as either, victim, bully, or bully/victim (a child that is both, bully and victim), an acceptable categorization for those involved in peer or school bullying (5).

Despite the importance of sibling bullying, a dearth of research has examined this form of bullying (2, 4, 6). Wolke and Skew (7) reviewed research that examined the frequency of sibling bullying and found that about half of the children were involved in some form of sibling bullying (as bully, as victim, or as bully/victim) at a frequency of more than four times in 6 months. Of these children, 16–20% reported frequent sibling bullying involvement (i.e., once a week or more). Wolke et al.'s (4) review suggests that sibling bullying is the most frequent form of abuse. Children suffer from sibling bullying more than from abuse by parents, adult strangers, or peers (4, 7).

Research shows an association between sibling bullying and school bullying. Studies found that 50% of the children who reported sibling victimization also suffered from victimization at school (8, 9). Duncan (10) showed the reverse of this association such that children who suffered from school bullying reported higher levels of involvement with bullying at home, either as victim or as bully.

One of the negative ramifications of sibling bullying involvement is depression (11). In a longitudinal research study, Bowes et al. (11) found that children who were victims of sibling bullying at age 12 were at a double risk for depression, anxiety, and self-harm, compared to children who did not suffer from sibling bullying. In addition, results also showed that the higher the frequency of the sibling bullying, the higher the risk for psychological difficulties for the victim. Klomek et al. (12) found that adolescents who were victims of school bullying were at an increased risk for depression but also for suicidal ideation, and suicidal attempts. To the best of our knowledge, there are no previous studies, which have examined suicidal ideation among those involved in sibling bullying, compared to suicidal ideation among those who are not involved in sibling bullying.

Only a few studies have examined the association between familial characteristics and sibling bullying, while using the definition of sibling bullying (4). The existing research suggests an association between familial characteristics and involvement in sibling bullying. For example, children who had many conflicts with their parents, who were reared in more violent homes, who underwent parental abuse or whose mothers suffered from depression, were more likely to be involved in sibling bullying than children not involved in sibling bullying (7, 11, 13–17) but attachment was not examined. Attachment theory focuses on the long-term relationship dynamics between people, starting from the developing relationship between child and parent in the child's first years of life (18, 19). The theory assumes this primary relationship to form the foundation for how the child perceives his relationship to the social world that surrounds him (20).

In recent decades, data from a range of research emphasized the association between attachment styles and the social and emotional development of children and adolescents. These associations, however, were not previously examined in relation to sibling bullying. There are a handful of studies, which examined the association between attachment style and sibling aggressiveness or violence. Results from these studies indicate that attachment styles toward one's mother and father can dictate the relationships between siblings and influence an individual's aggressive behavior (21–23). There is a high likelihood that siblings with insecure attachments toward their parents will respond with aggression, will engage in repeated conflicts, and will involve themselves in sibling bullying (6, 24, 25). Likewise, a small number of studies examined the association between attachment styles and involvement in school bullying (24, 26–29).

In summary, the associations between sibling bullying and suicidal ideation as well as the associations between sibling bullying and attachment to parents have not been previously examined. Moreover, the variables that moderate the association between sibling bullying and depression/suicidal ideation have yet to be examined. Therefore, the goal of the present research is to fill in these gaps. Our research hypotheses are as follows: (1) the likelihood for depression and suicidal ideation will be higher among children involved in sibling bullying compared to children not involved in sibling bullying; (2) children involved in sibling bullying will display less secure attachment styles toward their mothers and fathers compared to children not involved in sibling bullying; and (3) secure attachment styles toward one's mother and father will moderate the association between involvement in sibling bullying and depression/suicidal ideation in the following way: among children with secure attachments with their mothers/fathers, there will be a weaker association between sibling bullying involvement and depression/suicidal ideation than among children with insecure attachments with their mothers/fathers.

MATERIALS AND METHODS

Participants

Three hundred nineteen children and adolescents, ages 10–17, participated in the study. All participants were students in 5th through 12th grades in elementary schools, junior high schools, and high schools in Israel. Forty-nine participants were removed from the study due to incompletion of their questionnaires. Two hundred seventy-nine participants remained for the final analyses. These included 115 boys and 164 girls, in grades 5 to 12 (mean age—13.5, SD = 1.9).

Research Measures

Five self-report and anonymous questionnaires were completed by participants.

Demographic Questionnaire

This questionnaire included questions regarding age, gender, grade level, and sibling composition (i.e., number, gender).

Sibling and Peer Bullying

The bullying questionnaire was used to measure the participants' involvement in sibling and peer bullying. As in the original questionnaire (30), the first part of this questionnaire asked questions regarding school bullying and included 11 questions about bullying behaviors and 11 questions about victimization. Furthermore, this questionnaire is comprised of questions relating to type of bullying (e.g., physical bullying, "Hit, slapped or pushed you," "Took your money"; verbal bullying, "Threatened to hit or harm you"), place of bullying (inside/outside of school, at home, at social media, *via* the cellphone), and the characteristics of the bully (individual/group, gender). In the second part of this questionnaire, we appropriated the questions for sibling bullying. The questions remained identical to how they were presented in the original questionnaire, just adapted for siblings. The frequency items were coded on a 4-point scale ranging from 1 to 4 (1 = *not at all*, 2 = *less than once a week*, 3 = *More than once a week*, 4 = *Most days*). An adolescent was considered involved in bullying if he/she marked frequent involvement (*more than once a week* or more) in any type of bullying or victimization involvement (physical, verbal, social, etc.). Earlier research shows good reliability ($\alpha = 0.79$) for this questionnaire (31). In the present study, the reliability of this questionnaire was high, with an internal consistency score (alpha Cronbach) of $\alpha = 0.91$ for the school bullying sub-scale, and an internal consistency score (alpha Cronbach) of $\alpha = 0.90$ for the school victimization sub-scale. Likewise, the internal consistency score (alpha Cronbach) for the sibling bullying sub-scale was $\alpha = 0.90$, and the internal consistency score (alpha Cronbach) for sibling victimization was $\alpha = 0.91$.

Depression

In order to assess clinical depression, we used The *Mood and Feelings Questionnaire* [MFQ; (32)], a widely used questionnaire for identifying symptoms of depression among children and adolescents aged 8–18. The questionnaire includes 33 questions relating to the child's/adolescent's emotions, cognitions, and behaviors in the last 2 weeks. The questions require the child/adolescent to rank his/her answers on a scale of 0–2 (0 = *incorrect*, 1 = *sometimes correct*, 2 = *correct*). A sum score of 26 or above determines clinical depression, as suggested in research literature (33). Early findings show good validity and reliability ($\alpha = 0.87$) for this questionnaire (34). The reliability of this questionnaire in the present study was high ($\alpha = 0.96$).

Suicidal Ideation

Four items from the MFQ, all of which indicate suicidal ideation, were used to assess suicidal ideation. Three of the items reflect passive suicidal thinking ("I thought that there's no reason to live," "I thought about death," and "I thought that my family is better off without me"), and one item reflects active suicidal thinking ("I thought to kill myself"). The differentiation between passive and active suicidal thinking is consistent with the Columbia Suicide Severity Rating Scale (35). Answers range on a scale from 0 to 2 (0 = *incorrect*, 1 = *sometimes correct*, 2 = *correct*). As accepted in research literature, each positive answer is indicative of suicidal ideation. The use of questions concerning suicidal ideation from a depression questionnaire has been done in earlier research (33). The reliability of these four questions in the present study was good ($\alpha = 0.85$).

Attachment to Parents

Participants' parent-child attachments were assessed with *The Attachment Security Style Scale* (36). This questionnaire measures one's attachment style by using a Harter 4-point scale ("*There are children that … other children …*"). The child/adolescent is required to mark which of the statements is true regarding his/her relationship with his/her parent (e.g., "there are those that are not certain that they can trust their mother, but there are those for whom it is easy to trust their mothers"). Then, the child/adolescent is requested to decide if the statement is very true or pretty true with regard to himself/herself. The participants completed 2 editions of 15 items each, 1 regarding the mother and 1 regarding the father. Ratings for each participant were summed to form an attachment security score ranging from 15 to 60, with higher scores indicating a more secure relationship. Earlier findings showed high reliability and validity for this questionnaire (36, 37). The internal consistency (alpha Cronbach) score for the attachment to mother section was $\alpha = 0.84$, while the internal consistency (alpha Cronbach) score for the attachment to father section was $\alpha = 0.87$.

Procedure

The pilot study included 91 children and adolescents who were recruited as a convenience sample. All parents signed an informed consent form. The children read an explanation of the study and, then, completed the questionnaires. The 228 additional participants were recruited *via* their schools. We first requested permission from the school principals. Once permission was granted, we sent printed and emailed letters to parents describing the study. Attached to the letter was a request for non-participation. 2 weeks later, during a class set aside for the study, the students who were approved for participation *via* their parents, completed the self-report questionnaires. The study was approved by the Israeli Ministry of Education and the ethical committee of the Interdisciplinary Center (IDC), Herzliya.

Statistical Analyses

Chi-squared (χ^2) tests were performed in order to examine dependency between sibling bullying involvement and school bullying involvement, depression, and/or suicidal ideation. Likewise, independent sample *T* tests were performed in order to examine if children who are involved in sibling bullying have less secure attachment styles (toward mother and father separately) compared to children who are not involved in sibling bullying. Eventually, a multiple logistic regression analysis was performed in order to examine if the level of secure attachment to one's parent (mother and father separately) moderated the association between sibling bullying involvement and depression/suicidal ideation. In this analysis, the level of secure attachment (to mother and father separately), sibling bullying involvement, and the interaction between them were simultaneously entered as predictors. In accordance with Aiken et al. (38) and before conducting the regression analysis, we centered the values of the aforementioned variables (i.e., sibling bullying involvement and attachment). Considering the regression model for suicidal ideation yielded significance, we conducted a further analysis to examine if one's attachment style moderates the association between involvement in sibling bullying and suicidal ideation while controlling for depression. All statistical analyses of the study data were performed on SPSS edition 21. Finally, considering that suicidal ideation was measured *via* four items from the MFQ for depression, we conducted a further analysis to be certain that the moderating model would remain significant, even after removing the four items from the depression measure and using them as a measure for suicidal ideation.

RESULTS

In the total sample, 86 participants were involved in sibling bullying (193 participants were not involved), while 92 participants were involved in school bullying (187 participants were not involved). **Table 1** displays the frequency of involvement in school bullying and sibling bullying. In addition, 11.8% of the participants in the present sample met criteria for clinical depression and 19.7% of the participants presented either passive suicidal ideation or active suicidal ideation.

The Association between Involvement in Sibling Bullying and Involvement in School Bullying

A significant association was found between sibling and school bullying [$\chi^2(1) = 25.73, p < 0.001$]. Of the 86 participants involved in sibling bullying, 48 (55.8%) were involved in school bullying. By contrast, of the 193 participants not involved in sibling bullying, 46 (23.8%) were involved in school bullying. In other words, these results suggest that there is a significant association between involvement in school bullying and involvement in sibling bullying. Children involved in sibling bullying were 2.3 times more likely to suffer from school bullying than children not involved in sibling bullying.

The Association between Involvement in Sibling Bullying and Depression and Suicidal Ideation

A significant association between sibling bullying involvement and depression was found [$\chi^2(1) = 15.34, p < 0.001$]. Of the 86 participants involved in sibling bullying, 20 (23.2%) met criteria for clinical depression. By contrast, of the 193 participants uninvolved in sibling bullying, only 12 (6.2%) met criteria for clinical depression. In other words, these results suggest that there is a significant association between involvement in sibling bullying and clinical depression. Children involved in sibling bullying were 3.7 times more likely to suffer from clinical depression than children not involved in sibling bullying.

In addition, a significant association between sibling bullying involvement and suicidal ideation was found [$\chi^2(1) = 10.436$, $p < 0.005$]. Of the 86 participants involved in sibling bullying, 26 (30.2%) experience suicidal ideation. In contrast, of the 193 participants uninvolved in sibling bullying, only 25 (12.9%) experienced suicidal ideation. In other words, these results suggest that there is a significant association between involvement in sibling bullying and suicidal ideation such that children involved in sibling bullying were 2.3 times more likely to suffer from suicidal ideation than children not involved in sibling bullying.

TABLE 1 | The frequency of involvement in school bullying and sibling bullying.

	Percentage of the total sample which are involved in bullying			
	Victims	**Bully**	**Bully victim**	**Any type of involvement**
Sibling bullying	9.7% (n = 27)	4.3% (n = 12)	16.8% (n = 47)	30.8% (n = 86)
School bullying	13.2% (n = 37)	10.4% (n = 29)	9.3% (n = 26)	32.9% (n = 92)

The Association between Sibling Bullying Involvement and Attachment Style

We found a significant difference in levels of secure attachment to mothers and fathers between those involved in sibling bullying and those not involved in sibling bullying [*Mother*: $t(232) = 4.09$, $p < 0.001$; *Father*: $t(224) = 3.32$, $p < 0.005$]. Participants involved in sibling bullying have less secure attachments to their mothers (M = 43.41) than do participants uninvolved in sibling bullying (M = 48.19). Likewise, participants involved in sibling bullying have less secure attachments to their fathers (M = 41.69) than do participants uninvolved in sibling bullying (M = 46.36).

Attachment to Mother As a Moderating Variable on the Association between Sibling Bullying Involvement and Depression/Suicidal Ideation

The regression model that examined attachment to mother as moderating the association between sibling bullying and depression, while controlling for gender, was found to be significant ($-2LL = 119.53$, $p < 0.001$, Nagelkerke $R^2 = 0.24$, Cox & Snell $R^2 = 0.11$). The analysis resulted in a positive association between gender and depression such, that girls had a 4.76 times higher chance for depression than did boys ($B = 1.56$, $Z = 2.37$, OR = 4.76, $p < 0.05$). Attachment style to mother was *almost* significantly associated with depression ($B = -0.08$, $Z = 1.96$, OR = 0.92, $p = 0.0504$). In addition, involvement in sibling bullying was found to be positively and significantly associated with depression ($B = 1.38$, $Z = 2.52$, OR = 3.97, $p < 0.05$) such, that participants involved in sibling bullying have a 3.97 times higher chance for depression than do participants uninvolved in sibling bullying. Finally, an interaction effect between level of secure attachment to mother and bullying involvement was found to be insignificant ($B = 0.02$, OR = 3.73, $Z = 0.29$, ns). After conducting the above analyses, we performed an additional multiple logistic regression analysis in order to examine if gender influences the way in which attachment style to mother moderates the association between sibling bullying involvement and depression. This model did not appear significant, a likely result of the sample size.

A multiple logistic regression analysis was also performed to examine if the level of secure attachment to the mother moderates the association between sibling bullying involvement and suicidal ideation. This model was found to be significant ($-2LL = 201.12$, $p < 0.005$, Nagelkerke $R^2 = 0.12$, Cox & Snell $R^2 = 0.07$). This analysis resulted in a positive association between gender and suicidal ideation such, that girls have a 2.66 times higher chance for suicidal ideation than do boys ($B = 0.98$, $Z = 2.36$, $OR = 2.66$, $p < 0.05$). Likewise, analysis results showed that a secure attachment style to one's mother is negatively and significantly associated with suicidal ideation ($B = -0.05$, $Z = -2.15$, $OR = 0.96$, $p < 0.05$). In other words, the more secure one's attachment is to his/her mother, the lower the chance for suicidal ideation. Involvement in sibling bullying was not found to be significantly associated with suicidal ideation ($B = 0.68$, $Z = 1.80$, $OR = 1.98$, ns). Finally, an interaction effect between attachment to mother and involvement in sibling bullying was found to be insignificant ($B = -0.01$, $Z = -0.13$, $OR = 1.88$, ns). In other words, attachment to one's mother did not moderate the association between sibling bullying involvement and suicidal ideation. After the above analyses, we performed an additional multiple logistic regression analysis in order to examine if gender influences the way in which attachment style to one's mother moderates the association between sibling bullying involvement and suicidal ideation. This model did not appear significant, a likely result of the sample size.

Attachment to Father As a Moderating Variable on the Association between Sibling Bullying Involvement and Depression/Suicidal Ideation

The multiple logistic regression model performed to examine if the level of secure attachment to one's father moderates the association between involvement in sibling bullying and depression was found to be significant ($-2LL = 114.49$, $p < 0.001$, Nagelkerke $R^2 = 0.26$, Cox & Snell $R^2 = 0.11$). This analysis resulted in a positive association between gender and depression such, that girls have a 5.5 times higher chance for depression than do boys ($B = 1.71$, $Z = 2.42$, $OR = 5.5$, $p < 0.05$). Attachment style to one's father was found to be negatively and significantly associated with depression ($B = -0.11$, $Z = -3.11$, $OR = 0.9$, $p < 0.005$). Meaning, the more secure one's attachment is to his/her father, the lower the chance for depression. In addition, involvement in sibling bullying was found to be positively and significantly associated with depression ($B = 1.73$, $Z = 2.96$, $OR = 5.67$, $p < 0.005$) such that participants involved in sibling bullying have a 5.67 times higher chance for depression than participants uninvolved in sibling bullying. Finally, an interaction effect between level of secure attachment to one's father and involvement in sibling bullying was found to be significant ($B = 0.09$, Wald $= 4.37$, $OR = 5.60$, $p < 0.05$). In other words, attachment to one's father moderates the association between sibling bullying involvement and depression such, that the more secure one's attachment is to his/her father, the weaker the association between sibling bullying involvement and depression (**Figure 1**).

After the above analyses, we performed another multiple logistic regression analysis in order to examine if gender influences the way in which attachment style to one's father moderates the association between involvement in sibling bullying and depression. This model did not appear significant, a likely result of the sample size.

In addition, in order to be certain that the moderating model for depression would remain significant after separating the variables for depression and suicidal ideation; we examined the depression measure after removing the four items used for the suicidal ideation measure. We kept the threshold value for the depression questionnaire at 26, as a stringent criterion for determining clinical depression. A multiple logistic regression analysis was performed in order to examine if the level of secure attachment to one's father moderates the association between involvement in sibling bullying and depression (without the four items used to measure suicidal ideation). This moderating model appeared significant, meaning that attachment to one's father moderates the association between sibling bullying involvement and depression such, that the more secure one's attachment is to his/her father, the weaker the association between involvement with sibling bullying and depression ($B = 0.11$, Wald $= 6.73$, $OR = 2.69$, $p < 0.05$).

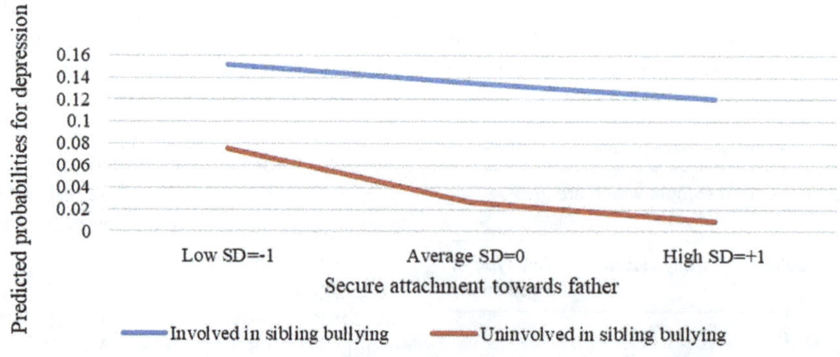

FIGURE 1 | Attachment to one's father as a moderating variable in the association between involvement in sibling bullying and depression.

The multiple logistic regression analysis, which examined if the level of secure attachment with one's father moderates the association between sibling bullying involvement and suicidal ideation, was found to be significant ($-2LL = 186.94$, $p < 0.001$, Nagelkerke $R^2 = 0.18$, Cox & Snell $R^2 = 0.11$). This analysis resulted in a significant and positive association between gender and suicidal ideation such that girls have a three times higher chance for suicidal ideation than do boys ($B = 1.11$, $Z = 2.53$, OR = 3.02, $p < 0.05$). Likewise, it was found that a secure attachment style to one's father is negatively and significantly associated with suicidal ideation ($B = -0.06$, $Z = -3.48$, OR = 0.94, $p < 0.001$). In other words, the more secure one's attachment is to his/her father, the lower the chance for suicidal ideation. Sibling bullying involvement was found to be significantly related to suicidal ideation ($B = 0.84$, $Z = 2.14$, OR = 2.31, $p < 0.05$), meaning that participants involved in sibling bullying have a 2.3 times higher chance for suicidal ideation than do participants uninvolved in sibling bullying. Finally, an interaction effect between level of secure attachment to one's father and involvement in sibling bullying was found to be significant ($B = 0.07$, Wald = 0.04, OR = 2.35, $p < 0.05$). In other words, attachment to one's father moderates the association between involvement in sibling bullying and suicidal ideation such, that the more secure the attachment is to one's father, the weaker the association between involvement in sibling bullying and suicidal ideation (**Figure 2**). After this analysis, we performed an additional multiple logistic regression analysis in order to examine if gender influences the way in which attachment to one's father moderates the association between involvement in sibling bullying and suicidal ideation. This model did not appear significant, again, a likely result of the sample size.

In order to examine if one's attachment style to his/her father moderates the association between involvement in sibling bullying and suicidal ideation beyond depression, we conducted a further analysis. In this analysis, we entered depression as a control variable and, as expected, an interaction effect between level of secure attachment to one's father and involvement in sibling bullying was found to be not significant ($B = 0.05$, Wald = 1.46, OR = 1.06, $p = 0.16$). Furthermore, sibling bullying involvement was not significantly associated with suicidal ideation ($B = 0.84$, $Z = 1.79$, OR = 2.12, $p = 0.07$). In other words, depression seems to play a central role in suicidal ideation and explains a large amount of its variance.

DISCUSSION

The findings of the present study suggest an association between involvement in sibling bullying and involvement in school bullying. The findings also suggest that involvement in sibling bullying is associated with depression and suicidal ideation. In addition, attachment to one's father (and not to one's mother) moderates the association between involvement in sibling bullying and depression/suicidal ideation among children/adolescents aged 8–18. However, the association between sibling bullying and suicidal ideation is not significant when depression is controlled for. In the same way, attachment to one's father does not appear to moderate the association between sibling bullying involvement and suicidal ideation when controlling for depression.

The findings, which support an association between sibling bullying involvement and school bullying involvement, are consistent with previous findings (7, 8). Earlier research assumes that behavioral structures learned at home and between siblings are transferred to relationships with peers (16). For example, studies have shown that children who are victims of sibling bullying are more likely to be victimized at school [e.g., Ref. (8)]. Victims of sibling bullying learn from their sibling interactions that they have little value and that they are powerless in the face of violence from others. As a result, they are likely to develop a submissive, non-assertive, and avoidant interpersonal style, which increases their chance for involvement in school bullying (10, 15). Likewise, school bullying can influence bullying at home. For example, research shows that school bullies display more negative emotions toward their brothers than do children who are uninvolved in bullying (39).

Our findings that individuals involved in sibling bullying are 3.6 times more likely for depression than are individuals not involved in bullying are consistent with previous studies (4, 11). One possible explanation for this association is that bullying between siblings is often a continuous situation, with those

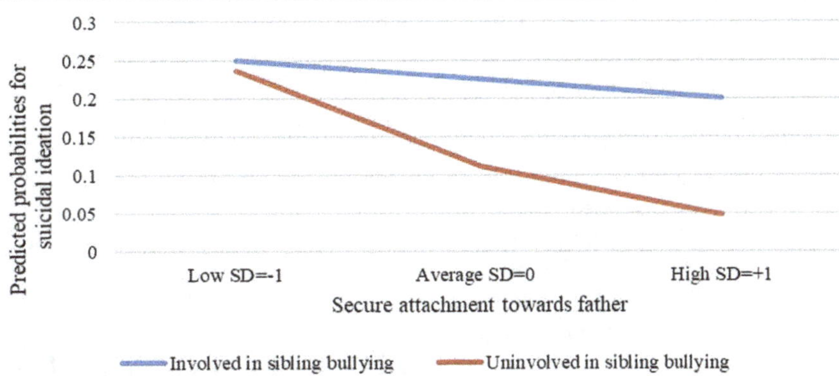

FIGURE 2 | Attachment to one's father as a moderating variable in the association between involvement in sibling bullying and suicidal ideation.

involved trapped in their own home environments without any possibility of avoiding or escaping the situation (11). A child is exposed to violence under his own roof while the parental figures which are responsible to protect, defend, support, and create guidelines are missing or not satisfactorily involved. A child involved in bullying is likely to develop a sense of helplessness and lack of security, which are likely to increase depression. Sibling bullying can therefore become a very harmful experience and present as a risk factor for emotional and psychological issues (11). The finding that participants involved in sibling bullying are at a 2.3 times higher risk for suicidal ideation than are participants uninvolved in sibling bullying, is the first of its kind in the field of sibling bullying. This finding is consistent with earlier studies which found an association between school bullying involvement and suicidal ideation (12, 40), independent of depression (41). The results which indicated an insignificant association between sibling bullying involvement and suicidal ideation once depression was entered into the model suggest that depression explains a large portion of this association.

The finding that participants involved in sibling bullying have less secure attachments to their mothers and fathers than do participants not involved in sibling bullying is in line with earlier findings regarding the association between involvement in school bullying and attachment styles (24, 29). The child's relationships with his/her parents are the first relationships the child will experience and through them he/she will learn what to expect from other relationships, how to behave in other relationships, and will develop useful (or not) interpersonal skills (18, 42). Children who suffer from difficulties in their attachment with their parents tend to not rely on others, display lower levels of empathy and concern for others, present low self-esteem and a need for affirmations from others, and show a wide range of adaptation difficulties across the life-span (6). Children and adolescents with these characteristics are at a high risk for many conflicts and bullying, including sibling bullying (6, 24, 25).

The finding that participants with a more secure attachment style with their fathers (not with their mothers) have a weaker association between involvement in sibling bullying and depression/suicidal ideation than participants with a less secure attachment style with their fathers, is consistent with the results Nikiforou et al.'s (28) study which found that attachment to one's mother was less contributing to victimization involvement than attachment to one's father. However, these results differ from the results of Klomek et al.'s (43) study, which suggest a significant association between attachment style to one's mother and the likelihood for victimization involvement at school. The difference between Klomek et al.'s (43) finding and the present study's finding may be explained by the fact that Klomek et al. (43) examined only peer victimization, while the present study examined all types of involvement in sibling bullying. It seems that attachment style to one's mother may have a different influence on the different roles involved in bullying (bully, victim, bully/victim). In addition, there seems to be a difference between involvement in bullying at home and in school.

Our findings are also consistent with the results of Desjardins and Leadbeater (44) which found that emotional support from the father (but not from mother) moderated the association between victims and depressive symptoms over time. It is possible that each parent provides different emotional support styles. Future research is needed to assess differences in the strategies that parents use to support their adolescents. Another potential explanation for why one's attachment style to his/her mother does not moderate the association between involvement in sibling bullying and depression/suicidal ideation may be that the adolescent feels the need to protect his/her mother's feelings (45). It may be that even if an individual holds a secure attachment with his/her mother, avoiding involving her out of fear for her emotional reaction narrows her ability to influence and moderate the association between involvement in sibling bullying and depression/suicidal ideation.

The present study has a few limitations. First, a majority (71.5%) of the research data was collected from one Israeli school and the sample size was relatively small. This limits our ability to generalize the findings. Second, the study is correlational, thus causality cannot be deduced. Third, all research variables were solely based on self-report questionnaires. Moreover, our measure for suicidal ideation was based on four items from the MFQ questionnaire for depression. Assessing suicidal ideation in this way limits our ability to assess and identify suicidal risk because we need to distinguish between suicidal ideation and suicidal behavior (35). Future studies should examine suicidal behavior and expand the measurement for suicidal ideation *via* a distinct tool. Finally, possible differences between different types of sibling bullying involvement (victim, bully, bully/victim) were not examined. Future research should examine if involvement in sibling bullying as a bully/victim is significantly different from involvement in sibling bullying as a bully or as a victim. Furthermore, the definition of the bully/victim type in the field of sibling bullying is still complicated, as it might include a sibling which both bullies and victimized by the same sibling(s). This raises questions regarding the criteria necessary for defining bullying, an imbalance of power. Future research should continue exploring the sibling bully/victim type.

Despite these limitations, the present study provides important clinical implications. The present study suggests that the assessment of sibling bullying involvement must be included as a risk factor in prevention protocols and in questionnaires, which identify depression and suicidality among adolescents. Likewise, parents, educators and children must be able to distinguish between fighting, violence, and sibling bullying, since involvement in sibling bullying is associated with psychopathology and perhaps, even, suicide ideation. In addition, it is critical for parents and, specifically, for fathers, to understand their role in their child's relationships with his/her siblings as well as the emotional aspects of such (44, 46). Future interventions and programs for the prevention of involvement in sibling bullying should enhance the father's emotional support capacity. It is important that future studies continue to examine the mother's role in the context of sibling bullying and depression/suicide ideation.

AUTHOR CONTRIBUTIONS

JB-Z conceptualized the topic as part of her MA studies in clinical psychology. JB-Z collected the data, analyzed the data, and drafted the first draft of the manuscript. AB-K supervised all stages of the work, including conceptualization, recruitment, analysis, and writing. JB-Z and AB-K are jointly accountable for the content of the work, ensuring that all aspects related to accuracy or integrity of the study are investigated and resolved in an appropriate way.

ACKNOWLEDGMENTS

This work was submitted in partial fulfillment of the requirements for the Master's Degree in MA Clinic Psychology, School Baruch Ivcher Psychology, Interdisciplinary Center, Herzliya, under the supervision of Anat Brunstein Klomek, Ph.D.

REFERENCES

1. Olweus D. Bully/victim problems among schoolchildren: basic facts and effects of a school based intervention program. In: Pepler D, Rubin K, editors. *The Development and Treatment of Childhood Aggression*. Hillsdale, NJ: Erlbaum (1991). p. 411–48.
2. Hoetger LA, Hazen KP, Brank EM. All in the family: a retrospective study comparing sibling bullying and peer bullying. *J Fam Violence* (2015) 30(1):103–11. doi:10.1007/s10896-014-9651-0
3. Olweus D. *Bullying at School: What We Know and What We Can Do*. Oxford, UK: Blackwell Publishers (1993).
4. Wolke D, Tippett N, Dantchev S. Bullying in the family: sibling bullying. *Lancet Psychiatry* (2015) 2(10):917–29. doi:10.1016/S2215-0366(15)00262-X
5. Haynie DL, Nansel T, Eitel P, Crump AD, Saylor K, Yu K, et al. Bullies, victims, and bully/victims: distinct groups of at-risk youth. *J Early Adolesc* (2001) 21(1):29–49. doi:10.1177/0272431601021001002
6. Kim J, Kim E. Bullied by siblings and peers the role of rejecting/neglecting parenting and friendship quality among Korean children. *J Interpers Violence* (2016):1–24. doi:10.1177/0886260516659659
7. Wolke D, Skew AJ. Bullying among siblings. *Int J Adolesc Med Health* (2012) 24(1):17–25. doi:10.1515/ijamh.2012.004
8. Wolke D, Samara MM. Bullied by siblings: association with peer victimization and behavior problems in Israeli lower secondary school children. *J Child Psychol Psychiatry* (2004) 45(5):1015–29. doi:10.1111/j.1469-7610.2004.t01-1-00293.x
9. Sapouna M, Wolke D, Vannini N, Watson S, Woods S, Schneider W, et al. Individual and social network predictors of the short-term stability of bullying victimization in the United Kingdom and Germany. *Br J Educ Psychol* (2012) 82(2):225–40. doi:10.1111/j.2044-8279.2011.02022.x
10. Duncan RD. Peer and sibling aggression: an investigation of intra- and extra-familial bullying. *J Interpers Violence* (1999) 14(8):871–86. doi:10.1177/088626099014008005
11. Bowes L, Wolke D, Joinson C, Lereya ST, Lewis G. Sibling bullying and risk of depression, anxiety, and self-harm: a prospective cohort study. *Pediatrics* (2014) 134(4):e1032–9. doi:10.1542/peds.2014-0832
12. Klomek AB, Sourander A, Niemelä S, Kumpulainen K, Piha J, Tamminen T, et al. Childhood bullying behaviors as a risk for severe suicide attempts and completed suicides. *J Am Acad Child Adolesc Psychiatry* (2009) 48(3):254–61. doi:10.1097/CHI.0b013e318196b91f
13. Button DM, Gealt R. High risk behaviors among victims of sibling violence. *J Fam Violence* (2010) 25(2):131–40. doi:10.1007/s10896-009-9276-x
14. Eriksen S, Jensen V. A push or a punch: distinguishing the severity of sibling violence. *J Interpers Violence* (2009) 24(1):183–208. doi:10.1177/0886260508316298
15. Menesini E, Camodeca M, Nocentini A. Bullying among siblings: the role of personality and relational variables. *Br J Dev Psychol* (2010) 28(4):921–39. doi:10.1348/026151009X479402
16. Tippett N, Wolke D. Aggression between siblings: associations with the home environment and peer bullying. *Aggress Behav* (2015) 41(1):14–24. doi:10.1002/ab.21557
17. Updegraff KA, Thayer SM, Whiteman SD, Denning DJ, McHale SM. Relational aggression in adolescents' sibling relationships: links to sibling and parent-adolescent relationship quality. *Fam Relat* (2005) 54(3):373–85. doi:10.1111/j.1741-3729.2005.00324.x
18. Bowlby J. *Attachment, Vol. 1 of Attachment and Loss*. New York: Basic Books (1969).
19. Bowlby J. Attachment and loss: retrospect and prospect. *Am J Orthopsychiatry* (1982) 52(4):664–78. doi:10.1111/j.1939-0025.1982.tb01456.x
20. Sroufe LA, Coffino B, Carlson EA. Conceptualizing the role of early experience: lessons from the Minnesota longitudinal study. *Dev Rev* (2010) 30(1):36–51. doi:10.1016/j.dr.2009.12.002
21. Grossmann K, Grossmann KE, Kindler H, Zimmermann P. A wider view of attachment and exploration: the influence of mothers and fathers on the development of psychological security from infancy to young adulthood. 2nd ed. In: Cassidy J, Shaver PR, editors. *Handbook of Attachment: Theory, Research, and Clinical Applications*. New York: Guilford Press (2008). p. 857–79.
22. Houston J, Grych J. Maternal attachment buffers the association between exposure to violence and youth attitudes about aggression. *Journal of Clinical Child & Adolescent Psychology* (2015) 45(5):605–13. doi:10.1080/15374416.2014.987380
23. Volling BL, Belsky J. The contribution of mother–child and father–child relationships to the quality of sibling interaction: a longitudinal study. *Child Dev* (1992) 63(5):1209–22. doi:10.2307/1131528
24. Eliot M, Cornell DG. Bullying in middle school as a function of insecure attachment and aggressive attitudes. *Sch Psychol Int* (2009) 30(2):201–14. doi:10.1177/0143034309104148
25. Whiteman SD, McHale SM, Soli A. Theoretical perspectives on sibling relationships. *J Fam Theory Rev* (2012) 3(2):124–39. doi:10.1111/j.1756-2589.2011.00087.x
26. Coleman PK. Perceptions of parent–child attachment, social self-efficacy, and peer relationships in middle childhood. *Infant Child Dev* (2003) 12(4):351–68. doi:10.1002/icd.316
27. Kõiv K. Attachment styles among bullies, victims and uninvolved adolescents. *Psychol Res* (2012) 2(3):160–5. doi:10.17265/2159-5542/2012.03.003
28. Nikiforou M, Georgiou SN, Stavrinides P. Attachment to parents and peers as a parameter of bullying and victimization. *J Criminol* (2013) 2013:e484871. doi:10.1155/2013/484871
29. Walden LM, Beran TN. Attachment quality and bullying behavior in school-aged youth. *Can J Sch Psychol* (2010) 25(1):5–18. doi:10.1177/0829573509357046
30. Sourander A, Brunstein Klomek A, Ikonen M, Lindroos J, Luntamo T, Koskelainen M, et al. Psychosocial risk factors associated with cyberbullying among adolescents: a population-based study. *Arch Gen Psychiatry* (2010) 67(7):720–8. doi:10.1001/archgenpsychiatry.2010.79
31. Klomek AB, Kleinman M, Altschuler E, Marrocco F, Amakawa L, Gould MS. Suicidal adolescents' experiences with bullying perpetration and victimization during high school as risk factors for later depression and suicidality. *J Adolesc Health* (2013) 53(1):S37–42. doi:10.1016/j.jadohealth.2012.12.008
32. Angold A, Costello EJ, Messer SC, Pickles A. Development of a short questionnaire for use in epidemiological studies of depression in children and adolescents. *Int J Methods Psychiatr Res* (1995) 5(4):237–49.
33. Costello EJ, Angold A. Scales to assess child and adolescent depression: checklists, screens, and nets. *J Am Acad Child Adolesc Psychiatry* (1988) 27(6):726–37. doi:10.1097/00004583-198811000-00011
34. Sund AM, Larsson B, Wichstrøm L. Depressive symptoms among young Norwegian adolescents as measured by the Mood and Feelings Questionnaire (MFQ). *Eur Child Adolesc Psychiatry* (2001) 10(4):222–9. doi:10.1007/s007870170011
35. Posner K, Brown GK, Stanley B, Brent DA, Yershova KV, Oquendo MA, et al. The Columbia–Suicide severity rating scale: initial validity and internal consistency findings from three multisite studies with adolescents and adults. *Am J Psychiatry* (2011) 168(12):1266–77. doi:10.1176/appi.ajp.2011.10111704
36. Kerns KA, Klepac L, Cole AK. Peer relationships and preadolescents' perceptions of security in the mother-child relationship. *Dev Psychol* (1996) 32(3):457–66. doi:10.1037/0012-1649.32.3.457

37. Granot D, Maysless O. Attachment security and adjustment to school in middle childhood. *Int J Behav Dev* (2001) 25(6):530–41. doi:10.1080/01650250042000366
38. Aiken LS, West SG, Reno RR. *Multiple Regression: Testing and Interpreting Interactions*. Thousand Oaks, CA: Sage Publications (1991).
39. Connolly I, O'Moore M. Personality and family relations of children who bully. *Pers Individ Dif* (2003) 35(3):559–67. doi:10.1016/S0191-8869(02)00218-0
40. Bannink R, Broeren S, van de Looij-Jansen PM, de Waart FG, Raat H. Cyber and traditional bullying victimization as a risk factor for mental health problems and suicidal ideation in adolescents. *PLoS One* (2014) 9(4):e94026. doi:10.1371/journal.pone.0094026
41. Kaltiala-Heino R, Rimpelä M, Marttunen M, Rimpelä A, Rantanen P. Bullying, depression, and suicidal ideation in Finnish adolescents: school survey. *BMJ* (1999) 319(7206):348–51. doi:10.1136/bmj.319.7206.348
42. Duncan RD. The impact of family relationships on school bullies and their victims. In: Espelage DL, Swearer SM, editors. *Bullying in American Schools*. Mahwah, NJ: Erlbaum (2004). p. 227–44.
43. Klomek AB, Kopelman-Rubin D, Al-Yagon M, Berkowitz R, Apter A, Mikulincer M. Victimization by bullying and attachment to parents and teachers among student who report learning disorders and/or attention deficit hyperactivity disorder. *Learn Disabil Q* (2016) 39(3):182–90. doi:10.1177/0731948715616377
44. Desjardins TL, Leadbeater BJ. Relational victimization and depressive symptoms in adolescence: moderating effects of mother, father, and peer emotional support. *J Youth Adolesc* (2011) 40(5):531–44. doi:10.1007/s10964-010-9562-1
45. Williams SK, Kelly FD. Relationships among involvement, attachment, and behavioral problems in adolescence: examining fathers' influence. *J Early Adolesc* (2005) 25(2):168–96. doi:10.1177/0272431604274178
46. Sarkadi A, Kristiansson R, Oberklaid F, Bremberg S. Fathers' involvement and children's developmental outcomes: a systematic review of longitudinal studies. *Acta Paediatr* (2008) 97(2):153–8. doi:10.1111/j.1651-2227.2007.00572.x

18

A Further Look at Therapeutic Interventions for Suicide Attempts and Self-Harm in Adolescents

Udita Iyengar[1†], Natasha Snowden[1†], Joan R. Asarnow[2], Paul Moran[3,4], Troy Tranah[5] and Dennis Ougrin[1,6]*

[1] Department of Child and Adolescent Psychiatry, Institute of Psychiatry, Psychology, and Neuroscience (IoPPN), King's College London, London, United Kingdom, [2] Semel Institute of Neuroscience and Behavior, David Geffen School of Medicine, University of California, Los Angeles, Los Angeles, CA, United States, [3] National Institute for Health Research Bristol Biomedical Research Centre, University Hospitals Bristol NHS Foundation Trust and University of Bristol, Bristol, United Kingdom, [4] Department of Population Health Sciences, Centre for Academic Mental Health, Bristol Medical School, University of Bristol, Bristol, United Kingdom, [5] Institute of Psychiatry, Psychology, and Neuroscience (IoPPN), London, United Kingdom, [6] South London and Maudsley National Health Service (NHS) Foundation Trust, London, United Kingdom

***Correspondence:**
Udita Iyengar
udita.iyengar@kcl.ac.uk

† These authors share first authorship

Background: Suicide attempts (SA) and other types of self-harm (SH) are strong predictors of death by suicide in adolescents, emphasizing the need to investigate therapeutic interventions in reduction of these and other symptoms. We conducted an updated systematic review of randomized controlled trials (RCTs) from our previous study reporting therapeutic interventions that were effective in reducing SH including SA, while additionally exploring reduction of suicidal ideation (SI) and depressive symptoms (DS).

Method: A systematic literature search was conducted across OVID Medline, psycINFO, PubMed, EMBASE, and Cochrane Library from the first available article to October 22nd, 2017, with a primary focus on RCTs evaluating therapeutic interventions in the reduction of self-harm. Search terms included *self-injurious behavior; self-mutilation; suicide, attempted; suicide; drug overdose.*

Results: Our search identified 1,348 articles, of which 743 eligible for review, yielding a total of 21 studies which met predetermined inclusion criteria. Eighteen unique therapeutic interventions were identified among all studies, stratified by individual-driven, socially driven, and mixed interventions, of which 5 studies found a significant effect for primary outcomes of self-harm and suicide attempts (31.3%), and 5 studies found a significant effect for secondary outcomes of suicidal ideation and depressive symptoms (29.4%) for therapeutic intervention vs. treatment as usual. Collapsing across different variations of Cognitive Behavior Therapy (CBT), and classifying Dialectical Behavior Therapy for Adolescents (DBT-A) as a type of CBT, CBT is the only intervention with replicated positive impact on reducing self-harm in adolescents.

Conclusion: While the majority of studies were not able to determine efficacy of therapeutic interventions for both primary and secondary outcomes, our systematic review suggests that individual self-driven and socially-driven processes appeared to show the greatest promise for reducing suicide attempts, with benefits of combined self-driven and systems-driven approaches for reducing overall self-harm. Further RCTs of all intervention categories are needed to address the clinical and etiological heterogeneity of suicidal behavior in adolescents, specifically suicidal ideation and depressive symptoms.

Keywords: suicide, self-harm, NSSI, depression, suicidal ideation, adolescent, RCT

INTRODUCTION

Suicide is a major global and public health concern (1). It is the second leading cause of death in people age 15–24 years (2) and there is a pressing need to identify effective interventions to reduce the risk of suicide. Non-fatal suicide attempts (SA) can be defined as self-directed injuries with implicit or explicit intent to kill oneself, while non-suicidal self-injury (NSSI) is direct destruction of one's body without intention to die (3). For the latter, it is useful to consider the definition of non-suicidal self-injury found in the DMS-5, which states that the preoccupied individual partakes in premeditated, self-directed damage to themselves in order to relieve negative experiences and does not exhibit suicidal intent through this behavior (4). Both suicide attempts (SA) and the broader category of "self-harm" (SH, which includes non-suicidal self-injury) are among the strongest predictors of death by suicide (5–7), and have therefore appropriately been the focus of therapeutic interventions for adolescents to decrease risk of suicide.

There has been significant progress in detection (8), identifying subtypes, understanding the long-term outcomes (9), and understanding help-seeking in adolescents with SH (10). There has also been recent progress regarding the treatment of self-harm in adolescents. We conducted the first meta-analysis of randomized controlled trials (RCTs) to specifically evaluate therapeutic interventions (TIs) in reducing SH in adolescents (11). A significant effect was found for tested interventions reducing SH compared to treatment as usual (TAU). While results evaluating the effects of therapeutic interventions on NSSI were generally consistent with those for overall self-harm, the effect size was weaker and escaped statistical significance. In contrast, there was little to no evidence of benefits of tested interventions in reducing suicide attempts. Our findings highlighted both the beneficial effects of therapeutic interventions for self-harm as a global category, the challenges of reducing the risk of future suicide attempts and the need for rigorous and replicable studies.

In addition to self-harm and suicide attempts, however, depression in adolescence is another key contributor to suicidal behavior (12, 13). A recent National Confidential Inquiry into Suicide and Homicide by People with Mental Illness (NCISH) report of suicide deaths in England and Wales between 2014 and 2015 indicated that out of 285 suicide deaths that occurred in youths aged 10–20, 52% had a history of SH, while 58% expressed thoughts of suicide or hopelessness (14). Depressive symptoms themselves have been found to be significant and independent contributors to elevated levels of deliberate self-harm in young people (15–18). Therefore, it would appear that the reduction of depressive symptoms and suicidal ideation (19) may be an important mechanism underpinning the effectiveness of certain treatments for suicide prevention.

We therefore sought to extend and update our initial meta-analysis focused on the reduction of self-harm and suicide attempts, while also examining the effect of a variety of unique therapeutic interventions on levels of depressive symptoms and suicidal thoughts. In this way, we acknowledge the relevance of these mechanisms to the field and aim to advance our previous study findings with a wider criterion and selection of interventions. Our primary outcomes were the reduction in self-harm including NSSI or suicide attempts (SAs), and our secondary outcomes were the reduction in suicidal ideation (SI), meaning thoughts and feelings related to suicide, as well as depressive symptoms (DS).

METHODS

Eligibility and Selection

We followed the same methodology as our previous systematic review [see (11)], using "self-harm" as an encompassing term, including previous suicide attempts, non-suicidal self-injury, and deliberate self-harm with undetermined intent. However, in addition to the original systematic review's reduction of self-harm and suicide attempts (primary outcomes) we also examined decrease of suicidal ideation and depressive symptoms (secondary outcomes) as markers of the efficacy of the therapeutic interventions.

Inclusion Criteria

Inclusion to the update depended on: study type, sample age, and frequency of self-harm occurring within the sample. We included only studies which were clinical, randomized trials of therapeutic interventions, defined as any theoretically coherent, manualized, psychological, psychosocial, or pharmacological intervention, compared to a placebo or control treatment (11). Further, we included only studies with a majority (>50%) child and adolescent population (<18 years old), engaged in either self-harm or had attempted suicide. Studies from all countries and languages were considered eligible, if they were accompanied by an English abstract.

Exclusion Criteria

Potential studies were excluded from the update if self-harm was a symptom of an overarching developmental condition (i.e., autism or intellectual disability). Finally, studies that did not meet the threshold score of >2 on the Jadad quality assessment tool (20), specifically used to ascertain methodological quality, coherence to blinding and allocation procedures, and amenability to participant attrition, were excluded from consideration.

Literature Search Strategy

A literature search was conducted through standard online databases (OVID Medline, psycINFO, PubMed, EMBASE, and Cochrane Library) in order to identify RCTs evaluating the efficacy of therapeutic interventions for adolescents with self-harm against control conditions. To maintain consistency with our first study, the same inclusion and exclusion criteria were utilized in this update. We excluded studies in which self-harm occurred as a result of stereotypic self-injurious behaviors such as those seen in moderate to severe forms of neurological disorders (e.g., Autism, Intellectual Disability), due to the complex neurological mechanisms which underlie the self-harm not otherwise seen outside of these conditions. All the aforementioned databases were searched from the first available article until October 22nd, 2017. Consistent with our original methodology, the following subject headings or MeSH keywords were used: *self-injurious behavior; self-mutilation; suicide, attempted; suicide; drug overdose.* When available, filters for study type and participant age were applied, with an additional manualized filter used for psycINFO to specifically identify clinical trials.

RESULTS

Study Selection

A total of 1,348 articles were found, with 743 of those studies eligible for review following duplicate removal (**Figure 1**). The screening procedure consisted of three phases: title, abstract and full text screening, with the latter two conducted independently by the two authors (UI and NS). Title screening was conducted by NS as a preliminary measure to ensure the exclusion of any not-pertinent studies and duplicates, reducing the number of eligible studies from 743 to 102. Within the abstract screening phase, 31 articles were eliminated as they failed to meet any one aspect of the inclusion criteria, producing a yield of 71 articles for full text screening. In the third and final phase, we excluded 50 studies, 16 of which had a sample with a mean age above 18 years, 23 which did not have a majority of adolescents who engaged in self-harming behaviors, 9 which were not RCTs, 1 which has been replaced by a paper with more recent follow-up data, and 1 which did not meet quality standards. We chose to remove one study included in the original systematic review (21), as its investigation of a treatment designed to increase linkage to outpatient services did not assess the same outcomes which we are addressing in this update. Disagreements in any phase of the screening process were resolved by consensus discussion between the authors (UI and NS).

Therapeutic Interventions

The final selection of 21 studies contained 18 unique therapeutic interventions. Two of the final 21 studies (22, 23) were replication trials assessing the efficacy of Developmental Group Psychotherapy (24), while another paper (25) was a follow-up to a previous pilot trial of Emotion Training Regulation (ERT) (26). As such, 18 unique interventions were identified among all studies. To facilitate analysis, the interventions can be stratified and evaluated by the underlying theoretical principles, including self-driven cognitive, behavioral and regulatory interventions (referred to as self-driven) and interventions which require engagement with family and social support (referred to as socially-driven). A brief description of the interventions and the study origins are listed in **Table 1**, with self-driven and socially-driven components identified for each respective study in **Table 2**. Results below are reported first by interventions which we believed had a primarily self-driven focus, followed by those with a primarily socially-driven focus, and finally, interventions which demonstrated aspects of both self-driven and socially-driven principles.

Primary Outcome Assessment

Table 3 provides a brief summary of primary outcomes of the studies for comparison of therapeutic intervention examined, and those that had significant group differences, significant overall differences, or null or negative findings. Of the 21 studies examined, 16 studies explored primary outcomes, out which 5 (31.3%) found significant group differences for intervention vs. treatment as usual (24, 28, 31, 32, 42), across all types of treatments.

Significant Differences in Therapeutic Interventions vs. Treatment as Usual

We first examined interventions that addressed individual problem solving, mentalization, cognitive behavior or skills deficits [these included treatments such as Cognitive Behavioral Therapy [CBT], Mentalization Based Therapy [MBT], Dialectical Behavioral Therapy [DBT]]. The only identified studies with a purely self-driven intervention model were those that evaluated Developmental Group Psychotherapy, an intervention which used cognitive-behavioral, problem-solving, dialectical, and psychodynamic group psychotherapy strategies. In a small initial trial among adolescents with repeated SH referred to child and adolescent mental health services in the UK, Developmental Group Psychotherapy compared to treatment as usual was associated with a significantly lower risk of repeating self-harm, with a lower latency period for repeated attempts, indicating an absolute risk reduction of 26% (24). The authors cautioned that this strong effect was likely due to a smaller sample, and urged replication studies with a larger sample. Indeed, two efforts at replication failed to find a significant advantage for the Developmental Group Psychotherapy intervention. These trials included one conducted in Australia with supervision from the original UK development team and somewhat different sampling criteria: youths referred for general child and adolescent mental health services identified with repeat self-harm (22). The other trial was a large trial ($N = 366$) conducted in the UK with members of the original development team and also failed to find an advantage for the Developmental Group Psychotherapy (23) over treatment as usual.

One study conducted in Australian outpatient mental health clinics used a socially driven intervention to evaluate a strength-based family education program, called Resourceful Adolescent Parent Program (RAP-P). Among patients recruited suicidal adolescents from emergency departments or public mental health services, the RAP-P program resulted in a significant improvement on a 9-item suicide index assessing suicide

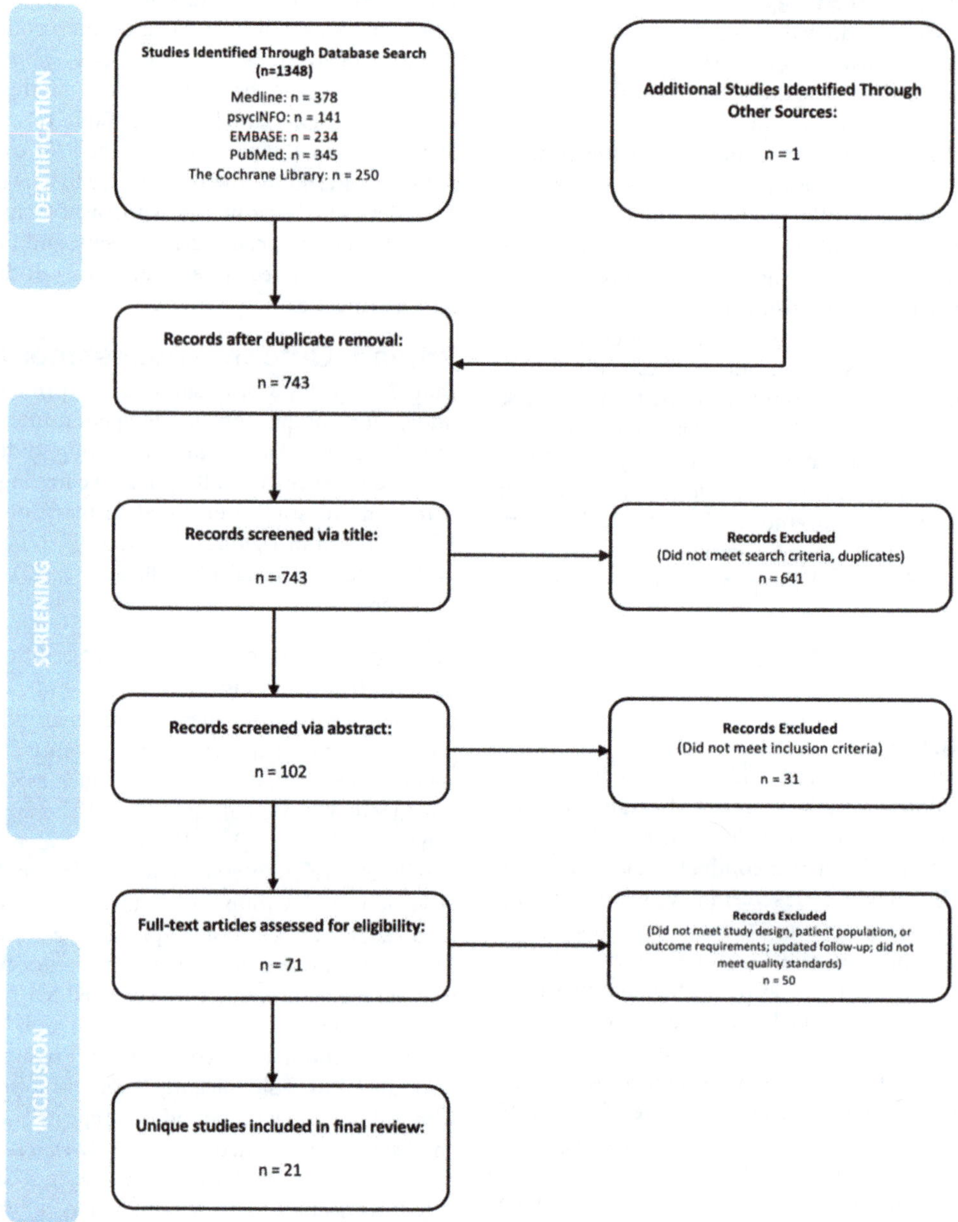

FIGURE 1 | Study flow diagram.

ideations, plans, threats, self-harm, and suicide attempts both at the 3-month post-treatment point, and at a 6-month follow-up compared to treatment as usual (41). This study was the only exclusively socially-driven intervention model to find a significant group difference on primary outcomes and it should be noted that the outcome variable was a broad measure of suicidality rather than a measure specifically of self-harm or suicide attempts.

Four trials examined more combined self-driven and system driven approaches. We begin with Mentalization-Based Treatment for adolescents (MBT-A), a manualized one-year psychodynamic psychotherapy rooted in attachment theory. MBT-A has a strong self-driven component consisting of weekly individual MBT-A sessions and compared to the other approaches in the combined approach group, the weakest of the socially-driven components; specifically, monthly family Mentalization-based family therapy. In an initial trial, Rossouw and Fonagy (32) found that adolescents selected for the presence of both self-harming behaviors and depression in the MBT- A condition had fewer self-harm episodes over the course of the treatment compared to treatment as usual youths and that the MBT-A group had a higher recovery rate and a reduction of self-harm at the end of the 12-month treatment. Thus, results from this initial trial support the efficacy of MBT-A for reducing overall self-harm. Results specifically for suicidal behavior were not reported.

TABLE 1 | Descriptions and Study Origins of Therapeutic Interventions of the Selected Randomized Controlled Trials.

TI name	Study origin	Description
CBT-SP	Alavi et al. (27)	A 3-phase Cognitive-Behavioral Therapy protocol adapted specifically for suicide prevention. Utilizes cognitive behavioral principles according to the Stanley et al. model, and is comprised of 12 weekly sessions, the first of which includes parents.
Integrated Cognitive Behavioral Therapy (I-CBT)	Esposito-Smythers et al. (28)	Utilizes cognitive behavioral techniques such as restructuring, problem-solving, affect regulation and communication skills to remediate maladaptive cognitions and provide skills training for the attending adolescent and parents. One-year long intervention consisting of three treatment phases, involving with weekly, bi-weekly, and monthly individual adolescent, family, and parent training sessions.
DBT-A	Mehlum et al. (29)	Streamlined Dialectical Behavioral Therapy protocol adapted for adolescents, incorporating a new skills module to address emotion dysregulation amongst adolescents and their families. Nineteen-week long intervention involving weekly individual therapy, multi-family skills training, and family therapy sessions.
Developmental Group Psychotherapy	Wood et al. (24)	Integrates techniques from problem solving and cognitive and dialectical behavioral interventions to resolve issues around relationships, school problems, peer relationships, depression and self-harm, hopelessness, and feelings about the future. Delivered through a maximum of 19 acute and long-term group sessions run in tandem, administered by a variety of trained personnel.
Skills-Based Treatment (SBT)	Donaldson et al. (30)	Intervention designed to target problem solving and affect management skills in self-harming adolescents through cognitive behavioral strategies such as restructuring and relaxation. Delivered by therapists trained in SBT for an undefined number of sessions (mean number of sessions: 9.25).
Emotion Regulation Training (ERT)	Donaldson et al. (26)	Designed to teach participants ways of coping with affective instability, daily stressors, and psychological vulnerability through psychoeducation and behavior modification. Treatment is conducted through 17 weekly multi-phase group sessions delivered by therapists trained in ERT.
Safe Alternative for Teens and Youth (SAFETY)	Asarnow et al. (31)	Emergency Department (ED) family-centered intervention informed by CBT and DBT aimed to reduce future suicide attempts by strengthening protective supports, teaching skills for managing stress reactions and formulating strategies for creating a safe environment for the adolescent. Treatment is conducted through 12 weekly individual and joint sessions for adolescents and their parents, delivered by two therapists, each working with the family.
Mentalization Based Therapy for Adolescents (MBT-A)	Rossouw and Fonagy (32)	An adapted form of Mentalization-based Treatment, a manualised intervention focusing on impulsivity and affect regulation, helping to enhance the patient's understanding of how to represent feelings in emotionally challenging situations. Year-long intervention with weekly individual and family based therapy (MBT-F) delivered by trained therapists.
Cognitive Analytic Therapy (CAT)	Chanen et al. (33)	Time limited, integrated model of development and psychopathology, equipping the patient with tools more effectively manage stressful situations which could lead to a repetition of pathological behavior. Conducted through 24 weekly sessions delivered by therapists trained in CAT.
Therapeutic Assessment	Ougrin et al. (34)	Manualised assessment protocol for self-harming adolescents facilitating the identification of the target problem, enhancing motivation for change, and exploring ways of relieving vicious cycles. Assessment takes place in one session and is delivered by a trained clinician.
Emergency Tokens	Cotgrove et al. (35)	Self-harming adolescents were allotted a token allowing hospital re-entry without question, to be used when adolescent was in need of escaping an intolerable (family) environment.
Home-based Family Intervention	Harrington et al. (36)	Short-term, intensive, focused, action orientated intervention used to address family dysfunction without lengthy treatment commitments or the need to present to a hospital setting. Conducted by psychiatric social workers during 5 home-based therapy sessions.
Family Intervention for Suicide Prevention (FISP)	Asarnow et al. (6)	Brief ED intervention which focuses on building a collaboration between adolescents and their parents by identifying and addressing the causes, reaction, and future actions related to the committed suicide attempt. Administered by a trained clinician.
Family-Based Crisis Intervention	Wharff et al. (37)	Brief intervention which provides the family with tools to manage current and future crises through psycho-education, cognitive behavioral skill building, therapeutic readiness and safety planning. Delivered during the adolescent's visit to the ED by a research clinician.
Attachment-Based Family Therapy (ABFT)	Diamond et al. (38)	Designed to improve problem solving, affect regulation and organization within the family. Number of sessions vary, depending on the adolescent's progress in resolving 5 specific tasks, and is delivered by a therapist trained in ABFT.
Youth Nominated Support Team-I	King et al. (39)	Supplements routine care by facilitating weekly contact between adolescents and their chosen support person (outside of the family), based on the notion that support people may minimize the impact of negative family environment. Support is provided to their adolescent by their nominated individual, who is asked to be in weekly contact with the adolescent. Support personnel are given 1.5–2 h of training.
Youth Nominated Support Team-II	King et al. (40)	Similar to YST-I, but with updated psychoeducation materials and the requirement that the nominated support person be an adult (rather than a peer). The support person has weekly check-ins with the adolescents for 3 months following hospitalization.
Resourceful Adolescent Parent Program (RAP-P)	Pineda and Dadds (41)	Strengths-based family psycho-education program, enhancing understanding of SH and SA, along with strategies to help minimize future self-injurious behavior, and information to facilitate access to support services. Sessions 2 h and held once a week or fortnightly.

Dialectical Behavioral Therapy for Adolescents, (DBT-A) addresses self-driven cognitive-behavioral and regulatory processes (e.g., emotion regulation, distress tolerance, and interpersonal effectiveness) and the social environment through inclusion of a weekly multi-family skills training group and as needed family therapy sessions. A first RCT evaluating DBT-A was conducted in Norwegian clinics and recruited youths with both at least two episodes of self-harm and symptoms of borderline personality disorder (43). This trial compared DBT-A to treatment as usual enhanced by a therapist agreement to provide at least 1 weekly session during the trial. Results indicated that the 19-weeks DBT-A reduced the frequency of self-harm with large effect sizes, compared to moderate and weak effect sizes in the TAU condition (29). The advantage of DBT-A for reducing self-harm extended to a 1-year post-treatment follow-up, with DBT-A youths continuing to demonstrate fewer episodes of self-harm compared to treatment as usual youths (42). The authors looked at a range of additional clinical outcomes including suicidal ideation, hopelessness, depression, borderline symptoms, and global functioning. Results indicated that while there was an initial advantage for DBT-A and DBT-A youths continued to show improved clinical and functioning outcomes at the 1-year post-treatment follow-up, with time the TAU youths caught up and looked similar to the DBT-A youths on these more general outcomes. This trial was not powered to evaluate outcomes regarding suicide attempts, thus such data were not reported.

The combined self-driven and socially-driven intervention model was used in two U.S. treatment development trials. Both trials used a 2-therapist model with one therapist focusing on the youth and the other the parent, and both studies showed evidence of benefits in reducing the risk of suicide attempts. First, Esposito-Smythers et al. (28) tested an integrated CBT (I-CBT) protocol for suicidality (along with co-occurring alcohol and drug related problems) and found that those randomized to I-CBT had fewer suicide attempts over the course of 18-months compared to those in the control condition. Second, Asarnow et al. (31) developed a DBT-informed cognitive-behavioral family treatment (referred to as SAFETY) which included attention to strengthening self-driven cognitive, behavioral and regulatory processes in the youth and parents, and family sessions aimed at promoting increased support and protection within the family and broader social environment. Results of this trial indicated a statistically significant advantage for SAFETY in decreasing suicide attempts over the 3-month treatment period, and reducing the risk of a first incident suicide attempt over a 6 to 12-month follow-up period. Weaker non-significant group differences were found for non-suicidal self-injury. While results of these trials are encouraging, it should be noted that both studies were relatively small treatment development trials, underscoring the need for cautious interpretation until replication is achieved.

Overall Group Differences Irrespective of Therapeutic Intervention

Overall symptom reduction across both treatment and control groups was found throughout several other studies included in this review, not specific to intervention type, including the Green et al. (23) trial of Developmental Group Psychotherapy intervention. In a specific clinical sample of Borderline Personality Disorder (BPD), three studies assessed the efficacy of cognitively-informed interventions. Chanen et al. (33) and Schuppert et al. (25, 26) investigated the efficacy of Cognitive Analytic Therapy (CAT) and Emotion Regulation Training (ERT), respectively, against TAU. Both CAT and ERT emphasize ways to react and respond to stressful situations with tools to more effectively manage stressful situations with aspects of self-driven processes. Both studies only observed the reduction of self-harm within the whole cohort with no statistically significant group differences, indicating that these therapies do not appear to perform any better than TAU in reducing self-harm within Borderline patients.

Null or Negative Findings

Several interventions included in this update demonstrated non-significant or negative findings. For instance, The Youth-Nominated Support Treatment (YST-I) is a socially driven treatment that focuses on improving support in youths' social support network and is added to TAU, with version II of the intervention focused on strengthening social support in youth-nominated supportive adults, rather than adults and peers. In both YST-I (39) and YST-II (40), no significant treatment effect was found in reduction of SA; authors emphasized the need for further research using this mode.

Cotgrove et al. (35) demonstrated non-significant findings regarding secondary prevention of suicide attempts in adolescents, examining re-admissions to Emergency Rooms. Adolescents were randomly allocated to a group receiving tokens guaranteeing re-admission to emergency services if they felt unable to cope within their environment. While there was no significant difference noted between adolescents with tokens and those without, those in the treatment condition had fewer repeat attempts than the control group, suggesting possible efficacy of a secondary prevention mechanism.

Two studies identified advantages of brief mental health interventions for linking youths to outpatient treatment after emergency presentation for suicidality and/or self-harm. Asarnow et al. (6) looked at a brief, cognitive-behavioral family-based Emergency Department (ED) intervention and found an advantage of the this intervention compared to treatment as usual for establishing linkage to outpatient care (the primary study outcome). Clinical outcomes were not evaluated close in time to the Emergency Department intervention. However, when clinical outcomes were evaluated roughly 2 months after discharge from the Emergency Department, no statistically significant advantage was found for this intervention in reducing suicide attempts. Importantly, there was also no evidence that linkage to outpatient treatment as usual after discharge from emergency services had any advantages relative to no post-discharge community treatment as usual.

Ougrin et al. (34) applied a brief therapeutic intervention incorporating elements of cognitive analytic therapy called Therapeutic Assessment (TA) following emergency presentation of self-harm. While there was no significant difference in the

TABLE 2 | Types of Therapeutic Intervention for the Selected Randomized Controlled Trials and Aspects of Individual or Social Components.

	Self-driven Components					Social Components			
	CBT	DBT	MBT	CAT	Problem Solving	Social Support	Family Involvement	Psycho-education	Communication skills
Alavi et al. (27)	•								
Asarnow et al. (6)							•		
Asarnow et al. (31)	•	•					•		
Cotgrove et al. (35)									
Chanen et al. (33)				•					
Diamond et al. (38)							•		
Diamond et al. (30)	•				•		•		
Esposito-Smythers et al. (28)	•						•		•
Green et al. (23)	•	•					•		•
Harrington et al. (36)							•		
Hazell et al. (22)	•	•			•				•
King et al. (39)						•		•	
King et al. (40)						•		•	
Mehlum et al. (42)		•					•		•
Ougrin et al. (34)				•			•		
Pineda and Dadds (41)							•	•	
Rossouw et al. (32)			•				•		
Schuppert et al. (26)		•							
Schuppert et al. (25)		•							
Wharff et al. (37)	•						•		
Wood et al. (24)	•	•			•				•

frequency of self-harm resulting in emergency presentations between the Therapeutic Assessment and treatment as usual groups, overall treatment engagement remained higher in the Therapeutic Assessment group than the control group. Collectively, the Asarnow et al. & Ougrin et al. studies underscore the value of brief mental health interventions for improving linkage to outpatient treatment after emergency presentation for self-harm and suicidality, as well as the importance of efforts to identify effective treatment strategies and implement them effectively within community programs.

Secondary Outcome Assessment: Suicidal Ideation, Depression, Other Clinical, and Functioning Outcomes

Significant Differences in Therapeutic Interventions vs. Treatment as Usual

Of the possible 21 studies, 17 studies explored secondary outcomes of depressive symptoms and suicidal ideation, of which 5 (29.4%) yielded significant differences by the intervention. Beginning with studies using primarily self-driven interventions, MBT-A was found to yield a significant reduction in depressive symptoms at the 12-month point (32). Both the treatment and control group showed reduced depressive symptoms, and a significant reduction over time was seen only in MBT-A youths condition. The largest mean difference between groups was seen at 9 months. Using a 12-week treatment period, Alavi et al. (27) evaluated the CBT-Suicide Prevention (CBT-SP) treatment developed for the Treatment of Adolescent Suicide Attempter's (TASA) study (44), results indicated significant reductions in both suicidal ideation and depressive symptoms at the end of the 3-month treatment period. These results are similar to those from the TASA trial, which was originally designed as an RCT but random assignment was discontinued due to patients' reluctance to accept randomization. The TASA trial found relatively low rates of suicidal events, including suicide attempts, interrupted suicide attempts, and levels of suicidal ideation requiring emergency evaluation or hospitalization (19) as well as declines in suicidal ideation and depressive symptoms over the 6-month treatment period (45).

For interventions focusing on social support and psychoeducation strategies, King's investigations of both versions of the Youth-Nominated Support Team intervention decreased suicidal ideation over time in both groups. Further, the first version of the intervention, YST-I, allowed both youth-nominated peers and adults in the Support Team and demonstrated a small to medium effect on the reduction of suicidal ideation only after altering analyses from intent-to-treat to actually treated; an effect that was seen only in female participants (39). Following with a study of the adapted YST-II intervention, which focused on youth-nominated adults, King again demonstrated a small to medium effect in the reduction of suicidal ideation, this time, only in those participants who had a history of multiple suicide attempts (40).

Another socially-driven intervention, Attachment-Based Family Therapy (ABFT), compared to TAU, was shown to

TABLE 3 | Selection of Randomized Control Trials and Results Investigating the Efficacy of Therapeutic Interventions (TI's) Versus Control Treatments on Self-Harming Adolescents.

Study	Sample Criteria (after attrition)		Inclusion Criteria (Self-harm definition)	Relevant Diagnostic Tools	Outcomes Investigated			Treatment Type		Periods of Assessment	Outcomes and Findings
	Treatment/ Control (n)	Demographics (mean age)			Self-Harm	Suicidal Ideation	Depressive Symptoms	Intervention	Control		
Alavi et al. (27) Iran	15/15	12–18 (16.1) 90% female	**Hospital presentation following suicide attempt within 3 months of study**	Scale for Suicidal Ideation (SSI) Hopelessness Inventory (BHI) Depression Inventory (BDI)		✓	✓	CBT for suicidal ideation	WL	12 weeks	Significant reduction in suicidal ideation, hopelessness, and depressive symptoms in treatment group
Asaranow et al. (6) USA	89/92	10–17 (14.7) 69% female	**Hospital presentation following suicide attempt or suicidal ideation** (intentional self-injury with/without intent to die)	Suicide attempts on the NIMH-DISC-IV Center for Epidemiological Studies Depression Scale (CES-D)	✓		✓	Family Intervention for Suicide Prevention (FISP)	TAU	~2 months	No significant reduction in self-harm or depressive symptoms, but improved linkage to outpatient care
Asarnow et al. (31) USA	20/22	11–18 (14.62) 88% female	**Suicide attempt within 3 months of study** or **≥3 episodes of self-harm within lifetime**	Columbia-Suicide Severity Rating Scale (C-SSRC) NIMH-DISC-IV Suicide History Interview (SHI) Service assessment for children and Adolescents (SACA)	✓			SAFETY (DBT informed CBT)	E-TAU	3 months	Significant differences between groups for SA at 30month timepoint, no difference between groups on NSSI.
Chanen et al. (33) Australia	44/42	15–18 (16.4) 76% female	**Fulfillment of 2/9 DSM-IV Criteria for Borderline Personality Disorder**	Semi-structured interview for paras-suicidal behavior developed by research group	✓			Cognitive Analytic Therapy	GCC	6, 12, 24 months	Reduction of parasuicidal behaviors seen within whole cohort, with no significant group differences
Cotgrove et al. (35) UK	47/58	≤16 (14.9) 85% female	**Hospital presentation following suicide attempt** (attempted suicide, deliberate acts of self-injury or self-poisoning)	Clinical records Questionnaire, unspecified		✓		Token for readmission to hospital + AAU	AAU	12 months	Fewer people (50%) with hospital readmission tokens re-attempt suicide than those without, but no significant effect found within treatment group
Diamond et al. (38) USA	35/31	12–17 (15.1) 83% female	**>31 SIQ score >20 BDI-II**	Suicide Ideation Questionnaire (SIQ-JR) Beck Depression Inventory (BDI-II) Scale for Suicidal Ideation (SSI)		✓	✓	Attachment-based Family Therapy	E-TAU	6, 12, 24 weeks	Significant reduction in SI within treatment group at all-time points; Significant reduction in DS within treatment group my mid-treatment, but loss of effect at post-treatment and follow-up

(Continued)

TABLE 3 | Continued

Study	Sample Criteria (after attrition)		Inclusion Criteria (Self-harm definition)	Relevant Diagnostic Tools	Outcomes Investigated			Treatment Type		Periods of Assessment	Outcomes and Findings
	Treatment/ Control (n)	Demographics (mean age)			Self-Harm	Suicidal Ideation	Depressive Symptoms	Intervention	Control		
Donaldson et al. (38) USA	21/18	12–17 (15) 82%female	**Hospital presentation following suicide attempt** (intentional non-fatal self-injury with intent to die)	Structured Follow-up Interviews SIQ CES-D	✓	✓	✓	Skills-Based Treatment (SBT)	SRT	3, 6 months	Overall reduction in likelihood of re-attempting suicide and an improvement in ideation and depressive symptoms, but no significant differences between groups at any point
Esposito-Smythers et al. (28) USA	20/20	13–17(15) 68% female	**Suicide attempt within 3 months of study or ≥41 on SIQ in the past month**	SIQ Columbia Impairment Scale (CIS) Reynolds Adolescent Depression Scale (RADS-2)	✓	✓	✓	I-CBT	E-TAU	18 months	Significant reduction in suicide attempts in treatment condition; overall improvement in cohort on ideation and depressive symptoms with no significant differences between groups
Green et al. (23) UK	179/180	12–17 89% female	**Hospital presentation following ≥2 episodes of self-harm within 12 months** (intentional self-inflicted injuries or overdose of toxic substances)	SIQ Mood and Feeling Questionnaire (MFQ) Health of Nation Outcomes Scales for Children and Adolescents (HoNOSCA)	✓	✓	✓	Developmental Group Psychotherapy	TAU	6,12 months	Overall improvement within cohort on self-harm, ideation and depressive symptoms, but no significant differences between groups at any point
Harrington et al. (36) UK	85/77	≤16 (14.5) 90% female	**Hospital presentation following deliberate self-poisoning** (ingestion of substances not for human consumption, or overdose)	SIQ Hopelessness Questionnaire McMaster Family Assessment Device		✓		Home-based Family Intervention + TAU	TAU	2, 6 months	No significant differences between groups at any point on rates of suicidal ideation
Hazell et al. (22) Australia	35/37	12–16 (14.5) 91% female	**≥3 episodes of self-harm, one happening within 1 month of study** (intentional self-inflicted injury irrespective of intent)	SIQ MFQ Schedule for Affective Disorders and Schizophrenia (K-SADS) HoNOSCA	✓	✓	✓	Developmental Group Psychotherapy	TAU	2, 6, 12 months	Overall improvement within cohort on self-harm, ideation, and depressive symptoms but no significant differences between by follow-up; Significantly higher proportion of treatment group engaged in self-harm until 6 months

(Continued)

TABLE 3 | Continued

Study	Sample Criteria (after attrition)		Inclusion Criteria (Self-harm definition)	Relevant Diagnostic Tools	Outcomes Investigated			Treatment Type		Periods of Assessment	Outcomes and Findings
	Treatment/ Control (n)	Demographics (mean age)			Self-Harm	Suicidal Ideation	Depressive Symptoms	Intervention	Control		
King et al. (39) USA	113/123	12–17 (15.3) 68% female	**Significant suicidal ideation or suicide attempt with 1 month of study / score of 20 or 30 on Self-harm subscale of the Child and Adolescent Functional Assessment Scale (CAFAS)**	SIQ-JR Spectrum of Suicide Behavior Scale Youth Self-Report (YSR) RADS CAFAS	✓		✓	YST-I + TAU	TAU	6 months	No significant difference in suicide attempts between groups. Small to medium effect on the reduction of suicidal ideation only after altering analyses from intent-to-treat to only in female participants
King et al. (40) USA	223/225	13–17 (15.6) 71% female	**Significant suicidal ideation or suicide attempt within 4 weeks of study**	SIQ-JR BHS Children's Depression Rating Scale Revised (CDRS-R)	✓		✓	YST-II + TAU	TAU	6 weeks, 3, 6, 12 months	No significant reduction in suicide attempts. Overall improvement on depressive symptoms (moderated by multiple attempts) lasting 6 weeks.
Mehlum et al. (42) Norway	39/38	(15.6) 83% female	**≥1 episode of self-harm within 16 weeks of study / Fulfillment of 2 criteria of BPD / fulfillment of 1 + 2 subthreshold criteria of BPD** (intention self-inflicted injury irrespective of intent)	Lifetime Parasuicide Count (LPC) Interview Suicide Intent Scale (SIS) SIQ-JR Short MFQ	✓	✓	✓	DBT-A	E-TAU	9, 15, 19, 71 weeks	Significant reduction in self-harm, ideation, and depressive symptoms at 19 weeks, but loss of significance at 1 year follow-up;
Ougrin et al. (34) UK	35/34	12–18 (15.5) 80% female	**Engaging in self-harm without prior involvement with psychiatric services** (intentional self-inflicted injury or self-poisoning irrespective of intent)	Health department records including: CAMHS, A&E, and Primary Care	✓			Therapeutic Assessment (TA)	AAU	24 months	No significant reduction in hospital presentations for self-harm, though treatment engagement increased significantly
Pineda and Dadds (41) Australia	22/18	12–17 (15.14) 75% female	**≥ 1 episode of suicidal behavior** (suicidal ideation, intent, suicide attempt, self-injury) within the last 2 months before referral to hospital; residing with at least 1 parent	Adolescent Suicide Questionnaire- Revised (ASQ-R)	✓			RAP-P	Routine Care	3, 6 months	Significant improvement in suicidal behavior at 3 and 6 months in RAP-P group, compared to control group.

(Continued)

TABLE 3 | Continued

Study	Sample Criteria (after attrition)		Inclusion Criteria (Self-harm definition)	Relevant Diagnostic Tools	Outcomes Investigated			Treatment Type		Periods of Assessment	Outcomes and Findings
	Treatment/ Control (n)	Demographics (mean age)			Self-Harm	Suicidal Ideation	Depressive Symptoms	Intervention	Control		
Rossouw et al. (32) UK	20/20	12–17 (14.7) 80% female	**≥1 episode of self-harm within past month** (intentional self-inflicted injury irrespective of intent)	Risk-Taking and Self-Harm Inventory (RTSHI) MFQ	✓		✓	MBT-A	TAU	3, 6, 9, 12 months	Significant reduction in self-harm and depressive symptoms for treatment group during treatment and at follow-up
Schuppert et al. (26) Holland	23/20	14–19(16.14) 88% female	**Fulfillment of 2/9 DSM-IV Criteria for Borderline Personality Disorder** including: Recurrent suicidal behavior, gestures, threats, or self-mutilation	Clinical interview Youth Self-Report (YSR) Internalizing & Externalizing	✓		✓	Emotion Regulation Training + TAU	TAU	3, 6 months	Reduction in self-harm and depressive symptoms seen within whole cohort with no significant group differences
Schuppert et al. (25) Holland	54/55	14–19 (15.98) 96% female	**Fulfillment of 2/9 DSM-IV Criteria for Borderline Personality Disorder** including: Recurrent suicidal behavior, gestures, threats, or self-mutilation	Clinical interview Youth Self-Report (YSR) Internalizing & Externalizing	✓		✓	Emotion Regulation Training + TAU	TAU	6, 12 months	Reduction in self-harm and depressive symptoms seen within whole cohort with no significant group differences (information obtained via e-mail)
Wharff et al. (37) USA	68/71	13–18 (15.5) 72% female	**Hospital presentation for suicidality** (suicidal self-identification, adult-noted suicidality, suicide attempt)	Reasons for Living Inventory for Adolescents (RFL-A)		✓		Family-Based Crisis Intervention	TAU	Post-test, 3 day, 1 week, 1 month	Overall reduction of ideation and depressive symptoms within whole cohort with no significant group differences; Intervention group significantly less likely to be re-hospitalized post treatment
Wood et al. (24) UK	32/31	12–16 (14.25) 78% female	**Hospital presentation following incident of self-harm** (intentional self-inflicted injury irrespective of intent)	MFQ SIQ HoNOSCA	✓	✓	✓	Developmental Group Psychotherapy	TAU	7 months	Significant reduction in likelihood of re-attempting suicide within treatment group; overall improvement within cohort but no treatment effect on ideation and depressive symptoms

TAU, Treatment As Usual; E-TAU, Enhanced Treatment As Usual; GCC, Good Clinical Care; AAU, Assessment As Usual; SDP, Standard Disposition Planning; SRT, Supportive Relationship Treatment; I-CBT, Integrated CBT.

have very strong effects in reducing suicidal ideation during all points of treatment with the strongest effect observed at 24 weeks, the final follow-up (38). This effect was seen within the total sample, and within a subsample of adolescents who met the diagnostic criteria for clinical depression. Additionally, a significant effect in the reduction of suicidal ideation was seen within the Home-Based Family intervention, but only when controlling for depression.

Overall Group Differences Irrespective of Therapeutic Intervention

Reductions over time in suicidal ideation were observed in nearly all studies, including those evaluating mentalization treatment, DBT-A, integrated CBT for suicidality and substance abuse, skills based treatment, youth-nominated support teams, and attachment based family treatment (28–30, 32, 38).

While a significant reduction in ideation was observed in 3 studies based on social or family models (38–40), none of these studies identified significant differences in the reduction of depressive symptoms between treatment and control groups at the final follow-up measure. The Attachment-Based Family therapy intervention appeared close to producing a nearly significant result at the 6 and 12-week measurements, but was unable to reach statistical significance altogether at the end of the trial (38).

When examining socially-driven interventions within an emergency service settings, Asarnow et al. (6) did not examine suicidal ideation or depressive symptoms close in time to the emergency intervention. However, when followed up roughly 2-months post -hospital discharge there were significant declines in depressive symptoms across groups. Of the socially-driven interventions administered during a presentation to emergency services or at the time of a psychiatric assessment, only Wharff investigated whether a Family-Based Crisis Intervention, a multi-module single session intervention would impact the adolescent's suicidal ideation (46). While an overall reduction in suicidal ideation was seen within the cohort, there was no significant treatment effect. In contrast to the other studies included this review, Wharff conducted pre-and post-test measures a mere 4-h apart.

Null or Negative Findings

Despite noting significant group differences in primary outcomes, Wood et al. (24) found no significant effect of Developmental Group Psychotherapy on reducing depressive symptoms and suicidal ideation. Consistent with what was noted for primary outcomes, neither of the two additional trials evaluating the same treatment (22, 23) saw treatment effects in secondary outcomes of reducing suicidal ideation or depressive symptoms.

Asarnow et al. (6) found no statistically significant advantage of the Emergency intervention in reducing depression levels, even though the intervention was associated with improved linkage to outpatient mental health services was observed. Indeed, there was no evidence that attendance in outpatient community treatment as usual was associated with lower depressive symptoms or suicidality.

DISCUSSION

We set out to examine the available literature for adolescents with a recent history of self-harm or suicide attempt, with the overall aim of clarifying which therapeutic interventions and approaches show evidence of benefits for reducing self-harm, suicide attempts, as well as suicidal ideation and depressive symptoms. Of the 18 unique interventions identified through this review, treatments that target individual, self-driven (cognitive-behavioral, self-regulatory processes) and socially-driven (family or social support network) processes appeared to show the greatest promise for reducing suicide attempts (28, 31), and there are data supporting the benefits of DBT-A and MBT-A (combined self-driven and systems-driven approaches), for reducing overall self-harm. If the somewhat different variations of CBT are considered together, and DBT-A is classified as a type of CBT, CBT is the only intervention type where initial positive findings have been replicated independently. It should be noted, however, that all of the CBT interventions with evidence for efficacy have strong family systems-driven components (I-CBT, SAFETY, DBT-A). Other interventions with initial positive outcomes, such as MBT-A require testing in adequately powered trials and replication.

The results of this review update are demonstrative of the effectiveness of DBT-A and CBT, the only interventions where initial positive findings have been replicated independently. These interventions are therefore an invaluable part of the clinical treatment of young people who present with self-harm and a history of suicide attempts.

Turning to the secondary outcomes of suicidal ideation and general measures of suicide risk, current research supports the efficacy of attachment based family treatment and the Resourceful Adolescent Parent Program. Results were not reported on suicide attempts specifically or self-harm in either trial, and replication is needed. While not all studies have reported on suicidal ideation when suicide attempts and self-harm were primary outcomes, both MBT-A and DBT-A have shown significant advantages in reducing both self-harm and suicidal ideation. Rossouw and Fonagy (32) reported an advantage for MBT-A compared to treatment as usual at end of the year-long treatment. Mehlum et al. (42) similarly reported an advantage for DBT relative to treatment as usual at end of treatment, which was at 16 weeks, although treatment as usual youths had caught up with the DBT-A youths by 71-weeks.

Results on depression outcomes tended to be similar to those for suicidal ideation, with a tendency for depression levels to diminish over time, and between group differences observed in the studies and time points where benefits on suicidal ideation were observed. The two studies that evaluated borderline symptoms (DBT-A and MBT-A) reported intervention benefits in reducing symptoms of Borderline Personality Disorder. Both suicidal ideation and depressive symptoms have been shown to precipitate non-suicidal self-injury and suicide attempts in adolescents (19, 47), and thus should not be overlooked as integral symptoms to address during treatment in future research.

Overall, the studies which showed significant effects in the reduction of outcomes at any point during treatment (without adjustments) were similar in several characteristics. First, these interventions mandated the family or support person's involvement in the adolescent's therapeutic journey in addition to the adolescent's individual therapy; five interventions included parental involvement throughout the duration of the intervention, through family training, family therapy, and/or family planning (28, 29, 31, 32, 38, 41). The Responsible Adolescent Parenting Program (2013) was the only exclusively socially-driven parenting intervention that yielded significant effects, suggesting a need for replication studies using this treatment. Finally, we noted that the effective interventions all share emotion regulation, problem solving, and communication skills as key tenets of the intervention. While dysregulated affect is shown to be a predictor of suicide attempts and non-suicidal self-injury (47), subsequent research is needed to assess whether problem-solving and communication skills would contribute to the reduction of self-harm, suicidal ideation, or depressive symptoms.

The current National Institute for Health and Care Excellence (NICE) guidelines (48) for the treatment of adolescents with self-harm, suggest tailored treatments incorporating elements of cognitive behavioral, psychodynamic and problem-solving therapies. Results of this review are generally consistent with these guidelines, and clinical guidance is needed to support optimal clinical care for this potentially life-threatening problem. However, it is important to note that the evidence is limited. We still lack replicated evidence of treatment efficacy for any of the reviewed interventions. It is also important to note that the sampling protocols and populations differed across studies, and these sampling differences could lead to differences in treatment efficacy and study results. For instance, the DBT-A trial selected youths based on the presence of repeated self-harm and symptoms of borderline personality disorder, the MBT-A trial selected youths for the presence of self-harm within the past month, the Integrated CBT model recruited youths with both suicidality (attempts or ideation) and substance abuse, the SAFETY trial selected youths based on the presence of suicide attempts or repeated self-harm, and the Peer Nominated Support Team trials recruited youths with previous suicide attempts or suicidal ideation. Because trials were conducted across different nations and health systems, "treatment as usual" will have varied considerably, and this could conceivably have affected the observed between group differences. Further, with few exceptions (32, 41) studies have not yet reported on treatment mediators and studies aimed at treatment mechanisms associated with reduced fatal and non-fatal self-harm risk would help guide the field. Research focusing on targeted interventions such as those aimed at reducing access to dangerous methods of self-harm (firearms, poisoning) could also help inform clinical care and data are accumulating supporting the value of such interventions.

Strengths and Limitations

The current review supplements the literature by conducting a systematic review on not only suicide attempts and self-harm, but also addresses the links between suicidal ideation and depressive symptoms in adolescents. While we were able to add a more comprehensive component to the systematic review, due to the complexity of the varied studies and primary and secondary outcomes, additional research is needed to identify effective treatment strategies, provide guidance regarding how to best personalize treatment and match youths and families to treatments that are most likely to be beneficial, and to develop cost-effective treatment delivery strategies. There are no published RCTs of pharmacological interventions for the reduction of self-harm. However, many young people who self-harm are offered pharmacological treatment to address co-occurring psychiatric symptoms. While an investigation of the possible influence of pharmacological interventions was out of the scope of the current review, future work addressing both psychosocial and psychopharmacological elements of treatment is needed. To date, there have been no RCTs evaluating the efficacy of psychopharmacological treatments for reducing self-harm, though this may also be a potential avenue for future research. In following the methodology of the previous analysis, studies which did not adhere to an RCT design were excluded, though may nonetheless be insightful in regards to reducing self-harm in young people. Additionally, as the search terms used to identify studies on self-harm were derived from the subject headings of the relevant databases and were limited to studies published in English, some studies representing unique cultural outlooks on self-harm may have been omitted. Indeed, the heterogeneity of the studies included in this review makes it difficult to account for additional influential factors, including the participants' previous engagement with therapy, their mental health histories and psychiatric co-morbidities, and the quantity and severity of their previous self-harm, among others. Future reviews may wish to pay particular attention to such elements in order to understand whether certain interventions work more effectively in some unique cases over others. A variety of additional factors, including small and highly selective samples limit the generalizability of the findings in some of the studies included in this review. Finally, the current failure to replicate certain interventions in different cultural contexts underscores the challenges for exporting treatment strategies across different cultures and settings, and the importance of building international consensus and developing care strategies that can work across diverse cultural contexts and health systems.

Future Directions for Effective Interventions

Considering future directions for studies aimed at decreasing self-harm and suicide attempts in adolescents, some treatments (such as DBT-A) led to significant reductions on outcomes more rapidly than others. Cost analyses could further inform knowledge about the viability of delivering certain interventions over others in routine clinical settings to large populations. Several of the evaluated interventions require multiple personnel (e.g., 2-therapist model used in the Integrated CBT model, the SAFETY intervention, and DBT-A with skills trainer and individual therapist). Likewise, whereas several of the interventions are completed in under 6 months, others require long and perhaps costly commitments to therapy, which may act as barriers to treatment adherence, particularly for adolescents who experience a lack of motivation to attend sessions as a symptom of depression (49, 50). These cost considerations will also have a major bearing on the likelihood of interventions being implemented in routine health setting. Additionally, some of the multi-component treatments, such as DBT-A which requires 1 h weekly psychotherapy plus 2 h of multi-family skills group may require a more intensive and burdensome treatment dose than needed for some youths and families. Stepped care approaches that match treatment intensity to assessed level of risk and need may prove helpful for identifying the most cost-effective treatment delivery strategies.

The results of a large, multi-center RCT investigating the effectiveness of Family Therapy in reducing self-harm in adolescents (51) were published following the intial literature review, and thus cannot be included in the results of the current update. However, these results, which demonstrated that Family Therapy was more costly and no more beneficial than treatment as usual, are nonetheless an important contribution to understanding which interventions are viable and effective in reducing self-harm in young people. In comparison to other therapies which include a strong family-based component as part of the treatment (such as DBT-A, MBT-A, and RAP-P among others), participants in the Family Therapy group were provided with 6–8 monthly sessions of therapy; far fewer than those participants which received any of the aforementioned treatments, indicating that the duration and intensity of the treatment may be an important factor in the success of an intervention aiming to reduce self-harm and preventing suicide attempts.

Other RCTs published following the completion of our search, include a study further strengthening the efficacy of DBT-A in reducing self-harm post-treatment, as well as a significantly lower number of suicide attempts and significantly fewer episodes of non-suicidal self-injurious behavior. Although no significant between-group differences were found at longer-term (12-month) follow-up in number of self-harm episodes, youths in the DBT-A were significantly more likely to show clinically significant change, defined as the absence of any self-harm, through the 12-month follow-up (52). Another study showed that young people with longer inpatient admissions were more likely to have multiple self-harm episodes, than young people treated with intensive community care (53).

Lastly, there were several unpublished protocol studies of RCTs for this subject population (54–58) and studies in progress (59–61), which we were unable to use for our systematic review. It is our hope that when these protocols are applied and published, such findings will greatly advance the field, and shed further light on effective treatments for adolescents at-risk for suicide.

Our updated systematic review suggests that given the heterogeneity of suicidal behavior, understanding which type of intervention is most effective for adolescents at risk of suicide can be a challenging but nonetheless paramount endeavor that requires further attention.

AUTHOR CONTRIBUTIONS

UI and NS conducted the update to the systematic review, including the literature search, and analysis, UI and NS wrote the draft of the paper, JRA, PM, and TT added clinical and critical insight to the overall paper structure, and DO supervised the procedure and the overall study.

FUNDING

The authors' time was paid for by Kings College London and South London and Maudsley NHS Foundation Trust.

JRA has received grant, research, or other support from the National Institute of Mental Health, the American Foundation for Suicide Prevention, the Substance Abuse and Mental Health Services Administration, the American Psychological Association (APA), the Society of Clinical Child and Adolescent Psychology (Division 53 of the APA), and the Association for Child and Adolescent Mental Health. She has served as a consultant on quality improvement for depression and suicide/self-harm prevention, serves on the Scientific Council of the American Foundation for Suicide Prevention, and the Scientific Advisory Board of the Klingenstein Third Generation Foundation.

PM is a co-applicant to the following grant: Mars B, Gunnell D, Joinson C, Moran P, Relton C, Hemani G, Heron J, Suderman M, Ford T. Pathways to self-harm: Biological mechanisms and genetic contribution. MRC. $297,867. 2017-2019 Co-applicant (to PM).

ACKNOWLEDGMENTS

The authors thank Dr. Emily Simonoff, Dr. Bruce Clarke and Mrs. Jo Fletcher who made this work possible. This study was supported by the NIHR Biomedical Research Centre at University Hospitals Bristol NHS Foundation Trust and the University of Bristol. The views expressed in this publication are those of the author(s) and not necessarily those of the NHS, the National Institute for Health Research or the Department of Health and Social Care.

REFERENCES

1. Prevention NAAFS. (2014). *Research Prioritization Task Force. A Prioritized Research Agenda for Suicide Prevention: An Action Plan to Save Lives.* Rockville, MD: National Institute of Mental Health and Research Prioritization Task Force.
2. Patton GC, Coffey C, Sawyer SM, Viner RM, Haller DM, Bose K, et al. Global patterns of mortality in young people: a systematic analysis of population

health data. *Lancet* (2009) 374:881–92. doi: 10.1016/S0140-6736(09) 60741-8
3. Butler AM, Malone K. Attempted suicide v. non-suicidal self-injury: behaviour, syndrome or diagnosis? *Br J Psychiatry* (2013) 202:324–5. doi: 10.1192/bjp.bp.112.113506
4. American Psychiatric Association. (2013). *Diagnostic and Statistical Manual of Mental Disorders, 5th edn.* Arlington, VA: American Psychiatric Publishing.
5. Hawton K, Harriss L. Deliberate self-harm in young people: characteristics and subsequent mortality in a 20-year cohort of patients presenting to hospital. *J Clin Psychiatry* (2007) 68:1574–83. doi: 10.4088/JCP.v68n1017
6. Asarnow JR, Porta G, Spirito A, Emslie G, Clarke G, Wagner KD, et al. Suicide attempts and nonsuicidal self-injury in the treatment of resistant depression in adolescents: findings from the TORDIA study. *J Am Acad Child Adoles Psychiatry* (2011) 50:772–81. doi: 10.1016/j.jaac.2011.04.003
7. Brent DA, Mcmakin DL, Kennard BD, Goldstein TR, Mayes TL, Douaihy AB. Protecting adolescents from self-harm: a critical review of intervention studies. *J Am Acad Child Adoles Psychiatry* (2013) 52:1260–71. doi: 10.1016/j.jaac.2013.09.009
8. Ougrin D, Boege I. Brief report: the Self Harm Questionnaire: a new tool designed to improve identification of self harm in adolescents. *J Adoles.* (2013) 36:221–5. doi: 10.1016/j.adolescence.2012.09.006
9. Moran P, Coffey C, Romaniuk H, Olsson C, Borschmann R, Carlin JB, et al. The natural history of self-harm from adolescence to young adulthood: a population-based cohort study. *Lancet* (2012) 379:236–43. doi: 10.1016/S0140-6736(11)61141-0
10. Rowe SL, French RS, Henderson C, Ougrin D, Slade M, Moran P. Help-seeking behaviour and adolescent self-harm: a systematic review. *Aust N Zeal J Psychiatry* (2014) 48:1083–95. doi: 10.1177/0004867414555718
11. Ougrin D, Tranah T, Stahl D, Moran P, Asarnow JR. Therapeutic interventions for suicide attempts and self-harm in adolescents: systematic review and meta-analysis. *J Am Acad Child Adoles Psychiatry* (2015) 54:97–107.e102. doi: 10.1016/j.jaac.2014.10.009
12. Shaffer D, Gould MS, Fisher P, Trautman P, Moreau D, Kleinman M, et al. Psychiatric diagnosis in child and adolescent suicide. *Arch Gener Psychiatry* (1996) 53:339–48. doi: 10.1001/archpsyc.1996.01830040075012
13. Gould MS, King R, Greenwald S, Fisher P, Schwab-Stone M, Kramer R, et al. Psychopathology associated with suicidal ideation and attempts among children and adolescents. *J Am Acad Child Adoles Psychiatry* (1998) 37:915–23. doi: 10.1097/00004583-199809000-00011
14. National Confidential Inquiry into Suicide and Homicide by People with Mental Illness. (2017). *Suicide by Children and Young People.* Manchester: University of Manchester, 2017.
15. Lundh L-G, Wångby-Lundh M, Paaske M, Ingesson S, Bjärehed J. Depressive symptoms and deliberate self-harm in a community sample of adolescents: a prospective study. *Depress Res Treat.* (2011) 2011:935871. doi: 10.1155/2011/935871
16. Singhal A, Ross J, Seminog O, Hawton K, Goldacre MJ. Risk of self-harm and suicide in people with specific psychiatric and physical disorders: comparisons between disorders using English national record linkage. *J R Soc Med.* (2014) 107:194–204. doi: 10.1177/0141076814522033
17. Yang F-Y, Lai CY, Yen C-F, Hsu Y-Y, Zauszniewski JA. The depressive symptoms, resourcefulness, and self-harm behaviors of adolescents. *J Nurs Res.* (2017) 25:41–9. doi: 10.1097/jnr.0000000000000127
18. Zubrick SR, Hafekost J, Johnson SE, Sawyer MG, Patton G, Lawrence D. The continuity and duration of depression and its relationship to non-suicidal self-harm and suicidal ideation and behavior in adolescents 12–17. *J Affect Disord.* (2017) 220:49–56. doi: 10.1016/j.jad.2017.05.050
19. Brent DA, Greenhill LL, Compton S, Emslie G, Wells K, Walkup JT, et al. The Treatment of Adolescent Suicide Attempters study (TASA): predictors of suicidal events in an open treatment trial. *J Am Acad Child Adoles Psychiatry* (2009) 48:987–96. doi: 10.1097/CHI.0b013e3181b5dbe4
20. Jadad AR, Moore RA, Carroll D, Jenkinson C, Reynolds DJM, Gavaghan DJ, et al. Assessing the quality of reports of randomized clinical trials: is blinding necessary? *Control Clin Trials* (1996) 17:1–12. doi: 10.1016/0197-2456(95)00134-4
21. Spirito A, Boergers J, Donaldson D, Bishop D, Lewander W. An intervention trial to improve adherence to community treatment by adolescents after a suicide attempt. *J Am Acad Child Adolesc Psychiatry* (2002) 41:435–42. doi: 10.1097/00004583-200204000-00016
22. Hazell PL, Martin G, Mcgill K, Kay T, Wood A, Trainor G, et al. Group therapy for repeated deliberate self-harm in adolescents: failure of replication of a randomized trial. *J Am Acad Child Adolesc Psychiatry* (2009) 48:662–70. doi: 10.1097/CHI.0b013e3181a0acec
23. Green JM, Wood AJ, Kerfoot MJ, Trainor G, Roberts C, Rothwell J, et al. Group therapy for adolescents with repeated self harm: randomised controlled trial with economic evaluation. *BMJ* (2011) 2011:342. doi: 10.1136/bmj.d682
24. Wood A, Trainor G, Rothwell J, Moore A, Harrington R. Randomized trial of group therapy for repeated deliberate self-harm in adolescents. *J Am Acad Child Adolesc Psychiatry* (2001) 40:1246–53. doi: 10.1097/00004583-200111000-00003
25. Schuppert HM, Timmerman ME, Bloo J, Van Gemert TG, Wiersema HM, Minderaa RB, et al. Emotion regulation training for adolescents with borderline personality disorder traits: a randomized controlled trial. *J Am Acad Child Adolesc Psychiatry* (2012) 51:1314–1323.e1312. doi: 10.1016/j.jaac.2012.09.002
26. Schuppert HM, Giesen-Bloo J, Van Gemert TG, Wiersema HM, Minderaa RB, Emmelkamp PM, et al. Effectiveness of an emotion regulation group training for adolescents—a randomized controlled pilot study. *Clin Psychol Psychother.* (2009) 16:467–78. doi: 10.1002/cpp.637
27. Alavi A, Sharifi B, Ghanizadeh A, Dehbozorgi G. Effectiveness of cognitive-behavioral therapy in decreasing suicidal ideation and hopelessness of the adolescents with previous suicidal attempts. *Iran J Pediatrics* (2013) 23:467–72. doi: 10.1016/j.neurenf.2012.04.266
28. Esposito-Smythers C, Spirito A, Kahler CW, Hunt J, Monti P. Treatment of co-occurring substance abuse and suicidality among adolescents: a randomized trial. *J Consult Clin Psychol.* (2011) 79:728–39. doi: 10.1037/a0026074
29. Mehlum L, Tormoen AJ, Ramberg M, Haga E, Diep LM, Laberg S, et al. Dialectical behavior therapy for adolescents with repeated suicidal and self-harming behavior: a randomized trial. *J Am Acad Child Adolesc Psychiatry* (2014) 53:1082–91. doi: 10.1016/j.jaac.2014.07.003
30. Donaldson D, Spirito A, Esposito-Smythers C. Treatment for adolescents following a suicide attempt: results of a pilot trial. *J Am Acad Child Adolesc Psychiatry* (2005) 44:113–20. doi: 10.1097/00004583-200502000-00003
31. Asarnow JR, Hughes JL, Babeva KN, Sugar CA. Cognitive-behavioral family treatment for suicide attempt prevention: a randomized controlled trial. *J Am Acad Child Adolesc Psychiatry* (2017) 56:506–14. doi: 10.1016/j.jaac.2017.03.015
32. Rossouw TI, Fonagy P. Mentalization-based treatment for self-harm in adolescents: a randomized controlled trial. *J Am Acad Child Adolesc Psychiatry* (2012) 51:1304–1313.e1303. doi: 10.1016/j.jaac.2012.09.018
33. Chanen AM, Jackson HJ, Mccutcheon LK, Jovev M, Dudgeon P, Yuen HP, et al. Early intervention for adolescents with borderline personality disorder using cognitive analytic therapy: randomised controlled trial. *Br J Psychiatry* (2008) 193:477–84. doi: 10.1192/bjp.bp.107.048934
34. Ougrin D, Boege I, Stahl D, Banarsee R, Taylor E. Randomised controlled trial of therapeutic assessment versus usual assessment in adolescents with self-harm: 2-year follow-up. *Arch Dis Child.* (2013) 98:772–6. doi: 10.1136/archdischild-2012-303200
35. Cotgrove A, Zirinsky L, Black D, Weston D. Secondary prevention of attempted suicide in adolescence. *J Adoles.* (1995) 18:569. doi: 10.1006/jado.1995.1039
36. Harrington R, Kerfoot M, Dyer E, McNiven F, Gill J, Harrington V, et al. Randomized trial of a home-based family intervention for children who have deliberately poisoned themselves. *J Am Acad Child Adolesc Psychiatry* (1998) 37:512–8.
37. Wharff EA, Ginnis KB, Ross AM, White EM, White MT, Forbes PW. Family-Based Crisis Intervention With Suicidal Adolescents: A Randomized Clinical Trial. *Pediatr Emerg Care* (2017). doi: 10.1097/PEC.0000000000001076. [Epub ahead of print].
38. Diamond GS, Wintersteen MB, Brown GK, Diamond GM, Gallop R, Shelef K, et al. Attachment-based family therapy for adolescents with suicidal ideation: a randomized controlled trial. *J Am Acad Child Adoles Psychiatry* (2010) 49:122–31. doi: 10.1016/j.jaac.2009.11.002

39. King CA, Kramer A, Preuss L, Kerr DC, Weisse L, Venkataraman S. Youth-nominated support team for suicidal adolescents (Version 1): a randomized controlled trial. *J Consult Clin Psychol.* (2006) 74:199–206. doi: 10.1037/0022-006X.74.1.199
40. King CA, Klaus N, Kramer A, Venkataraman S, Quinlan P, Gillespie B. The youth-nominated support team–version ii for suicidal adolescents: a randomized controlled intervention trial. *J Consult Clin Psychol.* (2009) 77:880. doi: 10.1037/a0016552
41. Pineda J, Dadds MR. Family intervention for adolescents with suicidal behavior: a randomized controlled trial and mediation analysis. *J Am Acad Child Adoles Psychiatry* (2013) 52:851–62. doi: 10.1016/j.jaac.2013.05.015
42. Mehlum L, Ramberg M, Tørmoen AJ, Haga E, Diep LM, Stanley BH, et al. Dialectical behavior therapy compared with enhanced usual care for adolescents with repeated suicidal and self-harming behavior: outcomes over a one-year follow-up. *J Am Acad Child Adoles Psychiatry* (2016) 55:295–300. doi: 10.1016/j.jaac.2016.01.005
43. Tørmoen A, Grøholt B, Haga E, Brager-Larsen A, Miller A, Walby F, et al. Feasibility of dialectical behavior therapy with suicidal and self-harming adolescents with multi-problems: training, adherence, and retention. *Arch Suic Res.* (2014) 18:432–44. doi: 10.1080/13811118.2013.826156
44. Stanley B, Brown G, Brent DA, Wells K, Poling K, Curry J, et al. Cognitive-behavioral therapy for suicide prevention (CBT-SP): treatment model, feasibility, and acceptability. *J Am Acad Child Adoles Psychiatry* (2009) 48:1005–13. doi: 10.1097/CHI.0b013e3181b5dbfe
45. Vitiello B, Brent DA, Greenhill LL, Emslie G, Wells K, Walkup JT, et al. Depressive symptoms and clinical status during the Treatment of Adolescent Suicide Attempters (TASA) Study. *J Am Acad Child Adoles Psychiatry* (2009) 48:997–1004. doi: 10.1097/CHI.0b013e3181b5db66
46. Wharff EA, Ginnis KM, Ross AM. Family-based crisis intervention with suicidal adolescents in the emergency room: a pilot study. *Soc Work* (2012) 57:133–43. doi: 10.1093/sw/sws017
47. Wilkinson P, Kelvin R, Roberts C, Dubicka B, Goodyer I. Clinical and psychosocial predictors of suicide attempts and nonsuicidal self-injury in the Adolescent Depression Antidepressants and Psychotherapy Trial (ADAPT). *Am J Psychiatry* (2011) 168:495–501. doi: 10.1176/appi.ajp.2010.10050718
48. National Center for Clinical Excellence. (2011). *Self-Harm in Over 8s: Long-Term Management. (Clinical Guideline CGI 33).* Available online at: https://www.nice.org.uk/guidance/cg133
49. Mohr DC, Ho J, Duffecy J, Baron KG, Lehman KA, Jin L, et al. Perceived barriers to psychological treatments and their relationship to depression. *J Clin Psychol* (2010) 66:394–409. doi: 10.1002/jclp.20659
50. Sturm R, Sherbourne CD. Are barriers to mental health and substance abuse care still rising? *J Behav Health Serv Res.* (2001) 28:81. doi: 10.1007/BF02287236
51. Cottrell DJ, Wright-Hughes A, Collinson M, Boston P, Eisler I, Fortune S, et al. Effectiveness of systemic family therapy versus treatment as usual for young people after self-harm: a pragmatic, phase 3, multicentre, randomised controlled trial. *Lancet Psychiatry* (2018) 5:203–16. doi: 10.1016/S2215-0366(18)30058-0
52. Mccauley E, Berk MS, Asarnow JR, Adrian M, Cohen J, Korslund K, et al. Efficacy of dialectical behavior therapy for adolescents at high risk for suicide: a randomized clinical trial. *JAMA Psychiatry* (2018) 75:777–85. doi: 10.1001/jamapsychiatry.2018.1109
53. Ougrin D, Corrigall R, Poole J, Zundel T, Sarhane M, Slater V, et al. Comparison of effectiveness and cost-effectiveness of an intensive community supported discharge service versus treatment as usual for adolescents with psychiatric emergencies: a randomised controlled trial. *Lancet Psychiatry* (2018) 5:477–85. doi: 10.1016/S2215-0366(18)30129-9
54. Rees CS, Hasking P, Breen LJ, Lipp OV, Mamotte C. Group mindfulness based cognitive therapy vs. group support for self-injury among young people: study protocol for a randomised controlled trial. *BMC Psychiatry* (2015) 15:154. doi: 10.1186/s12888-015-0527-5
55. Van Spijker BA, Calear AL, Batterham PJ, Mackinnon AJ, Gosling JA, Kerkhof AJ, et al. Reducing suicidal thoughts in the Australian general population through web-based self-help: study protocol for a randomized controlled trial. *Trials* (2015) 16:62. doi: 10.1186/s13063-015-0589-1
56. Wright-Hughes A, Graham E, Farrin A, Collinson M, Boston P, Eisler I, et al. Self-Harm Intervention: family Therapy (SHIFT), a study protocol for a randomised controlled trial of family therapy versus treatment as usual for young people seen after a second or subsequent episode of self-harm. *Trials* (2015) 16:501. doi: 10.1186/s13063-015-1007-4
57. Haddock G, Davies L, Evans E, Emsley R, Gooding P, Heaney L, et al. Investigating the feasibility and acceptability of a cognitive behavioural suicide prevention therapy for people in acute psychiatric wards (the 'INSITE'trial): study protocol for a randomised controlled trial. *Trials* (2016) 17:79. doi: 10.1186/s13063-016-1192-9
58. Pepping CA, Lyons A, Mcnair R, Kirby JN, Petrocchi N, Gilbert P. A tailored compassion-focused therapy program for sexual minority young adults with depressive symotomatology: study protocol for a randomized controlled trial. *BMC Psychol.* (2017) 5:5. doi: 10.1186/s40359-017-0175-2
59. Asarnow JR, and Clarke G. (2017). *Randomized Controlled Trial of Stepped Care for Suicide Prevention in Adolescents and Young Adults.* Available online at: https://clinicaltrials.gov: NIMH
60. Boudreaux E, and Kiefe C. (2017). *A System of Safety: Preventing Suicided Through Healthcare System Transformation.* Available online at: https://clinicaltrials.gov
61. Kemp K. (2017). *Implementing a Brief Suicide Intervention for High Risk Youth With Front-Line Juvenile Justice Staff.* Available online at: https://clinicaltrials.gov

19

Nonsuicidal Self-Injury: A Systematic Review

*Annarosa Cipriano, Stefania Cella and Paolo Cotrufo**

Observatory on Eating Disorders, Department of Psychology, University of Campania "Luigi Vanvitelli", Caserta, Italy

Correspondence:
Paolo Cotrufo
paolo.cotrufo@unicampania.it

Objective: Nonsuicidal self-injury (NSSI) refers to the intentional self-inflicted destruction of body tissue without suicidal intention and for purposes not socially sanctioned. Our paper presents an up-to-date overview on nonsuicidal, self-injurious behaviors.

Method: In accordance with PRISMA guidelines, a systematic literature search was conducted across two databases, PubMed and PsycARTICLES, regarding the main features of NSSI with a focus on epidemiological and etiologic data, diagnostic criteria, and functions. All English articles, published between 1998 and 2016, were considered, and screened against a priori inclusion/exclusion criteria. The search terms include: self-harm, self-injury, NSSI, epidemiology, comorbidity, gender, functions and DSM. We also examined the references of the retrieved articles.

Results: NSSI is most common among adolescents and young adults, and the age of onset is reported to occur between 12 and 14 years. Comorbidity with borderline personality disorder (BPD) and eating disorders is often reported. DSM-5 includes NSSI as a condition requiring further study. This review gives an overview of the prevalence rates (7.5–46.5% adolescents, 38.9% university students, 4–23% adults) and main causes that appear to stem from childhood trauma, comorbidity with many other disorders and several functions of NSSI, and the potential independence of a NSSI disorder.

Conclusion: Over the years, interest in NSSI grew to such an extent that an ongoing debate was instigated on whether NSSI should be considered as a diagnosis in its own right and given its own category. This paper provides an up-to-date overview on self-injury, what is known about it and what remains to be done. Clearly, our understanding of the main issues of NSSI has increased in last two decades. However, future researches is needed to examine the developmental trajectories, cultural backgrounds and shed light on the risk factors and functions as well as clarify its role as an independent diagnostic entity.

Keywords: deliberate self-harm, self-injury, nonsuicidal self-injury, NSSI, DSM-5

INTRODUCTION

Nonsuicidal Self-Injury (NSSI) behavior is a growing clinical and public health problem. NSSI is defined as the direct and deliberate destruction of one's own bodily tissue in the absence of lethal intent and for reasons not socially sanctioned (Favazza, 1996; Nock, 2010). Common forms of NSSI include behaviors such as cutting, burning, scratching, and self-hitting (Briere and Gil,

1998; Laye-Gindhu and Schonert-Reichl, 2005; Whitlock et al., 2006; Klonsky and Muehlenkamp, 2007) and most self-injurers report using multiple method (Favazza and Conterio, 1988; Favazza, 1992). Evidences focused on the psychological intentions underlying NSSI demonstrated that the behavior serves a variety of function, both interpersonal and intrapersonal, that are not mutually exclusive (Suyemoto, 1998; Nock and Prinstein, 2004; Klonsky, 2007). Initial research on self-injurious behavior focused on studies in clinical settings (Pattison and Kahan, 1983), primarily with female subjects (Favazza and Conterio, 1989; Favazza et al., 1989; Herpertz, 1995; Suyemoto and MacDonald, 1995).

Epidemiological studies have endured due to the over-inclusive definition of behavior, with and without suicidal intent, as well as the dearth of consistent assessment measures. Earlier estimates ranged from 40 to 82% among adolescents in psychiatric inpatient settings (Darche, 1990; DiClemente et al., 1991) and stated that ~4% of the general population have a history of NSSI (Briere and Gil, 1998). Most recently researchers noticed that self-injurious behavior is more prevalent even among adolescents and young adults. The first attempt to describe this behavior can be seen in the book *"Man against himself"* by Menninger (1938), in which the author defined self-injurious behavior as a sort of "partial suicide." There has been an absence of generally agreed upon terminology and, over the years, several different terms to define self-injurious behaviors have appeared in literature: syndrome of delicate self-cutting (Pao, 1969), deliberate self-harm (Pattison and Kahan, 1983), self-wounding (Tantam and Whittaker, 1992), moderate self-mutilation (Favazza and Rosenthal, 1993), self-mutilation (Ross and Heath, 2002); some of which include suicidal behaviors, risk taking, and an indirect form of self-harm (Favazza, 1996). The lack of consensus regarding terminology and definition has made the understanding of such behaviors very difficult. Self-injury is a common but—as yet—poorly understood phenomenon (Klonsky and Muehlenkamp, 2007).

Self-injury has long been linked to other disorders as well, including post-traumatic stress disorder (Briere and Gil, 1998; Bolognini et al., 2003), depressive disorders (Darche, 1990), obsessive-compulsive disorder (Bolognini et al., 2003), anxiety disorder (Darche, 1990; Simeon and Favazza, 2001), borderline personality disorder (BPD) (Klonsky et al., 2003; Nock et al., 2006), and eating disorder (Iannaccone et al., 2013). Many researchers and clinicians have argued for the adoption of a NSSI disorder: some of the earliest attempts to define such a syndrome being made by Graff and Mallin (1967); Pao (1969), and Rosenthal et al. (1972). Those first attempted failed (Favazza and Rosenthal, 1990) due to the inclusion of suicide attempts in the definitions. Kahan and Pattison (1984) differentiated self-harming behaviors from suicide and proposed a separate diagnostic disorder: the deliberate self-harm syndrome (DSH). Later, Favazza and Rosenthal (1990) suggested that habitual and repetitive self-injurious behavior could be considered as an impulse control disorder: the repetitive self-mutilation syndrome. Muehlenkamp (2005) also proposed that repetitive NSSI should be regarded as a separate diagnostic disorder. More recently, Wilkinson and Goodyer (2011) proposed that giving NSSI its own diagnostic category would improve communication and increase research on etiology, its treatment and outcome. There have been many arguments over NSSI, but given the high prevalence of self-injurious behaviors among clinical and community samples of adolescents (Muehlenkamp et al., 2012; Swannell et al., 2014), and associated clinical and functional impairment, the Childhood and Mood Disorders work-group of the DSM-5 proposed the inclusion of NSSI as a separate diagnostic disorder (Shaffer and Jacobson, 2009). Despite its criteria undergoing several revisions, due to a lack of research on the full set proposed criteria, inadequate sample size and unacceptably low inter-rater reliability results in the DSM-5 field trials (Regier et al., 2013), the NSSI disorder (NSSID) was only included as a condition requiring further study, in section 3 of DSM-5, and it represents an important step forward in recognizing NSSI as a disorder in its own right (Selby et al., 2015) and in promoting further research. Given the contrasts and conflicting data present in literature on NSSI, the aim of the present study is to systematize this broad field of research, focusing on (1) proposed diagnostic criteria for the DSM-5, (2) epidemiology, (3) comorbidity, (4) etiology, and (5) functions.

MATERIALS AND METHODS

Data Source and Search Strategy

The present study followed the Preferred Reporting Items for Systematic Reviews and Meta-Analysis (PRISMA, Liberati et al., 2009). PubMed and PsycARTICLES databases were searched for eligible studies published in English between 1998 and 2016. The following combinations of search terms were employed: 1. *self-harm* OR, *self-injury* OR, *nonsuicidal self-injury* OR, *NSSI*, 2. epidemiology, 3. comorbidity, 4. gender, 5. Functions, 6. DSM. Additionally, we also examined the references of the articles identified in the search.

Study Selection

Figure 1 shows the selection of included studies. In total, the initial database search yielded 12340 abstract, of which 6356 duplicate were removed. Articles were first screened by title and abstract by two independent reviewers. Of the remaining studies, the full text was obtained and inspected independently by the same two authors to ensure that the inclusion/exclusion criteria were met.

Inclusion/Exclusion Criteria

To be included in this review, studies had to: (a) be published between 1998 and 2016, (b) reported empirical data, (c) provide a definition of self-injury and of their method of assessment, (d) not focus on treatment for NSSI, (e) be published in the English language. There were no restrictions on participant.

Reason for exclusion were: (a) samples could be not categorized as universal, (b) studies were based on the same results already found in another publication, (c) the full text was not available.

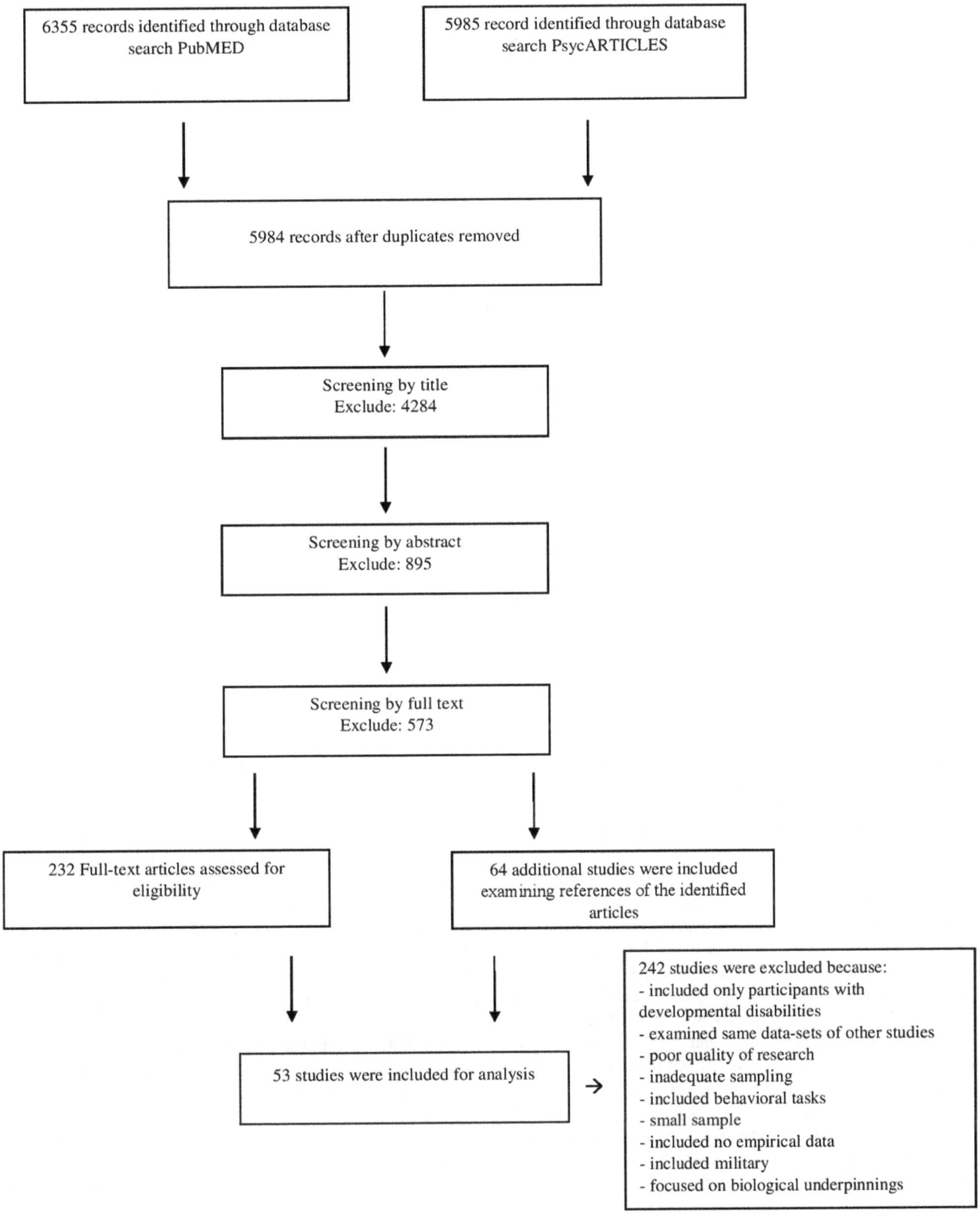

FIGURE 1 | PRISMA flow diagram of study selection.

RESULTS

We identified 53 studies that met the inclusion criteria for this review. **Table 1** provide a summary of the data obtained from each study.

Diagnostic Criteria

Recent research on NSSI disorder (American Psychiatric Association, 2013) found that a high percentage of those who self-injure met the DSM-5 proposed criteria (Glenn and Klonsky, 2013; Washburn et al., 2015). In a community sample of 3,097 Swedish adolescents, Zetterqvist et al. (2013) found that 6.7% met the criteria, whereas in a sample of adolescent impatients prevalence was 50% (Glenn and Klonsky, 2013). Empirical data on a potential NSSI disorder have collected among clinical and community samples of adolescents and adults, using different version of proposed criteria (Shaffer and Jacobson, 2009; American Psychiatric Association, 2012, 2013). In a combination samples of inpatient and intensive outpatient subjects 85.5% met Criterion A (Washburn et al., 2015). Two hundred and five of adolescents reported frequent and multiple forms of NSSI (Zetterqvist et al., 2013). For Criterion B, high endorsement was found in clinical sample of adolescents and adults (In-Albon et al., 2013; Zetterqvist et al., 2013; Washburn et al., 2015), as well as in general adult samples (Andover, 2014; Gratz et al., 2015). Almost all of adolescents (99.5%) who fulfilled criteria for NSSI disorder reported engaging NSSI to relieve both intrapersonal and interpersonal difficulties (Zetterqvist et al., 2013), likewise most patients engaged in NSSI with the expectation to lead relief from either a negative feeling or cognitive state (82.0%) or resolution of an interpersonal problem (57.1%) (Washburn et al., 2015). Automatic functions are reported significantly more often than social functions, in adolescents and adults (Zetterqvist et al., 2013; Andover, 2014). In Washburn et al. (2015), it was also rare to meet Criterion B without also meeting Criterion C: C1 (American Psychiatric Association, 2013) was the most commonly endorsed symptom, but patients also reported high endorsement (62.4%) for all three symptoms.

Clinicians and expert NSSI researchers described experiencing negative feeling or through prior to the NSSI behavior as a prototypic symptom, following by preoccupation and urge to engage with a less agreement (Lengel and Mullins-Sweatt, 2013). Criterion D—behavior act for purposes not socially sanctioned—had an agreement of 88% as being relevant characteristic to the disorder (Lengel and Mullins-Sweatt, 2013). The presence of clinically significant distress or impairment (Criterion E) is considered difficult to assess, NSSI behavior would lead relief rather than impairing. NSSID group reported more distress and impairment in functioning than non-NSSID group (Zetterqvist et al., 2013; Andover, 2014; Gratz et al., 2015). Several studies have assessed Criterion F using indirect methods (e.g., In-Albon et al., 2013; Andover, 2014).

Epidemiology

Prevalence rates of NSSI in adolescents fall between 7.5 and 46.5%, rising to 38.9% among university students and 4–23% among adults (Briere and Gil, 1998; Gratz et al., 2002; Whitlock et al., 2006; Lloyd-Richardson et al., 2007; Hilt et al., 2008a; Plener et al., 2009; Cerutti et al., 2012; Andover, 2014). Although self-injurious behavior is a widespread phenomenon, data vary considerably across samples. The age onset of NSSI most often occurs in early adolescence, between 12 and 14 years (Nock et al., 2006; Muehlenkamp and Gutierrez, 2007; Cerutti et al., 2011), but findings have also reported NSSI behavior in children under the age of 12 (Barrocas et al., 2012). The most common method was self-cutting (over 70%) followed by head banging, scratching, hitting and burning (Briere and Gil, 1998; Laye-Gindhu and Schonert-Reichl, 2005; Gratz, 2006; Whitlock et al., 2006). However, most individuals who engage in NSSI employ more than one method (e.g., Whitlock et al., 2011) acting on the arms, legs, wrists and stomach (Whitlock et al., 2006; Lloyd-Richardson et al., 2007; Klonsky, 2011; Sornberger et al., 2012). The results from some studies suggested that women displayed more NSSI behaviors than males, in both clinical and non-clinical samples (Ross and Heath, 2002; Laye-Gindhu and Schonert-Reichl, 2005; Whitlock et al., 2006, 2011; Claes et al., 2007; Muehlenkamp and Gutierrez, 2007; Yates et al., 2008; Plener et al., 2009; Sornberger et al., 2012; Muehlenkamp et al., 2013). A meta-analysis by Bresin and Schoenleber (2015) demonstrated that women are slightly more likely than men to engage in NSSI.

Differences concern also the type of method chosen: self-cutting is most common among women, that were more likely than men to engage in methods of NSSI that generally involve blood (Sornberger et al., 2012), whereas hitting, burning and banging are most common among men (Laye-Gindhu and Schonert-Reichl, 2005; Claes et al., 2007). On the other hand, equal rates of NSSI between the genders have been reported within samples of adolescents, college students, and adults (Briere and Gil, 1998; Nock et al., 2006; Lloyd-Richardson et al., 2007; Hilt et al., 2008a; Cerutti et al., 2011, 2012; Kirchner et al., 2011; Kaess et al., 2013), as well as clinical samples of adults (Briere and Gil, 1998). Although no race differences were noted in NSSI rate among adolescents and university samples (Gratz et al., 2002; Hilt et al., 2008a), data on ethnic/minority groups are scarce. Within ethnically diverse sample, multiracial college students reported high prevalence rates (20.8%), followed by Caucasian (16.8) and Hispanic (17%) (Kuentzel et al., 2012). However, research on non-Caucasian subjects was limited to few countries. Among Chinese students prevalence rates of NSSI ranged 24.9–29.2% (Wan et al., 2015; Tang et al., 2016), likewise Zoroglu et al. (2003) reported that 21.4% of Turkish adolescents engage NSSI.

NSSI and Other Disorders

According to research literature, NSSI is often associated with several maladaptive outcomes. Most notably, there is an association between NSSI and the diagnosis of BPD (Briere and Gil, 1998; Nock et al., 2006; Glenn and Klonsky, 2013; Gratz et al., 2015). Although listed as a diagnostic criterion for BPD (DSM-5, American Psychiatric Association, 2013), NSSI may also occur in individuals who do not receive BPD diagnosis, and not every individual who receives BPD diagnosis engages in self-harm behaviors (e.g., In-Albon et al., 2013). Differences between NSSI-group and BPD-group would suggest to define NSSI as syndrome in its own right (Selby et al., 2012; Turner et al., 2015). Even

TABLE 1 | Study characteristics.

References	Sample	Sample size (female %)	Mean age	Assessing tools	Prevalence	Endorsed criteria (%)
DIAGNOSTIC CRITERIA						
Andover, 2014	Community	548 (46.5)	35.70 (*SD* = 12.23)	FASM–Self report questionnaire developed on DSM-5 proposed criteria	23[c]	A: 20.8 B1: 60.8 B2: 8.8 B3: 26 C1: 82.4 C2: 37.6 C3: 19.4 E: Distress 8.08–Impairment 60.8
Barrocas et al., 2012	School	665 (55)	11.6 (*SD* = 2.4)	SITBI–FASM	8% (1.5% NSSI disorder)[a]	A: 1.5 B4: 1.5 C: 1.5
Glenn and Klonsky, 2013	Psychiatric inpatient and partial hospitalization	198 (74)	15.13 (*SD* = 1.38)	ISAS	50% (78% of the self-injuring sample)[a]	A: 50 B1: 98
Gratz et al., 2015	Community	107 (80)	23.86 (*SD* = 4.87)	CANDI	37[c]	A: 77 B: 79 C: 81 D: 91 E: 41 F: 80
In-Albon et al., 2013	Psychiatric Inpatient	73 (100)	13–18 years	DSM-5 criteria reformulated as questions in a clinical interview	56.2[b]	A: 20.8 B1: 97.4 B2: 46.2 B3: 89.7 B4: 87.2 C: Distress 100–Impairment 69.2
Washburn et al., 2015	Clinical inpatients, partial hospitalization and intensive outpatients	511 (90)	17.3 (*SD* = 6.2)	ABASI	74[c]	A: 85.5 B1: 82 B2: 57.1 B3: 34.8 C1:91.3 C2: 72.8 C3: 71.6 E: 98.2 F: 98.2
Zetterqvist et al., 2013	Community students	3,060 (48.8)	15–17 years	FASM SITBI-SF-SR	6.7% (18.8% of NSSI sample)[b]	A: 85.5 B1: 98.5 B2: 73.2 B3: 37.3 B4: 99.5 C: Distress 76.8–Impairment 92.2

References	Sample	Sample size (female%)	Mean age	Assessing tools	Prevalence (%)	Country
EPIDEMIOLOGY						
Andover, 2014	Community	548 (46.5)	35.70 (*SD* = 12.23)	FASM–Self report questionnaire developed on DSM-5 proposed criteria	23[c]	USA
Barrocas et al., 2012	School	665 (55)	11.6 (*SD* = 2.4)	SITBI–FASM	8 (1.5 NSSI disorder)[a]	USA
Briere and Gil, 1998	Community Clinical Self-mutilative	927 (50) 390 (52) 93 (96)	46 (*SD* = 17) 36 (*SD* = 10) 35 (*SD* = 9)	Self-administered questionnaire	4.0 21.0 100	USA

(Continued)

TABLE 1 | Continued

References	Sample	Sample size (female %)	Mean age	Assessing tools	Prevalence (%)	Country
Cerutti et al., 2011	School	234 (49.1)	16.47 (*SD* = 1.7)	DSHI–Italian Version	41.9	Italy
Cerutti et al., 2012	College	365 (62.79)	23.34 (*SD* = 4.06)	DSHI	38.9	Italy
Claes et al., 2007	Psychiatric inpatients	399 (66.4)	30.8 (*SD* = 12.2)	SIQ SHI	41.04	Belgium
Gratz et al., 2002	College	133 (67)	22.73 (SD = 6.17)	DSHI	38	USA
Gratz, 2006	College	249 (100)	23.29 (*SD* = 5.96)	DSHI	37	USA
Hilt et al., 2008a	School	508 (51)	–*	Self-report Questionnaire	7.5	USA
Kaess et al., 2013	Psychiatric inpatients	125 (50.4)	17.1 (*SD* = 3.1)	FASM	60	Germany
Kirchner et al., 2011	School	1171 (55.8)	3.96 (*SD* =1.32)	YSR Spanish version	11.4	Spain
Klonsky, 2011	Community	439 (61)	55.5 (*SD* = 16.6)	Structured interview	5.9	USA (Exclude Alaska and Hawaii)
Kuentzel et al., 2012	College	5,680 (70.12)	22.2 (*SD* = 6.35)	Self-report questionnaire	12.8	USA
Laye-Gindhu and Schonert-Reichl, 2005	Community	424 (55.6)	15.34 (*SD* = 1.06)	Self-Harm questionnaire	15	Canada
Lloyd-Richardson et al., 2007	Community	633 (57)	15.5 (*SD* = 1.18)	FASM	46.5	USA
Muehlenkamp and Gutierrez, 2007	School	540 (62.3)	15.53 (*SD* = 1.42)	SHBQ	23.2	USA
Muehlenkamp et al., 2013	College	1,243 (59.8)	21.52 (*SD* = 4.15)	NSSI-AT	14.72	USA
Nock et al., 2006	Psychiatric inpatients	89 (74.15)	14.7 (*SD* = 1.4)	FASM	100	USA
Plener et al., 2009	School	665 (57.1)	14.8 (*SD* = 0.66)	SHBQ–OSI	26	Germany
Ross and Heath, 2002	School	440 (50.2)	–*	Semi structured Interview	14.8	Canada
Sornberger et al., 2012	School	7,126 (50.8)	14.92 (*SD* = 1.61)	Self-administered questionnaire	24.5	USA
Whitlock et al., 2006	College	2,875 (56.3)	18–24 years	Self-report questionnaire	17	USA
Whitlock et al., 2011	College	11,529 (57.6)	Under 25 years	Self-report questionnaire	15.3	USA
Yates et al., 2008	Community	155 (51.61)	26 years	SIBQ	16.8	USA
Zoroglu et al., 2003	School	839 (61.1)	15.9 (*SD* = 1.8)	Self-report questionnaire	21.4	Turkey

References	Sample	Sample size (female %)	Mean age	Assessing tools	Prevalence (%)	Comorbidity
NSSI AND OTHER DISORDERS						
Briere and Gil, 1998	Community Clinical Self-mutilative	927 (50) 390 (52) 93 (96)	46 (*SD* = 17) 36 (*SD* = 10) 35 (*SD* = 9)	Self-administered questionnaire	4.0 21.0 100	Post-traumatic stress disorder, unspecified dissociative disorder, borderline personality disorder and dissociative identity disorder, dissociation and depression

(Continued)

TABLE 1 | Continued

References	Sample	Sample size (female %)	Mean age	Assessing tools	Prevalence (%)	Comorbidity
Cerutti et al., 2012	College	365 (62.79)	23.34 (*SD* = 4.06)	DSHI	38.9	Dissociation, depersonalization, and borderline personality symptoms
Claes et al., 2001	Psychiatric inpatients	134 (100)	Mean age	SIQ	44.6	Eating disorders, anxiety disorder and depression
Claes et al., 2007	Psychiatric inpatients	399 (66.4)	30.8 (*SD* = 12.2)	SIQ SHI	41.04	Personality disorders, depressive disorder, and obsessive-compulsive disorder
Eichen et al., 2016	College	508 (100)	20.61 (*SD* = 1.97)	FASM	13.8	Eating disorders, depressive disorder, anxiety disorder and difficulties with emotion regulation
Giletta et al., 2012	School	1,862 (49)	15.69 (*SD* = 0.87)	Self-report questionnaire	24	Depressive symptoms and substance use
Glenn and Klonsky, 2013	Psychiatric inpatient and partial hospitalization	198 (74)	15.13 (*SD* = 1.38)	ISAS	50% (78% of the self-injuring sample)[a]	Alcohol/substance use disorder, anxiety disorder, mood disorder, ADHD/disruptive behavior disorder, bulimia, borderline personality disorder and emotion dysregulation
Gratz et al., 2015	Community	107 (80)	23.86 (*SD* = 4.87)	CANDI	37[c]	Emotion dysregulation, borderline personality disorder, mood disorder, anxiety disorder, substance use disorder.
Hilt et al., 2008a	School	508 (51)	–*	Self-report Questionnaire	7.5	Maladaptive eating Habits and substance use
Iannaccone et al., 2013	Psychiatric inpatients and outpatients	65 (100)	27.46 (*SD* = 8.29)	Self-report questionnaire	50.9	Eating disorders, impulsivity, anxiety and depression
In-Albon et al., 2013	Psychiatric Inpatient	73 (100)	13–18 years	DSM-5 criteria reformulated as questions in a clinical interview	56.2[b]	Mood disorders, post-traumatic stress disorder, borderline personality disorder, anxiety disorders, oppositional deviant disorder, and bulimia nervosa
Jenkins et al., 2015	Clinical and control group	1,097 (53.6)	35.1 (*SD* = 10.3)	DSHI	18	Intermittent explosive disorder, personality disorders, mood and anxiety disorders, eating disorders, substance use disorder
Muehlenkamp and Gutierrez, 2007	School	540 (62.3)	15.53 (*SD* = 1.42)	SHBQ	23.2	Depressive symptoms
Nock et al., 2006	Psychiatric inpatients	89 (74.15)	14.7 (*SD* = 1.4)	FASM	100	Major depressive disorder, post-traumatic stress disorder, anxiety disorder, conduct and oppositional defiant disorder, substance abuse disorders and personality disorders (borderline, avoidant and paranoid personality disorders were most common)
Plener et al., 2009	School	665 (57.1)	14.8 years (*SD* = 0.66)	SHBQ–OSI	26	Depressive symptoms
Ross and Heath, 2002	School	440 (50.2)	–*	Semi structured Interview	14.8	Anxiety and depressive symptomatology
Selby et al., 2012	Clinical outpatients	571 (53)	Adults	Chart data	11.4[a]	Mood disorders, anxiety disorder, and Cluster A personality disorders
Turner et al., 2015	NSSI sample	100 (90)	31.57 (*SD* = 10.13)	DSHI	100	Mood and anxiety disorders, substance use disorders, eating disorders, psychotic disorders, and personality disorders.

(Continued)

TABLE 1 | Continued

References	Sample	Sample size (female %)	Type of sample	Assessing tools	Prevalence (%)	Key findings
ETIOLOGY						
Arens et al., 2012	College	407 (65)	20.33 (*SD* = 1.39)	DSHI	20	Childhood maltreatment
Auerbach et al., 2014	Clinical	194 (74.22)	15.53 (*SD* = 1.34)	SITBI	80.92	Child abuse
Briere and Gil, 1998	Community Clinical Self-mutilative	927 (50) 390 (52) 93 (96)	46 (*SD* = 17) 36 (*SD* = 10) 35 (*SD* = 9)	Self-administered questionnaire	4.0 21.0 100	Childhood trauma
Cerutti et al., 2011	School	234 (49.1)	16.47 (*SD* = 1.7)	DSHI–Italian Version	41.9	Dissociation and stress full life events
Goldstein et al., 2009	College	319 (65)	18.89 (*SD* = 2.30)	Self-report questionnaire	29.5	Depressive symptoms, physical abuse, emotional abuse, openness, sensation seeking and substance use
Gratz et al., 2002	College	133 (67)	22.73 (*SD* = 6.17)	DSHI	38	Dissociation, insecure paternal attachment, parental emotional neglect, childhood sexual abuse and childhood separation
Gratz, 2006	College	249 (100)	23.29 (*SD* = 5.96)	DSHI	37	Childhood maltreatment, low positive affect intensity/reactivity and emotional inexpressivity
Gratz and Chapman, 2007	College	97 (0)	22.67 (*SD* = 5.00)	DSHI	44	Physical abuse and emotion dysregulation
Jacobson et al., 2015	College	427 (73.3)	20.5 (*SD* = 4.5)	FASM	6	Emotional expressiveness
Kaess et al., 2013	Psychiatric inpatients	125 (50.4)	17.1 (*SD* = 3.1)	FASM	60	Adverse childhood experiences
Paivio and McCulloch, 2004	College	100 (100)	21 (*SD* = 1.66)	SIBQ	41	Child maltreatment
Tang et al., 2016	School	4,405 (49.67)	14.7 (*SD* = 1.9)	FASM	29.2	Stress full life events
Wan et al., 2015	School	14,211 (52.8)	5.1 (*SD* = 1.9)	FASM	24.9	Childhood abuse
Whitlock et al., 2006	College	2,875 (56.3)	18–24 years	Self-report questionnaire	17	Emotional, physical and sexual abuse
Yates et al., 2008	Community	155 (51.61)	26	SIBQ	16.8	Child sexual and physical abuse
Zoroglu et al., 2003	School	839 (61.1)	15.9 (*SD* = 1.8)	Self-report questionnaire	21.4	Physical, emotional and sexual abuse, neglect and dissociation

References	Sample	Sample size (female %)	Mean age	Assessing tools	Prevalence	Functions
FUNCTIONS						
Andover, 2014	Community	548 (46.5)	35.70 (*SD* = 12.23)	FASM–Self report questionnaire developed on DSM-5 proposed criteria	23[c]	Automatic positive, automatic negative, social negative and social positive
Calvete et al., 2015	School	1,864 (51.45)	15.3 (*SD* = 1.97)	FASM	55.6	Automatic positive, automatic negative, social negative and social positive
Claes et al., 2007	Psychiatric inpatients	399 (66.4)	30.8 (*SD* = 12.2)	SIQ SHI	41.04	Automatic and social
Giletta et al., 2012	School	1862 (49)	15.69 (*SD* = 0.87)	Self-report questionnaire	24	Internal and interpersonal
Glenn and Klonsky, 2013	Psychiatric inpatient and partial hospitalization	198 (74)	15.13 (*SD* = 1.38)	ISAS	50%[a] (78% of the self-injuring sample)	Affect regulation, marking distress, self-punishment and anti-dissociation

(Continued)

TABLE 1 | Continued

References	Sample	Sample size (female %)	Mean age	Assessing tools	Prevalence	Functions
Hilt et al., 2008b	Community	94 (100)	10–15 years	FASM	56.4	Automatic positive, automatic negative, social negative and social positive
Kaess et al., 2013	Psychiatric inpatients	125 (50.4)	17.1 (*SD* = 3.1)	FASM	60	Automatic, interpersonal and peer identification
Klonsky, 2011	Community	439 (61)	55.5 (*SD* = 16.6)	Structured interview	5.9	Affect regulation, self-punishment and interpersonal
Laye-Gindhu and Schonert-Reichl, 2005	Community	424 (55.6)	15.34 (*SD* = 1.06)	Self-Harm questionnaire	15	Affect regulation, self-punishment, distraction from problems, communicate with or influence others
Lloyd-Richardson et al., 2007	Community	633 (57)	15.5 years (*SD* = 1.18)	FASM	46.5	Automatic positive, automatic negative, social negative and social positive
Muehlenkamp et al., 2013	College	1,243 (59.8)	21.52 (*SD* = 4.15)	NSSI-AT	14.72	Emotional regulation and social
Nock and Prinstein, 2004	Psychiatric Inpatients	108 (70.37)	14.8 (*SD* = 1.4)	FASM	82.4	Automatic positive, automatic negative, social negative and social positive
Turner et al., 2012	NSSI sample	162 (100)	22.47 years (*SD* = 7.14)	QNSII–SASII	100	Emotion relief, feeling generation, self-punishment-, interpersonal communication, interpersonal influence
Turner et al., 2016	NSSI sample	60 (85)	23.25 (*SD* = 4.25)	DSHI	100	Affect regulation and interpersonal
Zetterqvist et al., 2013	Community students	3,060 (48.8)	15–17 years	FASM SITBI-SF-SR	6.7% (18.8% of NSSI sample)[b]	Automatic positive, automatic negative, social negative and social positive

Study by Lengel and Mullins-Sweatt (2013), on expert ratings, and meta-analysis by Bresin and Schoenleber were not included NSSI criteria used.
[a] *Shaffer and Jacobson (2009).*
[b] *American Psychiatric Association (2012).*
[c] *DSM-5 (American Psychiatric Association, 2013).*
**Data not reported. Alexian Brothers Assessment of Self-Injury (ABASI); Clinician-Administered Nonsuicidal Self-Injury Disorder Index (CANDI); Deliberate Self Harm Inventory (DSHI); Inventory of Statements About Self-Injury (ISAS); Functional Assessment of Self-Mutilation (FASM); Nonsuicidal Self-Injury-Assessment Tool (NSSI-AT); Ottawa Self-Injury Inventory (OSI); Questionnaire for Nonsuicidal Self-Injury (QNSSI); Self-Harm Behavior Questionnaire (SHBQ); Self-Injurious Behavior Questionnaire (SIBQ); Self-Injurious Thoughts and Behaviors Interview-Short Form-Self-Report (SITBI-SF-SR); Self-Injurious Thoughts and Behaviors Interview (SITBI); Self-Injury Questionnaire (SIQ); Self-Harm Inventory (SHI); Suicidal Attempt Self-Injury Interview (SASII); Youth Self Report (YSR).*

though NSSI and suicidal behavior are distinct, suicide attempts and suicide ideation were found in both clinical and non-clinical samples of adolescents (Nock et al., 2006; Plener et al., 2009).

Exploring the association between NSSI and psychiatric diagnoses, several researchers have reported self-injurious behavior in a wide range of other disorders, such as post-traumatic stress disorder (PTSD), dissociative disorder, conduct disorder, obsessive-compulsive disorder, intermittent explosive disorder, anxiety and mood disorder, substance use disorder, bulimia, and dissociative identity disorder (Briere and Gil, 1998; Nock et al., 2006; Claes et al., 2007; Selby et al., 2012; Glenn and Klonsky, 2013; In-Albon et al., 2013; Gratz et al., 2015; Jenkins et al., 2015; Turner et al., 2015). Furthermore, in a study on DSH behavior among young Italian adults, individuals with a history of DSH, compared with individuals with no history of DSH, reported higher levels of dissociations and depersonalization (Cerutti et al., 2012). In addition, a relationship between NSSI and eating disorders often appears (Claes et al., 2001; Iannaccone et al., 2013; Eichen et al., 2016), although not all researchers confirm such an association (Selby et al., 2012). Cerutti et al. (2012) found that adults with NSSI history reported negative attitudes toward the body and lower levels of body protection. In both clinical and non-clinical samples, those who self-injury were more likely to report depressive symptomatology and anxiety (Ross and Heath, 2002; Muehlenkamp and Gutierrez, 2007; Giletta et al., 2012; Selby et al., 2012). Moreover, results provided significantly higher rates of both internalizing (Nock et al., 2006; Glenn and Klonsky, 2013; In-Albon et al., 2013) and externalizing disorders (Nock et al., 2006). Adolescents who engage in NSSI were more likely to present several health-risk behaviors, such as substance abuse, risky sexual behaviors, and maladaptive eating habits (Hilt et al., 2008a; Giletta et al., 2012). In a study that assess potential NSSI disorder (Gratz et al., 2015) participants who met the proposed criteria for NSSID (DSM-5, American Psychiatric Association, 2013) differed from NSSI-group and reported significantly more depression, anxiety and stress symptoms, and BPD disorder.

Etiology

The potential etiologic factors of NSSI may be divided into two major categories: individual (e.g., emotional dysregulation, psychiatric disorders) and environmental (e.g., childhood maltreatments, attachment disruption). Most research focused on early childhood traumatic experiences found that childhood maltreatments emerged as a predictor of NSSI within adolescents and college students (Paivio and McCulloch, 2004; Gratz, 2006; Arens et al., 2012; Auerbach et al., 2014; Wan et al., 2015). Exploration of environmental contributors revealed that childhood sexual abuse would present a strong link with NSSI development (Briere and Gil, 1998; Gratz et al., 2002; Gratz, 2006; Gratz and Chapman, 2007; Yates et al., 2008; Auerbach et al., 2014). However, other researchers have not found a strong association with sexual abuse (Zoroglu et al., 2003; Whitlock et al., 2006; Goldstein et al., 2009). In their study among college female students, Gratz (2006) found that both environmental and individual factors were strongly associated with NSSI, as well their interaction. Gratz et al. (2002) emphasized the role of parental relationship in the etiology of self-injurious behaviors: insecure paternal attachment and both maternal and paternal emotional neglect were significant predictors of NSSI within women, whereas NSSI in men was primarily predicted by childhood separation (usually from father). Furthermore, maternal rejection appeared the only significant predictor among psychiatric inpatients sample (Kaess et al., 2013).

Most recent studies have investigated the role of stress-full life events in the etiology of NSSI (Cerutti et al., 2011; Tang et al., 2016). Among Chinese adolescents, Tang et al. (2016) found that adverse life experiences were associated with moderate and severe NSSI and a lesser risk of engaging NSSI in those who had a good emotional regulation. Examining individual factors, results reported that NSSI frequency was strongly predicted by emotion dysregulation and affect intensity/reactivity within men (Gratz and Chapman, 2007), and by emotional inexpressivity within women (Gratz, 2006). Low emotional expressiveness would have a role in engagement in NSSI (Jacobson et al., 2015). Results of a regression analysis showed that difficulties to identify and express emotional experience appropriately (i.e., alexithymia) mediated the relation between childhood trauma (except sexual abuse) and NSSI (Paivio and McCulloch, 2004).

Functions

Engage in NSSI may serves several functions that are not mutually exclusive (Nock and Prinstein, 2004; Klonsky, 2011). The most common function seems to be the affect regulation (Nock and Prinstein, 2004; Laye-Gindhu and Schonert-Reichl, 2005; Claes et al., 2007; Muehlenkamp et al., 2013). Indeed, negative emotions, such as anger, anxiety, depression, and loneliness, tend to occur before the NSSI behavior, whereas an increase in positive emotions and a decrease in negative emotions would follow as well (e.g., Laye-Gindhu and Schonert-Reichl, 2005; Claes et al., 2007). Moreover, Giletta et al. (2012) found that engaging NSSI were strongly associated with depressive feelings among Italian, USA and Dutch samples. NSSI may represent a strategy for affect regulation (Laye-Gindhu and Schonert-Reichl, 2005). Nock and Prinstein (2004) proposed a functional model of NSSI, known as the Four Factor Model (FFM). FFM is grounded on behavioral theory, which focus on the antecedent and consequent influences that produce and maintain the behavior.

The FFM delineates two dichotomous dimensions of functional processes: contingencies interpersonal/social vs. intrapersonal/automatic, and reinforcement positive vs. negative. The four processes proposed by the model include: automatic negative reinforcement when NSSI serves to reduce aversive internal states, automatic positive reinforcement, when NSSI serves to generate positive feelings, social negative reinforcement, when NSSI serves to avoid interpersonal demands, and social positive reinforcement, when NSSI serves to gain attention, or increase social support (Nock and Prinstein, 2004). Much of the studies on the psychological reasons underlying the NSSI behavior has mainly focused on emotion regulation and tension reduction, but social functions of NSSI have also been described in both adolescents (Nock and Prinstein, 2004; Lloyd-Richardson et al., 2007; Hilt et al., 2008a,b; Turner et al., 2012; Muehlenkamp et al., 2013; Zetterqvist et al., 2013) and adults samples (Turner et al., 2012, 2016). Engaging NSSI "to stop bad feelings" was endorsed by 56.8% of German inpatients sample, in which automatic functions were predicted by adverse childhood experiences (Kaess et al., 2013). Self-punishment function was commonly endorsed by adolescents and adult among community and clinic samples (Briere and Gil, 1998; Laye-Gindhu and Schonert-Reichl, 2005; Lloyd-Richardson et al., 2007; Turner et al., 2012; Glenn and Klonsky, 2013; Kaess et al., 2013). Although males were more likely to engage NSSI for social reasons (Claes et al., 2007) and females to relieve negative emotional states and self-punishment (Briere and Gil, 1998; Glenn and Klonsky, 2013), no significant gender differences emerged about NSSI functions among adolescents samples (e.g., Lloyd-Richardson et al., 2007; Calvete et al., 2015). Zetterqvist et al. (2013) found that about 90% of adolescents those met proposed criteria for NSSI disorder most commonly reported automatic negative functions, followed by automatic positive ones, and about 27% reported social functions. Greater endorsement of intrapersonal functions than social was also found among adult with NSSI Disorder (Andover, 2014).

DISCUSSION

The purpose of this study was to review the existing literature on NSSI by providing a preliminary understanding of the main features. There is general consensus that NSSI begins in early adolescence, with a main age onset of 12 years old. Even though only few studies have investigated NSSI within children younger than 12 years old (Kirchner et al., 2011; Barrocas et al., 2012; Sornberger et al., 2012). Prevalence is even high among adult, mostly in samples of university students. Studies have demonstrated a high variability on prevalence rates. Some of this variability may partially explain by a growing interest in NSSI behavior. Nevertheless, the assessment methods chosen appears to heavily influence the estimates of prevalence: checklists would seem to provide higher estimates than single item questions (Muehlenkamp et al., 2012).

In order to overcome the mentioned assessment bias, future research will have to accurately investigate perceptions and interpretations of participants which may not reflect NSSI definition provided. NSSI is generally assumed to be more common among females than men. This assumption is not fully supported by existing literature. Self-injury is popularly associated with "cutting" and this could have influenced data, as females are more likely to self-cut than men. Literature has primarily focused on women samples and higher prevalence on NSSI among females could be due to an over representation of women (Claes et al., 2007). Data on non-Caucasian samples are scarce, but it may be due to an ethnocentric bias that tend to underestimate the culture impact on NSSI. Indeed, similar rates of prevalence among female adolescent and methods used, in Chinese samples, could be consider a reflection of Western culture's influence, and NSSI in minorities group, such as Native Americans (e.g., Kuentzel et al., 2012), could be related to culturally sanctioned rituals (ceremonial or religious). Due to paucity of studies on racial/ethnic differences in NSSI, its distribution and prevalence remain unclear.

Regarding etiology, the relation between sexual abuse and NSSI remains still contentious. Evidence suggests that additional risk factors, both environmental and individual, may play a role in the etiology of NSSI: a history of child maltreatment and stressful life experiences could represent a vulnerability that disrupt emotional regulation function. Therefore, several forms of maltreatment appear to be related to engaging NSSI in both clinical and non-clinical samples (e.g., Briere and Gil, 1998; Gratz et al., 2002; Gratz, 2006; Yates et al., 2008; Arens et al., 2012; Auerbach et al., 2014), whereas individual factors might play a role in the maintenance of the behavior (e.g., Gratz and Chapman, 2007; Jacobson et al., 2015). So, a potential interaction between risk factors should be explored. Emotional regulation was the most common reason for NSSI behavior: individuals who self-injury commonly reported negative experiences, such as depression, anxiety, and angry, before NSSI. To further support automatic function, NSSI would result in a negative emotions reduction. Although interpersonal functions have not received as much attention, both adolescents and adult endorsed social reasons to engage NSSI (e.g., Nock and Prinstein, 2004; Lloyd-Richardson et al., 2007; Hilt et al., 2008b; Zetterqvist et al., 2013). Moreover, lower prevalence of social functions could be explained by the fact that NSSI is a private act and who self-injury may be socially isolated and experience negative emotions that increase the likelihood of further acts to reduce tension state. The inclusion of a potential NSSI disorder in the DSM-5 is justified by the clinical benefits that would ensue from a better understanding of the behavior.

Empirical research on NSSI disorder has recently begun to provide relevant data. It is however limited by the use of the different methods employed in assessing NSSI, and not originally envisaged for this purpose. There are several important obstacles regarding diagnostic validity of NSSID. Firstly, delimitation from other disorders. Self-injurious behavior primarily existed in the DSM as a symptom of BPD but, although NSSI and BPD can co-occur, they also present themselves independently (In-Albon et al., 2013). Most studies, focused on NSSI disorder rather than BPD, have highlighted that NSSI is not indicative of BPD and that the diagnostic coincidence of NSSI disorder and BPD was similar to existed to a lesser degree than BPD and other disorders (Glenn and Klonsky, 2013). Moreover, the introduction of NSSI disorder recognizes the importance of differentiating NSSI from attempted suicide. Although both suicide attempts and NSSI conform to a continuum of self-harming behaviors, there are important clinically differences among behaviors in etiology, psychiatric impairment, functions, methods and course. The use of diverse criteria, different assessment methodologies and the absence of studies employing all the criteria as proposed in the DSM-5, have deterred advancement in this field.

Strengths and Limitations

The current review not only includes women engaged in self-injury but also men, and goes some way to addressing the misrepresentation present in previous literature, which could be explained by the fact that men behave differently to women in this context. This study only addresses the links between NSSI and biological roots and developmental\intellectual disabilities in part, and does not address NSSI treatment. Our review attempted to understand the main causes and functions of NSSI through studies on clinical and non-clinical populations but many aspects remain unclear, especially as regard NSSI etiology. Finally, we must consider the secretive nature of self-injury due to which prevalence rates may be seen to be ambiguous. Studies on NSSI treatment were not included.

Implications for Future Research

Despite the behavior is more likely to present in adolescence, the variation in age of onset and in prevalence rates among adolescents and adults suggest that there may be different developmental trajectories in NSSI and a lack of knowledge regarding the course of NSSI: further exploration should employ a longitudinal approach aimed at examining the risk factors and progression of a potential NSSI disorder. This implication is directly related to the need for additional research using a variety of adult group to obtain accurate prevalence rates, as data on adult samples have mostly collected in educational institutions.

Findings on gender differences provided contradictory data that could benefit from future research that also consider other variables, such as culture, school, and social contagion. More research would be helpful in understanding the course and patterns of NSSI and exploring NSSI among gender. Research should be extended to other cultures and ethnicities, in order to recognize the influence of cultural factors on these behaviors. Self-injurious behavior for culturally sanctioned purposes (e.g., religious ritual, tattoos and piercings) was not considered in the research field nor included among the proposed diagnostic criteria for NSSID in the DSM-5. The contextualization of behavior is required, as is an exploration of the similarities and differences in prevalence rates, methods and functions across cultures. Although findings suggest the role of abuse, neglect and disruption in attachment in the potential development of NSSI behavior, future research could explore other characteristics of maltreatment experiences, such as frequency, perpetrator, bond type between child, and abuser, and cumulative effects.

There may be several reasons for engaging in NSSI and future research should investigate the mechanism underlying NSSI, the role of gender differences and whether functions change during development in order to a more complete understanding of the behavior. Moreover, there are still several areas that require further investigation to give credence to NSSI as a disorder in its own right: it would be pertinent to provide a valid, clinical delineation of the disorder and develop a standardized tool for its assessment in order to improve research, to conduct longitudinal studies and cross-cultural and ethnic studies, but there is still further work to be done.

CONCLUSIONS

NSSI is a common phenomenon among adolescents and adults, associated with significant impairment. Over the years, interest in NSSI grew to such an extent that an ongoing debate was instigated on whether NSSI should be considered as a diagnosis in its own right and given its own category. As a result, it was included in section 3 of the DSM-5 as a condition requiring further studies. This paper provides an up-to-date overview on self-injury, what is known about it and what remains to be done.

AUTHOR CONTRIBUTIONS

AC and SC conducted the study, AC writes the first draft of the paper, PC designed the study and supervise the procedure and the paper.

REFERENCES

1. American Psychiatric Association (2012). *Suggested Criteria for DSM-5 Non- Suicidal Self-injury Disorder*. Washington, DC: American Psychiatric Association.
2. American Psychiatric Association (2013). *Diagnostic and Statistical Manual of Mental Disorders, 5th Edition*. Washington, DC: American Psychiatric Association.
3. Andover, M. S. (2014). Non-suicidal self-injury disorder in a community sample of adults. *Psychiatry Res.* 219, 305–310. doi: 10.1016/j.psychres.2014.06.001
4. Arens, A. M., Gaher, R. M., and Simons, J. S. (2012). Child maltreatment and deliberate self-harm among college students: testing mediation and moderation models for impulsivity. *Am. J. Orthopsychiatry* 82, 328–337. doi: 10.1111/j.1939-0025.2012.01165.x
5. Auerbach, R. P., Kim, J. C., Chango, J. M., Spiro, W. J., Cha, C., Gold, J., et al. (2014). Adolescent nonsuicidal self-injury: examining the role of child abuse, comorbidity, and disinhibition. *Psychiatry Res.* 220, 579–584. doi: 10.1016/j.psychres.2014.07.027
6. Barrocas, A. L., Hankin, B. L., Young, J. L., and Abela, J. R. (2012). Rates of nonsuicidal self- injury in youth: age, sex, and behavioural methods in a community sample. *Pediatrics* 130, 39–45. doi: 10.1542/peds.2011-2094
7. Bolognini, M., Plancherel, B., Laget, J., Stephan, P., and Halfon, O. (2003). Adolescents' self-mutilation – relationship with dependent behaviour. *Swiss J. Psychol.* 62, 241–249. doi: 10.1024/1421-0185.62.4.241
8. Bresin, K., and Schoenleber, M. (2015). Gender differences in the prevalence of nonsuicidal self-injury: a meta-analysis. *Clin. Psychol. Rev.* 38, 55–64. doi: 10.1016/j.cpr.2015.02.009
9. Briere, J., and Gil, E. (1998). Self-mutilation in clinical and general population samples: prevalence, correlates, and functions. *Am. J. Orthopsychiatry* 68, 609–620. doi: 10.1037/h0080369
10. Calvete, E., Orue, I., Aizpuru, L., and Brotherton, H. (2015). Prevalence and functions of non-suicidal self-injury in Spanish adolescents. *Psychotema* 27, 223–228. doi: 10.7334/psicothema2014.262
11. Cerutti, R., Manca, M., Presaghi, F., and Gratz, K. L. (2011). Prevalence and clinical correlates of deliberate self-harm among a community sample of Italian adolescents. *J. Adolesc.* 34, 337–347. doi: 10.1016/j.adolescence.2010.04.004
12. Cerutti, R., Presaghi, F., Manca, M., and Gratz, K. L. (2012). Deliberate self-harm behavior among italian young adults: correlations with clinical and nonclinical dimensions of personality. *Am. J. Orthopsychiatry* 82, 298–308. doi: 10.1111/j.1939-0025.2012.01169
13. Claes, L., Vandereycken, W., and Vertommen, H. (2001). Self-injurious behaviors in eating-disordered patients. *Eat. Behav.* 2, 263–272. doi: 10.1016/S1471-0153(01)00033-2
14. Claes, L., Vandereycken, W., and Vertommen, H. (2007). Self-injury in female versus male psychiatric patients: a comparison of characteristics, psychopathology and aggression regulation. *Pers. Indiv. Dif.* 42, 611–621. doi: 10.1016/j.paid.2006.07.021
15. Darche, M. A. (1990). Psychological factors differentiating self-mutilating and non-self-mutilating adolescent inpatient females. *Psychiatr. Hosp.* 21, 31–35.
16. DiClemente, R. J., Ponton, L. E., and Hartley, D. (1991). Prevalence and correlates of cutting behavior: risk for HIV transmission. *J. Am. Acad. Child Adolesc. Psychiatry* 30, 735–739. doi: 10.1016/S0890-8567(10)80007-3
17. Eichen, D. M., Kass, A. E., Fitzsimmons-Craft, E. E., Gibbs, E., Trockel, M., Taylor, B., et al. (2016). Non-suicidal self-injury and suicidal ideation in relation to eating and general psychopathology among college-age women. *Psychiatr. Res.* 235, 77–82. doi: 10.1016/j.psychres.2015.11.046
18. Favazza, A. R. (1992). Repetitive self-mutilation. *Psychiatr. Ann.* 22, 60–63. doi: 10.4236/health.2010.24055
19. Favazza, A. R. (1996). *Bodies under Siege: Self-mutilation and Body Modification in Culture and Psychiatry, 2nd Edn.* Baltimore, MD: John Hopkins University Press.
20. Favazza, A. R., and Conterio, K. (1988). The plight of chronic self-mutilators. *Commun. Ment. Health J.* 24, 22–30. doi: 10.1007/BF00755050
21. Favazza, A. R., and Conterio, K. (1989). Female habitual self-mutilators. *Acta Psychiatr. Scand.* 79, 283–289. doi: 10.1111/j.1600-0447.1989.tb10259.x
22. Favazza, A. R., DeRosear, L., and Conterio, K. (1989). Self-mutilation and eating disorders. *Suicide Life Threat. Behav.* 19, 352–361.
23. Favazza, A. R., and Rosenthal, R. J. (1990). Varieties of pathological self-mutilation. *Behav. Neurol.* 3, 77–85. doi: 10.3233/BEN-1990-3202
24. Favazza, A. R., and Rosenthal, R. J. (1993). Diagnostic issue in self-mutilation. *Hosp. Commun. Psychiatry* 44, 134–139. doi: 10.1176/ps.44.2.134
25. Giletta, M., Scholte, R. H., Engels, R. C., Ciairano, S., and Prinstein, M. J. (2012). Adolescent non-suicidal self-injury: a cross-national study of community samples from Italy, the Netherlands and the United States. *Psychiatry Res.* 197, 66–72. doi: 10.1016/j.psychres.2012.02.009
26. Glenn, C. R., and Klonsky, E. D. (2013). Nonsuicidal self-injury disorder: an empirical investigation in adolescent psychiatric patients. *J. Clin. Child Adolesc. Psychol.* 42, 496–507. doi: 10.1080/15374416.2013.794699
27. Goldstein, A. L., Glett, G. L., Wekerle, C., and Wall, A. (2009). Personality, child maltreatment, and substance use: examining correlates of deliberate self-harm among university students. *Can. J. Behav. Sci.* 41, 241–251. doi: 10.1037/a0014847
28. Graff, H., and Mallin, R. (1967). The syndrome of the wrist cutter. *Am. J. Psychiatry* 124, 74–80. doi: 10.1176/ajp.124.1.36
29. Gratz, K. L. (2006). Risk factors for deliberate self-harm among female college students: the role and interaction of childhood maltreatment, emotional inexpressivity, and affect intensity/reactivity. *Am. J. Orthopsychiatry* 76, 238–250. doi: 10.1037/0002-9432.76.2.238
30. Gratz, K. L., and Chapman, A. L. (2007). The role of emotional responding and childhood maltreatment in the development and maintenance of deliberate self-harm among male undergraduates. *Psychol. Men Masculinity* 8, 1–14. doi: 10.1037/1524-9220.8.1.1
31. Gratz, K. L., Conrad, S. D., and Roemer, L. (2002). Risk factors for deliberate self-harm among college students. *Am. J. Orthopsychiatry* 1, 128–140. doi: 10.1037/0002-9432.72.1.128
32. Gratz, K. L., Dixon-Gordon, K. L., Chapman, A. L., and Tull, M. T. (2015).

Diagnosis and characterization of DSM-5 nonsuicidal self-injury disorder using the clinician administered nonsuicidal self-injury disorder index. *Assessment* 22, 527–539. doi: 10.1177/1073191114565878

33. Herpertz, S. (1995). Self-injurious behavior: psychopathological and nosological characteristics in subtypes of self-injurers. *Acta Psychiatr. Scand.* 91, 57–68. doi: 10.1111/j.1600-0447.1995.tb09743.x
34. Hilt, L. M., Cha, C. B., and Nolen-Hoeksema, S. (2008b). Nonsuicidal self-injury in young adolescent girls: moderators of the distress-function relationship. *J. Consult. Clin. Psychol.* 76, 63–71. doi: 10.1037/0022-006X.76.1.63
35. Hilt, L. M., Nock, M. K., Lloyd-Richardson, E. E., and Prinstein, M. J. (2008a). Longitudinal study of nonsuicidal self-injury among young adolescents: rates, correlates, and preliminary test of an interpersonal model. *J. Early Adolesc.* 28, 455–469. doi: 10.1177/0272431608316604
36. Iannaccone, M., Cella, S., Manzi, S. A., Visconti, L., Manzi, F., and Cotrufo, P. (2013). My body and me: self-injurious behaviors and body modifications in eating disorders—preliminary results. *Eat. Disord.* 21, 130–139. doi: 10.1080/10640266.2013.761087
37. In-Albon, T., Ruf, C., and Schmid, M. (2013). Proposed diagnostic criteria for the DSM-5 of nonsuicidal self-injury in female adolescents: diagnostic and clinical correlates. *Psychiatry J.* 2013:159208. doi: 10.1155/2013/159208
38. Jacobson, C. M., Hill, R. M., Pettit, J. W., and Grozeva, D. (2015). The association of interpersonal and intrapersonal emotional experiences with non-suicidal self-injury in young adults. *Arch. Suicide Res.* 19, 401–413. doi: 10.1080/13811118.2015.1004492
39. Jenkins, A. L., McCloskey, M. S., Kulper, D., Berman, M. E., and Coccaro,E. F. (2015). Self-harm behavior among individuals with intermittent explosive disorder and personality disorders. *J. Psychiatr. Res.* 60, 125–131. doi: 10.1016/j.jpsychires.2014.08.013
40. Kaess, M., Parzer, P., Mattern, M., Plener, P. L., Bifulco, A., Resch, F., et al. (2013). Adverse childhood experiences and their impact on frequency, severity, and the individual function of nonsuicidal self-injury in youth. *Psychiatry Res.* 206, 265–272. doi: 10.1016/j.psychres.2012.10.012
41. Kahan, J., and Pattison, E. M. (1984). Proposal for a distinctive diagnosis: the deliberate self-harm syndrome (DSH). *Suicide Life Threat. Behav.* 14, 17–35. doi: 10.1111/j.1943-278X.1984.tb00334.x
42. Kirchner, T., Ferrer, L., Forns, M., and Zanini, D. (2011). Self-harm behavior and suicidal ideation among high school students. Gender differences and relationship with coping strategies. *Actas Esp. Psiquiatr.* 39, 226–235.
43. Klonsky, E. D. (2007). The functions of deliberate self-injury: a review of the evidence. *Clin. Psychol. Rev.* 27, 226–239. doi: 10.1016/j.cpr.2006.08.002
44. Klonsky, E. D. (2011). Non-suicidal self-injury in United States adults: prevalence, sociodemographics, topography and functions. *Psychol. Med.* 41, 1981–1986. doi: 10.1017/S0033291710002497
45. Klonsky, E. D., and Muehlenkamp, J. J. (2007). Self-injury: a research review for the practitioner. *J. Clin. Psychol.* 63, 1045–1056. doi: 10.1002/jclp.20412
46. Klonsky, E. D., Oltmanns, T. F., and Turkheimer, E. (2003). Deliberate self-harm in a nonclinical population: prevalence and psychological correlates. *Am. J. Psychiatry* 160, 1501–1508. doi: 10.1176/appi.ajp.160.8.1501
47. Kuentzel, J. G., Arble, E., Boutros, N., Chugani, D., and Barnett, D. (2012). Nonsuicidal self-injury in an ethnically diverse college sample. *Am. J. Orthopsychiatry* 82, 291–297. doi: 10.1111/j.1939-0025.2012.01167.x
48. Laye-Gindhu, A., and Schonert-Reichl, K. A. (2005). Nonsuicidal self-harm among community adolescents: understanding the whats and whys of self-harm. *J. Youth Adolesc.* 34, 447–457. doi: 10.1007/s10964-005-7262-z
49. Lengel, G. J., and Mullins-Sweatt, S. N. (2013). Nonsuicidal self-injury disorder: clinician and expert ratings. *Psychiatry Res.* 210, 940–944. doi: 10.1016/j.psychres.2013.08.047
50. Liberati, A., Altman, D. G., Tetzlaff, J., Mulrow, C., Gøtzsche, P. C., Ioannidis, J. P. A., et al. (2009). The PRISMA statement for reporting systematic reviews and meta-analyses of studies that evaluate health care interventions: explanation and elaboration. *Br. Med. J.* 339:b2700. doi: 10.1136/bmj.b2700
51. Lloyd-Richardson, E. E., Perrine, N., Dierker, L., and Kelley, M. L. (2007). Characteristics and functions of non-suicidal self-injury in a community sample of adolescents. *Psychol. Med.* 37, 1183–1192. doi: 10.1017/S003329170700027X
52. Menninger, K. (1938). *Man Against Himself.* New York, NY: Harcourt and Brace. Muehlenkamp, J. J. (2005). Self-injurious behavior as a separate clinical syndrome. *Am. J. Orthopsychiatry* 75, 324–333. doi: 10.1037/0002-9432.75.2.324 Muehlenkamp, J. J., Brausch, A., Quigley, K., and Whitlock, J. (2013). Interpersonal
53. features and functions of nonsuicidal self-injury. *Suicide Life Threat. Behav.* 2013, 43–67. doi: 10.1111/j.1943-278X.2012.00128.x
54. Muehlenkamp, J. J., Claes, L., Havertape, L., and Plener, P. L. (2012). International prevalence of adolescent non-suicidal self-injury and deliberate self-harm. *Child Adolesc. Psychiatry Ment. Health* 6, 1–9. doi: 10.1186/1753-2000-6-10
55. Muehlenkamp, J. J., and Gutierrez, P. M. (2007). Risk for suicide attempts among adolescents who engage in non-suicidal self-injury. *Arch. Suicide Res.* 11, 69–82. doi: 10.1080/13811110600992902
56. Nock, M. K. (2010). Self-injury. *Annu. Rev. Clin. Psychol.* 6, 339–363. doi: 10.1146/annurev.clinpsy.121208.131258
57. Nock, M. K., Joiner, T. E., Gordon, K. H., Lloyd-Richardson, E., and Prinstein, M. J. (2006). Nonsuicidal self-injury among adolescents: diagnostic correlates and relation to suicide attempts. *Psychiatry Res.* 144, 65–72. doi: 10.1016/j.psychres.2006.05.010
58. Nock, M. K., and Prinstein, M. J. (2004). A functional approach to the assessment of self mutilative behavior. *J. Clin. Consult. Psychol.* 72, 885–890. doi: 10.1037/0022-006X.72.5.885
59. Paivio, S. C., and McCulloch, C. R. (2004). Alexithymia as a mediator between childhood trauma and self-injurious behaviours. *Child Abuse Negl.* 28, 339–354. doi: 10.1016/j.chiabu.2003.11.018
60. Pao, P. (1969). The syndrome of delicate self cutting. *Br. J. Med. Psychol.* 42, 213–221. doi: 10.1111/j.2044-8341.1969.tb02071.x
61. Pattison, E. M., and Kahan, J. (1983). The deliberate self-harm syndrome. *Am. J. Psychiatry* 140, 867–872. doi: 10.1176/ajp.140.7.867
62. Plener, P. L., Libal, G., Keller, F., Fegert, J. M., and Muehlenkamp, J. J. (2009). An international comparison of non-suicidal self-injury (NSSI) and suicide attempts: Germany and the USA. *Psychol. Med.* 39, 1549–1558. doi: 10.1017/S0033291708005114
63. Regier, D. A., Narrow, W. E., Clarke, D. E., Kraemer, H. C., Kuramoto, S. J., Kuhl, E. A., et al. (2013). DSM-5 field trials in the United States and Canada, part II: test–retest reliability of selected categorical diagnoses. *Am. J. Psychiatry* 170, 59–70. doi: 10.1176/appi.ajp.2012.12070999
64. Rosenthal, R., Rinzler, C., Wallsch, R., and Klausner, E. (1972). Wrist-cutting syndrome: the meaning of a gesture. *Am. J. Psychiatry* 128, 1363–1368. doi: 10.1176/ajp.128.11.1363
65. Ross, S., and Heath, N. (2002). A study of the frequency of self-mutilation in a community sample of adolescents. *J. Youth Adolesc.* 31, 67–77. doi: 10.1023/A:1014089117419
66. Selby, E. A., Bender, T. W., Gordon, K. H., Nock, M. K., and Joiner, T. E. (2012). Non-suicidal selfinjury (NSSI) disorder: a preliminary study. *Personal. Disord.* 3, 167–175. doi: 10.1037/a0024405
67. Selby, E. A., Kranzler, A., Fehling, K. B., and Panza, E. (2015). Nonsuicidal self- injury disorder: the path to diagnostic validity and final obstacles. *Clin. Psychol. Rev.* 38, 79–91. doi: 10.1016/j.cpr.2015.03.003
68. Shaffer, D., and Jacobson, C. (2009). *Proposal to the DSM-V Childhood Disorder and Mood Disorder Work Groups to Include Non-Suicidal Self-Injury (NSSI) as a DSM-V disorder.* Washington, DC: American Psychiatric Association.
69. Simeon, D., and Favazza, A. R. (2001). "Self-injurious behaviors: Phenomenology and assessment," in *Self-Injurious Behaviors: Assessment and Treatment*, eds D. Simeon and E. Hollander (Washington, DC: American Psychiatric Publishing), 1–28.
70. Sornberger, M. J., Heath, N. L., Toste, J. R., and McLouth, R. (2012). Nonsuicidal self-injury and gender: patterns of prevalence, methods, and locations among adolescents. *Suicide Life Threat. Behav.* 42, 266–278. doi: 10.1111/j.1943-278X.2012.0088.x
71. Suyemoto, K. L. (1998). The functions of self-mutilation. *Clin. Psychol. Rev.* 18, 531–554. doi: 10.1016/S0272-7358(97)00105-0
72. Suyemoto, K. L., and MacDonald, M. L. (1995). Self-cutting in female adolescents. *Psychotherapy* 32, 162–171. doi: 10.1037/0033-3204.32.1.162
73. Swannell, S. V., Martin, G. E., Page, A., Hasking, P., and St John, M. J. (2014). Prevalence of nonsuicidal self-injury in nonclinical samples: systematic review, meta-analysis and meta-regression. *Suicide Life Threat. Behav.* 44, 273–303. doi: 10.1111/sltb.12070
74. Tang, J., Yang, W., Ahmed, N. I., Ma, Y., Liu, H., Wang, J., et al. (2016). Stressful life events as a predictor for nonsuicidal self-injury in southern Chinese adolescence. *Medicine* 95:e2637. doi: 10.1097/MD.0000000000002637
75. Tantam, D., and Whittaker, J. (1992). Personality disorder and self-wounding. *Br. J. Psychiatry* 161, 451–464. doi: 10.1192/bjp.161.4.451
76. Turner, B. J., Chapman, A. L., and Layden, B. K. (2012). Intrapersonal and interpersonal functions of non-suicidal self-injury: associations with emotional and social functioning. *Suicide Life Threat. Behav.* 42, 36–55. doi: 10.1111/j.1943-278X.2011.00069.x
77. Turner, B. J., Cobb, R. J., Gratz, K. L., and Chapman, A. L. (2016). The role of interpersonal conflict and perceived social support in nonsuicidal self-injury in daily life. *J. Abnorm. Psychol.* 125, 588–598. doi: 10.1037/abn0000141

78. Turner, B. J., Dixon-Gordon, K. L., Austin, S. B., Rodriguez, M. A., Rosenthal,
79. M. Z., and Chapman, A. L. (2015). Non-suicidal self-injury with and without borderline personality disorder: differences in self-injury and diagnostic comorbidity. *Psychiatry Res.* 230, 28–35. doi: 10.1016/j.psychres.2015.07.058
80. Wan, Y., Chen, J., Sun, Y., and Tao, F. B. (2015). Impact of childhood abuse on the risk of non-suicidal self-injury in mainland Chinese adolescents. *PLoS ONE* 10:e0131239. doi: 10.1371/journal.pone.013123
81. Washburn, J. J., Potthoff, L. M., Juzwin, K. R., and Styer, D. M. (2015). Assessing DSM-5 nonsuicidal self-injury disorder in a clinical sample. *Psychol. Assess.* 27, 31–41. doi: 10.1037/pas0000021
82. Whitlock, J., Eckenrode, J., and Silverman, D. (2006). Self-injurious behaviors in a college population. *Pediatrics* 117, 1939–1948. doi: 10.1542/peds.2005-2543
83. Whitlock, J., Muehlenkamp, J. J., Purington, A., Eckenrode, J., Barreira, J., Abrams, G. B., et al. (2011). Non-suicidal self-injury in a college population: general trends and sex differences. *J. Am. College Health* 59, 691–698. doi: 10.1080/07448481.2010.529626
84. Wilkinson, P., and Goodyer, I. (2011). Non-suicidal self-injury. *Eur. Child Adolesc. Psychiatry* 20, 103–108. doi: 10.1007/s00787-010-0156-y
85. Yates, T. M., Tracy, A. J., and Luthar, S. S. (2008). Nonsuicidal self- injury among "privileged" youths: longitudinal and cross-sectional approaches to developmental process. *J. Consult. Clin. Psychol.* 76, 52–62. doi: 10.1037/0022-006X.76.1.52
86. Zetterqvist, M., Lundh, L. G., Dahlström, Ö., and Svedin, C. G. (2013). Prevalence and function of non-suicidal self-injury (NSSI) in a community sample of adolescents, using suggested DSM-5 criteria for a potential NSSI disorder. *J. Abnorm. Child Psychol.* 41, 759–773. doi: 10.1007/s10802-013-9712-5
87. Zoroglu, S. S., Tuzun, U., Sar, V., Tutkun, H., Savaçs, H. A., Ozturk, M., et al. (2003). Suicide attempt and self-mutilation among Turkish high school students in relation with abuse, neglect and dissociation. *Psychiatry Clin. Neurosci.* 57, 119–126. doi: 10.1046/j.1440-1819.2003.01088.x

20

The Association Between Suicidal Behavior, Attentional Control and Frontal Asymmetry

Catherine Thompson[1] and Elsie Li Chen Ong[1,2]*

[1] School of Health Sciences, University of Salford, Salford, United Kingdom, [2] Division of Information and Technology Studies, Faculty of Education, The University of Hong Kong, Pokfulam, Hong Kong

***Correspondence:**
Catherine Thompson
c.thompson@salford.ac.uk

It can be difficult to identify those at risk of suicide because suicidal thoughts are often internalized and not shared with others. Yet to prevent suicide attempts it is crucial to identify suicidal thoughts and actions at an early stage. Past studies have suggested that deficits in attentional control are associated with suicide, with the argument that individuals are unable to inhibit negative thoughts and direct resources away from negative information. The current study aimed to investigate the association of suicidal behavior with neurological and behavioral markers, measuring attentional bias and inhibition in two Stroop tasks. Fifty-four participants responded to the color of color words in a standard Stroop task and the color of positive, negative, and neutral words in an emotional Stroop task. Electroencephalographic (EEG) activity was recorded from frontal areas during each task and at resting. Participants were separated into a *low-risk* and *high-risk* group according to their self-reported suicidal behavior. Participants in the high-risk group showed slower response times in the color Stroop and reduced accuracy to incongruent trials, but faster response times in the emotional Stroop task. Response times to the word "suicide" were significantly slower for the high-risk group. This indicates an attentional bias toward specific negative stimuli and difficulties inhibiting information for those with high levels of suicidal behavior. In the emotional Stroop task the high-risk group showed reduced activity in leftward frontal areas, suggesting limitations in the ability to regulate emotional processing via the left frontal regions. The findings support the argument that deficits in attentional control are related to suicidal behavior. The research also suggests that under certain conditions frontal asymmetry may be associated with suicidal behavior.

Keywords: suicide, attentional control, inhibition, frontal asymmetry, emotional Stroop, capability model

INTRODUCTION

Suicidal behavior refers to a wide range of suicide-related cognitions, emotions, and behaviors (1). It is a term that has been used to categorize behavior associated with ideas, intentions, motivations, plans, and attempts for suicide. Prediction and prevention of suicide is challenging because it is a personal and sensitive topic (2). Those who experience suicidal behavior may avoid discussing this with others and sharing their thoughts can often trigger feelings of stigmatization. This can also lead to difficulties in identifying those who are vulnerable to suicide because assessments are largely based on clinical interviews and self-report measures (3). This means clinicians have to rely on individuals self-disclosing information regarding their current suicidal thoughts and plans, and any history of past suicide attempts. Such disclosure may be unreliable if a person is unwilling to report their intentions (4) and individuals may deliberately deny or conceal their suicide tendency to avoid intervention or hospitalization (2, 5). This highlights the importance of developing alternative measures for identifying individuals with a suicide risk. One potential option would be to use measures of cognitive and neurological processing (5).

Deficits in cognitive processing and neurological activity have been found in suicidal individuals and these are specifically related to "executive function" (6–9). Executive function [also termed cognitive control, e.g., Ref. (10)] constitutes many components that allow an individual to plan and execute goal-directed behavior including the ability to regulate emotions, exert inhibitory control, shift focus between multiple tasks, and flexibly modify behavior according to a situation (11–14). Deficits therefore relate to impairment of a broad range of cognitive functions such as memory, attention, and decision-making.

Miyake et al. (15) identify three key components of executive function: shifting, updating, and inhibition. Updating is the ability to maintain relevant information within working memory and to update this information in accordance with changes in task demands. Shifting refers to directing attentional resources away from task-irrelevant information and toward task-relevant information. Inhibition is the ability to override an automatic but irrelevant response. Attentional control (the ability to flexibly shift attentional resources in dynamic situations, maintain focus on relevant information, and inhibit irrelevant information) is implicated in each of these components. Deficits in attentional control are argued to be related to affective disorders as individuals have difficulties shifting resources away from negative thoughts and re-directing attention toward more positive information (16). The importance of executive control in the development and maintenance of affective disorders is outlined in an integrative cognitive-biological model of depression that proposes two key components (17, 18). Initially, low-level bottom–up processing of negative information results in attentional biases. Second, deficits in top–down control processes mean that an individual is unable to direct attention away from negative information.

Executive dysfunction is argued to have a direct impact on emotional regulation as it prevents individuals engaging in effective mood-regulation strategies and instead a person may utilize maladaptive strategies that serve to sustain negative biases. For instance, Joormann and Tanovic (10) make the argument that individuals with major depressive disorder may have difficulties changing the contents of working memory and moving the focus away from negative thoughts (updating). Deficits in shifting have also been associated with increased rumination in depressed individuals due to an inability to shift the focus of attention away from negative thoughts [e.g., Ref. (19)]. This increased focus on negative information serves to enhance and maintain negative mood states (20).

While the theoretical explanations for the links between executive function and affective disorders focus on depression, deficits in executive control have also been linked to the reduced ability to deal with emotional disturbances that are commonly found in suicidal patients (21, 22). For example, difficulties with response inhibition can make one more likely to act impulsively, while impairments in interference control can prevent the inhibition of irrelevant and intrusive thoughts, such as those relating to self-harm (13, 23). Richard-Devantoy and Courtet (24) proposed that suicidal individuals with impaired executive function are at a greater risk of attempting suicide due to their diminished ability to engage in protective cognitive strategies. This is because they are less able to accurately assess the consequences of their behavior, and less capable of inhibiting maladaptive emotional and behavioral responses. They found that individuals who had attempted suicide showed deficits in decision-making, problem solving, autobiographical long-term memory, and working memory. Loyo et al. (25) measured the links between executive functioning and suicidal behavior, taking measures of attentional control, abstract reasoning ability, and decision-making in 25 suicide attempters with depressive symptoms, 25 non-suicide attempters with depressive symptoms, and 24 non-depressed participants. Consistent with Richard-Devantoy and Courtet (24), they found that compared with the non-suicide attempters and non-depressed participants, suicide attempters showed greater deficits in a range of tasks including the Wisconsin Card Sorting Task and the Iowa Gambling Task. These findings suggest a relationship between executive dysfunction and suicidal behavior. Interestingly, a study by Keilp et al. (16) that compared executive function in depressed suicide attempters, depressed non-attempters, and healthy controls found that while the patient groups showed poor performance across a number of measures, those with a past suicide attempt showed specific deficits in tests of attentional control and working memory.

Further supporting evidence for the link between suicide and executive control comes from a study by Richard-Devantoy et al. (26) using a color-word interference test similar to the Stroop task. Participants were 17 healthy controls and 38 depressed individuals with no suicide attempts or ideation (thoughts of suicide), 16 depressed individuals with suicide ideation, 14 depressed low-lethality suicide attempters, and 17 depressed high-lethality suicide attempters. The task involved color naming, word reading, inhibition, and inhibition/switching trials and compared with healthy controls and those with suicide ideation, high-lethality suicide attempters took longer to respond to inhibition trials. Richard-Devantoy et al. (26) argued that the results have important implications for suicidal behavior because deficits in executive control may undermine the ability to deal with real-life emotional distractions. While individuals with adequate inhibition may exert control over inappropriate behaviors (such as self-harm) and are better able to resist suicidal urges, those with impaired inhibition may be less able to exercise control over these impulses, and may have difficulty resisting the urge to act on suicidal thoughts. Such deficits may therefore predict whether an individual will engage in suicidal behavior. The authors do however state that executive control is impacted by age and their findings are limited due to the fact that they used a group of older adults. Consequently it would be beneficial to assess executive dysfunction in a younger population.

Executive function is primarily controlled by the prefrontal cortex (PFC), which interacts closely with other brain regions such as the anterior cingulate and the amygdala (13, 27). It has been proposed that the frontal regions of the brain, predominantly the dorsal lateral and ventral lateral PFC (dlPFC, vlPFC), are responsible for guiding attention, maintaining information within the mind, shifting cognitive resources between different sources of information, and inhibiting the processing of task-irrelevant information (8, 9, 28–30). Compton et al. (28) measured PFC activity using functional Magnetic Resonance Imaging (fMRI) in a color Stroop and an emotional Stroop task. In a color Stroop task (31), participants are asked to name the color of words that possess a congruent (e.g., the word red printed in red) or incongruent semantic meaning (e.g., the word red printed in green). In an emotional Stroop task (32), participants are asked to name the color of emotional and neutral words. Both tasks require the inhibition of an automated, irrelevant response (reading the word), and the allocation of resources to process a relevant response (the name of the color); therefore, they allow for the measurement of attentional control. In general, studies show that responses are slower to incongruent trials compared with congruent trials in a standard color Stroop, revealing difficulties inhibiting the automatic processing of irrelevant information [known as the Stroop interference effect (33)]. Responses are also slower to emotional words compared with neutral words in an emotional Stroop task [also known as the emotional Stroop effect (34–36)]. This is particularly the case in patient groups when the emotional words are related to affective disorders [e.g., Ref. (37)]. Compton et al. (28) found that activity in the dlPFC increased for trials in which the word was incongruent to the color and for trials in which negative words were presented. It is argued that increased activity reflects greater investment of resources in order to inhibit automatic responses (regardless of whether these are emotionally significant); therefore, difficulties recruiting the dlPFC would lead to impaired inhibition.

Pan et al. (38) measured response inhibition using the Go/No-go task in adolescents with various degrees of suicidal thoughts and actions. The sample included 15 depressed adolescents with a history of suicide attempts, 15 depressed adolescents with no history of suicidal behavior, and 14 healthy controls. The Go/No-go task requires participants to press a button in response to a target stimulus (Go), but to inhibit the button press and do nothing in response to a non-target stimulus (No-go). In the healthy controls, fMRI recordings showed increased activation of the prefrontal, anterior cingulate, and parietal cortical regions. The anterior cingulate in particular is considered crucial for inhibitory control (8) and while the depressed individuals with no past history of suicidal behavior did not differ from the controls with regard to activity in this area, the depressed adolescents with a history of suicide attempts showed significantly reduced activity. This indicates impairments in inhibitory control for suicidal individuals and also shows the relationship between cognitive processing and cortical activity. The findings were consistent with those of Compton et al. (28) regarding the association between frontal activity and attentional control. They also suggest that this association may constitute a neurobiological basis for predisposition to suicidal behavior. It is proposed that executive control may moderate frontal cortical activity and neurological measures may therefore be used to predict suicidal behavior of individuals beyond the currently used self-report measures.

The majority of past research exploring the neurological basis of affective disorders has focused on clinical depression and there are comparatively fewer studies that measure executive function and neurological activity in suicidal populations. The initial argument that limited executive function and patterns of PFC activity may be related to affective disorders came from observations of patients who had experienced a stroke and were suffering from clinical depression [(39); see Ref. (40) for a review]. It was evident that following damage to the left prefrontal regions some patients became increasingly depressed, while damage to the right frontal regions resulted in increasing levels of manic symptoms. Schaffer et al. (41) explored this dissociation by measuring cortical activity in patients who were suffering from depression to varying extents. The aim was to identify any "asymmetry" of activity to support the claim that different patterns of frontal activation may be related to the severity of the disorder. Electroencephalogram (EEG) electrodes were placed on the frontal and parietal regions of the brain and similar to the clinical report of Gainotti (39), patients indicating more severe symptoms of depression showed greater activity in the right compared with the left. Importantly, this pattern was only found in the frontal regions, not the parietal regions.

These findings led to a rapid expansion of research surrounding lateralized frontal activation and EEG has been a common tool used to measure the correlates of relative hemispheric dominance (42, 43). It has been posited that the left hemisphere (LH) is dominant for processing positive emotions, whereas the right hemisphere (RH) is dominant for processing negative emotions. This means that if individuals have greater electrocortical activity in the right frontal region, they will have a disposition toward focusing on negative emotions and information. Supporting evidence for this came from Davidson and Fox (44) who were among the first to use asymmetric frontal cortical activity to make inferences about frontal asymmetry and emotions. They suggested that patterns of lateralized brain activity can be identified as early as infancy and to test this hypothesis they recruited 10-month old infants to view videotapes consisting of happy or sad facial expressions. Activity in frontal and parietal regions was recorded and it was found that increased activation in the left (relative to the right) corresponded to viewing happy faces while increased activation in the right (relative to the left) corresponded to viewing sad faces. The findings were also consistent with those of Schaffer et al. (41) as the differential pattern of activity was only found in the frontal regions, not the parietal regions.

Based on this research, Davidson et al. (45) and Davidson et al. (46) developed the *dispositional model*. The model holds a valence hypothesis that positive affect is associated with leftward frontal cortical activity, and negative affect is associated with rightward frontal cortical activity [e.g., Ref. (42)]. Since the introduction of this model research has been conducted to show the relationship between asymmetric frontal activation and depression (42, 43, 47–50). Overall the findings show that patients with a history of depression or with recurrent depression have relatively lower left frontal cortical activity (51), also known as left frontal hypoactivation [for reviews, see Ref. (52–54)]. This is in contrast to healthy controls that show the opposite pattern with greater leftward frontal cortical activity (50, 55). The level of reduced leftward activity also correlates with the level of symptoms reported, suggesting that this may provide a potential marker for assessing severity of disorders in patients (56).

The dispositional model makes the assumption that positive emotion is always associated with leftward frontal activation and negative emotion is always associated with rightward frontal activation. This has been challenged by Coan et al. (57) who proposed the *capability model*. This model supports the claim that individual differences in frontal asymmetry exist but argues that the differences will vary according to different situational contexts (40, 58). Therefore, while the dispositional model posits that rightward frontal activity will correspond to more negative emotional responses in all situations (e.g., in events that trigger joy, fear, or sadness), Coan and Allen (58) propose that differences in frontal asymmetry correspond to the different emotional demands of a situation. The capability model therefore suggests that asymmetrical differences are best thought of as interactions between individual differences and situational demands.

Despite the differences in these two models, neurological findings provide evidence that frontal asymmetry may serve as an indirect neurological indicator for predicting depression, or even suicide risk. For instance, using event-related fMRI, Jollant et al. (59) compared the neural activity of previously depressed men with past suicide attempts, previously depressed men with no suicide attempts, and healthy male controls. Across the three groups, only those with a history of suicide attempts showed frontal asymmetrical differences in response to emotional faces (angry, happy, and neutral). Specifically, they showed increased neural activation in the right lateral orbitofrontal cortex in response to angry faces relative to neutral faces. Jollant et al. argue that increased sensitivity to another person's disapproval (e.g., in the form of an angry facial expression) and a higher propensity to process and act on negative emotions may exacerbate suicidal behavior in suicidal individuals. This links to the proposal that increased processing of negative information (as demonstrated by increased activation) may serve to maintain negative attentional biases in individuals suffering from affective disorders (10, 17, 18).

Grimshaw and Carmel (60) provided an explanation for the inhibitory difficulties in depressed individuals arguing that they are unable to utilize the parts of the brain (i.e., the left PFC) responsible for inhibition, particularly the inhibition of negative information. Studies have supported this by showing that failure to recruit the left dlPFC when presented with irrelevant negative information is associated with depression (61, 62) and trait negative affect (63). Given the relationship between frontal asymmetry and inhibition, Grimshaw and Carmel (60) have proposed the *asymmetric inhibition model*. It is predicted that each frontal region specializes in the inhibition of different types of emotions, with the left dlPFC responsible for inhibiting negative stimuli, and the right dlPFC responsible for inhibiting positive stimuli. Therefore, frontal asymmetric activation reflects the ability to inhibit different types of emotional stimuli.

The current study aims to further investigate the relationship between frontal asymmetry, executive function (specifically attentional control), and suicidal behavior. While the majority of the previous research focuses on clinical samples there is an argument that early identification of those at risk of suicidal behavior is essential (64, 65). On the basis of this, the present work explores the links between suicidal behavior, attentional control, and asymmetry using a non-clinical population reporting relatively mild symptoms. Frontal asymmetry was recorded from individuals reporting high and low levels of suicidal behavior at resting state (both eyes closed and eyes opened) and during a color Stroop task and an emotional Stroop task. The dispositional model (45, 46) asserts that individuals who report higher levels of suicidal thoughts and behaviors will exhibit rightward frontal activity compared with those with low suicide risk regardless of the situation. However, the capability model (57) argues that the effect of suicidal behavior on asymmetric frontal brain activation will be more pronounced during emotionally demanding situations. By comparing frontal asymmetry at resting state and in emotional and non-emotional tasks it will be possible to test the predictions of these two models. Using the Stroop task also allows differences in attentional control to be compared according to levels of suicidal behavior. It is proposed that individuals reporting higher levels of suicidal behavior (high-risk) will show more difficulties in attentional control and will therefore be at a greater risk of suicide (and more likely to make a future suicide attempt) because they are less able to inhibit negative thoughts and direct attention toward task-relevant information. In contrast, those who experience low levels of suicidal behavior will have effective attentional control and will therefore be less likely to focus on irrelevant negative thoughts and actions. On the basis of this it was predicted that individuals with a high-risk would show a bigger Stroop interference effect in the color Stroop task compared with those in the low-risk group. For the emotional Stroop task, it was predicted that all participants would show the expected emotional Stroop effect, but that the high-risk group would show increased difficulty inhibiting negative words. According to the models of frontal asymmetry it was hypothesized that those who report high levels of suicidal behavior would also show relatively higher rightward frontal activation during the color Stroop task. Additionally, in the emotional Stroop task, leftward frontal activation would correspond to inhibition of negative stimuli whereas rightward frontal activation would correspond to inhibition of positive stimuli.

MATERIALS AND METHODS

Design

The study used a mixed measures design to investigate the effects of suicidal behavior in a Stroop task and an emotional Stroop task. Suicidal behavior was a between-participants variable with two conditions, high-risk and low-risk. In the color Stroop task a 2 (suicidal behavior) × 2 (congruency) design was used. Congruency referred to whether each color word was the same (congruent) or different (incongruent) to the color of ink in which the word was presented and this was a within-participants variable. In the emotional Stroop task a 2 (suicidal behavior) × 3 (emotion) design was used. Emotion was the valence of the words presented with positive, negative, and neutral words. This was a within-participants variable. The dependent variables were accuracy (total number of correct responses), and response times (milliseconds) to respond to the color of each word. A self-reported measure of depression was also recorded for each participant.

Frontal asymmetry (uV^2) was recorded during resting state and during the color Stroop and emotional Stroop tasks. In the resting state and color Stroop task asymmetry was compared between the high- and low-risk groups. In the emotional Stroop task asymmetry was compared between these two groups and across the three conditions of emotion.

Participants

Fifty-four undergraduate students (32 females) studying at The Open University in Hong Kong were recruited by convenience sampling. Age ranged from 18 to 27 years, with a mean of 21.65 years (SD = 2.10). Prospective participants were prescreened for previous history of neurological and mental health problems (e.g., currently taking medication known to affect cognitive performance, cognitive deficits, and diagnosis of PTSD).

Stimuli and Materials

Suicidal behavior was measured using the Suicidal Behavior Questionnaire-Revised [SBQ-R (66)]. This is a 4-item inventory that explores different dimensions of suicidal thoughts and actions. Item 1 measures lifetime suicide ideation and/or suicide attempts, item 2 assesses the frequency of suicidal thoughts in the previous 12 months, item 3 quantifies the threat of a suicide attempt, and item 4 is the self-reported likelihood of future suicidal behavior. Each question was answered using a Likert scale and the scale for each question differed slightly, with scales ranging from a minimum of 1 to a maximum of 6. Total scores, ranging from 3 to 18, represent overall suicide risk whereby higher scores represent greater risk. In an undergraduate student population the SBQ-R has demonstrated good internal reliability with Cronbach's alpha ranging from 0.76 (66) to 0.8 (67, 68). Individuals scoring a total of 7 or above were considered to be at a significant risk of suicidal behavior. A cut-off of 7 was selected on the basis of past findings from Osman et al. (66) who found a total score of 7 was most effective at distinguishing between those who had suicide ideation and/or had made a suicide attempt from those who had not experienced suicide behavior. This differs from clinical populations, and while Osman et al. (66) suggest a cut-off of 8, Rueda-Jaimes et al. (69) propose a cut-off of 11 for clinical populations.

The Stroop tasks were presented on a 19″ computer monitor using E-Prime. In the color Stroop task the words "red," "yellow," "blue," and "green" were presented in bold Times New Roman font, size 28. Each word was presented in the color red, yellow, blue, or green depending on the congruence of the trial. The emotional Stroop task was adapted from Herrington et al. (62) and consisted of positive, negative, and neutral words presented in one of the four colors (red, yellow, blue, and green). A total of 192 words were used from the Affective Norms for English Words [ANEW (70)], 64 positive (e.g., birthday, laughter, angel), 64 negative (e.g., bankrupt, suicide, funeral), and 64 neutral (e.g., handle, carpet, time). Valence of positive words ranged from 6.17 to 8.43 with a mean of 7.49, valence of negative words ranged from 1.61 to 3.69 with a mean of 2.47, and valence of neutral words ranged from 4.02 to 7.57 with a mean of 5.64.

Depression was measured using the Beck Depression Inventory-II [BDI-II (71)]. This self-report inventory measures different aspects of depression such as sadness and irritability. It is a 21-item inventory and all items are assessed on a 4-point rating scale from zero to three (0 indicates no symptoms and a score of 3 indicates severe symptoms). Each item focuses on a particular feeling or behavior and respondents are asked to indicate the extent to which they have experienced this in the previous two weeks. For instance, item 14 focuses on "worthlessness" with responses from 0 ("I do not feel I am worthless") to 3 ("I feel utterly worthless"). The total score ranges from 0 to 63 with higher scores indicating more severe depression symptoms. A score of 17 or above represents a risk of clinical depression, and scores higher than 31 are indicative of more severe depression. In the current investigation responses to item 9 were removed. This item refers to suicidal behavior and was removed to avoid any overlap with the SBQ-R.

Electroencephalogram activity was recorded using an Emotive EEG Neuroheadset with a sampling rate of 128 Hz (Emotiv Technology Inc., USA) that records from 14 sites (AF3, AF4, F3, F4, FC5, FC6, F7, F8, T7, T8, P7, P8, O1, O2) using a 16-channel Biosemi Active Two system. Two additional electrodes situated at the back of the ears (CMS, DRL) were selected as the reference of choice for all analyses and all sites were referenced to the average of these electrodes during recording, and re-referenced offline. Frontal electrodes were F3, F4, F7, F8, AF3, and AF4. Central electrodes were FC5, FC6, T7, and T8. Parietal electrodes were P7 and P8 and occipital electrodes were O1 and O2. The numbers also indicated the area of the right/left hemispheres of the brain an electrode was located, where even numbers represent the RH and odd numbers refer to the LH. Prior to use, all felt pads on top of the sensors were moistened with a saline solution.

Procedure

After providing written informed consent participants were seated in a dimly lit room and the EEG headset was affixed to the scalp with sites located according to the 10/20 system (72). The impedance at each site was checked to ensure good contact quality (large signal to noise ratio). Participants were instructed to remain seated in a relaxed state and EEG recordings were taken with the eyes closed for 2 min and the eyes open for 2 min to provide a resting state measure. Next, participants were asked to complete the color and the emotional Stroop tasks while wearing the EEG headset. The order of the tasks was counterbalanced across participants. For both tasks, a trial began with a fixation cross of 500 ms followed by the presentation of a word in the center of the computer screen. For each word participants were asked to identify the color of the text (red, yellow, blue, or green) as quickly as possible by pressing the corresponding key on the computer keyboard (R, Y, B, and G). A total of 60 trials were completed in the color Stroop task with 30 congruent and 30 incongruent trials. There were an equal number of words presented in red, yellow, blue, and green and all trials were presented in a random order. The emotional Stroop task consisted of three emotional blocks showing positive, negative, and neutral words. The order of the blocks was randomized and there were 64 trials in each block. An equal number of words were presented in each of the four colors within each block and all trials were presented in a random order.

EEG Data Processing

Activity was recorded across the entirety of each block to allow for a general pattern of hemispheric asymmetry to be gained. Consequently activity was taken for all elements within a trial (fixation, stimulus presentation, and response) and a precise measure of electrocortical activity in specific time epochs was not generated. Activity within each block was compared with a baseline measure taken over a period of 20 s in eyes-open resting state immediately prior to each block. All artifact screening, re-referencing, and spectral analysis were performed using EEGLAB toolbox (73) and custom scripts in MATLAB (74). Each data file was visually inspected to manually remove artifacts such as aberrant signals due to large non-blink eye movements, muscle movements, or signal discontinuities. Further EEG artifacts were removed using an independent component analysis [ICA; (73)] during offline signal processing. A bandpass filter of 2–45 Hz and a notch filter of 50 Hz were applied to the raw data with 128-Hz sampling frequency per channel. A Hamming window (1024 sample and 50% overlap) was also applied to the data in preparation for spectral analysis, from which the power and asymmetry estimates were derived.

The experiment was completed in blocks (eyes open resting, eyes closed resting, color Stroop, positive, negative, and neutral emotional Stroop) and activity was recorded and analyzed across each block. Frontal alpha asymmetry was calculated in 1-Hz frequency bins and averaged across the frequency bandwidths of interest: delta (1.5–3.5 Hz), theta (4–7.5 Hz), alpha (8–13 Hz), alpha1 (8–10 Hz), alpha2 (10–13 Hz), beta1 (13–20 Hz), and beta2 (20–28 Hz). Frontal alpha asymmetry was calculated for F3 (left frontal) and F4 (right frontal) electrodes using the Fast Fourier Transform (FFT) method. The alpha power values for F3 and F4 were natural log transformed (73) such that an asymmetry score comparing activity in the RH to activity in the LH in each block was computed [ln ALPHA = (ln[RH] – ln[LH])]. Frontal asymmetry indices were calculated by subtracting the natural log of the power of the LH electrode from that of the RH electrode [ln [right (F4)] – [left (F3)]] (75). Given the inverse relationship between alpha power and cortical activity (76), a positive alpha asymmetry index reflects relatively higher left frontal activity and lower right frontal activity, and a negative asymmetry index reflects relatively higher right frontal activity and lower left frontal cortical activity.

RESULTS

Two participants were excluded from the analysis due to poor EEG data or missing behavioral data. The remaining 52 participants (31 females) were all right handed and were not taking any medication known to affect brain activity or cognitive performance. The SBQ-R had a suitable level of internal reliability that was consistent with past studies [e.g., Ref. (66)], Cronbach's $\alpha = 0.74$. Participants were separated into high and low suicidal behavior groups according to their total score on the SBQ-R. Participants with a total score less than 7 were categorized as low-risk (median score = 5, range = 3–6), while participants with a score of 7 or above were categorized as high-risk (median score = 9.5, range = 7–15). There were a total of 22 participants (13 female, aged 20–23, mean age of 21.55) in the high-risk group and 30 (18 female, aged 20–25, mean age of 21.94) in the low-risk group. Six participants in the high-risk group and none of the participants in the low-risk group reported a past suicide attempt. To ensure that any group differences were not driven by those who had made a past suicide attempt, the results were analyzed once with all participants included, and a second time without attempters. Analysis without attempters is only reported where the results differed from that of the full sample.

The data did not meet parametric assumptions, and therefore a Mann–Whitney U test was used to confirm that the SBQ-R scores between the two groups were significantly different ($U = 0.001$, $z = -6.162$, $p < 0.001$, $r = 0.85$). Analysis of scores from the BDI-II (without item 9) also showed that participants in the high suicidal behavior group reported significantly higher levels of depression (median score = 28, range = 17–42) than those in the low suicidal behavior group [(median score = 8, range = 1–16), $U = 112.500$, $z = -4.034$, $p < 0.001$, $r = 0.57$].

Resting EEG

To investigate differences in alpha-asymmetrical activation in relation to suicidal behavior in the resting state, independent t-tests were conducted with suicidal behavior group as the between-participant variable and alpha-asymmetrical index as the dependent variable. Opposite to what was expected, the alpha-asymmetrical index was higher in the high-risk group ($M = 0.07\text{uV}^2$, SD = 0.49) than the low-risk group ($M = 0.51\text{uV}^2$, SD = 0.67) during the eyes-open resting state [$t(50) = -2.63$, $p = 0.01$, Cohen's $d = 0.75$]. This means that while both groups showed more activity in the left compared with the right, this was most pronounced for the high-risk group. There was no significant difference in alpha asymmetry between the high- and the low-risk groups during the eyes-closed resting state [$t(50) = -4.497$, $p = 0.141$, Cohen's $d = 0.42$].

Performance in the Stroop Task

All incorrect trials were removed and any correct response times that were more than 2.5 SD from the mean were classed as outliers and removed (a total of 4.84% of trials). Accuracy was analyzed using a generalized estimating equation (GEE) assuming a negative binomial distribution. All RTs were log transformed to ensure data met the assumptions of a normal distribution and RT data were analyzed using a 2 (suicidal behavior) × 2 (congruency) mixed measures ANOVA.

Analysis of accuracy in the color Stroop task showed a significant main effect of suicidal behavior [Wald χ^2 (1) = 4.385, $p < 0.05$, Cohen's $d = 0.61$]. Accuracy was higher for the low-risk group (M = 28.82, SD = 1.16) compared with the high-risk group (M = 27.35, SD = 1.71). There was also a significant effect of congruency [Wald χ^2 (1) = 24.053, $p < 0.001$, Cohen's d = 1.86], with higher accuracy in congruent (M = 29.4, SD = 0.76) compared with incongruent trials (M = 27.78, SD = 1.51). There was a significant interaction between suicidal behavior and congruency [Wald χ^2 (1) = 6.158, $p < 0.05$, Cohen's d = 0.73]. Differences between the low- and high-risk groups were only found in the incongruent trials (M of 28.19 and 27.35 respectively, SD of 1.12 and 1.76) and not the congruent trials (M of 29.44 and 29.36 respectively, SD of 0.89 and 0.67) (see **Figure 1A**).

For RT (see **Figure 1B**), there was a significant effect of suicidal behavior [F(1, 50) = 28.916, MSE = 27712.152, $p < 0.001$, partial η^2 = 0.366]. Participants reporting lower levels of suicidal behavior showed faster response times than those with higher levels (M of 700.95 and 878.72 ms respectively, and SD of 146.60 and 144.17). There was a significant effect of congruency [F(1, 50) = 157.325, MSE = 4360.631, $p < 0.001$, partial η^2 = 0.719], with faster response times to congruent (M = 704.17 ms, SD = 135.59) than incongruent trials (M = 848.05 ms, SD = 170.78). There was no interaction between suicidal behavior and congruence [F(1, 50) = 1.222, MSE = 4360.63, p = 0.274, partial η^2 = 0.084].

There was no significant difference in alpha-asymmetrical index between the high-risk group (M = 0.334uV2, SD = 0.50) and the low-risk group (M = 0.452uV2, SD = 0.85) in the color Stroop task [t(50) = −0.580, p = 0.564, Cohen's d = 0.18].

Performance in the Emotional Stroop Task

Analysis of the emotional Stroop task followed that of the color Stroop task. Accuracy was analyzed using a GEE and RT was analyzed with a 2 (suicidal behavior) × 3 (emotion) mixed measures ANOVA. A total of 4.21% of trials were removed due to low accuracy or because response times were more than 2.5 SD from the mean. All RTs were log transformed to satisfy distributional assumptions.

For accuracy (**Figure 2A**), the model revealed a significant main effect of suicidal behavior [Wald χ^2 (1) = 4.069, $p < 0.05$, Cohen's d = 0.58]. Accuracy was higher for the low-risk group (M = 61.88, SD = 2.39) compared with the high-risk group (M = 61.17, SD = 1.74). There was no main effect of emotion [Wald χ^2 (1) = 1.034, p = 0.309, Cohen's d = 0.28], and no interaction between suicidal behavior and emotion [Wald χ^2 (1) = 2.483, p = 0.115, Cohen's d = 0.45].

For RT (**Figure 2B**), there was a significant effect of suicidal behavior [F(1, 50) = 11.30, MSE = 8495.123, $p < 0.001$, partial η^2 = 0.184] with faster response times in the high-risk group (M = 593.31 ms, SD = 84.83) compared with the low-risk group (M = 679.76 ms, SD = 94.95). There was no significant effect of emotion [F(2, 100) = 1.824, MSE = 3969.585, p = 0.110, partial η^2 = 0.035] and no interaction between suicidal behavior and emotion [F(2, 100) = 0.608, MSE = 2413.522, p = 0.546, partial η^2 = 0.012].

To assess inhibition of suicide-related stimuli, response times were also considered across the two groups when responding to the word "suicide." A between-participants t-test was conducted that showed significantly longer response times for the high-risk group compared with the low-risk group [M of 725.20 and 652.78 respectively, SD of 126.32 and 116.12, t(50) = 2.17, p = 0.035, Cohen's d = 0.6].

A 2 (suicidal behavior) × 3 (emotion) mixed measures ANOVA was conducted to analyze alpha-asymmetrical index in the emotional Stroop task (where sphericity was violated Greenhouse–Geisser corrections are reported). This showed a significant effect of suicidal behavior [F(1, 50) = 4.024, MSE = 0.484, p = 0.05, partial η^2 = 0.074], with a more positive index in the low-risk

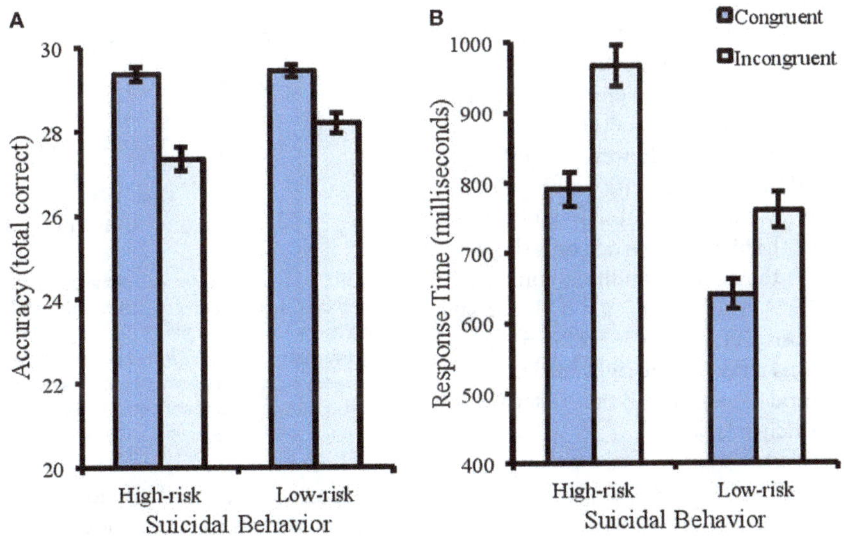

FIGURE 1 | Accuracy (total correct) and RT (ms) in the color Stroop task. Error bars represent standard error of the mean. **(A)** The interaction between suicidal behavior and congruency for accuracy. Reduced accuracy to incongruent trials compared with congruent trials was more apparent for the high-risk group. **(B)** Participants with a high risk of suicide were slower to identify the color of the words (regardless of congruency) than the low-risk group. Response times were also slower to incongruent trials compared with congruent.

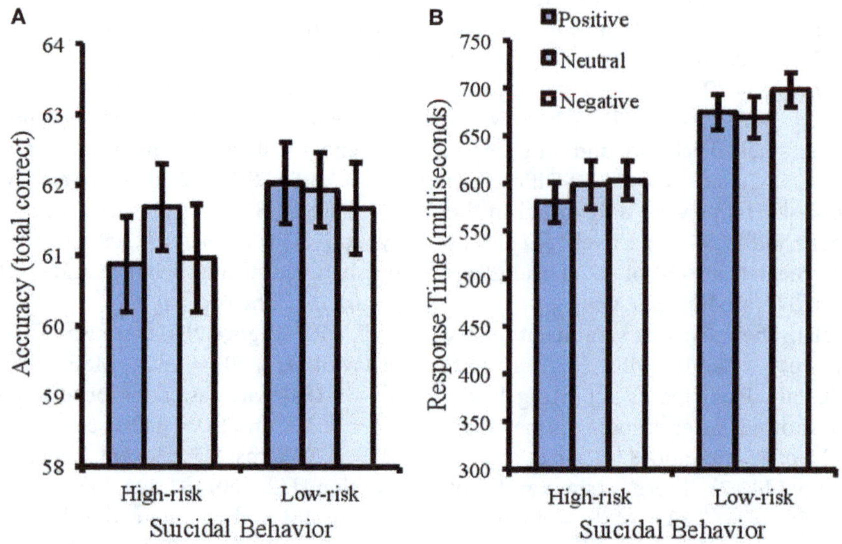

FIGURE 2 | Accuracy (total correct) and response times (ms) in the emotional Stroop task. Error bars represent standard error of the mean. There was a speed-accuracy trade-off in this task whereby the high-risk group responded faster **(B)** but were less accurate **(A)**.

group (M = 0.49uV^2, SD = 0.81) compared with the high-risk group (M = 0.10uV^2, SD = 0.61). With the removal of attempters from the high-risk group, this effect was no longer significant [$F(1, 44) = 2.955$, MSE = 0.501, $p = 0.093$, partial $\eta^2 = 0.063$]. There was also a significant effect of emotion [$F(1.358, 67.91) = 13.73$, MSE = 0.113, $p < 0.001$, partial $\eta^2 = 0.215$]. Planned contrasts were completed to compare asymmetry in the positive and negative conditions to that in the neutral condition. These revealed that the alpha-asymmetry index was significantly higher for negative words (M = 0.44uV^2, SD = 0.78) compared with neutral words [(M = 0.18uV^2, SD = 0.80), $F(1, 50) = 16.632$, MSE = 0.231, $p < 0.001$, partial $\eta^2 = 0.250$] and higher for positive words (M = 0.37uV^2, SD = 0.66) compared with neutral words [$F(1, 50) = 12.852$, MSE = 0.175, $p = 0.001$, partial $\eta^2 = 0.204$]; see **Figure 3**. There was no interaction between emotion and suicidal behavior [$F(1.358, 67.91) = 3.068$, MSE = 0.113, $p = 0.072$, partial $\eta^2 = 0.058$]. This interaction was however significant when attempters were removed from the high-risk group [$F(1.38, 60.902) = 5.312$, MSE = 0.079, $p < 0.05$, partial $\eta^2 = 0.11$]. This supported a trend showing that the high-risk participants showed a negative asymmetry index in the neutral condition compared with the positive [$F(1, 44) = 7.724$, MSE = 0.185, $p < 0.01$, partial $\eta^2 = 0.15$] and negative conditions [$F(1, 44) = 4.565$, MSE = 0.232, $p < 0.05$, partial $\eta^2 = 0.094$]. This reflects more rightward relative to leftward activity in the neutral condition and this pattern was not found for the low-risk participants.

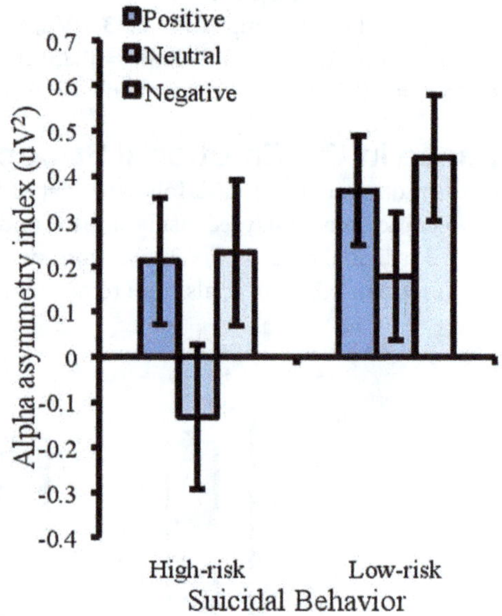

FIGURE 3 | Measures of frontal alpha asymmetry (uV^2) in the emotional Stroop task showing a more positive index for the low-risk group (a positive alpha asymmetry index reflects lower right frontal cortical activity and a negative asymmetry index reflects lower left frontal cortical activity). The asymmetry index was also higher for emotional trials compared with neutral. Error bars represent standard error of the mean.

DISCUSSION

Deficits in cognitive processing and neurological activity have been consistently linked to suicidal behavior in previous research (7, 9, 24) and the current study sought to extend this work by examining the association between frontal asymmetry, attentional control, and suicidal behavior. Frontal asymmetry was compared between individuals reporting high and low levels of suicidal behavior at resting state (both eyes closed and eyes opened), during a color Stroop task, and during an emotional Stroop task. It was predicted that individuals with a high risk of suicidal thoughts and actions would show general difficulties in attentional control, difficulties inhibiting negative stimuli, and reduced leftward-frontal activity.

In the color Stroop task, the high-risk group took significantly longer and were less accurate than the low-risk group to identify the color of each word, regardless of whether this was congruent or incongruent. They were also less accurate when responding to incongruent trials. This shows their difficulties with inhibiting irrelevant information. The results are consistent with previous research [e.g., Ref. (16, 26)], showing that suicidal individuals have more difficulty inhibiting distracting information. Inhibition is one of three components of executive function (15) that contributes to the control and regulation of behavior. It is a crucial element within attentional control and in many every-day tasks an individual needs to inhibit the automatic processing of irrelevant information and direct attention toward relevant information. It is argued that poor attentional control contributes to suicidal behavior as it prevents the disengagement from suicide-related thoughts making one less able to resist suicidal urges (26), and it limits the redirection of resources to more positive information therefore maintaining negative biases.

In contrast to the results of the color Stroop task, in the emotional Stroop task the high-risk group responded quicker than the low-risk group (although this was at the expense of accuracy). This pattern was found for all three types of words (positive, negative, and neutral) and would indicate that those reporting high levels of suicidal behavior are able to inhibit irrelevant information more effectively than those reporting low levels. The overall lack of any emotional Stroop effect within this task is also inconsistent with past findings showing that response times in an emotional Stroop task are generally slower to emotional words compared with neutral words (34, 35). It may be proposed that individuals with a high risk of suicidal behavior are slower to inhibit irrelevant information at a general level, yet when presented with emotional stimuli they may act more quickly and somewhat impulsively (this would be supported by the speed-accuracy trade-off whereby the high-risk group sacrificed accuracy for faster responses). The importance of impulsivity has been identified in the warning signs for suicidal behavior listed by the American Association of Suicidology and includes acting recklessly (77). The Association documented that the presence of impulsivity, inhibitory problems, and inflexible thinking processes may lead to an increased risk of suicidal behavior. Rudd (78) has also incorporated the measures of impulsivity into suicide risk assessment tools. This reflects the proposed importance of executive dysfunction in suicidal behavior with symptoms indicative of poor updating (sustained focus on negative information), shifting (inability to direct resources to task-relevant information), and inhibition (inability to suppress the processing of irrelevant, negative information).

While it may be argued that those with high levels of suicidal behavior can respond more quickly to emotional stimuli compared with neutral, one may question why this group did not show longer response times in the neutral condition of the emotional Stroop task (similar to the color Stroop). This effect illustrates key differences between these two tasks. In particular, in a color Stroop the to-be-ignored information in incongruent trials (the word) is in direct competition with the to-be-identified information (the color). This is not the case in the emotional Stroop task. Consequently the differing patterns of performance across the two tasks may indicate that individuals with a greater risk of suicide will have more difficulty inhibiting directly competing responses, but not information that has no semantic relationship to the task they are completing. Further support for this argument comes from the response times in identifying the color of the word "suicide" in the emotional Stroop task. Results showed that the pattern of performance in the task reversed and those in the high-risk group took longer to respond to the color of this word showing that they have difficulties inhibiting emotionally relevant information. It is proposed that such "personally" relevant information is more salient and despite being irrelevant to the task it competes for attentional resources in the same way that the directly competing word meaning does in the color Stroop.

The bias of attention to emotionally significant stimuli supports the findings of Chung and Jeglic (79) who also reported no emotional Stroop effect in individuals high in suicidal behavior but found evidence for a specific attentional bias to the word "suicide." Cha et al. (80) propose that a stimulus-specific Stroop interference effect (whereby only disorder-related words lead to longer response times) may be particularly useful for clinicians. They found that it was able to predict, above and beyond other clinical measures, those individuals who went on to make a suicide attempt within the following 6 months. Evidently, the current findings support this suggestion, in which a specific attentional bias may exceed the predictive ability of any general negativity bias. This can add to cognitive models that attempt to explain the development and persistence of affective disorders such as depression [e.g., Ref. (17, 18)]. It is theorized that an individual will be automatically distracted by negative information and the processing of this information will lead to an attentional bias. The results of the emotional Stroop task would suggest that these biases are disorder-specific, and while general deficits in top–down control predicted in the model will limit inhibitory processing at a general level (as demonstrated in the Stroop task) it will also manifest in specific impairments in the ability to inhibit disorder-related thoughts and behaviors.

In addition to measuring the importance of attentional control in suicidal behavior, the current study also aimed to determine whether patterns of frontal asymmetry could be used to identify those at risk of suicidal behavior. The dispositional model (45, 46) argues that positive affect is associated with leftward frontal cortical activity and negative affect is associated with rightward frontal cortical activity, whereas the capability model (57) predicts that frontal asymmetrical differences will be more pronounced under specific situational contexts [(57); see also Ref. (81)]. To examine frontal asymmetry in relation to both models, activity was measured during an emotionally challenging state (the emotional Stroop) to see if this may provide a more promising indicator of suicide risk than activity measured during resting state (as favored by the dispositional model) and during a challenging but non-emotional task (the color Stroop).

The EEG recordings in the eyes closed resting state gave no support for the dispositional model as individuals with high and low risk did not differ in their alpha asymmetry index. Although there was a significant group difference during the eyes open resting condition, the difference was opposite to the predictions made. Individuals in the high-risk group had more leftward frontal activity than the low-risk group indicating that this side of the brain is more active at baseline. It is interesting to note that increased leftward frontal activity is associated with the inhibition of negative information (60) and may reflect inhibition of general negative thoughts that an individual with suicidal behavior could be experiencing when not completing a demanding task (this would not be apparent in the low-risk group as it is predicted they would not experience upsetting thoughts and so would not need to engage in inhibition). However, when the EEG recordings were taken during the color Stroop task there was no significant difference in alpha-asymmetrical index between high- and low-risk groups. This reveals that measurements of frontal asymmetry taken during a demanding task are no more effective than those taken in a resting state with regard to identifying individuals high in suicidal behavior. The differences between activity in the Stroop and the eyes open resting state may also suggest that when engaged in a demanding neutral task high-risk participants in the current sample (reporting relatively mild suicidal behavior) are not having to devote additional resources to the inhibition of negative thoughts because the focus on the task itself prevents the processing of such information. Yet the results of asymmetry do not reflect performance in the Stroop task as the high-risk group performed less well than the low-risk group but showed no corresponding differences in frontal asymmetry. This may be due to the fact that stimuli in this task were neutral and therefore any increase in activity is unlikely to be related to specific inhibition of positive (right) or negative (left) information. This indicates a limitation to the use of asymmetry as a marker for affective disorders, including suicide. Compton et al. (28) found increased activity overall in the dlPFC for incongruent trials in a color Stroop and suggested that this shows greater investment in cognitive control processes in order to inhibit this information. Asymmetry does not provide a direct measure of activity and instead shows relative differences between the left and right. Arguably the measure is more relevant to the processing of emotional information if left and right areas are associated with inhibition of negative and positive stimuli respectively.

Consistent with proposals of the capability model, the results did reveal a significant difference in frontal asymmetry between the high- and low-risk groups during the emotional Stroop task. In particular, the low-risk group showed more leftward frontal activation compared with the high-risk group. This suggests greater recruitment of left frontal areas during completion of a task that requires inhibition of emotional information (although not specifically negative information as the models of asymmetry suggest). It should be noted that this effect disappeared when individuals reporting a past suicide attempt were removed from the analysis suggesting that the effect was driven by this subset of participants. This is supported by the findings of Jollant et al. (59) in which asymmetrical differences were only found in individuals with a history of suicide attempt. While behavioral performance in the Stroop tasks may be able to distinguish those at risk of mild levels of suicidal behavior (and would therefore be beneficial in identifying those at risk at an early stage) the same may not be concluded for measures of alpha asymmetry. In addition, the findings for asymmetry do not reflect performance in the task because those in the high-risk group were faster to make accurate responses. Once again this may indicate the limitations of using asymmetry as a marker because it reflects relative activity, it does not show whether an individual is putting more effort overall into the task. A study by Kaiser et al. (82) showed increased activation in the dorsal anterior cingulate cortex and the posterior cingulate cortex for depressed patients when completing a task requiring the inhibition of negative distracters. They proposed that increased activity demonstrates that individuals are devoting more cognitive resources to directing attention away from negative information; however, frontal asymmetry does not provide information about such overall patterns of activity.

Grimshaw and Carmel (60) suggest that inhibition of different emotional stimuli is linked to frontal alpha asymmetry and that individuals will exhibit leftward frontal cortical activity during inhibition of negative stimuli, and rightward frontal cortical activity during inhibition of positive stimuli. Although there is considerable evidence to suggest that frontal asymmetry reflects the inhibitory control of emotions [e.g., Ref. (60, 83); see Ref. (84)], the current findings provide only partial support for the asymmetric inhibition model. Individuals were showing more leftward frontal activation during inhibition of negative stimuli as predicted; however, they did not show an increase in rightward frontal activity when inhibiting positive stimuli. These results are similar to past findings (60, 62) that have shown that the links between cortical activity in the right dlPFC and control of positive distractors are different to those between the left dlPFC and the control of negative distractors. For example, Pérez-Edgar et al. (83) conducted a study investigating frontal asymmetry in relation to attentional bias and avoidance. Frontal EEG was measured from young adults at rest and under a socially threatening situation (preparing to give a short speech about their most embarrassing moment in public). Following this, participants performed a dot probe task in which they had to respond to probes appearing in the same spatial location as emotional faces. Results showed that although frontal alpha asymmetry in the resting state did not predict performance in the dot probe task, there was a strong link between behavioral performance and frontal asymmetry in the socially threatening condition. Specifically, an increase in rightward frontal alpha asymmetry in this condition was associated with increased attentional bias to angry faces and avoidance of happy faces but no association between leftward frontal asymmetry and emotions. This trend was replicated by Grimshaw and Carmel (60) who suggested that positive and negative stimuli may not exert the same level of influence on frontal alpha asymmetry.

One unexpected finding from the alpha asymmetry analysis was the trend toward a negative alpha asymmetry index in the neutral condition of the emotional Stroop task for the high-risk group. This trend did not reach significance until participants reporting a past suicide attempt were removed from the analysis, but the pattern of activation was markedly different to that of the other conditions. The finding shows that the high suicidal behavior group had relatively lower leftward activation in the neutral condition suggesting that they only recruited more left frontal areas when inhibiting emotional but not neutral information. Again, this was not evidenced by differences in performance in this task, providing limiting support for the use of asymmetry as a marker of suicidal behavior, and showing that the exact role of the right and left PFC is not yet apparent with regard to the inhibition of positive and negative distracters. Furthermore, Gable et al. (84) proposed that frontal asymmetry may reflect a wide range of cognitive mechanisms, not just inhibitory processes. For example, the dlPFC is activated during tasks requiring task switching (85), working memory (86), emotion regulation [for a review, see Ref. (30)], and attentional disengagement (87). All of these are implicated in vulnerability to psychopathologies associated with frontal asymmetry (88). These processes also require the executive control components of updating and shifting in addition to inhibition (10, 15, 89). Future work would benefit from recording performance and activity in a wider range of neuropsychological tasks [i.e., Ref. (90)].

The present results show some support for the association between attentional control, frontal asymmetry, and suicidal behavior. However, the findings do not fully support previous work and therefore may indicate that other factors may be involved. In particular, the current results may be influenced by depression. A measure of depression was taken from all participants and analysis showed clear differences between the two groups with the high-risk group reporting significantly higher symptoms of depression. It is well documented that depression is comorbid with suicide [e.g., Ref. (90)] and studies provide strong evidence for the links between depression and executive dysfunction [e.g., Ref. (10)] and depression and frontal asymmetry [e.g., Ref. (41)]. Consequently, the present findings may be showing differences due to depression, rather than suicide. However, researchers argue that the Stroop task is one of very few measures of executive control that is able to identify differences between levels of depression and suicidal behavior. Richard-Devantoy et al. (90) conducted a meta-analysis to explore the findings of studies investigating executive control in patients with mood disorders, patients with mood disorders and reporting a past suicide attempt, and healthy controls. Across a number of tasks designed to assess executive function they found that the patients performed worse than the healthy controls, yet performance in the Stroop task was also able to distinguish suicide attempters from non-attempters. Given the differences between the two groups in the color Stroop task, and the fact that the high-risk group showed a specific attentional bias to suicide-related information, rather than a general negativity bias [e.g., Ref. (37)], it is argued that the present study is assessing suicidal behavior additional to the effects of depression.

While it may be argued that this study assesses suicidal behavior, the results are limited due to the use of the SBQ-R (66). This is a relatively simplistic single-item assessment that groups a variety of quite distinct suicidal behaviors together. Many past studies in this field utilize more in-depth assessments and often use a mixture of clinical measures and interviews. Milner et al. (91) express concern over the use of single-item assessments due to the increased risk of Type-I and -II errors and after conducting an evaluation of such measures they found that many were unable to capture the precise nature of suicide-related thoughts and behaviors that were reported. While these limitations are acknowledged and future research would make use of more detailed measures, it is important to note that the aim of this study was to measure the association of attentional control, asymmetry, and suicidal behavior, rather than to measure whether deficits varied according to the severity of symptoms. The SBQ-R has benefits in this case due to the relative ease of administration.

Related to the measurement of suicide, future studies that explore variations in attentional control due to severity of suicidal behavior may employ a correlational design to allow for the prediction of suicide through measures of executive control. The small sample size and the relatively limited spread of suicidal behavior in the current study supported the use of group comparisons but arguably the findings have no predictive power. Given that past research focuses on more clinical samples, and often uses older patients [e.g., Ref. (26)] one key feature of the present work was to explore possible cognitive deficits associated with relatively mild symptoms of suicidal behavior. By showing that suicidal behavior in a non-clinical population is associated with deficits in attentional control (specifically difficulties inhibiting irrelevant information and an attentional bias to emotionally pertinent information) the current work expands on the past studies. For instance, when comparing executive function in depressed suicide attempters, depressed non-attempters, and healthy controls Keilp et al. (16) supported the findings of Richard-Devantoy et al. (90) by showing that performance in a Stroop task was a "relatively independent marker of suicide risk" (p546). In their study, deficits in attentional control (as evidenced through the Stroop task) were found in all individuals with a history of suicide attempt. In the current study the comparison of attempters and non-attempters was not possible as only 6 of those in the high-risk group reported a past suicide attempt, yet performance in the Stroop task did identify those more vulnerable to suicidal thoughts and behaviors. The findings demonstrate the effectiveness of the Stroop task in assessing vulnerability to suicide in non-clinical samples and support its use in the intervention and prevention of suicidal behavior.

Using EEG in a color Stroop task and an emotional Stroop task, the current study examined whether measures of cognitive and neurological processing can be used to identify individuals at risk of suicidal behavior. The study compared attentional control and frontal asymmetry between individuals reporting high and low levels of suicidal behavior. Results showed that individuals reporting higher levels of suicidal behavior are more likely to encounter difficulties in attentional control and will struggle to disengage attention from suicide-related information. The findings provide relatively limited support for the effectiveness of frontal asymmetry in identifying those vulnerable to suicide, and in line with the capability model of Coan et al. (57) general differences were only apparent in the emotional Stroop task. By exploring executive dysfunction in a non-clinical sample reporting relatively mild symptoms of suicidal behavior the current work lends support to those who advocate the use of the Stroop task in prevention of suicide, showing that its effectiveness extends beyond patient groups.

AUTHOR CONTRIBUTIONS

CT and EO conceived and designed the study. EO gained ethical approval and collected the data. CT and EO analyzed the data and drafted the manuscript.

REFERENCES

1. Silverman MM. The language of suicidology. *Suicide Life Threat Behav* (2006) 36(5):519–32. doi:10.1521/suli.2006.36.5.519
2. Nock MK, Park JM, Finn CT, Deliberto TL, Dour HJ, Banaji MR. Measuring the suicidal mind: implicit cognition predicts suicide behavior. *Psychol Sci* (2010) 21(4):511–7. doi:10.1177/0956797610364762
3. Wilson TD. Know thyself. *Perspect Psychol Sci* (2009) 4(4):384–9. doi:10.1111/j.1745-6924.2009.01143.x
4. Mann JJ, Currier D. A review of prospective studies of biologic predictors of suicidal behavior in mood disorders. *Arch Suicide Res* (2007) 11(1):3–16. doi:10.1080/13811110600993124
5. Mann JJ, Currier D, Stanley B, Oquendo MA, Amsel LV, Ellis SP. Can biological tests assist prediction of suicide in mood disorders? *Int J Neuropsychopharmacol* (2006) 9(4):465–74. doi:10.1017/S1461145705005687
6. Baddeley A. Working memory. *Science* (1992) 255(5044):556–9. doi:10.1126/science.1736359
7. Imbir KK, Jarymowicz MT. The effect of automatic vs. reflective emotions on cognitive control in antisaccade tasks and the emotional Stroop Test. *Polish Psychol Bull* (2013) 44(2):137–46. doi:10.2478/ppb-2013.0016
8. Løvstad M, Sigurdardottir S, Andersson S, Grane VA, Moberget T, Stubberud J, et al. Behavior Rating Inventory of Executive Function Adult Version in patients with neurological and neuropsychiatric conditions: symptom levels and relationship to emotional distress. *J Int Neuropsychol Soc* (2016) 22(6):682–94. doi:10.1017/S135561771600031X
9. Miller EK, Wallis JD. Executive function and higher-order cognition: definition and neural substrates. In: Squire LR, editor. *Encyclopedia of Neuroscience*. (Vol. 4), Oxford: Academic Press (2009). p. 99–104.
10. Joormann J, Tanovic E. Cognitive vulnerability to depression: examining cognitive control and emotion regulation. *Curr Opin Psychol* (2015) 4:86–92. doi:10.1016/j.copsyc.2014.12.006
11. Burgess PW, Veitch E, de Lacy Costello A, Shallice T. The cognitive and neuroanatomical correlates of multitasking. *Neuropsychologia* (2000) 38(6):848–63. doi:10.1016/S0028-3932(99)00134-7
12. Burton CZ, Vella L, Weller JA, Twamley EW. Differential effects of executive functioning on suicide attempts. *J Neuropsychiatry Clin Neurosci* (2011) 23(2):173–9. doi:10.1176/appi.neuropsych.23.2.173
13. Diamond A. Executive functions. *Annu Rev Psychol* (2013) 64:135–68. doi:10.1146/annurev-psych-113011-143750
14. Doty L. *Executive Function & Memory/Cognition Changes*. (2012). Available from: http://alzonline.phhp.ufl.edu/en/reading/executivefxlatest.pdf
15. Miyake A, Friedman NP, Emerson MJ, Witzki AH, Howerter A, Wager TD. The unity and diversity of executive functions and their contributions to complex "frontal lobe" tasks: a latent variable analysis. *Cogn Psychol* (2000) 41:49–100. doi:10.1006/cogp.1999.0734
16. Keilp JG, Gorlyn M, Russell M, Oquendo MA, Burke AK, Harkavy-Friedman J, et al. Neuropsychological function and suicidal behavior: attention control, memory and executive dysfunction in suicide attempt. *Psychol Med* (2013) 43:539–51. doi:10.1017/S0033291712001419
17. Auerbach RP, Webb CA, Gardiner CK, Pechtel P. Behavioral and neural mechanisms underlying cognitive vulnerability models of adolescent depression. *J Psychother Integr* (2013) 23(3):222–35. doi:10.1037/a0031417
18. Disner SG, Beevers CG, Haigh EAP, Beck AT. Neural mechanisms of the cognitive model of depression. *Nat Rev Neurosci* (2011) 12:467–77. doi:10.1038/nrn3027
19. Demeyer I, De Lissnyder E, Koster EH, De Raedt R. Rumination mediates the relationship between impaired cognitive control for emotional information and depressive symptoms: a prospective study in remitted depressed adults. *Behav Res Therapy* (2012) 50(5):292–7. doi:10.1016/j.brat.2012.02.012
20. Gotlib IH, Joormann J. Cognition and depression: current status and future directions. *Annu Rev Clin Psychol* (2010) 6:285–312. doi:10.1146/annurec.clinpsy.121208.131305
21. Desmyter S, van Heeringen C, Audenaert K. Structural and functional neuroimaging studies of the suicidal brain. *Prog Neuropsychopharmacol Biol Psychiatry* (2011) 35(4):796–808. doi:10.1016/j.pnpbp.2010.12.026
22. Jollant F, Lawrence NL, Olié E, Guillaume S, Courtet P. The suicidal mind and brain: a review of neuropsychological and neuroimaging studies. *World J Biol Psychiatry* (2011) 12(5):319–39. doi:10.3109/15622975.2011.556200
23. Carter CS, van Veen V. Anterior cingulate cortex and conflict detection: an update of theory and data. *Cogn Affect Behav Neurosci* (2007) 7(4):367–79. doi:10.3758/CABN.7.4.367
24. Richard-Devantoy S, Courtet P. Neurocognitive processes and decision making in suicidal behavior. In: Kaschka WP, Rujescu D, editors. *Biological Aspects of Suicidal Behavior*. Basel: Karger (2016). p. 88–100.
25. Loyo LMS, Martinez-Velazquez ES, Ramos-Loyo J. The influence of emotions on executive functions in suicide attempters. *Suicidology* (2013) 4:42–55.
26. Richard-Devantoy S, Szanto K, Butters MA, Kalkus J, Dombrovski AY. Cognitive inhibition in older high-lethality suicide attempters. *Int J Geriatr Psychiatry* (2015) 30(3):274–83. doi:10.1002/gps.4138
27. Anderson PJ. Towards a developmental model of executive function. In: Anderson V, Jacobs R, Anderson PJ, editors. *Executive Functions and the Frontal Lobes: A Lifespan Perspective*. New York: Taylor & Francis (2008). p. 23–56.
28. Compton RJ, Banich MT, Mohanty A, Milham MP, Herrington J, Miller GA, et al. Paying attention to emotion: an fMRI investigation of cognitive and emotional Stroop tasks. *Cogn Affect Behav Neurosci* (2003) 3(2):81–96. doi:10.3758/CABN.3.2.81
29. Miyake A, Friedman N. The nature and organization of individual differences in executive functions: four general conclusions. *Curr Direct Psychol Sci* (2012) 21(1):8–14. doi:10.1177/0963721411429458
30. Ochsner KN, Silvers JA, Buhle JT. Functional imaging studies of emotion regulation: a synthetic review and evolving model of the cognitive control of emotion. *Ann N Y Acad Sci* (2012) 1251:E1–24. doi:10.111/j.1749-6632.2012.06751.x
31. Stroop JR. Studies of interference in serial verbal reactions. *J Exp Psychol* (1935) 18(6):643–62. doi:10.1037/h0054651
32. Williams JM, Mathews A, MacLeod C. The emotional Stroop task and psychopathology. *Psychol Bull* (1996) 120(1):3–24. doi:10.1037/0033-2909.120.1.3
33. MacLeod CM. Half a century of research on the Stroop effect: an integrative review. *Psychol Bull* (1991) 109(2):163–203. doi:10.1037/0033-2909.109.2.163
34. Ben-Haim MS, Williams P, Howard Z, Mama Y, Eidels A, Algom D. The emotional Stroop task: assessing cognitive performance under exposure to emotional content. *J Vis Exp* (2016) (112):e53720. doi:10.379/53720
35. Cothran DL, Larsen R. Comparison of inhibition in two timed reaction tasks: the color and emotion Stroop Tasks. *J Psychol* (2008) 142(4):373–85. doi:10.3200/JRLP.142.4.373-385
36. Gilboa-Schechtman E, Revelle W, Gotlib IH. Stroop interference following mood induction: emotionality, mood congruence, and concern relevance. *Cognit Ther Res* (2000) 24(5):491–502. doi:10.1023/A:1005517326981

37. Gotlib IH, Krasnoperova E, Yue DN, Joormann J. Attentional biases for negative interpersonal stimuli in clinical depression. *J Abnorm Psychol* (2004) 113(1):127–35. doi:10.1037/0021-843X.113.1.121
38. Pan LA, Batezati-Alves SC, Almeida JR, Segreti A, Akkal D, Hassel S, et al. Dissociable patterns of neural activity during response inhibition in depressed adolescents with and without suicidal behavior. *J Am Acad Child Adolesc Psychiatry* (2011) 50(6):602–11. doi:10.1016/j.jaac.2011.03.018
39. Gainotti G. Emotional behavior and hemispheric side of the lesion. *Cortex* (1972) 8(1):41–55. doi:10.1016/S0010-9452(72)80026-1
40. Harmon-Jones E, Gable PA, Peterson CK. The role of asymmetric frontal cortical activity in emotion-related phenomena: a review and update. *Biol Psychol* (2010) 84(3):451–62. doi:10.1016/j.biopsyco.2009.08.010
41. Schaffer CE, Davidson RJ, Saron C. Frontal and parietal electroencephalogram asymmetry in depressed and nondepressed subjects. *Biol Psychiatry* (1983) 18(7):753–62.
42. Tomarken AJ, Davidson RJ, Wheeler RE, Doss RC. Individual differences in anterior brain asymmetry and fundamental dimensions of emotion. *J Pers Soc Psychol* (1992) 62(4):676–87. doi:10.1037/0022-3514.62.4.676
43. Tucker DM. Lateral brain function, emotion, and conceptualization. *Psychol Bull* (1981) 89(1):19–46. doi:10.1037/0033-2909.89.1.19
44. Davidson RJ, Fox NA. Asymmetrical brain activity discriminates between positive and negative affective stimuli in human infants. *Science* (1982) 218(4578):1235–7. doi:10.1126/science.7146906
45. Davidson RJ, Schwartz GE, Saron C, Bennett J, Goleman DJ. Frontal versus parietal EEG asymmetry during positive and negative affect. *Psychophysiology* (1979) 16:202–3.
46. Davidson RJ. Hemispheric asymmetry and emotion.In: Scherer K, Ekman P, editors. *Approaches to Emotion*. Hillsdale, NJ: Erlbaum (1984). p. 39–57.
47. Allen JJB, Kline JP. Frontal EEG asymmetry, emotion, and psychopathology: the first, and the next 25 years. *Biol Psychol* (2004) 67(1–2):1–5. doi:10.1016/j.biopsycho.2004.03.001
48. Allen JJB, Reznik SJ. Frontal EEG asymmetry as a promising marker of depression vulnerability: summary and methodological considerations. *Curr Opin Psychol* (2015) 4:93–7. doi:10.1016/jcopsych.2014.12.017
49. Heller W, Levy J. Perception and expression of emotion in right-handers and left-handers. *Neuropsychologia* (1981) 19(2):263–72. doi:10.1016/0028-3932(81)90110-X
50. Thibodeau R, Jorgensen RS, Kim S. Depression, anxiety, and resting frontal EEG asymmetry: a meta-analytic review. *J Abnorm Psychol* (2006) 115(4): 715–29. doi:10.1037/0021-843X.115.4.715
51. Gotlib IH, Ranganath C, Rosenfeld JP. Frontal EEG alpha asymmetry, depression, and cognitive functioning. *Cogn Emot* (1998) 12(3):449–78. doi:10.1080/026999398379673
52. Davidson RJ, Pizzagalli D, Nitschke JB, Putnam K. Depression: perspectives from affective neuroscience. *Annu Rev Psychol* (2002) 53:545–74. doi:10.1146/annurev.psych53.100901.135148
53. Miller EK, Cohen JD. An integrative theory of prefrontal cortex function. *Annu Rev Neurosci* (2001) 24:167–202. doi:10.1146/annurev.neuro.24.1.167
54. Miller GA, Crocker LD, Spielberg JM, Infantolino ZP, Heller W. Issues in localization of brain function: the case of lateralized frontal cortex in cognition, emotion, and psychopathology. *Front Integr Neurosci* (2013) 7:2. doi:10.3389/fnint.2013.00002
55. Stewart JL, Bismark AW, Towers DN, Coan JA, Allen JJ. Resting frontal EEG asymmetry as an endophenotype for depression risk: sex-specific patterns of frontal brain asymmetry. *J Abnorm Psychol* (2010) 119(3):502–12. doi:10.1037/a0019196
56. Saletu B, Anderer P, Saletu-Zyhlarz GM. EEG topography and tomography (LORETA) in diagnosis and pharmacotherapy of depression. *Clin EEG Neurosci* (2010) 41(4):203–10. doi:10.1177/155005941004100407
57. Coan JA, Allen JJB, McKnight PE. A capability model of individual differences in frontal EEG asymmetry. *Biol Psychol* (2006) 72(2):198–207. doi:10.1016/j.biopsycho.2005.10.003
58. Coan JA, Allen JJ. Frontal EEG asymmetry as a moderator and mediator of emotion. *Biol Psychol* (2004) 67(1–2):7–49. doi:10.1016/j.biopsycho.2004.03.002
59. Jollant F, Lawrence NS, Giampietro V, Brammer MJ, Fullana MA, Drapier D, et al. Orbitofrontal cortex response to angry faces in men with histories of suicide attempts. *Am J Psychiatry* (2008) 165(6):740–8. doi:10.1176/appi.ajp.2008.07081239
60. Grimshaw GM, Carmel D. An asymmetric inhibition model of hemispheric differences in emotional processing. *Front Psychol* (2014) 5(489):1–7. doi:10.3389/fpsyg.2014/00489
61. Engels AS, Heller W, Spielberg JM, Warren SL, Sutton BP, Banich MT, et al. Co-occurring anxiety influences patterns of brain activity in depression. *Cogn Affect Behav Neurosci* (2010) 10(1):141–56. doi:10.3758/CABN.10.1.141
62. Herrington JD, Heller W, Mohanty A, Engels AS, Banich MT, Webb AG, et al. Localization of asymmetric brain function in emotion and depression. *Psychophysiology* (2010) 47(3):442–54. doi:10.1111/j.1469-8986.2009.00958.x
63. Crocker LD, Heller W, Spielberg JM, Warren SL, Bredemeier K, Sutton BP, et al. Neural mechanisms of attentional control differentiate trait and state negative affect. *Front Psychol* (2012) 3(298):298. doi:10.3389/fpsyg.2012.00298
64. Palmer CJ. Suicide attempt history, self-esteem, and suicide risk in a sample of 116 depressed voluntary inpatients. *Psychol Rep* (2004) 95:1092–4. doi:10.2466/pr0.95.3f.1092-1094
65. Klonsky ED, May AM. Differentiating suicide attempters from suicide ideators: a critical frontier for suicidology research. *Suicide Life Threat Behav* (2014) 44(1):1–5. doi:10.1111/sltb.12068
66. Osman A, Bagge CL, Gutierrez PM, Konick LC, Kopper BA, Barrios FX. The Suicidal Behaviors Questionnaire-Revised (SBQ-R): validation with clinical and nonclinical samples. *Assessment* (2001) 8(4):443–54. doi:10.1177/107319110100800409
67. Aloba O, Ojeleye O, Aloba T. The psychometric characteristics of the 4-item Suicidal Behaviors Questionnaire-Revised (SBQ-R) as a screening tool in a non-clinical sample of Nigerian university students. *Asian J Psychiatr* (2017) 26:46–51. doi:10.1016/j.ajp.2017.01.017
68. Cotton CR, Peters DK, Range LM. Psychometric properties of the Suicidal Behaviors Questionnaire. *Death Stud* (1995) 19:391–7. doi:10.1080/07481189508252740
69. Rueda-Jaimes GE, Corzo-Casasadiego JD, Moreno-Quijano C, Camacho PA. Validity of the Suicide Behaviors Questionnaire-Revised in patients with short-term suicide risk. *Eur J Psychiatry* (2017) 31(4):145–50. doi:10.1016/j.ejpsy.2017.09.002
70. Bradley MM, Lang PJ. *Affective Norms for English Words (ANEW): Instruction Manual and Affective Ratings*. Technical report C-1. The Center for Research in Psychophysiology, Gainesville: University of Florida (1999).
71. Beck AT, Steer RA, Brown GK. *Manual for the Beck Depression Inventory-II*. San Antonio, TX: Psychological Corporation (1996)
72. Malmivuo J, Plonsey R. *Bioelectromagnetism: Principles and Applications of Bioelectric and Biomagnetic Fields*. New York: Oxford University Press (1995).
73. Delorme A, Makeig S. EEGLAB: an open source toolbox for analysis of single-trial EEG dynamics including independent component analysis. *J Neurosci Methods* (2004) 134(1):9–21. doi:10.1016/j.neumeth.2003.10.009
74. The MathWorks. *MATLAB and Statistics Toolbox Release*. Natick, MA: The MathWorks, Inc. (2007).
75. Allen J, Urry H, Hitt SK, Coan JA. The stability of resting frontal electroencephalographic asymmetry in depression. *Psychophysiology* (2004) 41(2): 269–80. doi:10.1111/j.1469-8986.2003.00149.x
76. Oakes TR, Pizzagalli DA, Hendrick AM, Horras KA, Larson CL, Abercrombie HC, et al. Functional coupling of simultaneous electrical and metabolic activity in the human brain. *Hum Brain Mapp* (2004) 21(4):257–70. doi:10.1002/hbm.20004
77. American Association of Suicidology. *Know the Warning Signs of Suicide*. (2017). Available from: http://www.suicidology.org/resources/warning-signs
78. Rudd MD. Fluid vulnerability theory: a cognitive approach to understanding the process of acute and chronic suicide risk. In: Ellis TE, editor. *Cognition and Suicide: Theory, Research, and Therapy*. Washington, DC: American Psychological Association (2006). p. 355–68.
79. Chung Y, Jeglic E. Use of the modified emotional Stroop task to detect suicidality in college population. *Suicide Life Threat Behav* (2016) 46(1):55–66. doi:10.1111/sltb.1274
80. Cha CB, Najmi S, Park JM, Finn CT, Nock MK. Attentional bias toward suicide-related stimuli predicts suicidal behavior. *J Abnorm Psychol* (2010) 119(3):616–22. doi:10.1037/a0019710

81. Stewart JL, Coan JA, Towers DN, Allen JJ. Resting and task-elicited prefrontal EEG alpha asymmetry in depression: support for the capability model. *Psychophysiology* (2014) 51(5):446–55. doi:10.111/psyp.12191
82. Kaiser RH, Andrews-Hanna JR, Spielberg JM, Warren SL, Sutton BP, Miller GA, et al. Distracted and down: neural mechanisms of affective interference in subclinical depression. *Soc Cogn Affect Neurosci* (2014) 10(5):654–633. doi:10.1093/scan/nsu100
83. Pérez-Edgar K, Kujawa A, Nelson SK, Cole C, Zapp DJ. The relation between electroencephalogram asymmetry and attention biases to threat at baseline and under stress. *Brain Cogn* (2013) 82(3):337–43. doi:10.1016/j.bandc.2013.05.009
84. Gable PA, Mechin NC, Hicks JA, Adams DL. Supervisory control system and frontal asymmetry: neurophysiological traits of emotion-based impulsivity. *Soc Cogn Affect Neurosci* (2015) 10(10):1310–5. doi:10.1093/scan/nsv017
85. Ambrosini E, Vallesi A. Asymmetry in prefrontal resting-state EEG spectral power underlies individual differences in phasic and sustained cognitive control. *Neuroimage* (2016) 124:843–57. doi:10.1016/j.neuroimage.2015.09.035
86. Petrides M. The role of the mid-dorsolateral prefrontal cortex in working memory. *Exp Brain Res* (2000) 133(1):44–54. doi:10.1007/s002210000399
87. Vanderhasselt MA, Kühn S, DeRaedt R. Healthy brooders employ more attentional resources when disengaging from the negative: an event-related fMRI study. *Cogn Affect Behav Neurosci* (2011) 11(2):207–16. doi:10.3758/s13415-011-0022-5
88. Snyder HR. Major depressive disorder is associated with broad impairments on neuropsychological measures of executive function: a meta-analysis and review. *Psychol Bull* (2013) 139(1):81–132. doi:10.1037/a0028727
89. Schmeichel BJ, Tang D. Individual differences in executive functioning and their relationship to emotional processes and responses. *Curr Direct Psychol Sci* (2015) 24(2):93–8. doi:10.1177/0963721414555178
90. Richard-Devantoy S, Berlim MT, Jollant E. A meta-analysis of neuropsychological markers of vulnerability to suicidal behavior in mood disorders. *Psychol Med* (2013) 44:1663–73. doi:10.1017/S0033291713002304
91. Milner AJ, Lee MD, Nock MK. Single-item measurement of suicidal behaviors: validity and consequences of misclassification. *PLoS One* (2015) 10(10):e0141606. doi:10.1371/journal.pone.0141606

21

The Zero Suicide Model: Applying Evidence-Based Suicide Prevention Practices to Clinical Care

Beth S. Brodsky[1,2], Aliza Spruch-Feiner[2] and Barbara Stanley[1,2]*

[1] Department of Psychiatry, Columbia University College of Physicians and Surgeons, New York, NY, United States,
[2] New York State Psychiatric Institute, New York, NY, United States

***Correspondence:**
Beth S. Brodsky
beth.brodsky@nyspi.columbia.edu*

Suicide is reaching epidemic proportions, with over 44,000 deaths by suicide in the US, and 800,000 worldwide in 2015. This, despite research and development of evidence-based interventions that target suicidal behavior directly. Suicide prevention efforts need a comprehensive approach, and research must lead to effective implementation across public and mental health systems. A 10-year systematic review of evidence-based findings in suicide prevention summarized the areas necessary for translating research into practice. These include risk assessment, means restriction, evidence-based treatments, population screening combined with chain of care, monitoring, and follow-up. In this article, we review how suicide prevention research informs implementation in clinical settings where those most at risk present for care. Evidence-based and best practices address the fluctuating nature of suicide risk, which requires ongoing risk assessment, direct intervention and monitoring. In the US, the National Action Alliance for Suicide Prevention has put forth the Zero Suicide (ZS) Model, a framework to coordinate a multilevel approach to implementing evidence-based practices. We present the Assess, Intervene and Monitor for Suicide Prevention model (AIM-SP) as a guide for implementation of ZS evidence-based and best practices in clinical settings. Ten basic steps for clinical management model will be described and illustrated through case vignette. These steps are designed to be easily incorporated into standard clinical practice to enhance suicide risk assessment, brief interventions to increase safety and teach coping strategies and to improve ongoing contact and monitoring of high-risk individuals during transitions in care and high risk periods.

Keywords: suicide, prevention, evidence-based, psychology, interventions

Suicide is a public health crisis reaching epidemic proportions and has claimed the lives of over 44,000 individuals in the US in 2015 (1) and 800,000 people worldwide in the past year. These figures reflect an increase in death by suicide by over 25% in the US (2), and 4% internationally in the last decade (3), despite increases in multitiered suicide prevention strategies and research. A 10-year systematic review of nearly 1,800 studies (4) highlighted the importance of increasing and coordinating the application of evidence-based suicide prevention strategies and concluded that research needs to lead to implementation across public health and clinical mental health systems.

In the US, the National Action Alliance for Suicide Prevention has put forth the Zero Suicide (ZS) Model, a framework and resources to coordinate a multilevel approach to implementing evidence-based practices for suicide prevention. Founded on the principle that death by suicide is preventable for patients in behavioral health systems, the ZS model offers an integrated, system-wide strategy for suicide prevention. Four components (Identify, Engage, Treat, and Transition) address aspects of clinical care, while the other three (Lead, Train, and Improve) concern administrative approaches.

The ZS elements of clinical care dictate that systematic protocols should involve ongoing risk screening and assessment, collaborative safety planning, access to evidence-based suicide-specific care, focus on lethal means reduction, consistent engagement efforts, and support during high risk periods. We will update the current state of knowledge regarding evidence-based and best clinical practice for suicide prevention, and describe how the ZS model informs application of these practices to clinical training and practice. We present a case vignette to illustrate 10 basic steps for best practice clinical suicide management, based on the ZS model.

THE ZS MODEL AND CLINICAL TRAINING

The Assess, Intervene and Monitor for Suicide Prevention model (AIM-SP) (5) model is proposed as a framework for implementing ZS in clinical care. "Assess" refers to the use of systematic screening and comprehensive risk assessment to identify at-risk patients. "Intervene" consists of conducting suicide-specific brief and psychosocial interventions. "Monitor" provides strategies for ongoing monitoring and increased contact during known high risk periods. AIM-SP provides guidelines for clinical training and best practice in suicide prevention that can be applied in a wide range of care settings.

Screening and Risk Assessment

Several approaches to suicide risk assessment have been developed and disseminated. The Columbia Suicide Severity Rating Scale (C-SSRS) is a validated and reliable instrument that measures current and past suicidal ideation, suicide attempts, preparatory behaviors as well as non-suicidal self-injury (NSSI), a deliberate self-harm behavior performed with no intent to die (6–8). The severity and intensity of suicidal ideation, lifetime suicide attempt and NSSI, as measured by the C-SSRS, were found to predict future suicide attempts among adolescent and young adult psychiatric emergency department (ED) patients (9). These findings contribute to the existing literature on the validity of the C-SSRS as a screening method for longitudinally predicting future suicidal behaviors (10, 11).

Other approaches consider risk factors besides suicidal ideation and behavior such as demographics, psychiatric and family history, diagnosis, trauma, and protective factors. The Suicide Assessment Five-step Evaluation and Triage (SAFE-T) (12) instrument guides clinicians to identify risk and protective factors, inquire into suicidal thoughts, plans, behavior and intent, determine risk level, and choose an appropriate intervention. SAFE-T incorporates the American Psychiatric Association Practice Guidelines for suicide assessment (13). Teaching the SAFE-T to ED nurses has been shown to enhance suicide inquiry, and increase knowledge regarding identifying risk and protective factors and determining risk level and appropriate intervention (14).

Psychosocial Treatment Interventions

Cognitive behavior therapy (CBT) and dialectical behavior therapy (DBT) are suicide-specific psychosocial treatments with evidence base in reducing suicidality in certain populations (4, 15). Randomized controlled trials (RCTs) indicate that the most effective psychosocial treatment interventions are cognitive behavioral therapies and others with interpersonal orientations that target precipitants to self-harm (16). Brief CBT, web-based CBT, CBT-/DBT-informed family treatment and DBT are effective in reducing suicidal ideation (17); preventing the onset of suicidal ideation (18); preventing post treatment suicide attempts and reattempts (19–22); decreasing hospitalizations and ED visits; and lowering medical risk of self-injurious acts (20). DBT skills training is efficacious in reducing NSSI acts (23). In addition, the suicide-specific intervention, Collaborative Assessment and Management of Suicidality (CAMS) in comparison with treatment as usual, was found to decrease suicidal ideation and related cognitions in inpatients receiving individual therapy from CAMS-trained clinicians (24, 25). The efficacy of these specific treatment interventions may vary when applied to special high risk populations (e.g., people with schizophrenia, or prison populations).

Additional research is needed to gain knowledge regarding the specific populations in which each psychosocial treatment is most efficacious, and the components of the treatments that most effectively reduce suicide-related symptoms. Obstacles to implementation such as lack of clinician training in these approaches need to be overcome through increased implementation research and dissemination efforts.

Brief Interventions

The safety plan intervention (SPI) (26) is a best practice brief intervention (27, 28) that incorporates evidence-based suicide risk reduction strategies such as lethal means reduction, brief problem solving and coping skills, increasing social support and identifying emergency contacts to use during a suicide crisis. In conducting a SPI, clinician and client collaborate to develop a six-step plan for staying safe. These include: identifying warning signs, individual coping skills, people and places for distraction, people to contact for help, professionals to contact for help, and steps for means safety.

Crisis response planning (29, 30) is a brief intervention (27) in which individuals use a small card to write out steps for self-identifying personal warning signs, coping strategies, enlisting social support, and accessing professional services. Within a sample of high-risk active duty soldiers, crisis response planning was found more effective than contracts for safety in preventing attempts, reducing suicide ideation and hospitalization (31).

Lethal Means Restriction

Suicides decreased following legislation pertaining to the restriction of firearms, pesticides, barbiturate prescriptions, detoxification of domestic gas, modification of analgesics packaging, mandated use of catalytic converters in automobiles, erection of barriers at common jumping locations, lowered toxicity of antidepressants (32), and restricted access to charcoal (33). The "Access to Lethal

Means" (CALM) training on strategies for talking to patients about means reduction increases gatekeeper confidence in ability to care for suicidal patients, and fosters positive changes in clinician practice. The SPI enhances clinical practice in means reduction. After receiving instructions to give the SPI to patients with positive suicide screens, nurses with no formal training were nevertheless more likely to ask about access to lethal means (34).

Follow-up and Monitoring

The practice of contacting people and providing support after discharge from the ED or after being identified as at risk for suicide reduces suicidal behaviors and deaths (4). The Brief Intervention and Contact (BIC), a 1-hour information session and follow-up contact after ED discharge was associated with a reduced number of suicide deaths in the 18 months following discharge in a five-country RCT (35). Multidisciplinary chain-of-care networks for suicide attempters following hospitalization in Norway have resulted in lower rates of repeat attempts (36). Active contact and follow-up was found effective in preventing repeat attempts over a year following admission to the ED for suicide attempts (37), and in-person and telephone follow-ups reduced suicidal thoughts and increased hope in suicide attempters (38). In a review of 11 empirical studies of follow-up interventions (i.e., phone, postal letter, postcards, in-person, e-mail, and texting), five demonstrated significant decreases in suicidal behavior (39). A combined safety planning/structured follow-up intervention (SPI-SFU) in the VA was viewed as acceptable and helpful in preventing future suicidal behavior and promoting treatment engagement (40, 41). Social support strategies can also be employed to follow-up with and monitor individuals following suicidal behaviors. In India, a peer support intervention led to a 36% decrease in suicide attempts (42). The Attempted Suicide Short Intervention Program (ASSIP) involves numerous elements including safety planning and semistandardized letters over a span of 2 years. Results from a randomized control trial (43) suggest that ASSIP effectively reduced the risk of suicide reattempts by 80%, and led to significantly less time spent in hospitals at follow-up.

APPLYING THE ZS/AIM MODEL TO CLINICAL TRAINING

The evidence base provides important information regarding the interventions that can help prevent suicide. A next crucial step is to apply evidence based suicide prevention interventions to the clinical training of health and mental health professionals.

Fluctuations in Suicide Risk

Evidence-based best practices address managing the fluctuation of suicide risk over time. A study using ecological momentary assessment (44) found that suicidal ideation, hopelessness, burdensomeness and loneliness varied considerably over the course of hours and days. Suicidal ideation has been found to recur with the emergence of depressive episodes (45). In a large community survey, suicidal ideation was reported to fluctuate irregularly prior to suicide attempt (46), and variability in suicidal ideation predicts future attempts (47).

Gaps in Training

Despite updated guidelines for suicide prevention training in the fields of psychology, social work and psychiatry (48, 49) in the US, formal training in suicide risk assessment and management remains limited (50). There is a gap in clinical "training as usual" that needs to be filled by evidence-based clinical approaches to identify, monitor and treat fluctuations in suicide risk. For example, historically, clinical approaches have relied on the use of "safety contracts" in which clinicians ask that patients sign contracts stating that they will either not act on or reach out for help when experiencing suicidal urges. However, there is little evidence that these contracts are effective (51).

Filling the Gap in Clinical Training

The AIM-SP model offers 10 steps for applying best suicide prevention practices to everyday clinical care (**Figure 1**). We present the case of Paul to illustrate 10 basic clinical interventions for the management of suicidal behavior in an ongoing outpatient treatment, which represents only one example as to how the model informs clinical care. The Assess, Intervene and Monitor framework for suicide prevention can be applied in other settings such as inpatient or prison environments, but many require modifications of these 10 steps.

Case Vignette

Paul is a 32-year-old single, college educated white male. He lives with a roommate and works as a graphic artist. He is talented, gets jobs easily, but has trouble keeping them. He experiences intense shame about the quality of his work. Paul periodically engages in non-suicidal self-injurious behaviors by cutting himself without suicidal intent on his upper arms with a knife. He has never tried to end his life but has had intermittent active suicidal ideation with a plan to jump from the roof of his building. On two occasions, he has gone to the roof and contemplated jumping but did not. Paul abuses alcohol, and binges on cocaine. He has aggressive episodes (e.g., gets into verbal confrontations with strangers). Paul reports being physically abused by his older brother until he was 10 years old. Paul had 3 years of outpatient therapy for depression and has been to the ED twice for NSSI behavior and active suicidal ideation. His ideation and urges to self-harm fluctuate.

How Can the 10 Clinical Steps Be Applied to an Ongoing Outpatient Treatment with Paul?

Assess

Step 1: Inquire explicitly about suicidal ideation and behavior, past and present

The first step in assessing Paul's suicide risk at any given moment is to explicitly ask whether he is having any suicidal thoughts. Paul's clinician should not assume that he is not suicidal if he does not report it. By neglecting to ask, Paul might feel that the clinician doesn't care or doesn't really want to know.

Clinicians are often reluctant to ask directly. In a 2014 survey of clinicians across New York State, 20% reported discomfort in asking about suicide, and 12% would not bring up the topic of suicide even if the patient's record or actions indicated risk (52).

Assess	Step 1: Inquire explicitly about suicide ideation and behavior, past and present.
	Step 2: Identify risk factors in addition to suicidal ideation and behavior.
	Step 3: Implement and maintain continued focus on safety.
Intervene	Step 4: Introduce and develop a collaborative safety plan intervention for managing suicidality, including lethal means restriction.
	Step 5: Initiate coping strategies and supports.
	Step 6: Integrate suicide-specific treatment targets in treatment planning process.
Monitor	Step 7: Increase flexibility and contact availability.
	Step 8: Initiate increased monitoring during periods of highest risk.
	Step 9: Involve family and other social supports.
	Step 10: Invoke clinician peer support and consultation .

FIGURE 1 | The AIM-SP model's 10 steps for applying best suicide prevention practices to everyday clinical care.

Clinicians feel unsure of how to intervene with someone who is at current risk for suicide, and they may erroneously believe that asking might introduce the idea.

A clinician can facilitate disclosure by building rapport and by establishing a collaborative agreement to monitor suicidal ideation. When asking directly, the clinicians should be matter-of-fact, but also warm, supportive and respectful. Knowing what to do can help the clinician balance concern with a sense of calm, to take the patient's experiences seriously without displaying anxiety. Such an approach can facilitate open communication and possibly avoid hospitalization.

Step 2: Identify risk factors in addition to suicidal ideation and behavior

Fifty percent of those who die by suicide do so after their first and only attempt (53). Thus, in addition to fluctuating suicidal ideation, urges, suicidal and NSSI behaviors, it is important to consider non-suicide based factors that contribute to risk. The following are population based risk factors:

Demographics: male, Caucasian, age 44–65 and 85+.

- Psychiatric diagnoses: major depression, bipolar disorder, schizophrenia, BPD, PTSD, substance use, and eating disorders.
- Abuse history.
- Recent activating events: Interpersonal loss, financial, or medical problems.
- History of treatment non-adherence.
- Access to lethal means.

Protective factors: support system, religious/spiritual beliefs (e.g., that suicide is a sin), family/children, fear of dying.

Paul has no history of suicide attempts, but has two "aborted attempts" in which he started to act but stopped himself before engaging in self-harm. He also engages in NSSI behavior. Paul fits into a high risk demographic (white male entering middle age), has been diagnosed with Major Depressive Disorder and Borderline Personality Disorder, and abuses substances. He also has impulsive aggressive personality traits, a history of childhood physical abuse, and access to means (knives, rooftop, pills).

Protective factors should also be assessed. Paul is smart and talented, and likeable when not in a stormy aggressive mood. Relationships with his mother and best friend are his stated reasons for living, and he has supportive family members in his life—his uncle and cousin.

Risk Factors Specific to Paul—Precipitants/Recent Activating Events

For Paul, nearing a deadline on an artistic project (shame about it not being good enough and fear of exposure) is a precipitating event that can trigger suicidal ideation. Depressed mood in and of itself is NOT a risk factor for Paul's suicidal ideation, but it does make him more vulnerable to being triggered. Increased use of alcohol and cocaine are warning signs for suicidal spikes.

Step 3: Implement and maintain continued focus on safety

Since suicidal urges fluctuate, an evidence-based clinical approach to suicide prevention necessitates ongoing assessment and continued focus on safety. Clinicians should explicitly inquire about suicidal thoughts, urges, or behaviors at each contact, and revisit and update plans for staying safe. Paul and his therapist agreed to check in about his suicidal thoughts and self-harm urges at each visit.

Intervene

Step 4: Introduce and develop a collaborative SPI for managing suicidality, including lethal means reduction

The SPI allows clinician and patient to develop a plan (26) for recognizing warning signs of spikes in and periods of higher risk and how to maintain safety. Safety planning increases mastery and self-efficacy for coping with suicidal urges. It can be used in both ongoing outpatient psychotherapy treatments as well as a single clinical contact such as during an ED visit. The SPI is a collaborative brief intervention that can be completed in one 30–45-min session, and then revisited/revised periodically. The six steps of the SPI are to identify: (1) warning signs, (2) internal coping strategies, (3) people and social settings that provide distraction, (4) people to contact for help, (5) professionals/agencies to contact, and (6) ways to make the environment safe.

When reviewing the last step, the clinician asks about access to and availability of means, especially those that are part of a suicide plan. These include: firearms, pills or other ingestible poisons, sharp objects such as knives/scissors/razors, proximity to high places such as rooftops/bridges, and the opportunity for hanging or asphyxiation.

Step 5: Initiate coping strategies and supports

The second step of the SPI is to generate a list of coping skills to use to manage suicidal urges independently. DBT distress tolerance skills for distraction and self-soothing (54) can be a helpful resource. See **Figure 2** for Paul's safety plan.

Step 6: Integrate suicide-specific treatment targets

Suicidal behavior is being increasingly understood as a symptom in its own right that needs to be specifically targeted in treatment (55). It is not enough to focus exclusively on non-suicidal treatment targets such as depressed mood or anxiety. Suicide–specific treatments (56) prioritize life threatening behaviors and offer a collaborative approach to engaging the patient in ongoing monitoring of suicidal thoughts, urges and behaviors. Paul's treatment focuses explicitly on his suicidal ideation, urges and NSSI behaviors.

Monitor

Step 7: Increase flexibility and contact availability

The ZS model recommends provision of increased contact during periods of suicidal crises. This can take the form of increased number of appointments, and availability for between session check-ins by phone or e-mail. Following discharge from an inpatient or ED setting, follow-up phone calls or other forms of non in-person contact (e.g., letters; texts) can provide some sense of continuity of care. The AIM-SP model Structured Follow Up and Monitoring Intervention outlines the following process for making follow-up calls: 1. assessing mood and safety; 2. reviewing and revising the individual's safety plan; 3. problem solving obstacles to follow-up care.

Step 8: Initiate increased monitoring during periods of highest risk

Knowing when to increase monitoring is key. Periods following a suicide attempt or suicide crisis, discharge from inpatient hospitalizations, an ED visit, transfer from higher to lower level of care, are well-known high-risk times. During care transitions, it is good practice to call other providers to give a "warm handoff".

Step 9: Involve family and other social supports

With permission, a clinician can involve members of the individual's support network to create a safety net. The clinician should obtain emergency contact information at initial contact,

Step 1. Warning signs	Isolating, feelings of self-hate and intense shame, urges to use cocaine
Step 2. Internal coping strategies	Video games, taking a bike ride
Step 3. People and social settings for distraction	Roommate, school friends, on-line chat rooms
Step 4: People to contact for help	Uncle, cousin, roommate
Step 5: Professionals/agencies to contact	Therapist, crisis hotline, ED
Step 6: Making the environment safe	Cleansing the environment of X-ACTO knifes (gave them to therapist) Limiting the amount of medication prescribed at any one time Deleting the phone number of drug dealer from his phone Having a plan in place to stay away from his rooftop when urges occur

FIGURE 2 | Paul's Safety Plan.

and encourage involving friends, family and other supports in treatment planning, means restriction and safety planning. Paul agreed to have his uncle and cousin involved in his care. They are a part of his safety plan and sometimes attend his therapy sessions. They help monitor Paul during high risk periods, check in with him regularly, and reach out to his clinician when necessary.

Step 10: Invoke clinician peer support and consultation

The clinician can also seek peer support for consultation and supervision regarding high risk patients. This includes maintaining contact and taking a team approach with other health providers involved with the patient, and reaching out when necessary to coordinate safety efforts.

SUMMARY

The ZS Initiative has been proposed by the United States National Alliance for Suicide Prevention and adopted by many health care systems in the US. We present the Assess, Intervene and Monitor for Suicide Prevention model (AIM-SP) to facilitate the implementation of the four clinical components, Identify, Engage, Treat, and Transition, of the ZS Model into an ongoing outpatient psychotherapy treatment. AIM-SP provides a framework for incorporating evidence-based and best suicide prevention approaches into clinical practice, and can inform training efforts to further disseminate evidence-based suicide prevention clinical practices. Future ZS efforts will include the application of this framework to other clinical and non-clinical medical settings, such as psychiatric inpatient services, psychiatric and medical EDs, primary care, and forensic settings.

AUTHOR CONTRIBUTIONS

BB: first author developed content, oversaw coauthor work, wrote majority of manuscript, and made final edits. AS-F: drafted and edited introduction and literature review, researched, and collated references. BS: developed and wrote AIM model and Safety Plan Intervention content, and made final edits.

REFERENCES

1. Center for Disease Control and Prevention (CDCP). *Web-Based Injury Statistics Query and Reporting System (WISQARS)*. (2017). Available from: http://www.cdc.gov/injury/wisqars/
2. Curtin SC, Werner M, Hedegaard H. *Data Brief 241: Increase in Suicide in the United States, 1999–2014*. Centers for Disease Control and Prevention (2016). Available from: https://www.cdc.gov/nchs/data/databriefs/db241_table.pdf#1
3. World Health Organization. *Global Health Estimates 2015: Deaths by Cause, Age, Sex, by Country and by Region, 2000–2015*. Geneva: Hinari (2016).
4. Zalsman G, Hawton K, Wasserman D, van Heeringen K, Arensman E, Sarchiapone M, et al. Suicide prevention strategies revisited: 10-year systematic review. *Lancet Psychiatry* (2016) 3(7):646–59. doi:10.1016/S2215-0366(16)30030-X
5. Stanley B. *Zero Suicide: Implementation and Evaluation in Outpatient Mental Health Clinics*. Las Vegas, NV: IASR/AFSP Suicide Research Summit (2017).
6. Claes L, Muehlenkamp J, Vandereycken W, Hamelinck L, Martens H, Claes S. Comparison of non-suicidal self-injurious behavior and suicide attempts in patients admitted to a psychiatric crisis unit. *Pers Individ Dif* (2010) 48:83–7. doi:10.1016/j.paid.2009.09.001
7. Posner K, Brown GK, Stanley B, Brent DA, Yershova KV, Oquendo MA, et al. The Columbia-Suicide Severity Rating Scale: initial validity and internal consistency findings from three multisite studies with adolescents and adults. *Am J Psychiatry* (2011) 168(12):1266–77. doi:10.1176/appi.ajp.2011.10111704
8. Gipson PY, Agarwala P, Opperman KJ, Horwitz A, King CA. Columbia-Suicide Severity Rating Scale: predictive validity with adolescent psychiatric emergency patients. *Pediatr Emerg Care* (2015) 31(2):88–94. doi:10.1097/PEC.0000000000000225
9. Horwitz AG, Czyz EK, King CA. Predicting future suicide attempts among adolescent and emerging adult psychiatric emergency patients. *J Clin Child Adolesc Psychol* (2014) 44(5):751–61. doi:10.1080/15374416.2014.910789
10. Chappell P, Feltner DE, Makumi C, Pharm D, Stewart M. Initial validity and reliability data on the Columbia-Suicide Severity Rating scale. *Am J Psychiatry* (2012) 169(6):662–3; author reply 663. doi:10.1176/appi.ajp.2012.12010123
11. Viguera AC, Milano N, Ralston L, Thompson NR, Griffith SD, Baldessarini RJ, et al. Comparison of electronic screening for suicidal risk with the Patient Health Questionnaire item 9 and the Columbia Suicide Severity Rating Scale in an outpatient psychiatric clinic. *Psychosomatics* (2015) 56(5):460–9. doi:10.1016/j.psym.2015.04.005
12. Jacobs D. *Suicide Assessment Five-Step Evaluation and Triage for Mental Health Professionals (SAFE-T)*. (2009). Available from: www.sprc.org
13. American Psychiatric Association. Practice guideline for the assessment and treatment of patients with suicidal behaviors. *Am J Psychiatry* (2003) 160 (11 Suppl):1–60.
14. Rico E. *Teaching and Evaluation of Suicidal Assessment, Five-Step Evaluation and Triage (SAFE-T) in the Emergency Department [Doctoral Projects]*. San Jose California: California State University (2016). 38 p.
15. Linehan MM, Armstrong HE, Suarez A, Allmon D, Heard HL. Cognitive behavioral treatment of chronically parasuicidal borderline patients. *Arch Gen Psychiatry* (1991) 48(12):1060–4. doi:10.1001/archpsyc.1991.01810360024003
16. Petrick ML, Gutierrez PM, Berlin JS, Saunders SM. Barriers and facilitators of suicide risk assessment in emergency departments: a qualitative study of provider perspectives. *Gen Hosp Psychiatry* (2015) 37(6):581–6. doi:10.1016/j.genhosppsych.2015.06.018
17. Goldstein TR, Fersch-Podrat RK, Rivera M, Axelson DA, Merranko J, Haifend Y, et al. Dialectical behavior therapy for adolescents with bipolar disorder: results from a pilot randomized trial. *J Child Adolesc Psychopharmacol* (2015) 25(2):140–9. doi:10.1089/cap.2013.0145
18. Guille C, Zhao Z, Krystal J. Web-based cognitive behavioral therapy intervention for the prevention of suicidal ideation in medical interns. *JAMA Psychiatry* (2015) 72(12):1192–8. doi:10.1001/jamapsychiatry.2015.1880
19. Brown GK, Have TT, Henriques GR, Xie SX, Hollander JE, Beck AT. Cognitive therapy for the prevention of suicide attempts: a randomized controlled trial. *JAMA* (2005) 294(5):563–70. doi:10.1001/jama.294.5.563
20. Linehan MM, Comtois KA, Murray AM, Brown MZ, Gallop RJ, Heard HL, et al. Two-year randomized controlled trial and follow-up of dialectical behavior therapy vs therapy by experts for suicidal behaviors and borderline personality disorder. *Arch Gen Psychiatry* (2006) 63(7):757–66. doi:10.1001/archpsyc.63.7.757
21. Rudd DM, Bryan CJ, Wertenberger EG, Peterson AL, Young-McCuaghan S, Mintz J, et al. Brief cognitive-behavioral therapy effects on post-treatment suicide attempts in a military sample: results of a randomized clinical trial with 2-year follow-up. *Am J Psychiatry* (2015) 172(5):441–9. doi:10.1176/appo.ajp.2014.14070843
22. Asarnow JR, Hughes JL, Babeva KN, Sugar CA. Cognitive-behavioral family treatment for suicide attempt prevention: a randomized controlled trial. *J Am Acad Child Adolesc Psychiatry* (2017) 56(6):506–14. doi:10.1016/j.jaac.2017.03.015

23. Linehan MM, Korslund KE, Harned MS, Gallop RJ, Lungu A, Neacsiu AD, et al. Dialectical behavior therapy for high suicide risk in individuals with borderline personality disorder: a randomized clinical trial and component analysis. *JAMA Psychiatry* (2015) 72(5):475–82. doi:10.1001/jamapsychiatry.2014.3039
24. Ellis TE, Rufino KA, Allen JG, Fowler JC, Jobes DA. Impact of a suicide-specific intervention within inpatient psychiatric care: the Collaborative Assessment and Management of Suicidality. *Suicide Life Threat Behav* (2015) 45:5. doi:10.1111/sltb.12151
25. Ellis TE, Rufino KA, Allen JG. A controlled comparison trial of the Collaborative Assessment and Management of Suicidality (CAMS) in an inpatient setting: outcomes at discharge and six month follow-up. *Psychiatry Res* (2017) 249:252–60. doi:10.1016/j.psychres.2017.01.032
26. Stanley B, Brown GK. Safety planning intervention: a brief intervention to mitigate suicide risk. *Cogn Behav Pract* (2012) 19(2):256–64. doi:10.1016/j.cbpra.2011.01.001
27. The Joint Commission. *Sentinel Event Alert 56: Detecting and Treating Suicide Ideation in All Settings*. Oakbrook Terrace, IL: The Joint Commission (2016).
28. SAMHSA. *Suicide Prevention Resource Center/American Foundation for Suicide Prevention Best Practices Registry for Suicide Prevention*. Waltham, MA: SAMHSA (2015).
29. Rudd MD, Mandrusiak M, Joiner TE Jr. The case against no-suicide contracts: the commitment to treatment statement as a practice alternative. *J Clin Psychol* (2006) 62(2):243–51. doi:10.1002/jclp.20227
30. Bryan CJ. *Managing Suicide Risk in Primary Care*. New York: Springer Publishing Company (2010). 216 p.
31. Bryan CJ, Mintz JM, Clemans TA, Leeson B, Burch ST, Williams SR, et al. Effect of crisis response planning vs. contracts for safety on suicide risk in U.S. Army Soldiers: a randomized clinical trial. *J Affect Disord* (2017) 212:64–72. doi:10.1016/j.jad.2017.01.028
32. Mann JJ, Apter A, Bertolote J, Beautrais A, Currier D, Haas A, et al. Suicide prevention strategies: a systematic review. *JAMA* (2005) 294(16):2064–74. doi:10.1001/jama.294.16.2064
33. Yip PS, Law CK, Fu KW, Law YW, Wong PW, Xu Y. Restricting the means of suicide by charcoal burning. *Br J Psychiatry* (2010) 196(3):241–2. doi:10.1192/bjp.bp.109.065185
34. Betz ME, Arias SA, Miller M, Barber C, Espinola J, Sullivan AF, et al. Change in emergency department providers' beliefs and practices after use of new protocols for suicidal patients. *Psychiatr Serv* (2015) 66(6):625–31. doi:10.1176/appi.ps.201400244
35. Fleischmann A, Bertolote JM, Wasserman D, De Leo D, Botega NJ, Da Silva D, et al. Effectiveness of brief intervention and contact for suicide attempters: a randomized controlled trial in five countries. *Bull World Health Organ* (2008) 86(9):703–9. doi:10.2471/BLT.07.046995
36. Dieserud G, Loeb M, Ekeberg Ø. Suicidal behavior in the municipality of Baerum, Norway: a 12-year prospective study of parasuicide and suicide. *Suicide Life Threat Behav* (2000) 30(1):61–73. doi:10.1111/j.1943-278X.2000.tb01065
37. Inagaki M, Kawashima Y, Kawanishi C, Yonemoto N, Sugimoto T, Furuno T, et al. Interventions to prevent repeat suicidal behavior in patients admitted into an emergency department for a suicide attempt: a meta analysis. *J Affect Disord* (2015) 175:66–78. doi:10.1016/j.jad.2014.12.048
38. Mousavi SG, Amini M, Mahaki B, Bagherian-Sararoudi R. Effect of phone call versus face-to-face follow-up on recurrent suicide attempts prevention in individuals with a history of multiple suicide attempts. *Adv Biomed Res* (2016) 5:184. doi:10.4103/2277-9175.190990
39. Luxton DD, June JD, Comtois KA. Can postdischarge follow-up contacts prevent suicide and suicidal behavior? A review of the evidence. *Crisis* (2013) 34(1):32–41. doi:10.1027/022
40. Stanley B, Chaudhury SR, Chesin M, Pontoski K, Bush MA, Knox KL, et al. An emergency department intervention and follow-up to reduce suicide risk in the VA: acceptability and effectiveness. *Psychiatr Serv* (2016) 67(6):680–3. doi:10.1176/appi.ps.201500082
41. Chesin MS, Stanley B, Haigh EAP, Chaudhury SR, Pontoski K, Knox KL, et al. Staff views of an emergency department intervention using safety planning and structured follow-up with suicidal veterans. *Arch Suicide Res* (2017) 21(1):127–37. doi:10.1080/13811118.2016.1164642
42. Patel V, Weiss HA, Chowdhary N, Naik S, Pednekar S, Chatterjee S, et al. Lay health worker led intervention for depressive and anxiety disorders in India: impact on clinical and disability outcomes over 12 months. *Br J Psychiatry* (2011) 199(6):459–66. doi:10.1192/bjp.bp.111.092155
43. Michel K, Valach L, Gysin-Maillart A. A novel therapy for people who attempt suicide and why we need new models of suicide. *Int J Environ Res Public Health* (2017) 14(3):E243. doi:10.3390/ijerph14030243
44. Kleinman EM, Turner BJ, Fedor S, Beale EE, Huffman JC, Nock MK. Examination of real-time fluctuations in suicidal ideation and its risk factors: results from two ecological momentary assessment studies. *J Abnorm Psychol* (2017) 126(6):726–38. doi:10.1037/abn0000273
45. Williams JMG, Crane C, Barnhofer T, Van der Does AJW, Segal ZV. Recurrence of suicidal ideation across depressive episodes. *J Affect Disord* (2006) 91(2–3):189–94. doi:10.1016/j.jad.2006.01.002
46. De Leo D, Cerin E, Spathonis K, Burgis SH. Lifetime risk of suicide ideation and attempts in an Australian community: prevalence, suicidal process, and help-seeking behavior. *J Affect Disord* (2005) 86(2–3):215–24. doi:10.1016/j.jad.2005.02.001
47. Witte TK, Fitzpatrick KK, Joiner TE Jr, Schmidt NB. Variability in suicidal ideation: a better predictor of suicide attempts than intensity or duration of ideation. *J Affect Disord* (2005) 88(2):131–6. doi:10.1016/j.jad.2005.05.019
48. Rudd MD, Cukrowicz KC, Bryan CJ. Core competencies in suicide risk assessment and management: implications for supervision. *Train Educ Prof Psychol* (2008) 2(4):219–28. doi:10.1037/1931-3918.2.4.219
49. Schmitz WM, Allen MH, Feldman BN, Gutin NJ, Jahn DR, Kleespies PM, et al. Preventing suicide through improved training in suicide risk assessment and care: an American Association of Suicidology task force report addressing serious gaps in U.S. mental health training. *Suicide Life Threat Behav* (2012) 42(3):292–304. doi:10.1111/j.1943-278X.2012.00090
50. Melton BB, Coverdale JH. What do we teach psychiatric residents about suicide? A national survey of chief residents. *Acad Psychiatry* (2009) 33:47–50. doi:10.1176/appi.ap.33.1.47
51. McMyler C, Pryjmachuk S. Do 'no-suicide' contracts work? *J Psychiatr Ment Health Nurs* (2008) 15(6):512–22. doi:10.1111/j.1365-2850.2008.01286.x
52. NYS-OMH. *Data from Zero Suicide Workforce Survey – Aggregate Results*. Washington, DC: National Action Alliance for Suicide Prevention (2015).
53. Roy A. Depressed patients who suicide at their first attempt have had few admissions. *Depress Anxiety* (1999) 9(2):75–7. doi:10.1002/(SICI)1520-6394(1999)9:2<75::AID-DA5>3.0.CO;2-D
54. Linehan MM. *DBT Skills Training Manual*. 2nd ed. New York: The Guilford Press (2015). 504 p.
55. Oquendo MA, Baca-Garcia E. Suicidal behavior disorder as a diagnostic entity in the DSM-5 classification system: advantages outweigh limitations. *World Psychiatry* (2014) 13(2):128–30. doi:10.1002/wps.20116
56. Linehan MM. *Cognitive-Behavioral Treatment of Borderline Personality Disorder*. New York: The Guilford Press (1993). 558 p.

Permissions

All chapters in this book were first published by Frontiers; hereby published with permission under the Creative Commons Attribution License or equivalent. Every chapter published in this book has been scrutinized by our experts. Their significance has been extensively debated. The topics covered herein carry significant findings which will fuel the growth of the discipline. They may even be implemented as practical applications or may be referred to as a beginning point for another development.

The contributors of this book come from diverse backgrounds, making this book a truly international effort. This book will bring forth new frontiers with its revolutionizing research information and detailed analysis of the nascent developments around the world.

We would like to thank all the contributing authors for lending their expertise to make the book truly unique. They have played a crucial role in the development of this book. Without their invaluable contributions this book wouldn't have been possible. They have made vital efforts to compile up to date information on the varied aspects of this subject to make this book a valuable addition to the collection of many professionals and students.

This book was conceptualized with the vision of imparting up-to-date information and advanced data in this field. To ensure the same, a matchless editorial board was set up. Every individual on the board went through rigorous rounds of assessment to prove their worth. After which they invested a large part of their time researching and compiling the most relevant data for our readers.

The editorial board has been involved in producing this book since its inception. They have spent rigorous hours researching and exploring the diverse topics which have resulted in the successful publishing of this book. They have passed on their knowledge of decades through this book. To expedite this challenging task, the publisher supported the team at every step. A small team of assistant editors was also appointed to further simplify the editing procedure and attain best results for the readers.

Apart from the editorial board, the designing team has also invested a significant amount of their time in understanding the subject and creating the most relevant covers. They scrutinized every image to scout for the most suitable representation of the subject and create an appropriate cover for the book.

The publishing team has been an ardent support to the editorial, designing and production team. Their endless efforts to recruit the best for this project, has resulted in the accomplishment of this book. They are a veteran in the field of academics and their pool of knowledge is as vast as their experience in printing. Their expertise and guidance has proved useful at every step. Their uncompromising quality standards have made this book an exceptional effort. Their encouragement from time to time has been an inspiration for everyone.

The publisher and the editorial board hope that this book will prove to be a valuable piece of knowledge for researchers, students, practitioners and scholars across the globe.

List of Contributors

Jacob Y. Stein, Liat Itzhaky and Zahava Solomon
I-CORE Research Center for Mass Trauma, Bob Shapell School of Social Work, Tel Aviv University, Tel Aviv, Israel

Yossi Levi-Belz
Department of Behavioral Sciences, Ruppin Academic Center, Emek-Hefer, Israel
Ruppin Academic Center, Emek Hefer, Israel

Trevor A. Pickering and Thomas W. Valente
Department of Preventive Medicine, Keck School of Medicine, University of Southern California, Los Angeles, CA, United States

Peter A. Wyman, Karen Schmeelk-Cone, Chelsey Hartley and Anthony R. Pisani
Department of Psychiatry, School of Medicine and Dentistry, University of Rochester, Rochester, NY, United States

Kelly L. Rulison
Department of Public Health Education, University of North Carolina at Greensboro, Greensboro, NC, United States

Charles Hendricks Brown and Mark LoMurray
Department of Psychiatry and Behavioral Sciences, Feinberg School of Medicine, Sources of Strength, Inc., Chicago, IL, United States

Emma Hofstra, Iman Elfeddali, Jacobus J. de Jong and Christina M. van der Feltz-Cornelis
Academic Department of Specialised Mental Health Care, GGz Breburg, Tilburg, Netherlands
Tranzo—Scientific Center for Care and Welfare, Tilburg University, Tilburg, Netherlands

Marjan Bakker
Department of Methodology and Statistics, Tilburg University,Tilburg, Netherlands

Chijs van Nieuwenhuizen
Tranzo—Scientific Center for Care and Welfare, Tilburg University, Tilburg, Netherlands
Institute for Mental Health Care, GGzE, Eindhoven, Netherlands

Tomoe Sakashita and Hirofumi Oyama
Department of Social Welfare, Faculty of Health Sciences, Aomori University of Health and Welfare, Aomori, Japan

Xiaojun Zhao
School of Education, Hebei University, Baoding, China

Changxiu Shi
School of Criminal Justice, China University of Political Science and Law, Beijing, China

Paniz Tavakoli
Children's Hospital of Eastern Ontario Research Institute, Ottawa, ON, Canada

Addo Boafo
Department of Psychiatry, University of Ottawa, Ottawa, ON, Canada
Children's Hospital of Eastern Ontario, Ottawa, ON, Canada

Allyson Dale and Kenneth Campbell
School of Psychology, University of Ottawa, Ottawa, ON, Canada

Rebecca Robillard
School of Psychology, University of Ottawa, Ottawa, ON, Canada
University of Ottawa Institute of Mental Health Research, Ottawa, ON, Canada

Stephanie L. Greenham
Children's Hospital of Eastern Ontario Research Institute, Ottawa, ON, Canada
Children's Hospital of Eastern Ontario, Ottawa, ON, Canada
School of Psychology, University of Ottawa, Ottawa, ON, Canada

Sergio Mérida-López and Natalio Extremera
Department of Social Psychology, University of Málaga, Málaga, Spain

Lourdes Rey
Department of Personality, Assessment and Psychological Treatment, University of Málaga, Málaga, Spain

Anna Szücs
Department of Psychiatry, Faculty of Medicine, University of Geneva, Geneva, Switzerland
Decision Neuroscience and Psychopathology Laboratory, Department of Psychiatry, School of Medicine, University of Pittsburgh, Pittsburgh, PA, United States

Katalin Szanto and Alexandre Y. Dombrovski
Decision Neuroscience and Psychopathology Laboratory, Department of Psychiatry, School of Medicine, University of Pittsburgh, Pittsburgh, PA, United States

Jean-Michel Aubry
Department of Psychiatry, Faculty of Medicine, University of Geneva, Geneva, Switzerland

Giorgio Falgares and Giovanna Manna
Department of Psychological, Pedagogical and Educational Sciences, University of Palermo, Palermo, Italy

Daniela Marchetti and Maria C. Verrocchio
Department of Psychological, Health and Territorial Sciences, University of Chieti–Pescara, Chieti, Italy

Pasquale Musso
Department of Languages and Educational Sciences, University of Calabria, Rende, Italy

Osmano Oasi
Department of Psychology, Catholic University of Sacred Heart, Milan, Italy

Daniel C. Kopala-Sibley
Department of Psychiatry, Mathison Centre for Mental Health Research and Education, Hotchkiss Brain Institute, University of Calgary, Calgary, AB, Canada
Alberta Children's Hospital Research Institute, University of Calgary, Calgary, AB, Canada

Sandro De Santis
Azienda Provinciale peri Servizi Sanitari, Provincia Autonoma di Trento, Trento, Italy

Shira Barzilay
Department of Psychiatry, Icahn School of Medicine at Mount Sinai, New York City, NY, United States

Zimri S. Yaseen and Igor Galynker
Department of Psychiatry, Icahn School of Medicine at Mount Sinai, New York City, NY, United States
Department of Psychiatry and Behavioral Health, Mount Sinai Beth Israel Medical Center, New York City, NY, United States

Mariah Hawes and Rachel Altman
Department of Psychiatry and Behavioral Health, Mount Sinai Beth Israel Medical Center, New York City, NY, United States

Bernard Gorman
Gordon F. Derner School of Psychology, Adelphi University, Garden City, NY, United States

Adriana Foster
Herbert Wertheim College of Medicine, Florida International University, Miami, FL, United States

Alan Apter
Feinberg Child Study Center, Schneider Children's Medical Center, Petach Tikva and Sackler Faculty of Medicine, Tel Aviv University, Tel Aviv, Israel

Paul Rosenfield
Department of Psychiatry, Mount Sinai St. Luke's, New York City, NY, United States

Gergö Hadlaczky, Sebastian Hökby, Anahit Mkrtchian, Danuta Wasserman and Vladimir Carli
National Centre for Suicide Research and Prevention of Mental Ill-Health, Department of Learning, Informatics, Management and Ethics, Karolinska Institutet, Stockholm, Sweden

Judit Balazs
Vadaskert Child Psychiatry Hospital and Outpatient Clinic, Budapest, Hungary
Institute of Psychology, Eötövös Loránd University, Budapest, Hungary

Núria Machín
Skylark Health Research Ltd., London, United Kingdom

Marco Sarchiapone
Department of Medicine and Health Science, University of Molise, Campobasso, Italy
National Institute for Health, Migration and Poverty, Rome, Italy
Kazakh National Medical University, Almaty, Kazakhstan

Merike Sisask
Estonian-Swedish Mental Health and Suicidology Institute, Tallinn, Estonia
School of Governance, Law and Society, Tallinn University, Tallinn, Estonia
Antônio Geraldo da Silva and António Pacheco Palha
Faculty of Medicine, University of Porto, Porto, Portugal

Leandro Fernandes Malloy-Diniz
Brazilian Society of Dual Pathology, Brasília, Brazil
Universidade Federal de Minas Gerais, Belo Horizonte, Brazil

Marina Saraiva Garcia
Molecular Medicine Department, Universidade Federal de Minas Gerais, Belo Horizonte, Brazil

Carlos Guilherme Silva Figueiredo and Renata Nayara Figueiredo
Associação Brasileira de Psiquiatria, Rio de Janeiro, Brazil

Alexandre Paim Diaz
Universidade do Sul de Santa Catarina, Palhoça, Brazil

Stefanie J. Schmidt
University Hospital of Child and Adolescent Psychiatry and Psychotherapy, University of Bern, Bern, Switzerland
Department of Psychiatry and Psychotherapy, University of Cologne, Cologne, Germany

Frauke Schultze-Lutter
University Hospital of Child and Adolescent Psychiatry and Psychotherapy, University of Bern, Bern, Switzerland
Department of Psychiatry and Psychotherapy, Medical Faculty, Heinrich-Heine University, Düsseldorf, Germany

Sarah Bendall and Barnaby Nelson
Orygen, The National Centre of Excellence in Youth Mental Health, University of Melbourne, Melbourne, VIC, Australia
Centre for Youth Mental Health, University of Melbourne, Melbourne, VIC, Australia

Nicola Groth and Nadja Inderbitzin
University Hospital of Child and Adolescent Psychiatry and Psychotherapy, University of Bern, Bern, Switzerland

Chantal Michel
University Hospital of Child and Adolescent Psychiatry and Psychotherapy, University of Bern, Bern, Switzerland
Developmental Clinical Psychology Research Unit, Faculty of Psychology and Educational Sciences, University of Geneva, Geneva, Switzerland

Benno G. Schimmelmann
University Hospital of Child and Adolescent Psychiatry and Psychotherapy, University of Bern, Bern, Switzerland
University Hospital of Child and Adolescent Psychiatry, University Hospital Hamburg Eppendorf, Hamburg, Germany

Daniela Hubl
University Hospital of Psychiatry and Psychotherapy, University of Bern, Bern, Switzerland

Yari Gvion
Bar-Ilan University, Ramat Gan, Israel

Berta Moreno-Küstner, Ana Ruíz-Ibáñez and Serafina Castro-Zamudio
Departamento de Personalidad, Evaluación y Tratamiento Psicológico, Universidad de Málaga, Málaga, Spain
Grupo Andaluz de Investigación Psicosocial (GAP) (CTS-945), Instituto de Biomedicina de Málaga (IBIMA), Málaga, Spain

José del Campo-Ávila and Gonzalo Ramos-Jiménez
Departamento de Lenguajes y Ciencias de la Computación, Universidad de Málaga, Málaga, Spain

Ana I. Martínez-García
Unidad de Gestión Clínica del Dispositivo de Cuidados Críticos y Urgencias del Distrito Sanitario Málaga-Coín-Guadalhorce, Málaga, Spain

José Guzmán-Parra
Grupo Andaluz de Investigación Psicosocial (GAP) (CTS-945), Instituto de Biomedicina de Málaga (IBIMA), Málaga, Spain
Unidad de Salud Mental del Hospital Regional Universitario de Málaga, Málaga, Spain

Monika Miklosi
Institute of Psychology, Eötvös Loránd University, Budapest, Hungary
Heim Pál Paediatric Hospital, Centre of Mental Health, Budapest, Hungary

Jozsef Halasz
Vadaskert Child Psychiatry Hospital, Budapest, Hungary
Alba Regia Technical Faculty, Obuda University, Szekesfehervar, Hungary

Lili Olga Horváth and Dóra Szentiványi
Institute of Psychology, Eötvös Loránd University, Budapest, Hungary
Doctoral School of Psychology, Eötvös Loránd University, Budapest, Hungary

Péter Vida
Institute of Psychology, Eötvös Loránd University, Budapest, Hungary
School of Ph.D. Studies, Semmelweis University, Budapest, Hungary

Jasmin Bar-Zomer and Anat Brunstein Klomek
Baruch Ivcher School of Psychology, Interdisciplinary Center (IDC), Herzliya, Israel

Udita Iyengar and Natasha Snowden
Department of Child and Adolescent Psychiatry, Institute of Psychiatry, Psychology, and Neuroscience (IoPPN), King's College London, London, United Kingdom

Joan R. Asarnow
Semel Institute of Neuroscience and Behavior, David Geffen School of Medicine, University of California, Los Angeles, Los Angeles, CA, United States

Paul Moran
National Institute for Health Research Bristol Biomedical Research Centre, University Hospitals Bristol NHS Foundation Trust and University of Bristol, Bristol, United Kingdom
Department of Population Health Sciences, Centre for Academic Mental Health, Bristol Medical School, University of Bristol, Bristol, United Kingdom

Troy Tranah
Institute of Psychiatry, Psychology, and Neuroscience (IoPPN), London, United Kingdom

Dennis Ougrin
Department of Child and Adolescent Psychiatry, Institute of Psychiatry, Psychology, and Neuroscience (IoPPN), King's College London, London, United Kingdom
South London and Maudsley National Health Service (NHS) Foundation Trust, London, United Kingdom

Annarosa Cipriano, Stefania Cella and Paolo Cotrufo
Observatory on Eating Disorders, Department of Psychology, University of Campania "Luigi Vanvitelli", Caserta, Italy

Catherine Thompson
School of Health Sciences, University of Salford, Salford, United Kingdom

Elsie Li Chen Ong
School of Health Sciences, University of Salford, Salford, United Kingdom
Division of Information and Technology Studies, Faculty of Education, The University of Hong Kong, Pokfulam, Hong Kong

Beth S. Brodsky and Barbara Stanley
Department of Psychiatry, Columbia University College of Physicians and Surgeons, New York, NY, United States
New York State Psychiatric Institute, New York, NY, United States

Index

R

S

T

V

W

www.ingramcontent.com/pod-product-compliance
Lightning Source LLC
LaVergne TN
LVHW082143200926
848484LV00008B/2101